TREATMENT OF
SKIN DISEASES

Dr. Kashieca Yap

ALLIED
HEALTH
PRESS

Treatment of Skin Diseases

Author: **Dr. Kashieca Yap**

Allied Health Press
4164 Lakeshore Road
Burlington ON L7L 1A4
Canada
www.alliedhealthpress.com
Email: orders@arclereducation.com

ISBN: 978-1-77956-796-3

General Disclaimer:

This book is a summation of information from different sources and encompasses a wide range of medical conditions, the latest therapy methods, principals and techniques that are used in current practice, at the time of publication. This book offers general information with educational purposes, it is not to be applied or relied on for any diagnostic or treatment purposes. Please do not use the data/matter as a substitute for professional diagnosis and treatment. Please consult your healthcare provider or a licensed physician before making any healthcare queries or treatment choices. The medical information and research findings presented in this book are for educational purposes only and should not be used for the treatment of specific individual patients, as individual cases may vary. The author(s), editors(s) and publisher cannot be held accountable and make no guarantees that the information provided in this book will apply to each and individual patient. This book is meant to serve as a basic guideline and other relevant literature sources should be used for more specific information. This text can be a vital resource for students, trainees, and practitioners, covering essential topics. This book encompasses a wide range of medical conditions and the latest therapy options used in current practice. Through the utilization of many different medical studies this book provides the basics of different medical conditions, which can be used as a basic guide from where medical students, trainees and practitioners can extract necessary information. Further, some of the books have graphic images to explain anatomy for medical/educational purposes only. Hence, the book is intended for students or teachers/staff or individuals with a mature outlook looking to learn or enhance their knowledge.

Allied Health Press publishes wide variety of books and eBooks. For more information about Allied Health Press and its products, visit our website at www.alliedhealthpress.com

ABOUT THE AUTHOR

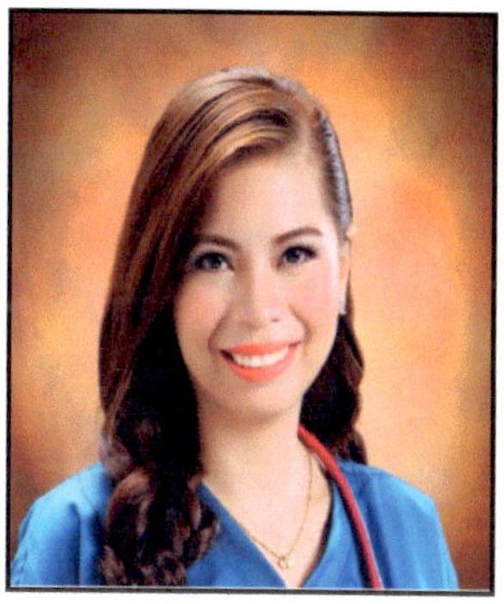

Kashieca Yap, M.D., is a devoted medical doctor and medical writer. She currently works as a general practice physician in a rural town, where she handles adult and pediatric cases, infectious diseases, and chronic medical conditions. Kashieca also lectures on mental health, clinical pharmacology, physiology, and psychiatry and is an enthusiastic researcher and medical writer. She obtained her medical degree from Cebu Doctor's University College of Medicine and further developed her clinical skills at a large public hospital. Alongside her professional endeavors, Kashieca dedicates her time to volunteering at NGOs and medical missions, reaching out to people in geographically isolated areas. Her unwavering passion for medicine and her strong desire to serve people is a testament to her compassion and skill as a healthcare professional.

Brief Table of Contents

Detailed Table of Contents

CHAPTER 3

CHAPTER 4

CHAPTER 12

Pediatric Dermatology 381

CHAPTER 13

Geriatric Dermatology 415

LIST OF FIGURES

LIST OF ABBREVIATIONS

AD	Atopic Dermatitis
ADSC	Adipose-Derived Stem Cell
AGE	Advanced Glycation End-Product
AHR	Aryl Hydrocarbon Receptor
AhR	Arylhydrocarbon Receptor
AI	Artificial Intelligence
AIT	Allergen Immunotherapy
AMP	Antimicrobial Peptide
ANA	Antinuclear Antibodies
ASIA	Autoimmune/Inflammatory Syndrome Induced by Adjuvants
BCC	Basal Cell Carcinoma
BFRB	Body-Focused Repetitive Behavior
BSA	Body Surface Area
CAF	Cancer-Associated Fibroblast
CALM	Café-Au Lait Macule
CA-MRSA	Community-Acquired MRSA
CAP	Cold Atmospheric Plasma
CBC	Complete Blood Count
CFS	Clinical Frailty Scale
CGRP	Calcitonin Gene-Related Peptide
CHB	Congenital Heart Block
CHG	Chlorhexidine Gluconate
CINDU	Chronic Inducible Urticaria
CNN	Convolutional Neural Network
CPD	Cyclobutane Pyrimidine Dimer
CREB	cAMP Response Element Binding Protein
CRP	C-Reactive Protein

CSU	Chronic Spontaneous Urticaria
CT	Computed Tomography
CTD	Connective Tissue Disease
CVD	Chronic Venous Disease
DAS	Derriford Appearance Scale
DEJ	Dermal-Epidermal Junction
DIF	Direct Immunofluorescence
DKK1	Dickkopf1
DLQI	Dermatology Life Quality Index
DMARD	Disease-Modifying Antirheumatic Drug
DPT	Drug Provocation Test
EDS	Ehlers-Danlos Syndrome
ELISA	Enzyme-Linked Immunosorbent Assay
ENA	Extractable Nuclear Antigens
ESR	Erythrocyte Sedimentation Rate
GACI	Generalized Arterial Calcification of Infancy
HFMD	Hand, Foot, and Mouth Disease
Hh	Hedgehog
HIFU	High Intensity Focused Ultrasound
HLA	Human Leukocyte Antigen
HPA	Hypothalamus-Pituitary-Adrenal
HPV	Human Papillomavirus
IACS	International Alliance for the Control of Scabies
IBD	Inflammatory Bowel Disease
ICI	Immune Checkpoint Inhibitor
ICSI	Intralesional Corticosteroid Injection
IGSRT	Image Guided Superficial Radiation Therapy
ILC2	2 Innate Lymphoid Cell
ILD	Interstitial Lung Disease
IMRT	Intensity-Modulated Radiation Therapy
IPL	Intense Pulsed Light
IR	Immune Repertoire
IVIG	Intravenous Immunoglobulin
JAKi	Janus Kinase Inhibitors
KGF	Keratinocyte Growth Factor

KOH	Potassium Hydroxide
LC-OCT	Line-Field Confocal Optical Coherence Tomography
LLLT	Low-Level Laser Therapy
MASCD	Machine-Aided Skin Cancer Detection
MBSR	Mindfulness-Based Stress Reduction
MCAS	Mast Cell Activation Syndrome
MCTD	Mixed Connective Tissue Disease
MIBG	Metaiodobenzylguanidine
MND	Median Nail Dystrophy
MPS-1	Metallopanstimulin-1
MRI	Magnetic Resonance Imaging
MRSA	Methicillin-Resistant *Staphylococcus aureus*
MSC	Mindful Self-Compassion
NF1	Neurofibromatosis Type 1
NIH	National Institutes of Health
NMSC	Non-Melanoma Skin Cancer
NNCS	non-Neuronal Cholinergic System
NSAID	Nonsteroidal Anti-Inflammatory Drug
NTCI	Nuclear Transport Checkpoint Inhibitor
OCT	Optical Coherence Tomography
ODS	Overall Dry Skin
OSCE	Objective Structured Clinical Examination
PDRN	Polydeoxyribonucleotide
PDT	Photodynamic Therapy
PPD	Phenylenediamine
PRP	Platelet-Rich Plasma
RA	Rheumatoid Arthritis
RCM	Reflectance Confocal Microscopy
RDC	Rheumatology/Dermatology Clinic
RF	Rheumatoid Factor
RONS	Reactive Oxygen and Nitrogen Species
SACS™	Studio Alterazioni Cutanee Stomali
SAF	Skin Autofluorescence
SCF	Stem Cell Factor
SCFA	Short-Chain Fatty Acid
scRNA-seq	Single-Cell RNA Sequencing

SFTD	Store-and-Forward Teledermatology
SIRS	Systemic Inflammatory Response Syndrome
SIT	Specific Immunotherapy
SJS	Stevens-Johnson Syndrome
SLE	Systemic Lupus Erythematosus
Smo	Smoothened
SSc	Systemic Sclerosis
SSI	Surgical Site Infection
SSSS	Staphylococcal Scalded Skin Syndrome
TBSE	Total Body Skin Examination
TEN	Toxic Epidermal Necrolysis
TEWL	Transepidermal Water Loss
TGF	Transforming Growth Factor
TNFα	Tumor Necrosis Factor-Alpha
T-VEC	Talimogene Laherparepvec
UV	Ultraviolet
VASI	Vitiligo Area Scoring Index
VEGF	Vascular Endothelial Growth Factor
XP	Xeroderma Pigmentosum

PREFACE

Skin is the most apparent extrinsic body barrier. It functions by shielding us from the external environment, perceiving touch, and temperature, and maintaining fluid balance. Skin health is an indicator of internal health and has an impact on quality of life in deeply significant ways. Cutaneous disease ranges from annoying to fatal. Inflammation, infection, pigmentary alterations, hair and nail disorders, and neoplastic neoplasms all pose varied diagnostic and therapeutic challenges. Progress in diagnostic imaging, molecular biology, and drug targeting during the last two decades completely revolutionized the capacity to diagnose and treat diseases. However, the very velocity of change is daunting without a guide that situates the enormity of new information within tested clinical principles.

An understanding of skin anatomy and physiology forms the basis of all clinical decision-making. The capacity to diagnose disease patterns requires a penetrating understanding of the interactive cooperation of cells, vessels, nerves, and appendages. In addition, the choice of an optimal therapeutic intervention depends on an awareness of the underlying pathology and the patient's general health status. The book begins with a short overview of skin structure and methods used by clinicians for its examination. It follows through the main categories of dermatoses, offering current knowledge and practical advice. The emphasis is on the application of diagnostic insight to individualized treatment plans that allow healing, reduce complications, and promote patient well-being.

The book, *Treatment of Skin Diseases*, provides a balanced overview of crucial principles and state-of-the-art treatments in dermatology. It is intended to meet the needs of those who want an introductory overview as well as a reliable handbook for clinical use. Recent evidence from clinical trials and consensus guidelines is integrated with expert opinion where possible to allow readers to make fully informed choices. Illustrations and clinical photographs shown with the text add to the discussion, allowing identification of significant findings in the clinic or at the bedside. By the integration of theoretical understanding and practical illustration of cases, this book attempts to fill the gap between academic and clinical practice.

The book opens with Chapter 1, "Introduction to Dermatology and Skin Structure."

Here, readers will find a concise review of epidermal layers, dermal components, and skin appendages. Emphasis is placed on how normal anatomy influences disease presentation and how to perform a focused skin examination. Illustrations clarify the relationship between structure and function, preparing the reader for more specialized topics.

Chapter 2, "Diagnostic Techniques in Dermatology," covers a range of instruments, such as dermoscopy, confocal microscopy, histopathology, and molecular diagnostics. For every diagnostic process, the respective indications, advantages, and limitations are discussed. Guidelines are given on how to select the best tests in specific clinical situations, how to interpret test results, and how to avoid common pitfalls.

Chapter 3, "Inflammatory Skin Diseases," discusses diseases like eczema, psoriasis, and lichen planus. It outlines the mechanisms of immune activation, followed by the therapeutic approaches involving topical therapy, phototherapy, and systemic immunomodulatory medications. Case presentations provide information on decision-making in therapy when the disease is refractory or is complicated by comorbidities.

Chapter 4, "Infectious Skin Diseases," addresses bacterial, fungal, viral, and parasitic infections. The key organisms are described, with emphasis on developing resistant strains and worldwide epidemiology. Diagnostic algorithms aid in differentiating infectious from non-infectious eruptions. Treatment protocols include topical and systemic antimicrobial therapies, with an emphasis on stewardship and minimizing side effects.

Chapter 5, "Acne and Rosacea," summarizes pathophysiology in terms of hormonal signals, sebum secretion, and microbial colonization. Medical and procedural treatment is detailed, from topical retinoids to laser therapy. Prevention of scarring and psychosocial management are emphasized.

Chapter 6, "Pigmentary Disorders," addresses disorders of hyperpigmentation and hypopigmentation, such as melasma, vitiligo, and post-inflammatory change. Mechanisms of melanocyte function are described, and treatment varies from topical depigmenters and photoprotection to surgical procedures such as melanocyte transplantation.

Chapter 7, "Hair and Nail Disorders," encompasses alopecia areata, androgenetic alopecia, nail dystrophies, and infection. The reader will become proficient at differentiating between scarring and non-scarring alopecia and between nail plate abnormalities and selecting therapy that promotes regrowth and reconstructs nail strength.

Chapter 8, "Autoimmune and Connective Tissue Disorders," addresses lupus erythematosus, scleroderma, and dermatomyositis. The systemic disease necessitates interdisciplinary cooperation. Cutaneous disease may frequently give the initial clue, and therapy consists of immunosuppressive agents and skin-directed therapies.

Chapter 9, "Skin Tumors and Malignancies," covers benign nevi, actinic keratoses, basal cell and squamous cell carcinomas, and melanoma. Risk factors, screening guidelines, and biopsy algorithms are outlined. Surgical and nonoperative treatment options are contrasted, and follow-up is outlined for the detection of recurrence or metastasis.

Chapter 10, "Vesiculobullous Diseases," discusses bullous pemphigoid, pemphigus vulgaris, and related disorders. The chapter emphasizes the autoantibody mechanism of blistering, early diagnosis, and the choice of corticosteroid and steroid-sparing regimens. Screening for such complications as infections and metabolic side effects is also discussed.

Chapter 11, "Urticaria and Drug Reactions," differentiates acute from chronic urticaria and includes angioedema. Hypersensitivity reactions are categorized by type, and desensitization protocols are presented for those patients on life-saving medications. Emergency management of life-threatening reactions, such as anaphylaxis, is addressed in a stepwise manner.

Chapter 12, "Pediatric Dermatology," covers conditions observed in children and infants, such as atopic dermatitis (AD), hemangiomas, and genetic disorders. Treatment modalities suitable for growth take into consideration differences in skin thickness, absorption, and development. Strategies in education for involving the family are emphasized to support long-term management.

Chapter 13, "Geriatric Dermatology," addresses changes in the form and function of the skin with age. Issues presented are xerosis, pruritus, vascular lesions, and healing of wounds. Polypharmacy and comorbidity in older patients influence treatment options. Directions are provided on dose reduction and monitoring of side effects.

Chapter 14, "Cosmetic and Procedural Dermatology," addresses minimally invasive procedures such as chemical peels, laser resurfacing, and injectable treatments. Indications, contraindications, and patient selection criteria direct practitioners to deliver safe and effective aesthetic procedures. Post-procedure care and complications management are also addressed.

Chapter 15, "Dermatologic Emergencies and Treatment," outlines evidence-based management of urgent and emergent clinical presentations such as Stevens-Johnson syndrome, toxic epidermal necrolysis, and angioedema. Triaging techniques, supportive care strategies, and coordination with critical care services are addressed within the chapter. Efficient techniques of rapid intervention that reduce morbidity and mortality in these emergent states are discussed.

This book summarizes current dermatologic disease management modalities for dermatology residents, practicing dermatologists, and medical students. It is also valuable for primary care physicians, physician assistants, and nurse practitioners who encounter skin diseases frequently as a part of general practice. Researchers and clinicians in allied fields will be particularly interested in the chapters on diagnostic innovation and therapeutic advancement. By combining current evidence with clinical expertise, this book allows educational development as well as everyday patient care, either as a core text or an instant bedside reference.

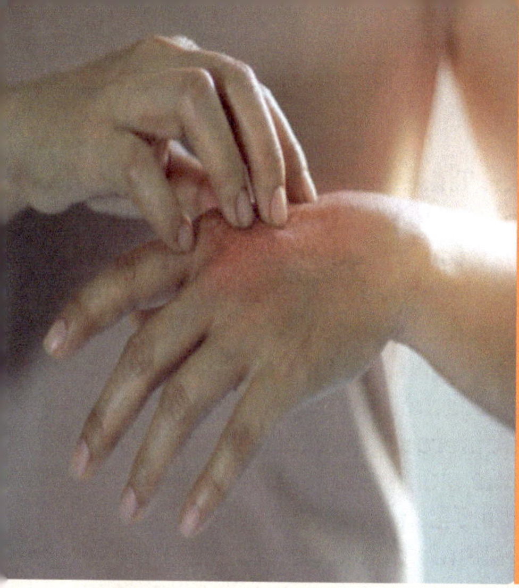

Chapter 1

INTRODUCTION TO DERMATOLOGY AND SKIN STRUCTURE

Contents

Introduction

The largest human body organ is the skin, which is a sophisticated interface between the external environment and the internal world. Its complex histology consists of three main layers: the epidermis, dermis, and hypodermis, each with unique functions in homeostasis and protection against environmental injury. It is important to understand this layered composition in order to appreciate the clinical presentations of dermatological disorders, which often results from derangements of these layers. The epidermis forms a first line of defense against pathogens and prevents water loss. The dermis contributes elasticity and strength in the form of connective tissue, blood vessels, and nerve endings. The hypodermis, consisting largely of fat tissue, serves as padding and storage of energy. A detailed understanding of this anatomy forms the basis of a scientific practice of diagnosing and treating skin conditions, emphasizing the biological complexity underlying dermatologic practice (Varnosfaderani et al., 2024). Beyond structural concerns, skin physiology encompasses multifunctional activities vital to survival. It controls body temperature by the secretion of sweat and modulation of blood flow, provides sensory perception through nerve receptors, and is involved in immunological defense by being the home to specialized cells. Additionally, skin cells, particularly keratinocytes, synthesize

Vitamin D when exposed to ultraviolet (UV) light, highlighting its involvement in metabolic functions. The appearance and condition of the skin can frequently mirror systemic disease, and therefore dermatological assessment becomes an integral part of general care. Advances in imaging techniques, such as photoacoustic imaging, have enhanced the ability to assess skin physiology at the macroscopic and microscopic levels, with information on vascular and metabolic functions that is unrivaled (Park et al., 2023). Increased understanding guides the development of targeted therapies and improves diagnostic accuracy in clinical dermatology. Systemic examination of skin lesions and classification of disease are the pillars of dermatology, allowing proper diagnosis and effective planning of treatment. Skin diseases exhibit an amazing diversity of appearance and are typically classified according to etiology, morphology, and pathophysiology. Broad categories include inflammatory diseases, infections, neoplasia, and hereditary diseases, with numerous subtypes within each. The overall clinical assessment of skin lesions includes scrutinizing the color, diameter, shape, distribution, and texture of the lesions and is supported by patient history and appropriate diagnostic studies. This structure allows for differential diagnosis of multifaceted cases and informs therapeutic choices. Furthermore, knowledge of the skin's functions puts into perspective how some diseases damage protective barriers or immune processes, supporting the value of combining anatomical, physiological, and pathological information in dermatological practice (Varnosfaderani et al., 2024).

Definition and Scope of Dermatology

The skin carries out a complex interplay of protective, regulatory, and sensory roles, thus its exploration is pertinent to general medicine and specialist health care. Dermatology, as a medical specialty, involves the thorough examination and care of skin and appendages such as hair, nails, and glands. This specialty not only treats cosmetic and physiological problems but also encompasses a wide spectrum of conditions ranging from benign lesions to malignant and metastatic tumors. It even extends to the learning of skin anatomy, physiology, and pathology, forming the foundation for the diagnosis and treatment of numerous diseases manifesting on or beneath the skin surface. Dermatologists participate in interdisciplinary endeavors, taking into account systemic diseases with cutaneous expression. This further enhances the process of diagnosis and treatment in clinical practice beyond conditions exclusively cutaneous in nature (Western University, 1961). The scope of dermatology is practical, ranging from the diagnosis and classification of skin disorders, which are of varied etiology, presentation, and severity. Skin diseases can be caused by infectious agents, immune disorders, genetic predisposition, or environmental factors, and thus require a sophisticated approach to successful intervention. The clinical method involves careful history taking, physical examination, and the application of diagnostic aids to differentiate among many types of skin lesions such as macules, papules, plaques, and nodules. Dermatological equipment advancements have enhanced lesion documentation and tracking, as seen with equipment such as the Studio Alterazioni Cutanee Stomali (SACS™) instrument, which enhances precision in assessing complex lesions, including peristomal skin issues, and encourages consistency in clinical evaluations among different healthcare providers (Kapsandoy et al., 2015). These advances reflect the evolving nature of dermatology, with a particular interest in precise evaluation techniques in the management of disease. Dermatology's domain is also widened by its emphasis on therapeutic modalities to accommodate each function or disorder of the skin. Understanding skin physiology—barrier function, thermoregulation, and immune function—enables clinicians to diagnose the pathogenic mechanisms of skin diseases. The specialty combines medical, surgical, and cosmetic treatments in response to the dynamic role of dermatology in the treatment of acute and chronic disorders. The dermatological field extends into preventive medicine and education of patients to limit risk factors causing skin injury. Furthermore, the discipline continually seeks investigation of psychosocial implications of skin disease, forging holistic patient care. Synthesis of anatomical knowledge, physiological insight, diagnostic precision, and therapeutic skill defines dermatology's diverse spectrum and fundamental role in medical science (Kapsandoy et al., 2015; Western University, 1961).

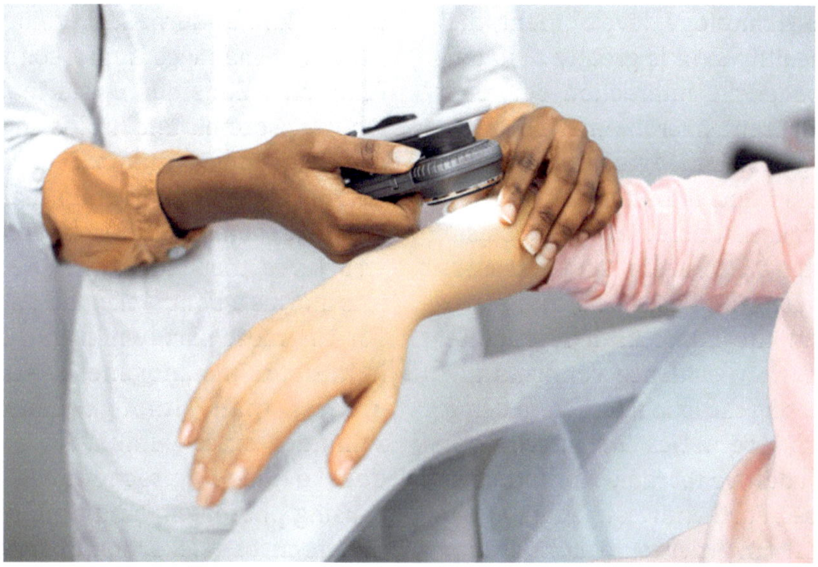

Source: https://medical.rossu.edu/sites/g/files/krcnkv261/files/styles/atge_3_2_crop_md/public/2022-04/Dermatology.jpg?h=f9d06ff2&itok=ktvUIeL9.

Importance of Skin Health

The complex interplay between the anatomical organization of the skin and its physiological functions emphasizes the need to maintain skin health. The skin, being the body's largest organ, acts as the initial barrier against pathogens, UV radiation, and physical injury from the external world. Anything but passive, this protective role involves complex mechanisms such as immune surveillance and the control of microbial populations living on the skin surface. Abrogation of such processes can compromise the integrity of the skin and put it at risk for infection and inflammatory disease. Furthermore, skin health affects general well-being since disruptions can stimulate or aggravate larger body area pathologies. Understanding the complex organization of the skin layers, made possible by dermatological advances, encourages early detection and treatment of most skin disorders, ranging in severity from benign lesions to malignancy. The focus on skin health, thus, goes beyond appearances, being a focal point of utmost importance in preventive medicine as well as general healthcare management (Bekbolatova et al., 2024). Technological advancements in the recent past have revolutionized the way skin health is managed through more accurate and tailored interventions. Artificial intelligence (AI) has been particularly promising in dermatology by enhancing diagnostic accuracy and refining treatment regimens. Machine learning software can process huge amounts of data from skin imaging and medical history to identify small changes that signify pathology. This integration aids in the early detection of skin lesions and differentiation of benign and malignant disease, therefore reducing morbidity. AI also helps to relieve clinicians from monotonous jobs, allowing increased focus on subtle clinical decisions and patient care. Such innovation speaks to issues of today's healthcare provision, such as the limitation of resources and mounting patient volumes, in the long run leading to enhanced skin disease management and improved patient outcomes (Bekbolatova et al., 2024). Beyond the technology development, the sustainability of healthy skin is greatly dictated by the mutually beneficial interaction between the skin and its inherent microbiome. The rich variety of microorganisms modifies the immune processes of the skin and maintains its barrier integrity. Disruptions in microbial homeostasis have been connected with several skin diseases, including eczema, acne, and psoriasis, and place the microbiome in the clinic as a legitimate therapeutic target. New evidence confirms the promise for modulating the skin microbiota using specific probiotics, prebiotics, or microbiota transplantation as additive therapies for difficult-to-treat skin diseases. Further investigation in this area will be necessary in order to further develop new, non-surgical treatments that resuscitate normal skin homeostasis and provide long-term therapeutic benefits to skin health. Therefore, skin health is a complex issue that demands an integrated knowledge of anatomy, physiology, microbial ecology, and novel clinical approaches (Aggarwal et al., 2022).

Overview of Skin Structure

The skin is not merely a wrapper; it is a stratified wonder with various components collaborating in unforeseen fashions. On top of it all, there is the epidermis, a squamous cell wall that typically acts as the body's initial defense against external threats. Keratinocytes in this region continue to proliferate and differentiate into the hardened outer stratum corneum—a sort of tough shield created layer upon layer. Ironically enough, inside this same external layer are cells such as melanocytes, Langerhans cells, and Merkel cells that continually reappear and take care of things such as pigmentation, immune notifications, and tactile sensing. A little lower down, the dermis, with its web of elastin and collagen fibers, provides strength and support; interspersed throughout it are structures such as hair follicles, sweat glands, and small blood vessels that assist with temperature regulation and sensation, introducing complexity and utility to our skin. Underneath its simple structure, the skin also manages some complex biochemical functions. Consider epidermal differentiation, where proteins and lipids are synthesized in a sort of chaos that has to be ordered for a barrier to form and retain moisture. The lipids organize themselves into layered, nearly lamellar structures that aid in the prevention of water loss and, as a bonus, exclude unwanted microbes. For the most part, when UV light hits the skin, it initiates melanogenesis—a photoprotective process that, although beneficial, is also a reminder since cumulative sunlight exposure does damage mitochondrial DNA, for years causing photoaging and even skin cancer. These biochemical tricks demonstrate that the skin is not passive but actively defends our body against all sorts of external hazards. In clinical practice, particularly in dermatologic surgery, it is important to be familiar with these layers. In areas such as the eyelid, for example, where the skin is so thin but so critical to the comfort and operation of the eyes, surgeons have to be particularly careful. Procedures like Mohs micrographic surgery, which tend to provide full tumor removal with the preservation of as much healthy tissue as possible, rely on that intimate inner familiarity. It is interesting how even slight variations in reconstructive methods can make a big difference here, considering the eyelid's role in keeping the eye moist, safe, and clear. This layered understanding, both structurally and biochemically—proves essential for tailoring surgical interventions that respect both form and function.

1.1. Skin Anatomy

Under the body's surface lies an complex system vital to protection and homeostasis. The skin has three major layers: the epidermis, dermis, and hypodermis, each playing separate yet interactive roles. The epidermis plays a mostly barrier role, which is made of stratified squamous epithelial cells, called keratinocytes, that are continuously replaced through keratinization. This external layer blocks pathogens from entering and reduces water loss. Below it, the dermis supplies structural support and elasticity, containing collagen and elastin fibers, blood vessels, nerve endings, hair follicles, and sweat glands. The inner hypodermis is composed primarily of fat tissue, padding the body and acting as an energy reservoir. This layered structure supports not only mechanical defense but also essential immunologic and sensory functions, highlighting the skin's function as an active interface between the organism and the environment. At the cellular level, the skin is highly adaptive to internal physiological conditions and external environmental stimuli. Keratinocytes predominate the epidermis, with a process of maturation that leads to the development of a tough, protective layer. Langerhans cells are antigen-presenting cells, combining cutaneous immunity with systemic immune processes. Melanocytes play a role in pigment formation, protecting deeper tissues from ultraviolet (UV) radiation-induced damage. In addition, the dermis provides vascular networks essential for the delivery of nutrients and thermoregulation, highlighting the skin's function in homeostasis. Notably, stress and systemic health conditions affect the skin condition. Chronic stress increases cortisol, interfering with collagen synthesis and inhibiting skin repair mechanisms, which demonstrates a bi-directional relationship between psychological states and skin physiology (Gradowicz-Prajsnar, 2023). Knowledge of these cellular components is necessary to understand the pathogenesis of many dermatological disorders. The anatomy of the skin is inherently associated with its functional potential and susceptibility to disease. Its complex vascular supply, sensory innervation, and immunological components expose it to numerous disorders categorized based on etiology, morphology, and pathophysiology. Inflammatory, infectious, or neoplastic lesions of the skin indicate underlying disruptions in these anatomical structures. The notion of skin as a neuro-immuno-endocrine organ underscores its systemic relationship. For instance, rheumatologic diseases not only involve the joints but also exhibit characteristic cutaneous features, reflecting subtle systemic interaction (Spender, 1892). This highlights the need for a comprehensive anatomical and physiological insight in dermatology to dictate both diagnostic evaluation and treatment modalities directed toward maintaining skin integrity and function. The complexity of the layers of the skin necessitates an interdisciplinary clinical approach that is specific to multifactorial disease processes (Figure 1.1).

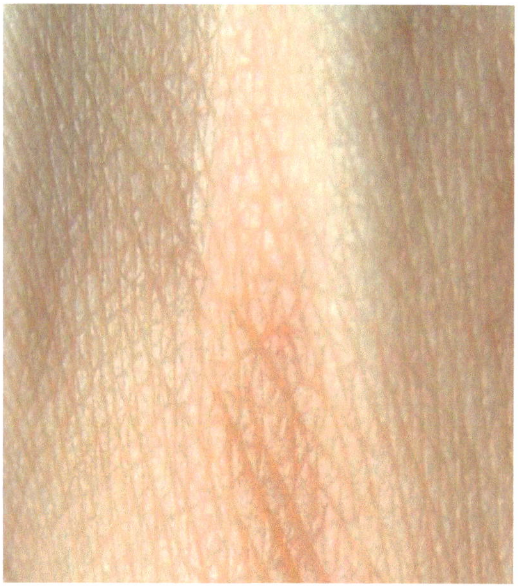

Figure 1.1. The skin of a human hand.

Source: Wikimedia Commons. (2006). *Human Skin Structure.* https://upload.wikimedia.org/wikipedia/commons/1/13/Human_skin_structure.jpg.

1.1.1. Layers of the Skin: Epidermis, Dermis, and Hypodermis

Under the microscope, the skin is a stratified, complex structure that performs several protective and regulatory roles vital to human health. The outermost surface, the epidermis, acts essentially as a barrier against environmental attack in the form of pathogens, UV light, and toxic chemicals. Its structure is made up primarily of keratinocytes that are constantly being replaced through the process of keratinization, leading to the accumulation of the stratum corneum, which is central to its barrier function. It also has melanocytes, which contribute pigmentation and partial protection against UV damage, and Langerhans cells which help in immune surveillance. The thickness and hydration of the epidermis may differ considerably between various body locations, depending on age, sex, and physical activity, with dynamic adaptability to internal and external forces (Chirikhina, 2022). These differences highlight the important function of the epidermis in the skin's overall health and demonstrate the need for knowledge about its structure in dermatology. Underneath the epidermis, there is the dermis, a thick and complex layer that gives mechanical strength and resilience to the skin. Well supplied with elastin and collagen fibers, the dermis mechanically supports the epidermis and accommodates blood vessels, nerves, hair follicles, sweat and sebaceous glands. The appendages are important for thermoregulation, sensation, and metabolic activity, playing their part in the general physiological functions of the skin. The vascular network of the dermis is significant in immune response and healing of wounds, allowing for quick delivery of immune cells to areas of compromise. The density and organization of collagen fibers in the dermis are also important determinants of elasticity and mechanical stress resistance of the skin, often impaired in most dermatological disorders. New imaging methods have made it possible to map dermal thickness and composition in detail, emphasizing its variability and importance in healthy skin as well as pathological conditions (Chirikhina, 2022).

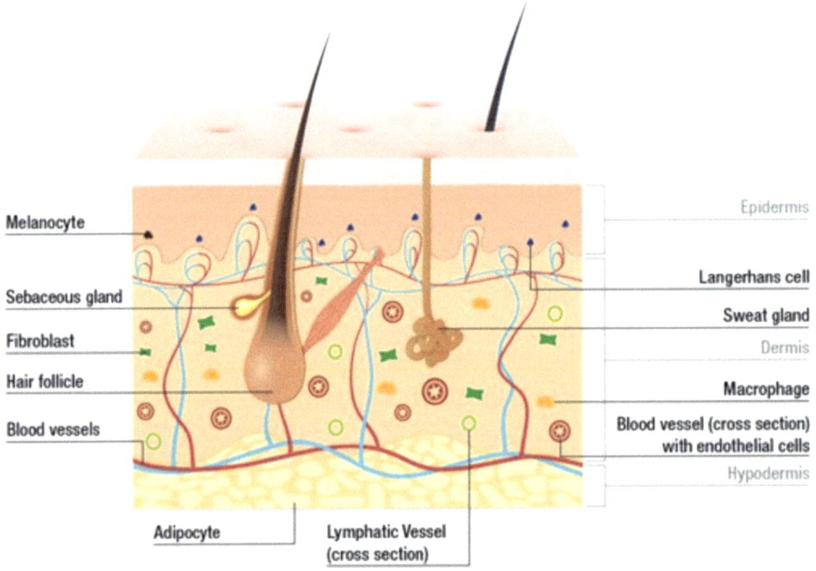

Figure 1.2. Layers of the skin.

Source: Hofmann E, Schwarz A, Fink J, Kamolz L-P, Kotzbeck P. Modelling the Complexity of Human Skin In Vitro. *Biomedicines*. 2023; 11(3):794. https://doi.org/10.3390/biomedicines11030794

Even deeper is the hypodermis, or subcutaneous tissue, that acts as an interface between the skin and underlying muscles or bones. This layer is mostly made up of adipose tissue, offering insulation, energy storage, and protection against mechanical trauma. The hypodermis also facilitates the anchoring of the dermis to internal structures, enabling structural support essential for maintaining skin integrity and mobility. Beyond its mechanical functions, this fat-rich layer plays a dynamic role in endocrine signaling and systemic metabolism. Current progress in skin modeling, including that associated with the establishment of skin-on-chip technology, underscores the need to reproduce the hypodermis in addition to the epidermis and dermis to more effectively mimic the human skin's physiological environment for pharmacological and toxicological assessment. Integrating the hypodermis and its interactions with immune and vascular elements into these models is a major step toward mimicking more accurately and reliably experimental platforms for dermatology research (Figure 1.2).

1.1.2. Skin Appendages: Hair, Nails, and Glands

Outside the major layers of skin, specialized structures called skin appendages are important for preserving overall integumentary function. Appendages such as hair, nails, and glands all contribute uniquely to protective, sensory, and regulatory functions. Hair follicles, rooted deep within the dermis, are not just cosmetic and tactile, but also assist with thermoregulation and protect deeper tissues from UV radiation. The development and structure of hair are affected by complex physiological mechanisms including stem cells and hormonal regulation. Similarly, nails made up largely of keratin confer structural support and defend terminal digits from mechanical trauma while facilitating fine motor function. Together, these appendages represent the dynamic skin interface with the outside world, highlighting the criticality of their integrity in dermatologic wellness (Terrell, 1987). Glands connected with the skin add additional complexity and multifunctionality to these appendages. Sebaceous glands, closely associated with hair follicles, produce sebum, an oily substance that keeps skin hydrated and intact, thus preventing excessive water loss and microbial invasion. On the other hand, sweat glands, classified as eccrine or apocrine, play a crucial role in thermoregulation through sweating and allow for excreting metabolic waste. Pathological change or dysfunction of these glands may result in a broad spectrum of dermatologic disorders ranging from acne vulgaris caused by overactivity of the sebaceous glands, to hyperhidrosis from dysregulation of the eccrine glands. Knowledge of the physiology and the potential for pathological involvement of these appendages is crucial for clinicians who are treating skin lesions or diseases that directly involve or indirectly impact these structures (Wilson, 1871). Abnormalities in skin appendages tend to manifest as clinically meaningful dermatoses requiring an educated path to diagnosis and treatment. Ailments in hair, nail, and gland structures may result from genetic, inflammatory, infectious, or neoplastic sources, ranging from a spectrum of cosmetic issues to markers of systemic disease. An example is patterned hair loss representing underlying autoimmune processes, while nail dystrophies may point to systemic processes such as psoriasis or infection. Similarly, glandular pathology may take the form of cysts, tumors, or inflammatory lesions complicating the skin's main defenses. Hence, a close knowledge of skin appendage anatomy and physiology improves the dermatologist's capacity for contextual interpretation of skin lesions, merging morphological evaluation with clinical history to develop effective treatment plans (Terrell, 1987; Wilson, 1871) (Figure 1.3).

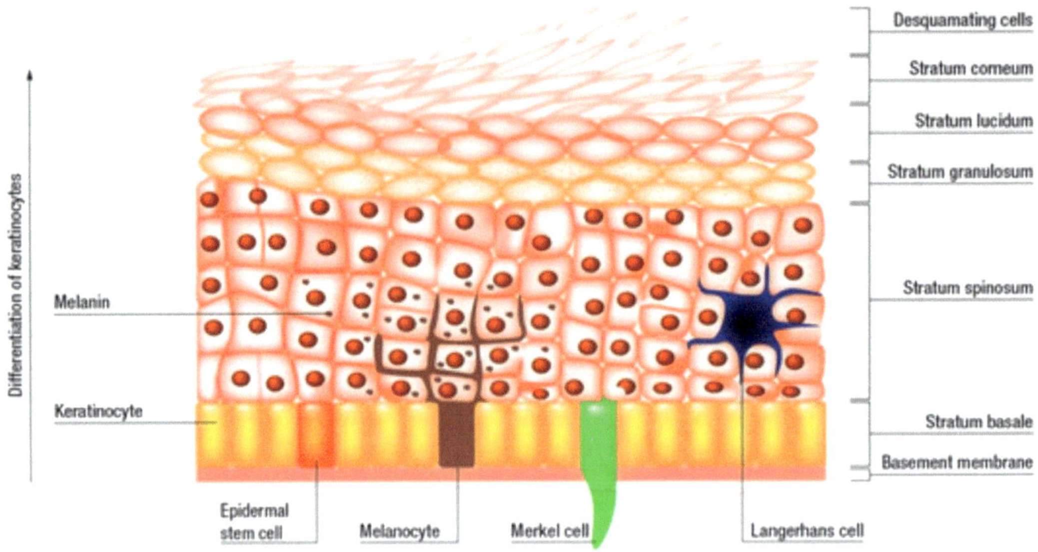

Figure 1.3. Skin appendages.

Source: Hofmann E, Schwarz A, Fink J, Kamolz L-P, Kotzbeck P. Modelling the Complexity of Human Skin In Vitro. *Biomedicines*. 2023; 11(3):794. https://doi.org/10.3390/biomedicines11030794

1.1.3. Vascular and Nervous Supply of the Skin

The complex relationship of the skin with its support structures is essential for its functioning and integrity. Of these, vascular supply is the most important in ensuring skin health through the provision of oxygen and nutrient supply and the removal of waste. The blood supply of the skin is supplied mainly by two discrete plexuses, the superficial papillary plexus in the dermis and the cutaneous plexus at the dermal-subcutaneous boundary. These intercommunicating network of blood vessels allow for thermoregulation by means of vasodilatation and vasoconstriction, permitting the skin to react dynamically to changes in the environment and in physiology. In addition, the dense vascular network plays a vital role in wound healing and inflammation, as it facilitates effective immune cell trafficking. Such sophisticated vascular organization highlights the skin's ability not just as a barrier but also as a responsive organ essential in systemic homeostasis. Also important is the nervous supply of the skin, which includes a complex system of sensory and autonomic fibers that facilitate perception and regulation. Sensory receptors situated within the skin respond to a range of stimuli, including pain, temperature, pressure, and vibration, conveying this information for interpretation by the central nervous system. Nociception and temperature are contributed to by small unmyelinated C fibers and myelinated A-delta fibers, underlining the skin's protective function through rapid sensory input. Autonomic nerve fibers also control such functions as sweating and vascular tone, further emphasizing the integrated physiological processes of the skin. This innervation is of paramount significance not only for sensation but also for the maintenance of the microenvironment of the skin, influencing processes like inflammation and repair. The understanding of the neural pathways sheds light on the pathophysiology of neuropathic skin disorders and sensory impairment, bridging clinical dermatology and neuroscience. The interaction between vascular and nervous supplies in the skin displays a system that preserves both its structural and functional capacities. This cooperation endows the skin with the power to react against internal and external insults such as alterations in temperature, damage, and infection. Interferences with either supply may present as cutaneous diseases, for example, peripheral neuropathy may lead to diminished sensation and secondary ulcerations, and vascular diseases may produce ischemic skin changes and compromised healing. Therefore, understanding the significance of such networks guides clinical practice in skin lesions and diseases, emphasizing the necessity of an integrated knowledge of cutaneous anatomy and physiology in dermatology. While existing knowledge in cerebrovascular domains is mainly under neuroanatomy, analogies in fluid dynamics and homeostasis could provide additional understanding of skin vascular regulation, as discussed in other organ systems' literature (Gutiérrez-Cerrajero et al., 2023) (Figure 1.4).

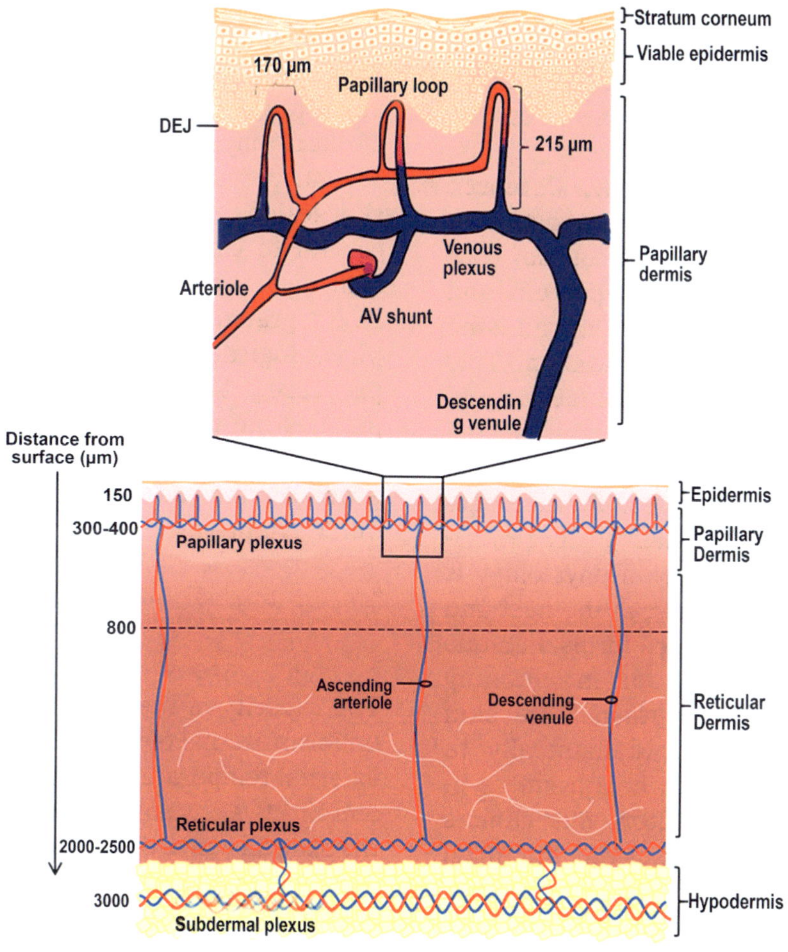

Figure 1.4. Schematic of blood circulation in the skin.

Source: Shah, P., Patel, D., Shah, R., & Shah, M. (2022). Schematic of blood circulation in the skin. In Artificial intelligence in dermatology: A review. *ResearchGate.*

1.2. Skin Physiology

Appreciation of the dynamic response of the skin to both external and internal stimuli is necessitated in the understanding of the complex physiological processes of the skin. Physiologically, skin encompasses several mechanisms to promote homeostasis, including barrier function, immune protection, thermoregulation, and perception. These mechanisms are completely reliant on the cellular and molecular composition of the skin, encompassing keratinocytes, melanocytes, immune cells, and extracellular matrix components. The ability of skin to regenerate and repair itself highlights its central position in the defense of the body against environmental stress and pathogens. Moreover, stress with a physiological basis impacts skin functioning immensely; elevated cortisol with stress that is chronic inhibits protein and collagen synthesis, thereby compromising skin strength and repair mechanism. This interaction between psychological factors and skin physiology exemplifies the multifaceted nature of skin health, especially in conditions like acne vulgaris, where stress may exacerbate disease severity and delay healing (Gradowicz-Prajsnar, 2023). Integral to skin physiology is the complex interaction between the host and its resident microbiome, which forms a unique microenvironment critical for maintaining cutaneous immune homeostasis. The skin microbiome also responds dynamically to endogenous factors like the health status of the host and exogenous factors like climate and hygiene. A derangement of this microbial community, known as dysbiosis, has been associated with numerous skin diseases. Thereby, illustrating the homeostatic balance required for skin physiologic function. For instance, in leprosy, *Mycobacterium leprae* infection leads to microvascular dysfunction and disturbed hydration status, which then disrupts microbial composition and diversity of the skin. This illustrates the way in which physiological disturbance at the microvascular level can have a decisive impact on the microbial environment of the skin, demonstrating the interrelatedness of skin physiology, microbial ecology, and pathogenesis of disease (Teng & Esti, 2021). Physiological functions of the skin also involve thermoregulation and sensory processing, both of which are dependent on its vascular supply and nerve endings contained in the dermis. Both systems cooperate to control body temperature by the production of sweat and vasodilation or vasoconstriction of blood vessels in the skin. Sensory receptors in the skin perceive diverse stimuli—temperature, pressure, pain—so that the body can respond adaptively to environmental demands. Alteration of these physiological processes manifests as several dermatological disorders with related skin lesions. Knowledge of these processes is central to the diagnosis and management of skin diseases, highlighting the importance of an integrated approach that takes into account physiological, immunological, and microbial processes. Such an integrative perspective justifies the development of specific therapies that target the underlying pathophysiologic processes instead of just addressing cosmetic outer symptoms.

1.2.1. Role of Skin in Thermoregulation

The capacity of the human body to maintain a uniform internal temperature despite fluctuating external temperatures is necessary for survival and effective physiological processes. At its core is the skin, an active organ whose role is intimately involved in the process of thermoregulation. The multilayered nature of the skin, comprising the epidermis, dermis, and hypodermis, allows it to develop a barrier as well as facilitate heat exchange with the environment. Many blood vessels in the dermis regulate blood flow, dilating for heat release by radiation and constricting for warmth conservation. Furthermore, the sweat glands, scattered on the skin surface, secrete sweat that evaporates to cool the body, showing the skin's evaporative cooling mechanism. This complex process emphasizes the skin's important role in thermal homeostasis to achieve cellular and systemic stability when exposed to thermal stress (Goh, 2023). Other than vascular modulation and sweating, the skin also has specialized nerve endings for detecting temperature changes and feeding back to the central nervous system. This feedback induces autonomic responses that regulate the body's thermoregulatory mechanisms, such as heat production by shivering or vasomotor regulation. The hypodermis with its high adipose tissue content is also responsible for acting as insubstantial insulation for the body and reducing heat loss. Also, pilomotor muscle distribution and activity in the skin may produce "goosebumps," a reaction to capture an insulating air layer close to the skin's surface. These physiological responses combined emphasize the manner in which skin anatomy is intimately connected with thermoregulation, emphasizing its essential role in internal balance maintenance (Vladlenov, 2022).

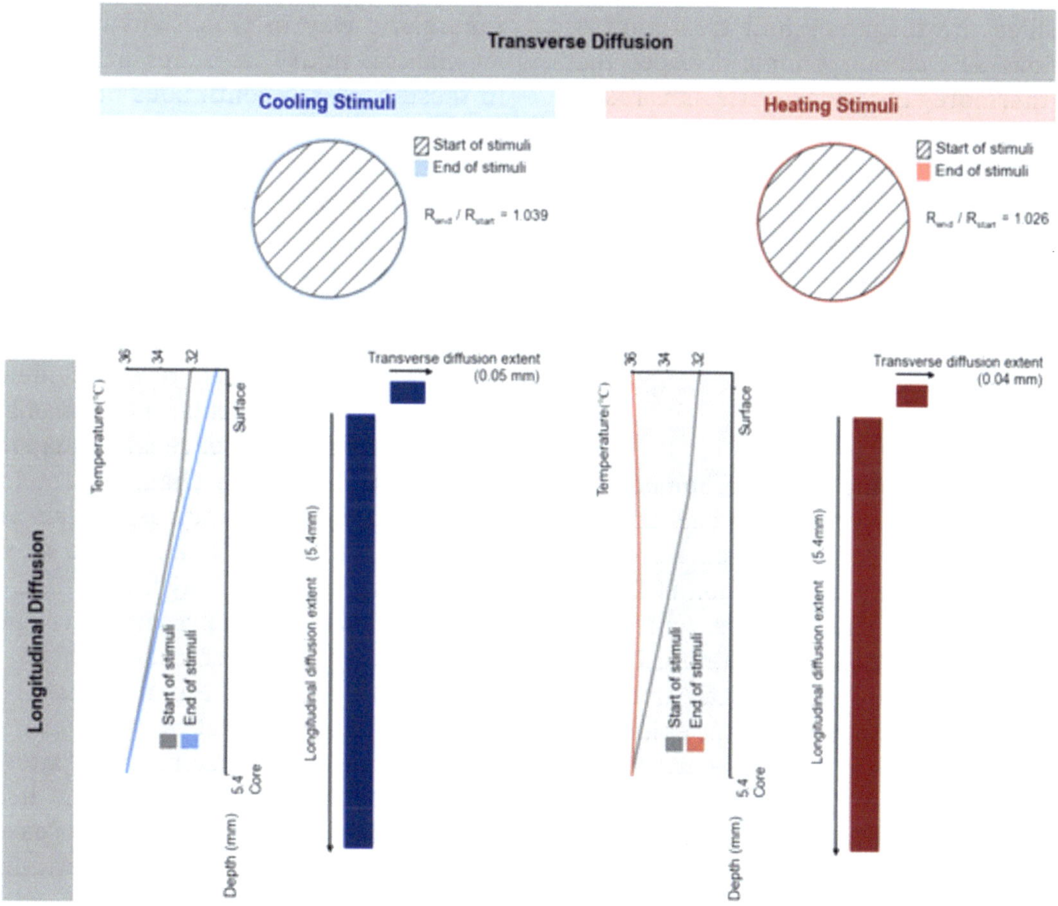

Figure 1.5. Temperature regulation in skin.

Source: Zhou Y, Yu H, Luo M, Zhou X. Skin Heat Transfer and Thermal Sensation Coupling Model under Steady Stimulation. *Buildings*. 2024; 14(2):547. https://doi.org/10.3390/buildings14020547

The clinical relevance of skin's function in thermoregulation transcends normal physiology to dermatological health and disease. Vascular response or sweat gland dysfunctions may create conditions like hyperhidrosis or anhidrosis, which compromise the ability of the body to regulate its temperature. Likewise, inflammatory processes within the skin, possibly amplified through microbial stimuli or immune dysregulation, can interrupt normal thermoregulatory mechanisms, disturbing homeostasis and patient comfort (Goh, 2023). Appreciation of how the skin organizes such complex processes is germane in dermatology, as it guides the diagnosis and treatment of skin lesions as well as systemic diseases that involve thermoregulatory aspects. As a result, understanding skin structure and function not only clarifies fundamental biological principles but also informs clinical approaches in the management of diseases affecting the skin's thermoregulatory function (Vladlenov, 2022) (Figure 1.5).

1.2.2. Skin's Barrier Function and Permeability

The skin is essential in the process of homeostasis by serving as a strong interface between the internal milieu and the external environment. The role of performing this function is largely due to its barrier characteristics, which bar the unauthorized passage of pathogens and injurious agents while retaining vital moisture. The outermost surface of the skin, the epidermis, which is mainly made up of keratinocytes, controls this selective permeability through an orchestrated process of keratinization. As keratinocytes move from the basal layer toward the surface, they differentiate, leading to the development of a dense, hard stratum corneum. The protein-rich and lipid-rich layer provides the skin with mechanical integrity and a water barrier, hence safeguarding underlying tissues against mechanical, chemical, and microbial injuries. Disruption of this barrier function predisposes individuals to a host of skin disorders, highlighting its critical role in dermatological well-being (Szot et al., 2024). Central to the barrier function of the skin is its dynamic ability to adapt to environmental stressors, reflected by groups in repeated contact with difficult conditions, i.e., athletes. Extended interaction with sweat, clothing friction, and contact with diverse microbial agents weaken the skin barrier, enhancing permeability and susceptibility to infection. Mechanical disruption to the epidermis tends to trigger a cascade leading to dermatoses, which points out the synergistic way in which environmental and mechanical injury degrades barrier function. In these contexts, continuous observation and preventive procedures become necessary in order to maintain skin homeostasis and prevent the onset of skin disease. The interaction of environmental factors and disruption of the skin barrier underlines the complicated relationship between physiology and externalities in dermatology (Szot et al., 2024). Apart from its structural elements, recent evidence has underscored the molecular mechanisms of skin permeability and barrier repair. Aquaporins are specialized membrane channel proteins with expression in keratinocytes, which promote regulated water and small solute movement, maintaining epidermal hydration and barrier homeostasis. These proteins are involved in a number of processes, such as wound repair, modulation of immune response, and proliferation of keratinocytes, all having direct effects on barrier recovery after injury. Dysregulation of aquaporins has also been implicated in inflammatory skin diseases with impaired barrier function, demonstrating their role in both skin physiology and pathology. Knowledge of these molecular actors provides new perspectives on therapeutic strategies to restore barrier integrity and control skin diseases (Tricarico et al., 2022) (Figure 1.6).

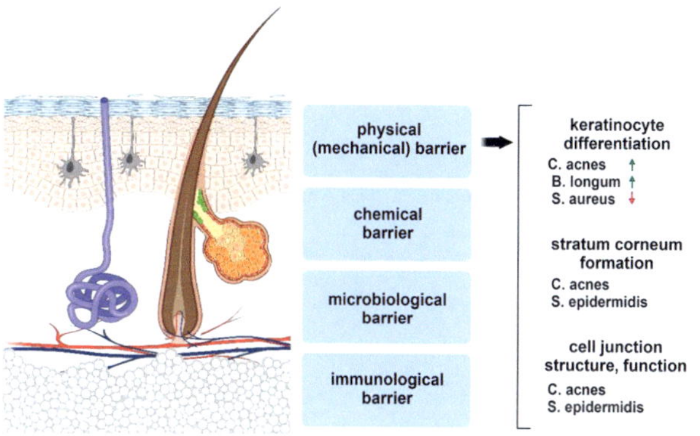

Figure 1.6. The human skin forms a complex barrier. The skin microbiota affects various properties of this complex interface, even the formation of anatomically intact and functionally mature tissue. The figure shows the bacterial strains with a proven effect on the particular physical barrier component. A green arrow indicates a positive, while a red a negative effect.

Source: Xu, X., Liu, S., Xu, H., & Zhang, X. (2023). Artificial intelligence in skin disease diagnosis: a review. *International Journal of Molecular Sciences, 24*(20), 15962.

1.2.3. Immune Response and Skin Health

Central to preserving skin integrity is the interactive process between the cutaneous immune system and epidermal cells that together present a strong barrier to environmental damage and pathogens. The immune response is tightly regulated so that defense and tissue homeostasis are maintained, avoiding excess inflammation that can result in chronic skin disease. In this context, the aryl hydrocarbon receptor (AHR) has been identified as a key molecular mediator that regulates skin immunity through the modulation of keratinocyte differentiation and cytokine production. AHR signaling pathway activation is involved in the maintenance of skin barrier integrity and the orchestration of immune cell responses, thus avoiding dysregulated inflammation that is typical of psoriasis and atopic dermatitis (AD). Knowing the molecular basis of AHR's function therefore gives insightful information regarding likely therapeutic targets intended to reconstitute immune homeostasis in a host of dermatologic disorders (Michał et al., 2024). In addition to AHR, the immune regulating mechanisms of the skin are substantially determined by the non-neuronal cholinergic system (NNCS), which has an important role to play in cutaneous physiology and immune modulation. Acetylcholine synthesized by keratinocytes and resident immune cells targets nicotinic and muscarinic receptors to modulate inflammatory processes, wound healing, and vascular tone in the skin microenvironment. This cholinergic signaling is finely regulated to control the production of pro-inflammatory cytokines and restore barrier function, thereby preventing microbial invasion and tissue damage. Dysregulation of the NNCS has been shown to contribute to worsening inflammatory skin conditions such as rosacea and bullous diseases, highlighting the role played by it in ensuring immune homeostasis. The neural-immune crosstalk conveyed through the NNCS presents promising lines of intervention to modulate localized immune reactions for enhancing skin health outcomes (Qu et al., 2024). The convergence of these complex immune pathways demonstrates that cutaneous immunity is not a rigid defense but a delicately calibrated system sensitive to both exogenous and endogenous inputs. The ability of skin cells to detect environmental toxins through AHR and to balance inflammatory signals through cholinergic mechanisms demonstrates the advanced interaction of immune and physiological processes necessary for skin homeostasis. Dysregulation of these regulatory networks can initiate a range of skin lesions from acute inflammatory reactions to chronic skin diseases. Hence, an overall understanding of immune-skin interactions is critical in the clinical strategy for the diagnosis and treatment of skin lesions, focusing on therapeutic interventions that restore immune balance to preserve skin integrity and function (Michał et al., 2024; Qu et al., 2024) (Figure 1.7).

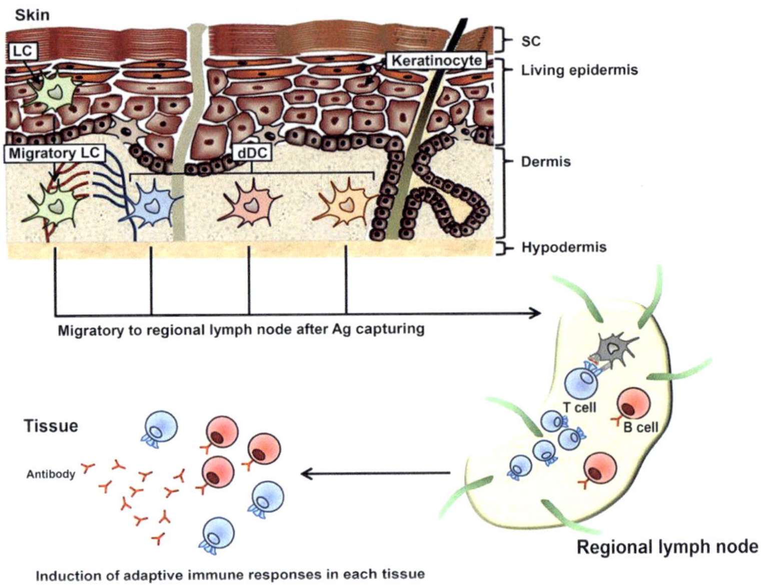

Figure 1.7. Skin immune system.

Source: Okada, N. (2013). Skin immune system: The skin is enriched with various immunocompetent cells such as LCs. In The skin as a novel immune organ for the induction of tolerance. *ResearchGate.*

1.3. Classification of Skin Diseases

Appreciation of the complex structure and multifaceted functions of the skin is necessary to classify various skin diseases. Skin diseases present with a range of lesions and signs that represent underlying pathophysiological mechanisms. Classification of the diseases allows for proper diagnosis, directs treatment, and determines prognosis. Skin diseases have traditionally been classified according to etiology, morphology, and clinical presentation. Etiological classification separates diseases into infectious, inflammatory, neoplastic, genetic, and degenerative types. Morphologic classification emphasizes the type of lesion, e.g., macules, papules, petechiae, pustules, ecchymoses, vesicles, or ulcers. This strategy helps clinicians differentiate among disorders that can clinically resemble one another but differ enormously in etiology and treatment. Because the skin acts as a barrier and immune organ, numerous diseases also interact with systemic elements, calling for an integrated perspective of dermatologic assessment to provide complete care. The clinical presentation of skin diseases also includes chronic and acute forms, adding to the complexity of diagnosis, and management plans. Diseases such as chronic venous disease (CVD) exemplify this complexity, wherein long-standing vascular changes lead to diverse cutaneous presentations ranging from telangiectasias to ulcerations (Miguel et al., 2021). The progressive course of such disorders highlights the necessity of a dynamic, rather than a static, classification scheme addressing disease stage and severity, as opposed to solely based on lesion descriptions. Further, improvements in imaging and molecular diagnostics are starting to narrow classifications by allowing better identification of subtypes and pathogenetic mechanisms. These advances hold the promise of enhanced personalization of treatment and underscore the shortcomings of traditional categories that address mostly visible or histologic phenotypes rather than underlying biological mechanisms. Advances in technology more recently augmented the classification system by combining spectral imaging and artificial intelligence (AI) to detail skin lesions with increased specificity (Neil et al., 2020). Multi- and hyperspectral imaging presents comprehensive optical signatures of skin tissue, enabling differential discrimination between benign vs. malignant lesions and between infectious vs. inflammatory pathology. Used in association with AI-guided image analysis, these technologies bring non-invasive, real-time diagnostic perception that goes beyond classification limits. It is this particular modality that has tremendous promise in the application of surgery, where minute margins and appropriate diagnosis are an important consideration. Though clinical uptake is premature, the synergy of spectral data and machine learning has the potential to transform the taxonomy of skin diseases into a more quantitative and objective science that ties classification tightly to pathophysiology and personalized patient care.

1.3.1. Infectious Skin Diseases: Bacterial, Viral, and Fungal

The skin is the body's first line of defense, with continuous exposure to numerous microorganisms, some of which can penetrate this protective barrier and result in infections. Infectious cutaneous disease occurs when pathogenic bacteria, viruses, or fungi colonize and interfere with the homeostasis of the skin, causing a range of clinical presentations. Bacterial infections, including impetigo, are the most prevalent infectious dermatoses, especially in children, and tend to flourish in environments where hygiene and socioeconomic status are impaired. They usually manifest with erythematous, crusted lesions mainly on the face and extremities, which is a reflection of the skin's susceptibility in certain anatomical areas. Epidemiological research stresses the increased rate of bacterial skin infections in low socioeconomic status children and in rural settings, as their exposure patterns and immune status shape the risk and severity of infection (Mahajan et al., 2019). The insight stresses the interaction between environmental, social, and biological factors in the pathogenesis of bacterial skin infections. Viruses are another very important group of infectious agents of the skin causing specific pathologies that may extend from benign warts to more severe viral exanthems. Viral cutaneous infections most commonly result from direct contact or reactivation in the dermal layers of latent viruses. *Human papillomavirus* (HPV), for instance, causes hyperproliferative lesions whose clinical manifestations depend on the viral subtype and immune response of the host. Other viral diseases, such as *Herpes simplex* and *Varicella zoster*, demonstrate how viruses take advantage of the skin microenvironment, presenting recurrent or disseminated lesions that are indicative of systemic disease. The interaction of viral pathogens with the skin's innate defense is a complex one that indicates that both barrier function and immune surveillance have an important role to play in managing these infections (Gall and Riely, 2025). As a result, a thorough dermatological evaluation should include viral causes in the evaluation of infectious skin lesions. Fungal cutaneous infections, or dermatophytoses, are a separate category marked by superficial invasion of keratinized tissues such as the stratum corneum, hair, and nails. *Dermatophytes* and *Candida species* are the usual pathogens responsible for these infections, the latter usually appearing in intertriginous zones (candidal intertrigo).

The clinical course of fungal infections varies from light scaling and erythema to acute chronic disease, usually depending on humidity, immunological status, and the integrity of the skin barrier. There is a high frequency of candidal infections in preschool children, emphasizing the need for high suspicion and targeted antifungal treatment (Mahajan et al., 2019). Moreover, chronic colonization by fungi in the skin's microflora ecological niche renders it difficult to distinguish commensal colonization from pathologic overgrowth (Gall and Riely, 2025). Knowledge about these fungal patterns is critical in managing and preventing recurrent infectious dermatoses in risk groups (Figure 1.8).

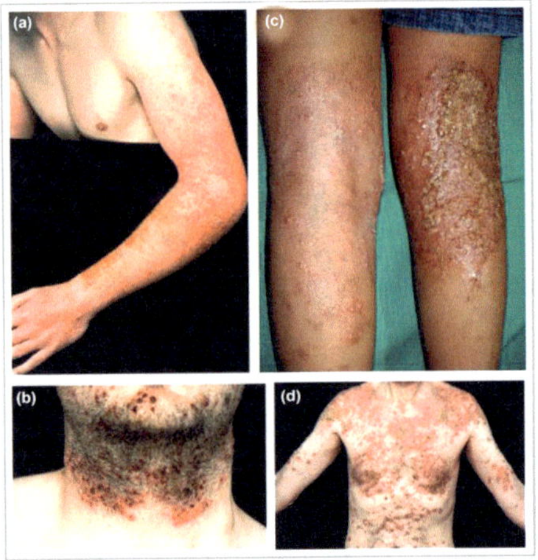

Figure 1.8. Clinical features of bacterial skin infection in atopic dermatitis (AD). Clinical features of *S. aureus* infection in atopic dermatitis lesions include (a) weeping, honey-colored crusts; (b) folliculitis; (c) pustulation; and (d) Beta-hemolytic streptococcal infection may present with well-defined bright red erythema.

Source: H. Alexander, A.S. Paller, C. Traidl-Hoffmann, L.A. Beck, A. De Benedetto, S. Dhar, G. Girolomoni, A.D. Irvine, P. Spuls, J. Su, J.P. Thyssen, C. Vestergaard, T. Werfel, A. Wollenberg, M. Deleuran, C. Flohr, The role of bacterial skin infections in atopic dermatitis: expert statement and review from the International Eczema Council Skin Infection Group, *British Journal of Dermatology*, Volume 182, Issue 6, 1 June 2020, Pages 1331–1342, https://doi.org/10.1111/bjd.18643

1.3.2. Non-Infectious Skin Diseases: Inflammatory and Autoimmune

The skin, the body's largest organ, is of first importance in defending against environmental insults and the regulation of homeostasis. Occasionally, disturbances in immune control cause non-infectious inflammatory responses that substantially compromise skin integrity. These inflammatory skin diseases are the result of complex interactions between environmental stimuli and genetic predisposition, leading to increased immune responses without associated infection. Psoriasis and atopic dermatitis are classic examples of this, where immune-mediated inflammation produces erythema, scaling, and pruritus. Understanding the pathophysiology of these disease states requires knowledge of skin anatomy and immunologic events, as the dermis and epidermis themselves are active participants in immune surveillance and response. This differentiation is critical for treating clinicians of skin lesions where the infection is absent but inflammation defines the presentation, a concept central to the broader realm of skin disease classification and enabling certain therapeutic strategies. Autoimmune dermatoses constitute a group of non-infectious inflammatory disorders that are differentiated on the basis of autoantibody production and immune-mediated injury. Diseases such as lupus erythematosus and pemphigus vulgaris are characterized by the autoimmune attack on constituents of the skin with resultant chronic inflammation and characteristic cutaneous features in the form of vesicles, plaques, and photosensitivity changes. The self-perpetuating nature of autoimmunity in these conditions complicates diagnosis and management and necessitates global strategies that consider both systemic and cutaneous involvement. These conditions illustrate the two functions of the skin as an immunoregulatory organ and as a barrier, emphasizing the importance of early diagnosis and intervention to prevent irreversible damage. Adding general skin physiology and lesion assessment into the evaluation is critical because autoimmune processes manifest with subtle clinical patterns, which are imitative of other dermatologic processes.

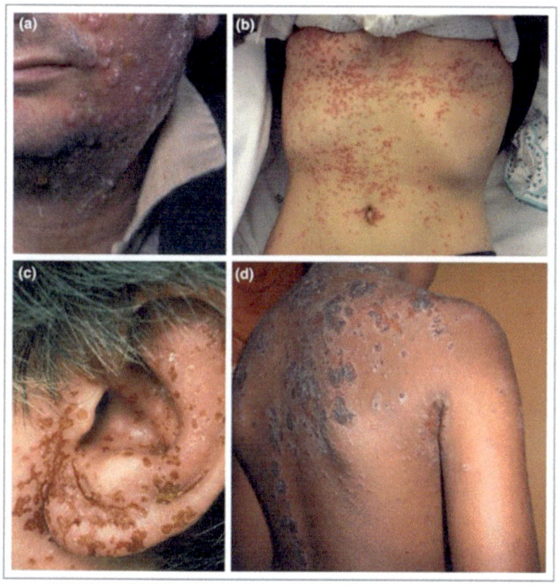

Figure 1.9. Inflammatory skin disease.

Source: H. Alexander, A.S. Paller, C. Traidl-Hoffmann, L.A. Beck, A. De Benedetto, S. Dhar, G. Girolomoni, A.D. Irvine, P. Spuls, J. Su, J.P. Thyssen, C. Vestergaard, T. Werfel, A. Wollenberg, M. Deleuran, C. Flohr, The role of bacterial skin infections in atopic dermatitis: expert statement and review from the International Eczema Council Skin Infection Group, *British Journal of Dermatology*, Volume 182, Issue 6, 1 June 2020, Pages 1331–1342, https://doi.org/10.1111/bjd.18643

Although infectious etiologies tend to predominate in dermatologic presentations, appropriate consideration of the subtle evaluation of non-infectious inflammatory and autoimmune conditions is crucial. Inappropriate treatment or delayed diagnosis from misdiagnosis can result in considerable morbidity, emphasizing increased clinical awareness. Though not a result of infectious pathogens, conditions may elicit systemic symptoms as well as complex psychosocial effects similar to those in infectious diseases (Zwart et al., 2024). Additionally, inflammatory responses can also manifest with aggressive behavior and psychological distress, which contribute to the overall disease burden (Gutiérrez-Cerrajero et al., 2023). Therefore, a multidisciplinary treatment strategy with a focus on accurate lesion categorization, immune modulation strategies, and patient-centered care is the solution to healing these stubborn dermatoses within dermatology practice and an understanding of skin anatomy (Figure 1.9).

1.3.3. Neoplastic Skin Diseases: Benign and Malignant Tumors

Neoplastic cutaneous diseases are a large group of dermatological pathology defined by cutaneous cell proliferation leading to tumor development. The tumors can be broadly divided into benign and malignant types. Benign neoplasms, as in the case of seborrheic keratoses and dermatofibromas, are usually slowly growing and have a low ability to invade local tissues, being of little risk to overall health. By contrast, malignant tumors such as basal cell carcinoma (BCC), squamous cell carcinoma, and melanoma are characterized by their dangerous potential, local destructive behavior, and risk of metastasis. Knowledge of the morphological and histological distinctions between benign and malignant skin neoplasms is critical to proper diagnosis and management. Differentiation also affects therapy and prognosis, and it accordingly represents an important element in the dermatology practice that requires adequate clinical and histopathological assessment. The etiology of neoplastic skin cancers is multicausal and includes genetic mutations, environmental insults, like UV light exposure—

and intrinsic inflammatory processes that lead to dysregulation of cells. Chronic inflammation, for example, is an essential factor in tumor promotion by encouraging a culture permissive to DNA damage and abnormal cellular growth. Although the precise etiology of most skin tumors is still not well known, correlations with immune status, genetic predisposition, and viral infections have been made. Treatment for skin neoplasms typically starts with an extensive clinical evaluation and can be followed by a biopsy for histopathologic diagnosis. Advances in molecular dermatology have further increased the accuracy of categorization of such tumors in precise terms, hence making treatment planning individualized. This meeting of clinical, pathological, and molecular data is a demonstration of the multidisciplinary emphasis of modern dermatologic oncology, with the evolving nature of neoplastic skin disease evaluation. From a practical perspective, the overall strategy in the evaluation of skin lesions requires observant attention for signs of neoplastic change.

Prompt recognition of malignant neoplasms is important because delayed detection can be associated with larger tissue spread and greater morbidity. Therapeutic approaches depend on the tumor type, size, location, and comorbidities of the patient, from topical treatments and cryotherapy for benign lesions to surgical removal, radiation, and systemic therapy for malignancies. Functional endoscopic methods and imaging modalities are frequently used to define tumor extent, particularly when deeper structures are potentially involved, as surgical planning requires accurate anatomical knowledge. While neoplastic skin conditions impact varied patient populations, men have been reported to present with greater incidence rates of some tumor forms, which may mirror possible biological and environmental factors. This epidemiological information is used in public health policy with regard to prevention and early intervention to ultimately enhance patient outcomes through multidisciplinary treatment (Dogjani et al., 2022; Bonciu et al., 2023) (Figure 1.10).

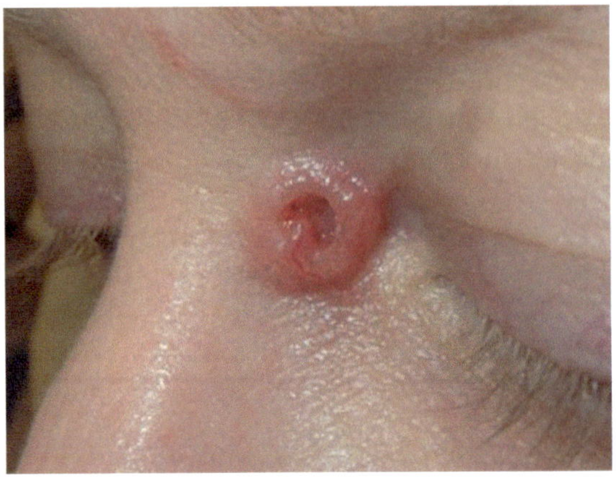

Figure 1.10. Neoplastic skin lesions.

Source: Peeling, R. W., & Hook, E. W. (2006). Syphilis. In *Encyclopedia of Infectious Diseases* (pp. 489–495). Springer.

1.4. Functions of the Skin

The largest organ in the human body takes on a role of enormous influence far beyond the physical self, acting as an essential bridge between internal and external systems. Perhaps its most critical function is one of defense, shielding the interior from mechanical damage, microbial infection, and detrimental UV light. The stratified skin arrangement in the form of epidermis, dermis, and hypodermis is an impermeable barrier that excludes noxious organisms but allows as little water as possible to be retained. This selective permeability ensures not only bodily fluid homeostasis but also homeostasis, highlighting the regulatory role of skin. Besides, the specialized skin cells allow for immune surveillance to identify the threat to the integrity of the body and make a response. This active protection adds to the depth of the skin and its invaluable position as the body's first defense, paramount in the maintenance of health and the prevention of disease processes in dermatology (Esteva et al., 2021). Besides the protective role, the skin is also important in the sensory process, having a large number of diverse nerve endings that detect pressure, temperature, and pain. Through these sensory receptors, the skin can act as a significant communication medium between the outside world and the central nervous system, allowing for reflex response and conscious perception. This sensory function is not only important for environmental adaptation but also for the feeling of noxious stimuli, thereby preventing harm. Moreover, the skin is actively involved in thermoregulation through vasodilation, vasoconstriction, and sweating to maintain an internal homeostasis. The complicated balance of these physiological processes guarantees that the skin supports overall systemic homeostasis, highlighting its multifunctional nature in health, which is fundamental in appreciating the various dermatological diseases and their implication in systemic homeostasis (Esteva et al., 2021). In addition, skin has a significant metabolic role via vitamin D synthesis during exposure to UV light, a process that is central to calcium homeostasis and bone metabolism. This biochemistry demonstrates the contribution of the skin to overall physiological processes beyond the immediate surrounding environment. Additionally, the skin participates in excretion through sweat glands, allowing for the elimination of metabolic waste products such as urea and salts. This excretory function aids in detoxification and regulation of electrolyte homeostasis. The development of medical technology, especially in digital health platforms, is continuously improving surveillance over these skin functions, which enhances diagnostic precision and individualized treatment strategies for skin diseases. Taken together, these various functions highlight the skin's essential role in overall health, which is central to successful dermatological practice and management of patients (Figure 1.11).

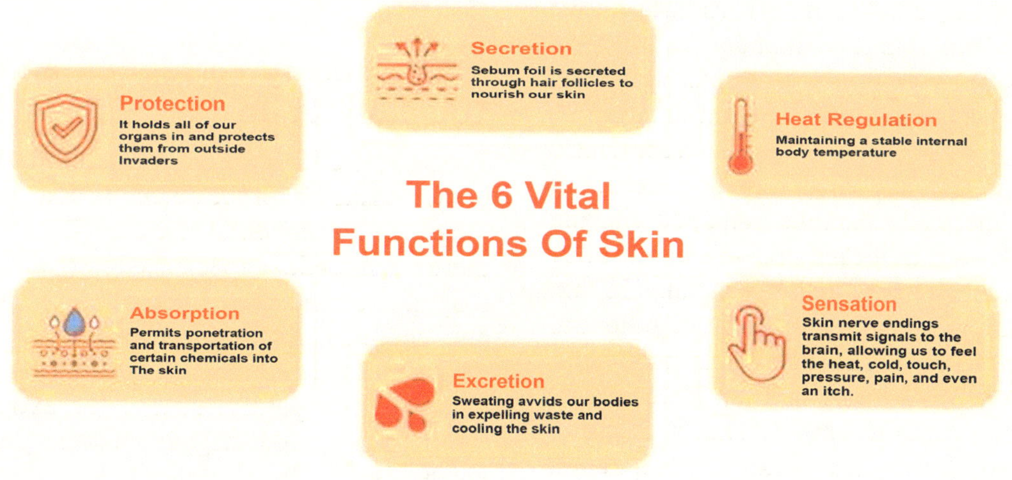

Figure 1.11. Vital functions of skin.

Source: DermaMed Solutions. (n.d.). Skin condition close-up. *Shopify*. https://external-content.duckduckgo.com/iu/?u=https%3A%2F%2Fcdn.shopify.com%2Fs%2Ffiles%2F1%2F0030%2F3064%2F6896%2Ffiles%2FS2_2484ff63-19be-427c-a66c-0bb9f80cd144_600x600.png%3Fv%3D1682439873&f=1&nofb=1&ipt=d7e83f077121c898f707b444762edbe26731fe24cfa3c1c36cc738b8764510be.

1.4.1. Protection Against Environmental Hazards

The skin is not just a physical barrier but also the body's first defense against a host of external insults, such as UV radiation, toxins, pathogens, and chemical irritants. Its stratified nature, especially its outermost layer, the stratum corneum, is essential in denying entry to noxious substances while providing hydration and structural support. Also, skin cells synthesize melanin, which absorbs and dissipates UV radiation, thus preventing DNA damage and skin cancers. The skin's ability to perceive and react to environmental stimuli is controlled by its dense population of sensory receptors and immune cells, which trigger inflammatory or healing responses as needed. Recognition of these defense mechanisms highlights the dynamic function of the skin as greater than a mere covering and confirms its participation in total homeostasis and health. Stressors in the environment also induce oxidative stress within skin cells, leading to premature aging and various dermatologic disorders. Reactive oxygen species created by UV radiation and inhaled irritants induce damage to cellular structures such as lipids, proteins, and DNA that compromise the integrity and function of the skin. To counter this, skin possesses intrinsic antioxidant defense mechanisms, including enzymes superoxide dismutase and non-enzyme compounds such as vitamin E, which neutralize oxidative damage and facilitate cellular repair. Recent findings reveal the therapeutic potential of nanomaterials in enhancing skin protection by more effectively targeting antioxidants or therapeutic agents to amplify skin protection, offering new approaches against environmental insults. However, their application in dermatological treatments should be well thought out for safety because they have specific interactions with the biological tissue and can have potential toxicities (Joseph et al., 2023). The developments indicate an emerging horizon for dermatology as a science of protection against hazards from the environment that merges with advanced biotechnology. Apart from direct cutaneous exposure, the environment also acts on systemic well-being through subtle mechanisms related to the skin microbiome and immunological processes. Variable microbiota on the skin sustains homeostatic conditions that ward off pathogenic colonization and modulate local immune reactions. An interruption of the resulting microbiota from pollutants or allergens is responsible for provoking inflammatory diseases of the skin or intensifying systemwide allergic inflammation. Moreover, research on microbiota within the respiratory and intestines demonstrates the action of agents within the environment upon dysbiosis, encouraging hypersensitivity as well as immunoregulation-associated diseases like asthma (Hufnagl et al., 2020). These observations shed light on the interconnectivity of environmental exposure, microbial community, and function of the skin, highlighting the significance of maintaining the integrity of the skin not just for localized defense but also for its general function in immune homeostasis and prevention of disease.

1.4.2. Sensory Perception and Communication

The skin, the largest sense organ of the human body, is tasked with the detection of an extensive range of environmental stimuli. Within its layers, there are embedded specialized receptor cells that respond to mechanical pressure, temperature, and chemical stimuli. These receptors allow the body to sense environmental changes and dangers, like painful stimuli or extremes of temperature, and trigger instant protective mechanisms. The complex neural network of the skin provides for the speedy conduction of sensory information to the central nervous system for processing and interpretation. The dynamic sensory role also plays a part in nonverbal communication, as variations in color, texture, and development of lesions tend to activate underlying physiological or pathological conditions and provide visible cues to others. Knowledge about these mechanisms is crucial in dermatology because most skin diseases present through the channel of changed sensory perception or breakdown in communication routes, which affect diagnosis and treatment methods (Päkk et al., 2012). Psychological factors and stress can significantly affect sensory perception and communication in skin disease. For instance, in chronic inflammatory diseases such as AD, patients often describe exacerbations induced by psychological stress, which increases sensory symptoms such as itching and burning. Studies have shown that stress changes brain activity involved in sensory integration and processing, especially in motor and somatosensory association cortices, thus modifying the way patients perceive and react to stimuli. This neurocutaneous link highlights the necessity of the treatment of both peripheral and central elements in the response of skin to injury and inflammation. Further, alterations in neuropeptides such as calcitonin gene-related peptide (CGRP) in the nerve fibers of the skin have been linked with increased sensory sensitivity and emotional distress in patients with AD, proposing an complex bidirectional communication between the nervous system and the skin (Abdelhadi, 2023). The skin's communication function also involves more than sensory input and involves the active modulation of inflammatory and immune responses that are essential signals in defending homeostasis and fighting infection. Specialized cells in the epidermis assist in this interaction by sending chemical mediators and displaying antigens, which affect overall immune activity. In addition, cellular elements like epidermal club cells are also suspected of being involved in injury response and regeneration mechanisms, demonstrating the skin's ability to signal tissue damage and launch repair processes. This complex system of communication enables the coordination of external environmental signals with internal body responses, enabling the skin to be both a sensory interface and an active participant in the body's defense system. The advancement of the mechanisms of these interactions is important in the development of therapeutic approaches aimed at improving sensory perception and recovering communication pathways damaged by skin conditions (Päkk et al., 2012) (Figure 1.12).

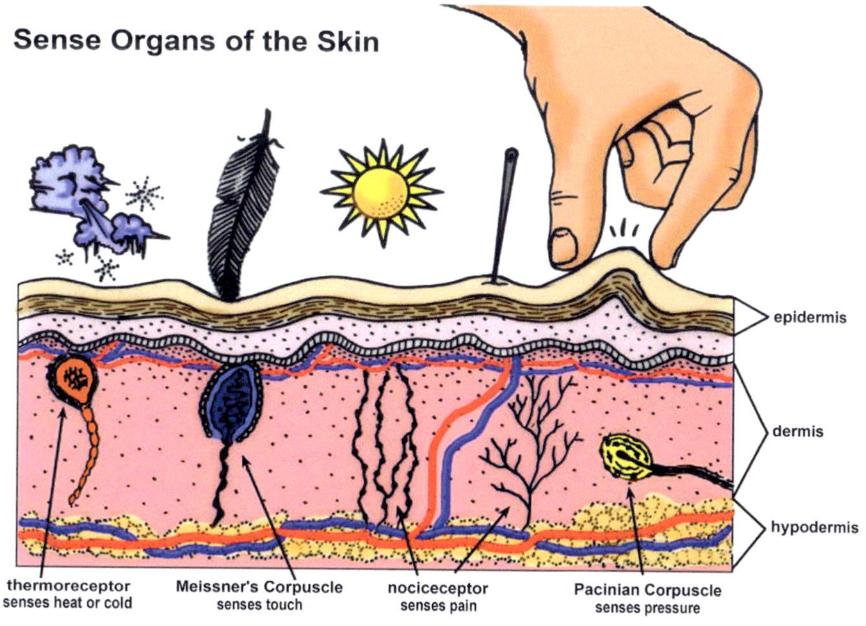

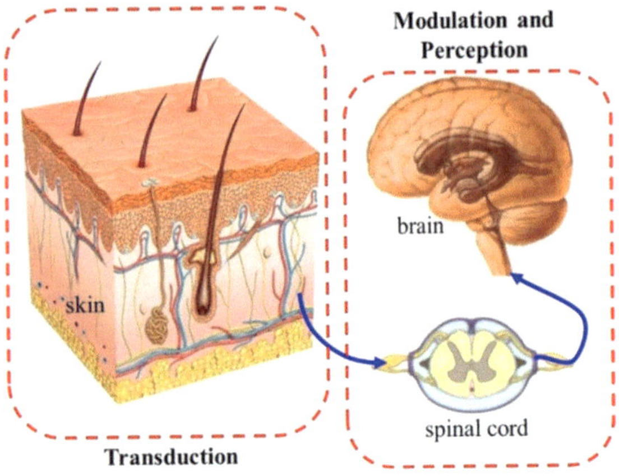

Figure 1.12. Sense organs of the skin.

Source: Ji D, Shi Y, Chen J, Zhao Z, Zhao G. Mathematical Model for Skin Pain Sensation under Local Distributed Mechanical Compression for Electronic Skin Applications. *Micromachines*. 2022; 13(9):1402. https://doi.org/10.3390/mi13091402

1.4.3. Metabolic Functions, Including Vitamin D Synthesis

The skin is an active interface between the internal and external environment, with significant functions beyond protection. One such important contribution of the skin is the metabolic functions required for systemic homeostasis. Among these, vitamin D synthesis is a critical process that relates skin physiology to general health. When exposed to ultraviolet B (UVB) radiation, 7-dehydrocholesterol in the epidermis absorbs UVB photons and is converted to pre-vitamin D3, which then goes through thermal isomerization to become vitamin D3 (cholecalciferol). The process highlights the skin as an endocrine organ that produces a molecule that has an effect on calcium metabolism, bone health, and immune regulation. Therefore, disruptions to skin structure or function, as seen in many dermatologic diseases, can compromise cutaneous vitamin D production, again drawing attention to the overlap between skin disease and systemic metabolic consequences (Gutiérrez-Cerrajero et al., 2023). Vitamin D production via the skin represents a complex relationship between environmental exposure and physiological control. The precursor molecule, 7-dehydrocholesterol, is found mostly in the spinous and basal layers of the epidermis, so intact epidermal architecture is required for efficient vitamin D production. Disturbances in keratinocyte differentiation or epidermal barrier function, frequent in disorders such as ichthyoses, can disturb this metabolic activity. These disorders tend to be associated with hyperkeratosis and defective barrier formation, which can diminish UVB penetration and restrict vitamin D synthesis. Apart from structural aspects, pigmentation and aging also affect cutaneous vitamin D production since melanin absorbs UV radiation and decreases photoconversion efficiency, and aged skin has lower concentrations of 7-dehydrocholesterol. Thus, knowing the skin's microanatomical and functional characteristics helps one better understand the metabolic difficulties encountered during dermatological disorders (Gutiérrez-Cerrajero et al., 2023).

In addition to vitamin D production, the skin is involved in other metabolic processes including lipid production, thermoregulation, and the catabolism of xenobiotics. The epidermis produces a variety of lipids important in maintaining barrier function and hydration, such as ceramides and cholesterol derivatives, essential in keeping cutaneous homeostasis intact. Impairment of these metabolic pathways may worsen skin diseases with barrier dysfunction, making disease treatment more complicated. In addition, the skin contributes to xenobiotic metabolism through cytochrome P450 enzymes that enable detoxification and antigen presentation. These metabolic processes collectively demonstrate the skin's multifaceted involvement in overall physiology, highlighting the importance of skin integrity and function in health and disease. Consequently, clinical management of skin lesions and disease prefers to incorporate such metabolic aspects to optimize patient outcomes (Gutiérrez-Cerrajero et al., 2023).

1.5. Common Skin Lesions

Skin lesions are an assortment of abnormal skin appearance changes that often arise from infections, inflammatory processes, or neoplasia. Their clinical presentation may vary from subtle color change to open growths, and clinical detection hence forms the core of dermatological diagnosis. The most commonly seen lesions are macules, papules, nodules, vesicles, pustules, and plaques, each with specific morphological characteristics. For example, macules are non-palpable and flat lesions characterized by color changes without elevation, whereas papules consist of small elevated lesions typically less than centimeter in size.

The heterogeneity of skin lesions is a reflection of the complex anatomy and physiology of the skin such that derangements at various levels of the dermis and epidermis present in diverse ways. This variability calls for a methodical process to characterize lesions on the basis of size, shape, color, texture, and location in order to accurately diagnose and treat them. Merging clinical examination with new diagnostic technology improves lesion characterization and informs therapy (Said et al., 2024).

The causes of prevalent skin lesions are extensive, including infectious causes in the form of bacteria, viruses, fungi, and parasites and autoimmune and allergic responses. Among infections, bacterial impetigo and viral warts are frequent, appearing as pustules and papillomatous lesions respectively. Inflammatory lesions like eczema and psoriasis show scaling plaques, indicating immune dysregulation affecting epidermal turnover and barrier function. Neoplastic lesions, such as benign nevi and malignant melanomas, need to be carefully assessed because they tend to progress and metastasize. The visual similarity of benign and malignant lesions emphasizes the importance of thorough skin examination and may require advanced diagnostic modalities such as dermoscopy or histopathology. Understanding the pathophysiology underlying these lesions enables the clinician to distinguish acute inflammatory from chronic or malignant processes and thus optimize patient outcomes (Gutiérrez-Cerrajero et al., 2023).

Improved diagnostic technology has greatly improved the detection and classification of complex skin lesions. Artificial intelligence and machine learning now supplement traditional clinical assessment with enhanced sensitivity in the detection of early malignant changes, particularly melanoma. Advanced algorithms use dermoscopic images to evaluate slight changes in lesion morphology, color patterns, and border abnormalities, which are difficult to identify visually. These computer algorithms synthesize pattern recognition and feature extraction to facilitate efficient, non-invasive screening, thus permitting early interventions.

The utilization of such tools is proof of the interdisciplinary interfacing of dermatology and computer science. It is most likely to reduce diagnostic errors and improve the prognosis of patients with skin cancer. Clinical experience, however, cannot be avoided since the interpretation of these technologies must be made in the context of the patient's comprehensive dermatological history and physical examination (Said et al., 2024) (Figure 1.13).

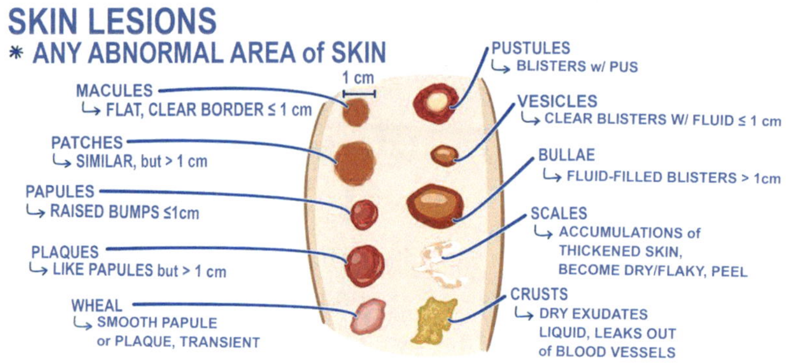

Figure 1.13. Skin lesions.

Source: Osmose IT. (n.d.). *Image of Skin Condition*. https://osmose-it.s3.amazonaws.com/JKZLnEDEQq_MpX6rNMahX6SyRDWZPsIn/_.jpg.

1.5.1. Types of Skin Lesions: Macules, Papules, and Nodules

The skin, being the body's largest organ, performs a critical function of protecting deeper structures and maintaining homeostasis. Insight into the several presentations of dermatologic changes is important in dermatology, since skin lesions are usually outward signs of generalized or local disease processes. Of the countless types of lesions, macules are flat, bordered patches of color change smaller than 1 cm. Unlike raised lesions, macules are not palpable on elevation or depression. Such small changes in pigmentation can be indicative of a range of conditions, from benign freckles to developing inflammatory or infectious disease. Their clinical value is in their discrimination function, to enable clinicians to differentiate benign from potentially hazardous skin alterations and therefore guide further examination or therapy. In contrast to macules, papules are small solid, projecting lesions typically less than 1 cm in diameter. Papules arise from superficial dermatosis and also often signify a localized inflammatory process or neoplastic process. Because they can be palpable, papules are easily visible on clinical examinations and may present in a myriad of morphologies and distributions. Examples include acne vulgaris as well as many forms of dermatitis. The pathophysiologic mechanism behind papule development is cellular growth and infiltration within epidermal or dermal layers, which indicates a chronic dynamic response to infection or injury. Papules are essential to understand since they often act as precursors or part of more complex patterns of lesions, requiring critical clinical assessment to distinguish between benign and malignant etiologies. Nodules are distinguished from macules and papules based on size and depth; they are larger, commonly more than 1 cm in diameter, and penetrate into the deeper dermis or subcutaneous tissue. These hard, mobile or fixed lesions can occur from a host of etiologies encompassing inflammatory, infectious, or neoplastic etiologies. Nodules tend to indicate a more severe or more chronic pathology than papules since their depth indicates deeper tissue involvement. Clinically, nodules may be related to disorders like rheumatoid nodules, lipomas, or even malignancies like squamous cell carcinoma (Sundaresan et al., 2022). Their recognition and description are important in dermatology as they usually demand biopsy and subsequent histopathological examination to determine the diagnosis and proper treatment modalities, illustrating the interface of clinical observation and molecular and cellular insight (Gutiérrez-Cerrajero et al., 2023) (Figure 1.14).

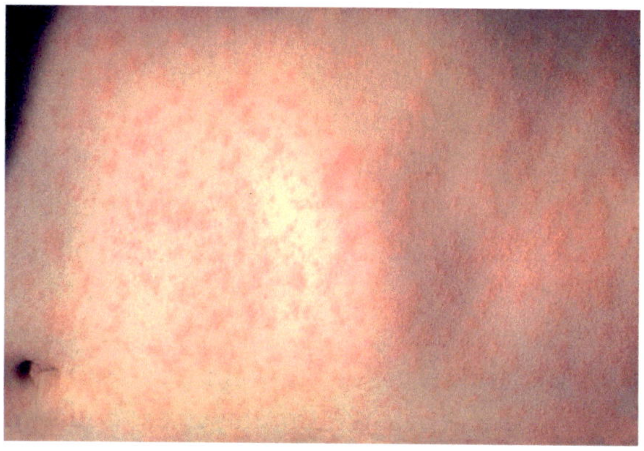

Figure 1.14. Macules.

Source: By Photo Credit:Content Providers(s): CDC/Dr. Heinz F. Eichenwald - This media comes from the Centers for Disease Control and Prevention's Public Health Image Library (PHIL), with identification number #3168| +/− Originally from en.wikipedia; description page is/was here., Public Domain, https://commons.wikimedia.org/w/index.php?curid=4393873

1.5.2. Characteristics and Significance of Skin Lesions

Skin lesion expression typically serves as a significant indicator of one's underlying health status, necessitating a complete understanding of their characteristics to facilitate appropriate diagnosis and management. Lesions are defined by morphology, distribution, size, color, and texture, all of which contribute to the clinical assessment and the differentiation between benign and malignant processes. The importance of skin lesions is that they not only represent localized manifestations but can also be windows to systemic diseases. Identification of certain patterns of lesion presentation helps clinicians establish the etiology of disease, influence diagnostic strategies, and guide prognosis. These sorts of extensive characterization need a multidisciplinary understanding of skin anatomy and pathophysiology, which increases the accuracy of dermatological assessment and helps to result in better patient outcomes by facilitating early and effective intervention (Varnosfaderani et al., 2024). In general skin physiology, lesions represent disturbances in the integumentary system's normal protective and regulatory roles. The complex function of the skin, ranging from barrier defense to immunologic surveillance, is disturbed when lesions occur, often revealing the site and nature of injury or infection. Morphologic features like papules, plaques, vesicles, and ulcers are linked with specific pathomechanisms like inflammation, neoplasia, or immune dysregulation. The temporal evolution of lesions provides hints of disease progression or resolution, underscoring their diagnostic and therapeutic roles. Knowledge of the microenvironmental stimuli and cellular interactions that contribute to lesion development also presents opportunities for novel therapy and emphasizes the strategic interplay between cutaneous expression and systemic wellness (Gali et al., 2023). Technical improvements in diagnostic techniques have greatly improved the clinical management of skin lesions, enabling more advanced, non-invasive techniques of evaluation. Methods like dermoscopy, high-resolution imaging, and computer analysis using AI now complement routine examination, providing enhanced sensitivity and specificity in classifying lesions. AI is able to provide pattern recognition and predictive modeling, making diagnosis faster and minimizing human errors (Varnosfaderani et al., 2024). Not only do such technological advancements intensify the understanding of lesion morphology but also support earlier identification of malignant transformations, thus improving prognosis in patients. Accordingly, the assimilation of innovative technologies into dermatological practice is a turning point in the management of skin lesions, highlighting their importance in the broader context of skin health and disease management (Gali et al., 2023).

1.5.3. Diagnostic Methods for Evaluating Skin Lesions

The first stage in the evaluation of skin lesions is usually a good clinical examination, where palpation and visual inspection help gain essential information about the morphology, distribution, and course of the lesion. The dermatoscope, an inexpensive hand-held instrument similar to a camera, provides magnification and illumination and aids to visualize structures beneath the skin. This non-surgical method helps differentiate benign from malignant lesions by magnifying characteristic features such as pigment networks, vascular patterns, and lesion margins. Outside the naked-eye examination, digital imaging and artificial intelligence algorithms have increasingly complemented clinical expertise by processing lesion images to estimate malignancy risk with promising accuracy.

Such AI-based instruments simplify the diagnostic process, particularly in environments where expert availability is low, as part of the general trend in healthcare toward utilizing digital innovation to enhance clinical decision-making and patient-tailored care (Varnosfaderani et al., 2024). Where clinical examination and dermatoscopy indicate uncertainty or possible malignancy, histopathological examination is still the gold standard for certain diagnoses. A biopsy, which can be excisional, incisional, or punch, permits microscopic inspection of skin tissue to directly view cellular architecture and pathological alterations. Histopathology yields essential information about the nature, size, and depth of the lesion, enabling proper classification and directing proper treatment modalities. Supportive methods like immunohistochemistry improve diagnostic accuracy by detecting specific cellular markers. Over the last few years, technological improvements in imaging modalities, such as functional photoacoustic imaging, have provided more non-invasive methods for evaluating microvascular and metabolic properties of skin lesions. The technology allows for the quantification of parameters such as oxygen saturation and blood flow, potentially used to distinguish between benign and malignant tissue without invasive techniques (Park et al., 2023). Apart from conventional methods, new diagnostic techniques use multidisciplinary technologies to enhance early detection and surveillance of skin lesions. Confocal microscopy, for instance, generates *in vivo* cellular resolution images, enabling real-time, non-invasive skin layer examination. Further, molecular diagnostic approaches, such as genetic and proteomic analysis, provide information about the pathogenesis of complexcomplex lesions, enabling targeted therapy. These next-generation diagnostics supplement the bedrock of clinical exam and biopsy with solutions to their limitations, including invasiveness and turnaround time. With advancing research, combining AI with emerging imaging and molecular diagnostics has great promise to extend diagnostic accuracy and clinical efficacy in dermatology, developing more personalized and targeted evaluation of skin lesions (Park et al., 2023; Varnosfaderani et al., 2024).

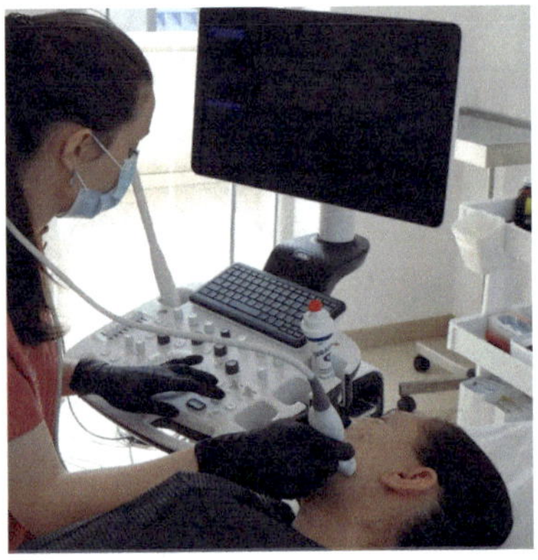

Source: Delia Thiess Clinic. (n.d.). *Ecografie Cutanată.* https://deliathiess.com/wp-content/uploads/2024/04/Ecografie-cutanata-e1713967092335-1024x1024.webp.

1.6. General Approach to Skin Lesions

A complete assessment of skin lesions is a critical part of clinical dermatology, requiring a systematic approach that includes patient history, morphology of the lesion, and diagnostic methods. Foremost, taking a thorough patient history, such as lesion appearance, evolution, concomitant symptoms, and possible exposure to environmental or infectious factors, prevents potential pitfalls in diagnosis. This information informs follow-up clinical evaluation, wherein lesions are examined according to features such as size, color, form, border, texture, and distribution. Morphological division, identifying macules, papules, nodules, vesicles, and plaques, and so on—is useful for limiting differential diagnoses. Additionally, integrating clinical findings with the anatomy and physiology of skin is crucial, because the understanding of which layers of the skin are involved can be a clue to lesion pathogenesis. This organized assessment allows for focused diagnostic testing, increasing precision and patient care. After clinical inspection, the use of diagnostic adjuncts is an important part of the workup of skin lesions. Dermoscopy (or dermatoscopy), an imaging method that does not involve puncture, offers increased visualization of subsurface structures, increasing diagnostic accuracy in conditions like melanoma and benign nevi. Where uncertainty does exist, biopsy continues as the gold standard and allows histopathological evaluation to secure diagnoses and inform treatment pathways. Novel technologies, further synergized through AI and machine learning, show the potential to support enhanced diagnostic sensitivity by interpreting complex visual data patterns that are beyond human ability (Bekbolatova et al., 2024; Varnosfaderani et al., 2024). These developments reflect the increasing interaction between clinical expertise and technological advancements, establishing the necessity for dermatologists to keep current with both conventional and modern modes of diagnosis. Ultimately, integrating these devices maximizes results by facilitating early diagnosis and proper management of possibly serious cutaneous disease. The overall strategy of treating skin lesions goes beyond diagnosis to include factors such as etiologic considerations, variables specific to the patient, and treatment goals. Successful management requires an individualized approach guided by lesion type, underlying pathology, and possible systemic involvement. Education of the patient is essential and involves addressing issues of sun protection, hygiene, and awareness of warning signs that require reevaluation. Treatment measures vary from topical therapy to systemic drugs and excision surgery, selected according to the severity of the lesion and malignancy or infection risk. In addition, follow-up on a regular basis enables observation of lesion development and therapeutic response, adjusting management as necessary. Multidisciplinary input can also be added to further improve patient care, especially in refractory or complicated cases. This integrated approach to skin lesions supports the overall dermatological objective of maintaining skin integrity and function while reducing morbidity, in line with changing clinical best practices (Bekbolatova et al., 2024; Varnosfaderani et al., 2024).

1.6.1. Clinical Assessment and History Taking

Good clinical evaluation and history taking are the cornerstones of dermatology practice, determining greatly diagnosis and treatment of skin disease. Physical examination precedes detailed patient history that gives crucial information regarding the onset, duration, course, and aggravating and relieving factors of the skin lesion. Such a history helps clinicians situate skin features within a larger systemic or environmental context. In addition, the history tends to uncover comorbidities, use of medications, allergies, occupational exposures, and family history of skin disease, all of which fine-tune differential diagnoses. Knowledge of patient habits and psychosocial issues also directs individualized counseling and therapeutic compliance plans. Clinicians need to take a methodical approach to avoid missing important information, thereby enhancing detection and outcome. This careful history taking also enables a robust patient-provider relationship, with trust and adherence essential to continued skin disease management (Chukwu & Mankila, 2018). Physical examination of skin lesions requires not only scrupulous observation but also accurate documentation and interpretation of morphological features. Practitioners examine the color, size, shape, distribution, location, and texture of lesions. Through palpation, they can check for induration, temperature, or tenderness. These observations help distinguish between primary and secondary lesions and between benign and malignant lesions. The skin examination is often supplemented by aids like dermoscopy, which improves visualization of the features below the surface. Note is taken of related findings such as mucosal involvement or lymphadenopathy, which reveal patterns of systemic involvement. Close examination of the skin is a window into internal health states and disease processes (Wallis, 2017). The physical examination therefore complements the history in the construction of a complete clinical picture, informing further diagnostic and therapeutic actions. It is crucial to synthesize assessment findings and patient history in the creation of an efficient management plan depending on individual requirements. Dermatological nurses, as active participants in the healthcare team, have a key role to play in cementing patient knowledge of their condition and treatments and so promoting compliance and outcomes. Their knowledge allows them to recognize gaps in patient understanding and overcome issues of cultural divergence or complexity of treatment that may impair adherence. Furthermore, continuous patient education and counseling empower patients to become actively involved in their care, enhancing recovery and enhancing quality of life. The continued therapeutic relationship fostered between patient and caregiver plays a critical role in sustaining motivation and trust, essential in the management of chronic or recurrent skin disorders (Chukwu & Mankila, 2018). Therefore, combining comprehensive clinical evaluations with empathetic communication maximizes patient-centered dermatological care.

1.6.2. Laboratory Tests and Imaging Techniques

Laboratory advances have significantly improved the process of diagnosis in dermatology, such that there is a more accurate assessment of skin disease and lesions. The tests frequently encompass measurements of the skins biophysical properties like hydration, transepidermal water loss (TEWL), and thickness of the skin layers, which are important for determining skin barrier integrity and function. Tools such as high-resolution ultrasound imaging allow quantitation of these layers, demonstrating heterogeneity at various anatomical locations and demographics such as age and sex. These quantitative measurements not only enable mapping of the state of the skin but also assess pathological changes associated with disease advancement or treatment response. The integration of such detailed laboratory analyses allows clinicians to develop an increased understanding of dermatological health beyond visual inspection, thereby informing targeted management approaches for a wide range of skin conditions (Chirikhina, 2022). Concurrent with laboratory testing, non-invasive imaging has transformed the in-vivo analysis of skin morphology and pathology. Optical coherence tomography (OCT), for example, provides micrometer-scale spatial resolution and real-time cross-sectional imaging to a depth of as much as 2 millimeters within the skin. This makes OCT very beneficial for imaging microstructural detail without the removal of tissue and hence contributing to diagnostic and interventional dermatology. Other recent advances involve the use of OCT to precisely guide biopsies, outline lesion borders before excision, and track topical drug delivery.

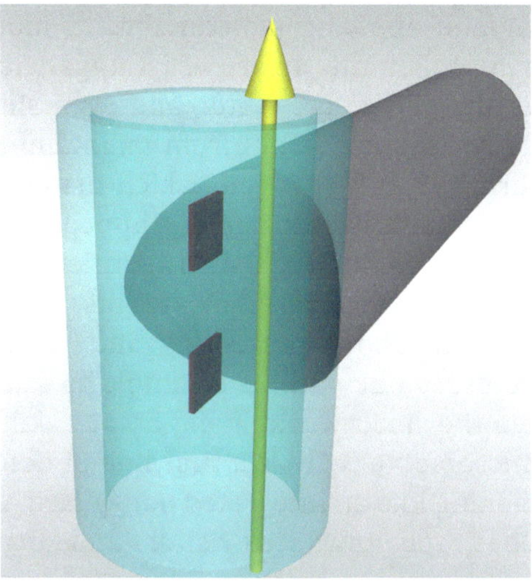

Figure 1.15. Illustration of transepidermal water loss (TEWL).

Source: By Xorx - This image was created with POV-Ray., CC BY-SA 4.0, https://commons.wikimedia.org/w/index.php?curid=73492948

The application of contrast-enhanced OCT further enhances the detection of malignant melanoma cells by differentiating them from normal keratinocytes, signifying a major advance in early cancer diagnosis and patient prognosis. As such, OCT exemplifies the integration of cutting-edge imaging into dermatological practice, augmenting clinicians' ability to detect, characterize, and manage skin diseases effectively (Xu , 2021). In addition to imaging resolution and method, the acquisition of quantitative information from diagnostic modalities provides valuable criticality for the evaluation of skin health in a variety of populations. Values of skin optical attenuation coefficients obtained from OCT images have been demonstrated to be anatomically-, age-, and phototype-dependent, indicating underlying physiological variation. For instance, the epidermis typically has greater attenuation than the dermis, and darker skin has unique optical characteristics that can impact diagnostic interpretation. In addition, lab studies demonstrate that skin hydration declines with age, impacting barrier function and susceptibility to dermatologic disease. Identification of skin sites and conditions through the use of machine learning algorithms and imaging data allows for automatic classification and the potential for enhanced diagnostic accuracy and tailored treatment planning. Together, these advances highlight the value of synergizing laboratory and imaging methodologies to improve dermatological science and clinical practice (Xu, 2021; Chirkhina, 2022) (Figure 1.15).

1.6.3. Treatment Options and Management Strategies

Management of a skin disease has to be managed with intensive insight into the cause and overall medical condition of the patient. There must be appropriate management towards the type of lesion of the skin because, even within systemic disorders, therapy ranges from topically applied medication to extensive operations. For instance, pharmacotherapy stands at the pinnacle of treating diffuse diseases such as Type 2 diabetes mellitus, for which oral hypoglycemia agents are not only commonplace but also represent conventional treatment. However, one must watch out for cutaneous adverse drug effects induced by these drugs from mild erythema to perhaps life-threatening conditions like Stevens-Johnson syndrome. Early detection and withdrawal of the offending drug are required to prevent complications. Thus, dermatologists must be particularly sensitive to drug-induced skin presentation to ensure the optimal result in patients without leading to severe adverse effects, particularly in susceptible subjects like elderly individuals (Kowalska et al., 2024). Surgical excision is a significant cornerstone of most skin cancers, even more BCC, and consequently, often present in locations like the external ear. The anatomical complexity of the region calls for a multidisciplinary treatment to consider complete resection of the tumor with preservation of function and aesthetics. Mohs micrographic surgery is generally employed since it possesses a tissue-sparing advantage and cure rates that are high. However, when invasive tumors involve critical adjacent structures such as the parotid gland or external auditory canal, treatment modalities need to be escalated. These types of cases can include extensive resections including partial pinnectomy or parotidectomy with complex reconstructive procedures like free flap repair. Multidisciplinary consultation guarantees the selection of optimal modalities unique to tumor size as well as patient quality of life (Kloczko et al., 2024). In addition to selecting some treatments, plans should also include education, prevention, and surveillance to enable long-term skin health. Informing the patients about risk factors, earliness of skin lesions, and the importance of following prescribed therapies will go a significant way in managing the disease and reducing recurrence rates. Preventive measures, like sun protection and avoiding known drug allergens, are important aspects in the management of susceptibility to neoplastic as well as inflammatory skin disorders. Follow-up that is persistent is used to detect early signs of failure of treatment or side effects, thereby enabling timely adjustment of treatment protocols. Last but not least, the inclusion of these holistic practices allows for an integrated style of dermatology care in line with the multifaceted nature of skin function as well as the diversity of manifestations of skin diseases.

1.7. Skin Health and Maintenance

Our skin is a living puzzle that requires attention on multiple levels. You have got your outer epidermis, middle dermis, and deeper hypodermis—all playing roles such as buffering us from the sun's damaging rays, maintaining our temperature, and even allowing us to feel the texture. Daily maintenance may be as basic as washing gently to preserve the natural barrier and applying moisturizers to monitor water loss. For the most part, things such as proper diet, adequate water, and even slightly reduced stress keep skin from maintaining its cell turnover and collagen, which many claim are the secrets to an ageless appearance. It appears that combining both scientific concepts and daily practices truly indicates just how skin care is also about protecting and repairing what crosses our path. It is simple to take for granted the small world living on our skin, but this microbiome truly is a first line of defense. Functioning like an integrated bodyguard, these microbes repel unwanted visitors and keep our immune system in balance. Recently, there has been excitement over applying peptide-based antimicrobials as a new means of combating skin infections. For instance, certain bioactive peptides, originally derived naturally from fish skin, have been reported to be used in combination with probiotic byproducts to get in the way of bacteria—breaking up their membranes and even their very functions (Gu et al., 2025). Not only does this approach reduce the risk of infection, but it may also relieve our reliance on traditional antibiotics, which, by and large, might serve to mitigate problems with resistance in the long term. It is an organized move in the direction of strategies that shield the skin yet do not disturb its natural allies. Taking care of your skin is not all about maintaining its structure and microbiologic friends in top shape; it is also about catching danger before it gets to work. New non-invasive technology allows physicians to examine the skin in a similar way engineer's scan for structural defects; consider infrared cameras or equipment picking up subtle acoustic signals that suggest minor damage (Quresh et al., 2025). With AI now providing an additional pair of eyes, such tools can decode complex skin information, allowing for better anticipation of future problems. In most instances, these innovations are pushing dermatology towards individualized care—an approach as adaptable and dynamic as our own skin (Figure 1.16).

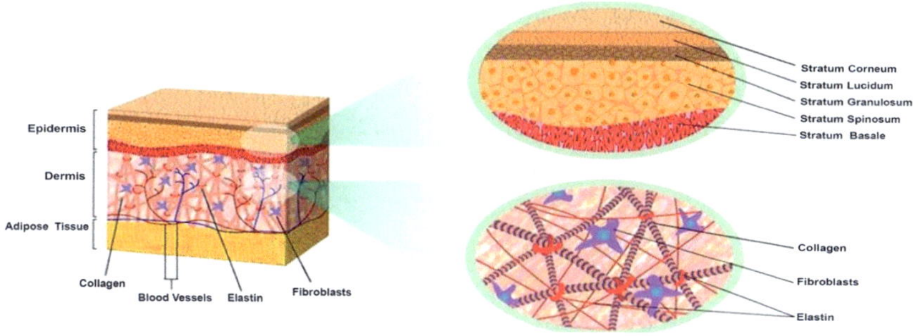

Figure 1.16. Diagram showing the structure of healthy skin, in which the different layers are visible: epidermis, dermis and adipose tissue. Collagen fibers, elastin and fibroblasts are also represented in the diagram.

Source: Sibilla, S., Godfrey, M., Brewer, S., Budh-Raja, A., & Genovese, L. (2015). An overview of the beneficial effects of hydrolyzed collagen as a nutraceutical on skin properties: Scientific background and clinical studies. *The Open Nutraceuticals Journal, 8*, 29–42.

1.7.1. Importance of Hydration and Nutrition

There is more to optimal skin health than coincidence; it is the result of a combination of what is occurring within and around our body. Water and proper nutrition really keep everything in line for how our skin will perform. Our skin is the first line of defense for the body against the world at large, yet it requires sufficient water in not only the outer layers but also deep within the dermis to maintain its shape. Maintaining skin adequately hydrated keeps it pliable and supple, avoiding dryness and even reducing the chances of inflammation. Apart from simple water consumption, our cells also require a continuous flow of valuable nutrients to repair and regenerate themselves. Without these valuable resources, skin starts to age too quickly and can be less effective at fending off environmental stress—hydration is more than a cosmetic solution; it's a fundamental part of how our skin stays stabilized and resilient in the long run. Some nutrients are also helpful, each with a different function to make the skin better. Vitamins A, C, and E, for instance, are crucial antioxidants that eliminate free radicals and facilitate the repair of minor damage to the skin. Omega-3 fatty acids, meanwhile, appear to quiet inflammation and improve the skin's holding capacity for moisture by maintaining its lipid barrier. Dietary patterns rich in these staples have also typically been related to enhanced elasticity and even lower prevalence of common skin problems like acne or dermatitis. This nutritional foundation prevents aging signals and gives a natural shine that cosmetics alone cannot replicate. Essentially, a balanced, nutrition-rich diet is quite basic in maintaining both the appearance and integrity of the skin (Safitri et al., 2025). The significance of hydration is not limited to what we consume, either—it is also linked to what we apply to our skin. For example, in conditions like AD, topical moisturizers become a central component of the strategy for maintaining hydrated skin. There have been some clinical trials indicating that creams packed with anti-inflammatory active ingredients, combined with occlusive and humectant ingredients, can do a great deal to enhance moisture content and reduce symptom severity. This type of external targeted hydration helps to repair damaged skin barriers, relieve dryness and itching and overall enhance overall function. The combination of shea butter, bacterial lysates, and other botanical extracts in these items demonstrates the potential for combining nutrition-conceptual thinking with cutaneous direct care. Ensuring that we hydrate properly both through what we ingest and what we apply on our skin is important, particularly for individuals that are working to overcome inflammatory skin issues (Prakoeswa et al., 2024) (Figure 1.17).

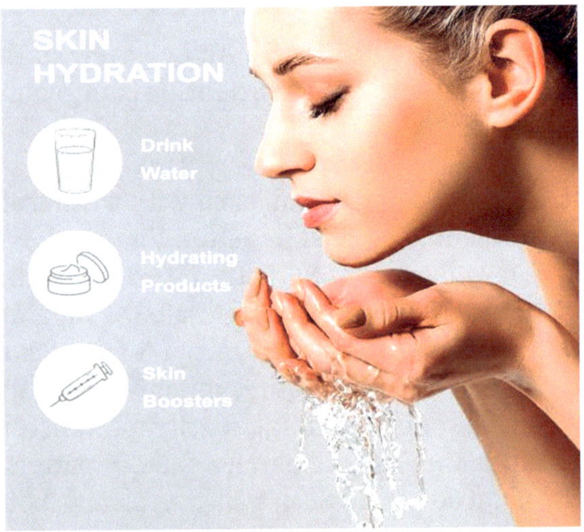

Figure 1.17. Skin hydration.

Source: Mulberry House Clinic. (2023). *Skin Hydration Tips for a Healthy Glow.* https://www.mulberryhouseclinic.co.uk/wp-content/uploads/2023/09/skin-hydration-tips.jpeg.

1.7.2. Sun Protection and Its Effects on Skin Health

Skin is constructed in layers that all do their own little job of keeping us safe; it is a design that indicates we must maintain it in one piece against any kind of external attack. UV light, for instance, can interfere with our DNA, trigger oxidative stress, and even accelerate cellular aging. Occasionally you have physical barriers, such as dressing, or you may employ chemical shields like sunscreens; these tactics combine in ways that keep the damage at bay. Sunscreens, filled with UV filters, do not simply block the rays—instead, they absorb, reflect, or scatter them (thus reducing the risk of photodamage and other skin ills). And, of course, in the majority of instances, skin care is also about maintaining important proteins such as collagen and elastin that make it strong. When you tally up these impacts, you not only deflect unpleasant sunburns in the short term but, in the longer term, lower the risk of skin cancers and photoaging, making skin care very serious indeed. Cosmetic blends and skin well-being have gone in a new direction nowadays, as individuals become more attuned to what is safe and what really works. Fragrances, which are added to most skincare products, tend to influence consumer preference and performance. Natural plant-based essential oils, such as citrus and lavender—add a pleasant scent while also providing such benefits as antimicrobial and anti-inflammatory benefits. Nevertheless, it must be kept in mind that the same thing may smell wonderful yet cause sensitizations or allergies in some individuals. In general terms, a brilliant formulation that compromises between these essential natural ingredients will have to consider both their preservation efficacy and safety profile. Technically, doing so not only makes consumers more content but keeps the skin's barrier intact along with overall wellness (Jugreet et al., 2021). We now understand that genetics and body-wide processes are major factors in how well skin copes with daily stresses. In most instances, inherited conditions can make a person more susceptible to environmental challenges, so careful monitoring through individualized check-ups becomes crucial. New guidelines indicate that early detection of skin changes and quick action result in improved outcomes. In addition, added attention, occasionally even monitoring for neuropsychiatric warning signs and other systemic signs in genetic disease, has led us towards an increasingly team-based treatment practice. This individualized technique, combining environmental resistance with individual genetic knowledge, truly emphasizes the necessity for a general, cautious plan. Eventually, combining these pieces of knowledge with day-to-day preventive measures creates a forward-thinking paradigm for maintaining skin strength against numerous kinds of dangers (Northrup et al., 2021).

1.7.3. Skincare Routines: Products and Practices

The skin is a layered, complex system in which the outside shell (epidermis) and the underlying network (dermis) each have their own thing while cooperating to make you look your best. Everyday care begins with a light clean that removes oils and impurities without harming that natural barrier. Choosing the correct products is about selecting those that work for you ideally so your skin's surface, or stratum corneum, remains resilient. For instance, a moisturizer full of water-attracting humectants and emollient-like compounds can prevent water from escaping. Occasionally, your skin's requirements change due to hormones or metabolism—for example, pregnant women tend to experience changes such as hyperpigmentation and coarser texture (AlAdwan et al., 2025). In general, having a routine that feels tailored and supported by real-world data is essential for long-term skin health. Today, much of what we believe we know about caring for skin comes directly from the internet. Social media streams are abuzz with tips, tricks, and gaudy product advertisements that influence how many people select their routines—often by potentially confusing facts and fiction. A lot of this information is received from friends and social media influencers more than from professionals and can make people use products in ways they were not designed to be used (Ramya et al., 2025). In most cases, even though there is high awareness about basic skincare, the gap between knowing the theory and putting it into practice can result in mistakes that might irritate the skin or weaken its barrier. It turns out, combining a bit of expert advice with what you read online helps bring balance to your routine. There has also been a discernible shift toward natural and environmentally friendly skincare, something that matches our increasing caring about the earth and our general well-being. Everybody appears to be grabbing products that promote plant extracts and reduce synthetic additives. But just because it is called natural does not mean it is going to be gentle, either. Natural products may still trigger allergies or irritation. Results will always depend on the individual skin composition. Dermatologists will usually recommend a closer examination of ingredient lists even when products tout a natural feel. In general, this preference for nature pairs well with conventional dermatologic knowledge, allowing you to create a routine that not only makes you appear good but also nourishes the long-term health of your skin (Ramya et al., 2025). Amidst a buzzword-filled world and reliance on fix-it-quick schemes, a careful, customized strategy is still most important.

CLOSER LOOK

Melanocyte

Melanocytes are melanin-containing neural crest cells that are present in the deepest layer (the stratum Basale) of the skin epidermis, the middle of the eye (the uvea), inner ear, vaginal epithelium, meninges, bones, and heart tissues in most mammals and birds. Melanin is a pigmented substance mostly contributing to the color of skin. After synthesis, melanin is stored in specific organelles known as melanosomes that can be delivered to adjacent keratinocytes to cause pigmentation. Darker skin types therefore contain more melanosomes than lighter skin colors. In terms of function, melanin acts as a shield against UV radiation. Melanocytes also play a part in the immune system.

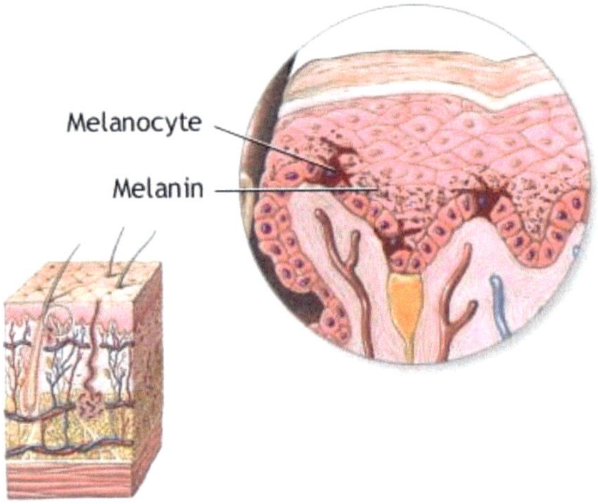

Source: Arcadian. (2006). *Structure of the Human Skin* https://upload.wikimedia.org/wikipedia/commons/d/dd/Illu_skin02.jpg.

Melanocytes create melanin, a pigment in the skin, eyes, hair, nasal passages, and inner ear, through a process known as melanogenesis. Melanogenesis results in long-term pigmentation, which contrasts with the pigmentation resulting from oxidation of previously present melanin.

There exist basal and stimulated levels of melanogenesis; typically, individuals who are light-skinned possess low basal levels of melanogenesis. UV-B radiation exposure triggers enhanced melanogenesis. Melanogenesis serves to defend the hypodermis, the layer beneath the skin, against harm caused by UV radiation. Melanin is black in color, which enables it to absorb most of the UV light and prevent it from being transmitted through the epidermis.

Because the action spectrum of melanogenesis and sunburn are almost the same, they are presumed to be caused by the same process. The concordance of the action spectrum with the DNA absorption spectrum suggests the formation of cyclobutane pyrimidine dimers (CPDs) – direct DNA damage.

Normally, 1000 to 2000 melanocytes are present per square millimeter of skin or about 5% to 10% of the cells of the basal layer of the epidermis. Even though their size may be variable, melanocytes are usually 7 μm long.

Both lightly and darkly pigmented skin have approximately equal numbers of melanocytes, with variation in skin color due to variation in the packing of eumelanin into keratinocyte melanosomes: those of dark-toned skin are "packed into peri-nuclear distributed, ellipsoid" melanosomes whereas those of light-tone skin are "assembled into clustered small, circular melanosomes." There is also variation in the amount and relative proportions of eumelanin and pheomelanin. Melanization and tanning are hormone-controlled and involve the MSH and ACTH peptides derived from the precursor proopiomelanocortin (Maurício et al., 2023).

SUMMARY

The complex interplay between skin physiology and anatomy is the basis for its multifarious and essential functions ranging from a protective barrier to regulation of sensory perception and immunity. Knowledge regarding the classification of skin disease is also essential as this has implications for diagnostic precision and therapeutic plans. The complexity of the lesions also requires methodical investigation encompassing clinical assessment, histopathological investigation, and assessment for possible systemic participation. This type of comprehensive strategy not only sounds like the ideal form of disease control but also allows complications to be anticipated. Ultimately, progress in dermatology will have to continue to combine fundamental knowledge with new technologies to optimize patient results and promote integral health of the skin. Such complete integration makes the importance of the skin both as an organ and a diagnostic window to general health all the more apparent, solidifying its place at the forefront of medical science. Fresh advances in health care, in particular, the advent of AI and machine learning, hold hopeful new horizons for dermatology's future (Bekbolatova et al., 2024). The technologies hold considerable promise to facilitate clinical decision-making and allow more accurate identification and classification of skin diseases through the employment of advanced pattern recognition and image analysis. By optimizing iterative diagnosis processes, AI systems have the potential to free the clinician burden, and therefore the clinician can dedicate time to more complex cases and personalized care (Bekbolatova et al., 2024). Nevertheless, incorporation of such software necessitates careful consideration of ethical, legal, and practical concerns such as data privacy and algorithmic bias. As dermatology embraces these technologies, there will be an imperative to carefully balance human knowledge and AI to deliver optimal patient outcomes and maintain the standards of care in clinical practice. Parallel to developments in technology, natural products continue to make worthwhile contributions to dermatological therapeutics, especially in the treatment of inflammatory, neoplastic, and infectious skin conditions. These drugs most often have multi-functionalities such as anti-inflammatory, antioxidant, and antimicrobial activity, which match the pathophysiological targets of the majority of skin diseases. Despite promising in vitro and in vivo findings, large-scale clinical trials will be necessary to ascertain their efficacy and safety profiles with certainty. Additionally, the engineering of delivery systems can theoretically maximize their bioavailability and therapeutic effects. The combination of conventional remedies with modern drugs is an integrative process capable of saving healthcare expenditure and enhancing patient tolerance and therefore making natural products a superb adjuvant in the future treatment of dermatoses.

The complex anatomy and multi-faceted physiology of skin highlight its essential function as the body's largest organ, providing a robust protective shield against external insults while maintaining temperature control and sensory perception. The skin is composed of three principal layers, epidermis, dermis, and hypodermis, each possessing unique cells and functions, which collectively control an complex interplay between protection, immunity, and homeostasis. Proteomic analysis innovations have significantly added to skin biology understanding, revealing novel molecular profiles that underlie healthy skin and disease conditions. This information facilitates biomarkers and targets identification for diagnosis and treatment optimization. These advances demonstrate the dynamic nature of dermatology where molecular depth is accorded emphasis alongside traditional anatomical and physiological understanding to improve patient care (Dyring-Andersen et al., 2021). Differential categorization of skin diseases remains the foundation of clinical diagnosis and management, spanning a spectrum from inflammation and infection to neoplasia. The split is not founded merely on the morphologic presentation but also on an understanding of underlying mechanisms of pathophysiologic principles having a direct influence on treatment. The skin's multifarious functions, ranging from a physical barrier and immune mediator to participation in thermoregulation and sense perception—highlight its dynamic condition and vulnerability to heterogeneous lesions. Clinical evaluation, histopathological examination, and, increasingly nowadays, quantitative assessment form part of the complete management of skin lesions. These techniques are guaranteed to describe the lesion appropriately, which is needed for effective intervention and monitoring of disease progression (Dyring-Andersen et al., 2021). In practice, standardized tools such as the SACS™ demonstrate the growing importance of systematic assessment in skin lesion care, particularly in specialty groups like children. The reliability and validity of these instruments facilitate communication between caregiver and clinician, optimizing the accuracy of diagnosis and treatment. Of particular interest, whenever discord arises between novices and experts in wound care, the tendency to overestimate lesion severity as a bias for preserving safety functions as a protection mechanism, guaranteeing early referral and patient safety. These advances are reflective of a wider movement toward evidence-based, systematic practice in dermatology that provides for homogeneity and optimizes clinical performance in varied patient populations.

KEY TERMS FROM THIS CHAPTER

- Acne
- Atopic dermatitis (Ad)
- Benign lesions
- Central nervous system
- Dermatological disorders
- Dermis
- Eczema
- Environment
- General medicine
- Langerhans cells
- anatomical knowledge
- autonomic nerve fibers
- biochemical functions
- cutaneous immunity
- dermatology
- diagnostic accuracy
- elasticity
- fine motor function
- herpes simplex
- anatomy
- barrier function
- candida species
- dermatological assessment
- dermatophytes
- ecchymoses
- elastin fibers
- fungal infections
- immune function

REFERENCES

1. Abdelhadi, Saly Mustafa Mohamed (2023). Atopic dermatitis and distress. Karolinska Institutet. Thesis. https://hdl.handle.net/10616/48824 (accessed on 12 May 2025).
2. Accettola, E., Bogdan, A., Callahan, S., Chawda, et al. (2023). *Introduction to Health Assessment for the Nursing Professional: Part II*. https://core.ac.uk/download/622362029.pdf (accessed on 12 May 2025).
3. Aggarwal, N., Kitano, S., Puah, G. R. Y., Kittelmann, S., Hwang, I. Y., & Chang, M. W. (2022). Microbiome and human health: Current understanding, engineering, and enabling technologies. *Chemical Reviews, 123*, 31–72. https://doi.org/10.1021/acs.chemrev.2c00431.
4. Gutiérrez-Cerrajero, C., Sprecher, E., Paller, A. S., Akiyama, M., Mazereeuw-Hautier, J., Hernández-Martín, A., & González-Sarmiento, R. (2023). Ichthyosis. *Nature reviews. Disease primers, 9*(1), 2. https://doi.org/10.1038/s41572-022-00412-3 (accessed on 12 May 2025).
5. Alcaine, C., Angenent, M., Ciriza, J., Fernández-Carro, M., et al. (2022). Modeling an optimal 3D skin-on-chip within microfluidic devices for pharmacological studies. *Pharmaceutics, 14*, 1417. https://core.ac.uk/download/548591332.pdf (accessed on 12 May 2025).
6. Bekbolatova, M., Mayer, J., Ong, C. W., & Toma, M. (2024). Transformative potential of AI in healthcare: Definitions, applications, and navigating the ethical landscape and public perspectives. *Healthcare, 12*, 125. https://doi.org/10.3390/healthcare12020125.
7. Bonciu, A., Almasan, T., Cordunianu, A., Necula, V., Pelin, S., Ganea, G., Anghel, I., et al. (2023). Abstracts of the 7th Congress of the Romanian Rhinologic Society. *Romanian Journal of Rhinology, 13*, 201–228. https://doi.org/10.2478/rjr-2023-0029.
8. **Book reviews.** (2011). *Journal of Zoo and Wildlife Medicine, 42*(1), 169–170. https://www.semanticscholar.org/paper/97568b9fbfbc8f35b336e02c0d4c5a6fceb52857 (accessed on 12 May 2025).
9. Bulletin of Integrative Psychiatry. (2023). *Bulletin of Integrative Psychiatry, 98*. https://doi.org/10.36219/bpi.2023.3.
10. Cerebrospinal fluid. (2022). https://core.ac.uk/download/534903726.pdf (accessed on 12 May 2025).
11. Chirikhina, E. (2022). Human Face Mapping Based on TEWL, Hydration and Ultrasound. PhD Thesis London South Bank University School of Engineering https://doi.org/10.18744/lsbu.9349z(accessed on 12 May 2025).
12. Chukwu, R., & Mankila, J. (2018). *Dermatology Nurses' Job Description: Literature Review*. Bachelor's thesis Degree programme in Nursing PNURSS15 2018 https://core.ac.uk/download/161432240.pdf.
13. Clancy, N. T., Jones, G., Maier-Hein, L., Elson, D. S., & Stoyanov, D. (2020). Surgical spectral imaging. *Medical Image Analysis, 63*, 101699. https://doi.org/10.1016/j.media.2020.101699.
14. Dec, M., & Arasiewicz, H. (2024). Aryl hydrocarbon receptor role in chronic inflammatory skin diseases: A narrative review. *Advances in Dermatology and Allergology/Postępy Dermatologii i Alergologii, 41*, 9–19. https://www.semanticscholar.org/paper/e0a3ffbe06760a569cd4260e90d7d96789959947 (accessed on 12 May 2025).

15. Dogjani, A., Gjata, A., Draçini, X., Çeliku, E., Mesquita, C., Puyana, J. C., Zago, M., et al. (2022). The 6th Albanian Congress of Trauma and Emergency Surgery. *Albanian Journal of Trauma and Emergency Surgery, 6*, 1–132. https://doi.org/10.32391/ajtes.v6i2.6.307.

16. Dyring-Andersen, B., Fredman, G., Mann, M., Skov, L., et al. (2021). Towards precision dermatology: Emerging role of proteomic analysis of the skin. *Dermatology, 238*(3), 185–194. https://core.ac.uk/download/491527992.pdf (accessed on 12 May 2025).

17. Esteva, A., Chou, K., Yeung, S., Naik, N., Madani, A., Mottaghi, A., Liu, Y., et al. (2021). Deep learning-enabled medical computer vision. *npj Digital Medicine, 4*, Article 5. https://doi.org/10.1038/s41746-020-00376-2.

18. Galić, I., Habijan, M., Leventić, H., & Romić, K. (2023). Machine learning empowering personalized medicine: A comprehensive review of medical image analysis methods. *Electronics, 12*(21), 4411. https://doi.org/10.3390/electronics12214411.

19. Gall, L. S., & Riely, P. E. (2025). *Effect of Diet and Atmosphere on Intestinal and Skin Flora. Volume II–Literature Survey*. https://core.ac.uk/download/pdf/85249155.pdf (accessed on 12 May 2025).

20. Goh, J. P. Z. (2023). *Understanding Malassezia Secreted Proteases in Host-Microbial Crosstalk in Skin Health* [Doctoral dissertation, Nanyang Technological University]. https://doi.org/10.32657/10356/172557.

21. Gradowicz-Prajsnar B. Stress and skin diseases. Overview using acne vulgaris as an example. *Aesth Cosmetol Med.* 2023;12(6):207-212.

22. https://doi.org/10.52336/acm.2023.027

23. Hufnagl, K., Pali-Schöll, I., Roth-Walter, F., & Jensen-Jarolim, E. (2020). Dysbiosis of the gut and lung microbiome has a role in asthma. *Seminars in Immunopathology, 42*(1), 75–93. https://doi.org/10.1007/s00281-019-00775-y.

24. Colette Maurício, A., Alvites, R., & Gönül, M. (Eds.). (2023). Wound Healing - Recent Advances and Future Opportunities. IntechOpen. doi: 10.5772/intechopen.101005Joseph, T. M., Mahapatra, D. K., Esmaeili, A., Piszczyk, Ł., Hasanin, M. S., Kattali, M., Haponiuk, J. T., et al. (2023). Nanoparticles: Taking a unique position in medicine. *Nanomaterials, 13*(3), 574. https://doi.org/10.3390/nano13030574.

25. Kapsandoy, S. C. (2015). *Doctor of Philosophy*. https://core.ac.uk/download/276263195.pdf (accessed on 12 May 2025).

26. Ewa Kloczko, Mark Wilsher, Andreas Naparus, Kevin Kulendra, Navara Anjum, DS20 Challenges and considerations of Mohs surgery in the ear, *British Journal of Dermatology*, Volume 191, Issue Supplement_1, July 2024, Page i103, https://doi.org/10.1093/bjd/ljae090.215(accessed on 12 May 2025).

27. Kowalska, J., & Wrześniok, D. (2024). Skin-related adverse reactions induced by oral antidiabetic drugs—A review of literature and case reports. *Pharmaceuticals, 17*. https://www.semanticscholar.org/paper/d144b6928426edd2a37dc7af4ca3a15bb4b80c92 (accessed on 12 May 2025).

28. Mahajan, S. S. (2019). *Clinico Epidemiological Profile of Dermatological Manifestations in Preschool Going Children in A Tertiary Health Care Centre*. https://core.ac.uk/download/235670531.pdf (accessed on 12 May 2025).

29. National Aeronautics and Space Administration. (2025). *Aerospace Medicine and Biology: A Continuing Bibliography with Indexes (Supplement 314)*. https://core.ac.uk/download/pdf/42831714.pdf (accessed on 12 May 2025).

30. Ortega, M. Á., Fraile-Martínez, O., García-Montero, C., Álvarez-Mon, M. Á., Chen, C. W., Ruiz-Grande, F., Pekarek, L., et al. (2021). Understanding chronic venous disease: A critical overview of its pathophysiology and medical management. *Journal of Clinical Medicine, 10*, 3239. https://doi.org/10.3390/jcm10153239.

31. Päkk, P. (2012). *Nakkuste Poolt Põhjustatud Epidermise Rakkude Talitusliku Aktiivsuse Muutused Kaladel* [Functional activity changes in epidermal cells of fish caused by infections]. https://core.ac.uk/download/366811901.pdf (accessed on 12 May 2025).

32. Park, B., Oh, D., Kim, J., & Kim, C. (2023). Functional photoacoustic imaging: From nano- and micro- to macro-scale. *Nano Convergence, 10*, Article 1. https://doi.org/10.1186/s40580-023-00377-3.

33. Qu, H., Kao, C., & Hakonarson, H. (2024). Implications of the non-neuronal cholinergic system for therapeutic interventions of inflammatory skin diseases. *Experimental Dermatology, 33*(10), e15181. https://www.semanticscholar.org/paper/1f69bb1076eca633912e19be769a2209220d03c3 (accessed on 12 May 2025).

34. Said, K. K., & Rhaimi, C. B. (2024). Melanoma skin cancer detected based on artificial intelligence: Survey. *International Science and Technology Journal*. https://www.semanticscholar.org/paper/3b9ffa58e19adb185b1362bc8f3eeebfe6ed39d8 (accessed on 12 May 2025).

35. Schmidt-Posthaus, H., Pugovkin, D., & Wahli, T. (2005). Iridophoroma in a European grayling (*Thymallus thymallus*) in Switzerland. https://www.semanticscholar.org/paper/320871b2259ca2516d1f81113042e3b4e3dd21d8 (accessed on 12 May 2025).

36. Senbekov, M., Saliev, T., Bukeyeva, Z., Almabayeva, A., Zhanaliyeva, M., Aitenova, N., Toishibekov, Y. M., et al. (2020). The recent progress and applications of digital technologies in healthcare: A review. *International Journal of Telemedicine and Applications, 2020*, 1–18. https://doi.org/10.1155/2020/8830200.

37. Spender, J. (1892). On some of the rarer complications of rheumatoid arthritis. *British Medical Journal, 1*, 905–907. https://www.semanticscholar.org/paper/14beeef61843179bc642a291df09aa6eaed70afa (accessed on 12 May 2025).

38. Sundaresan, S., Çetin, F., Birge, Ö., Sharan, M., Mathur, R., Kumar, M., Rana, K., et al. (2022). *Clinical Diagnosis and Management of Squamous Cell Carcinoma*. IntechOpen eBooks. https://doi.org/10.5772/intechopen.94812.

39. SZOT, Anna, KMAK, Bożena and GÓRSKA, Magdalena. The most common dermatoses of athletes. Journal of Education, Healthand Sport. 2024;67:54887. eISSN 2391-8306. https://dx.doi.org/10.12775/JEHS.2024.67.54887 https://apcz.umk.pl/JEHS/article/view/54887(accessed on 12 May 2025).

40. Teng, V. C., & Esti, P. K. (2021). Skin microbiome dysbiosis in leprosy cases. *International Journal of Research in Dermatology, 7*(5), 741–747. https://doi.org/10.18203/issn.2455-4529.IntJResDermatol20213355(accessed on 12 May 2025).

41. Terrell, J. (1987). Clinical dermatology: An illustrated textbook. *Archives of Dermatology, 123*, 958. https://www.semanticscholar.org/paper/0adc9442939073941217c2df03bad8df7bbef829 (accessed on 12 May 2025).

42. Tolar, J., & Tolar, M. (2015). A living band-aid for epidermolysis bullosa. *Blood transfusion = Trasfusione del sangue, 13*(1), 1–2. https://doi.org/10.2450/2014.0289-14 (accessed on 12 May 2025).

43. Tricarico, P., Mentino, D., De Marco, A., Del Vecchio, C., Garra, S., Cazzato, G., Foti, C., et al. (2022). Aquaporins are one of the critical factors in the disruption of the skin barrier in inflammatory skin diseases. *International Journal of Molecular Sciences, 23*. https://www.semanticscholar.org/paper/bca1201083597822720043a2c1211630a15ae140 (accessed on 12 May 2025).

44. Varnosfaderani, S. M., & Forouzanfar, M. (2024). The role of AI in hospitals and clinics: Transforming healthcare in the 21st century. *Bioengineering, 11*, 337. https://doi.org/10.3390/bioengineering11040337.

45. Vladlenov, D. (2022). *Scientific Foundations in Medicine and Pharmacy*. International Science Group. https://doi.org/10.46299/isg.2022.mono.med.2.

46. Wallis, J. (2017). *Investigating the Body in the Victorian Asylum: Doctors, Patients, and Practices.* https://core.ac.uk/download/478101749.pdf (accessed on 12 May 2025).

47. Western University. (1961). *University of Western Ontario Medical Journal, 31*(1), 231. https://core.ac.uk/download/61662848.pdf (accessed on 12 May 2025).

48. Wilson, E. (1871). Lectures on dermatology. *British Medical Journal, 1*, 163–164. https://www.semanticscholar.org/paper/aa294b03480116ea79b6642f3321b9a6d52a8eb1 (accessed on 12 May 2025).

49. Xu, Qiuyun, "The Advanced Applications For Optical Coherence Tomography In Skin Imaging" (2021). *Wayne State University Dissertations*. 3526. https://digitalcommons.wayne.edu/oa_dissertations/3526 (accessed on 12 May 2025).

50. Zaid, N. A. M., Sekar, M., Bonam, S. R., Gan, S. H., Lum, P. T., Begum, M. Y., Mat Rani, N. N. I., et al. (2022). Promising natural products in new drug design, development, and therapy for skin disorders: An overview of scientific evidence and understanding their mechanism of action. *Drug Design, Development and Therapy, 16*, 23–66. https://doi.org/10.2147/DDDT.S326332.

51. Zwart, D., ten Berg, M., de Wit, N. J., Fernholm, R., Hautz, W. E., et al. (2024). The future of diagnosis: Navigating uncertainty. *Diagnosis, 11*(S1), A95–A131. https://doi.org/10.1515/dx-2023-0178.

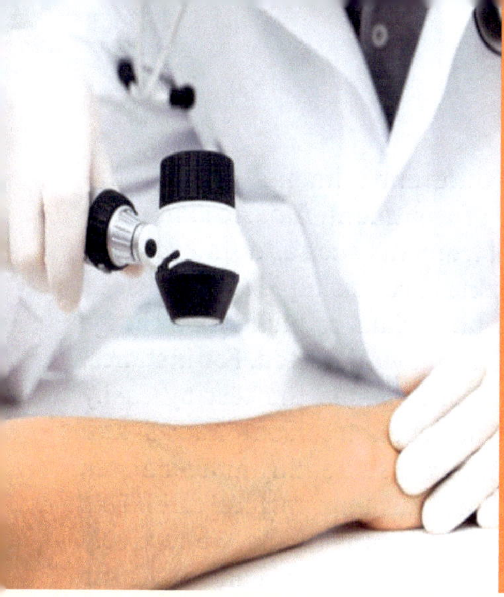

Chapter 2

DIAGNOSTIC TECHNIQUES IN DERMATOLOGY

Contents

Introduction

Skin is more than a covering—it is the body's largest organ and usually suggests difficulty near and far. Even minor variations in its appearance often indicate greater, underlying problems, so careful, diligent inspection is essential in routine practice. Skin conditions are varied, from innocuous moles to advanced inflammatory or tumorous conditions, and the minuscule differences in their appearances make it sometimes a headache figuring it out. In bygone eras, a simple exam, and a talk about the history of the patient were the predominant methods; today, technology and laboratory tests predominantly bring a clearer vision, delivering more precise specificity. Combining plain old observation with fancy high-tech diagnostics has revolutionized the field, so knowing a range of techniques is darn important for optimal patient care. Dermoscopy now becomes one of those nifties, noninvasive techniques that sort of bridges the gap between simple looking and going deep into tissue minutiae. It amplifies what is beneath the surface, allowing physicians to catch characteristics that would otherwise evade a naked eye. Most of the time, studies indicate that it will sort out cases in which lesions appear too uniform, consider, for instance, the various etiologies responsible for palmoplantar hyperkeratosis, which can be kind of impossible to distinguish based on appearance alone (Chaduvula et al., 2023). Despite this, however, dermoscopy presents only a tantalizing glimpse and does not eliminate the necessity of a biopsy when the issue remains unclear; rather, it allows doctors to sort out which patients may require that additional step. Combining dermoscopy with old-fashioned checks provides a more complete, though slightly less predictable, method for diagnosing the skin. On the other hand, histopathology remains the first choice when clinical appearances and dermoscopy just do not quite get it right. A skin biopsy, granted, somewhat invasive, allows clinicians to focus on the microscopic design of the tissue and cellular components and thereby gain crucial insight into the very nature of a disorder. By and large, where treatment decisions rest on knowing exactly what is occurring, histopathology is a must (consider nail psoriasis, where although dermoscopy provides clues, a biopsy is needed to establish things (Sari et al., 2019)). Put in other supportive tests such as Wood's lamp tests, patch tests, or skin scrapings, and you have a sort of patchwork of methods that collectively aid in identifying infections, allergies, or parasites. All these approaches overlap to create an integrated system necessary for arriving at a correct diagnosis and treating skin ailments efficiently.

Importance of Dermatological Diagnostics

Accurate diagnosis is at the center of proper treatment, particularly when it is skin problems that are notoriously a catch-all. Various skin problems sometimes have the same shade, texture, or appearance that easily bewilders a simple diagnosis. Even slight dissimilarities might mean entirely different ailments that require their own type of treatment. A basic skin exam coupled with instruments such as dermoscopy—even if they at times are as simple as a judicious glance—allows physicians to pick up on things that otherwise may go undetected. For instance, dermoscopy has often stood the test by easily distinguishing between innocent marks and those that may indicate something more sinister, guiding immediate and appropriate care. This added focus not only improves how effectively treatments are working but often alleviates the anxiety that comes with an unresolved skin spot. Devices such as dermoscopy and even a Wood's lamp really disrupted how skin problems get examined these days. They provide a noninvasive and rather keen means of identifying problems involving changes in pigment or infection. These devices assist in separating the likes of benign hypopigmentation conditions, such as Pityriasis alba—from conditions that are more socially stigmatized such as vitiligo or even leprosy, which can strike particularly hard in darker-skinned individuals (Irene et al., 2023). By allowing physicians to visualize characteristics such as scattered white, unstructured spots and magnifying up close, these techniques do not merely increase diagnostic rates; they also open the door to patient-specific treatment plans that soothe unfounded fears.

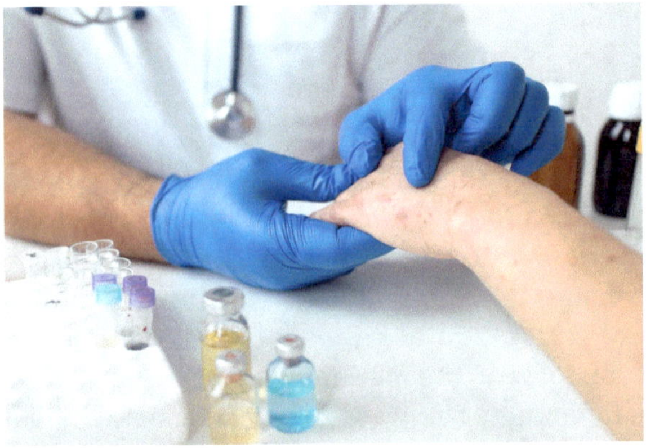

Source: HexaMed Healthcare. (n.d.). *Dermatology Clinic Image.* https://hexamedhealthcare.com/img/polyclinic/dermatology1.jpg.

In most instances, additional diagnostic tools have become nearly essential companions to the routine physical examination when deciphering the multitude of facial expressions of skin disease. Oftentimes, settling on an absolute diagnosis for skin issues still requires taking a closer look with a biopsy and some work done in the lab. Methods such as skin scrapings or patch testing provide other avenues to identify issues from annoying parasites to allergic contact dermatitis. In the majority of cases, these tests identify what is causing the symptoms so that every condition gets sorted out in the right manner and that the treatment is not derailed by a false assumption (White, 2025). Notably, the blend of these diverse approaches is near-married to improved patient care—by combining strategies, clinicians provide a more complete perspective that challenges evidence-based practice and results in care that is more refined to meet the individual needs of each.

Overview of Common Diagnostic Techniques

Physicians do not simply have one trick for examining skin conditions—hand and eye are supplemented by special instruments. They begin by merely observing the skin, picking up on slight changes in color, roughness, or unusual scaling. Dermoscopy, for example, zooms in on the surface of the skin so that pale pigment networks and fine blood vessel patterns are visible—the sort of details you would never notice with the naked eye. This non-invasive technique is usually welcomed since it separates benign spots from concerning lesions, and it is frequently utilized to identify evidence of inflammation or infection. In most instances, studies (Irene et al., 2023) indicate that dermoscopy beelines directly to such problems as distinguishing Pityriasis alba from conditions such as vitiligo or even leprosy, which consequently guides the appropriate treatment and alleviates patient anxiety. Another handy technique illuminates the scene, literally. Wood's lamp examination, comprised of a flash of ultraviolet (UV) light, can expose changes in skin pigments as well as microbial fluorescence. The glow can be particularly diagnostic when fungi, such as dermatophytes, respond by glowing under the lamp, allowing for rapid screening. Usually, physicians pair this with skin scrapings (they scrape off a small amount of skin) to look under the microscope for annoying mites or fungi. Whether human patients or even pets, these methods work together to address common issues such as parasitic infestations and surface infections. With most, combining up direct visualization with a small collection sample provides more balanced information, making clinicians come to a conclusion more quickly regarding treatments (White, 2025). On other occasions, when the suspicion remains about a diagnosis, one must use more direct means. A skin biopsy—cutting a tiny piece of tissue for closer study under a microscope—maps out the cellular facts, reveals inflammatory patterns, and even detects nascent cancer in its earliest stages. Histopathology, as many still refer to this detailed excursion into skin structure, remains the first resort when less involved tests fall short. In addition to this, patch testing (where small amounts of suspected allergens are applied to the skin) aids in uncovering allergic contact dermatitis if a local reaction appears. All of these tools combined provide dermatologists with a comprehensive toolkit, enabling them to construct precise diagnoses and formulate treatment plans that truly suit the patient's needs.

2.1. Skin Examination Methods

Occasionally, the skin examination begins with a really simple look-and-feel examination. You just look and lightly touch to notice any subtle changes of color, texture, or bumps, even when the differences are virtually infinitesimal. Physicians do this by palpating and looking, attempting to distinguish between a benign spot and one that may be suspicious. Good lighting and even a handheld lens as small as a pen will make those little details stand out, and a patient's history, as it turns out, helps connect what you see with potential internal or environmental problems. Although this strategy might seem obvious, it requires a great deal of attention to the details because it lays the groundwork for later, more complicated tests. In all but a few instances, mastering these basics continues to be central to skin care, even as technology advances.

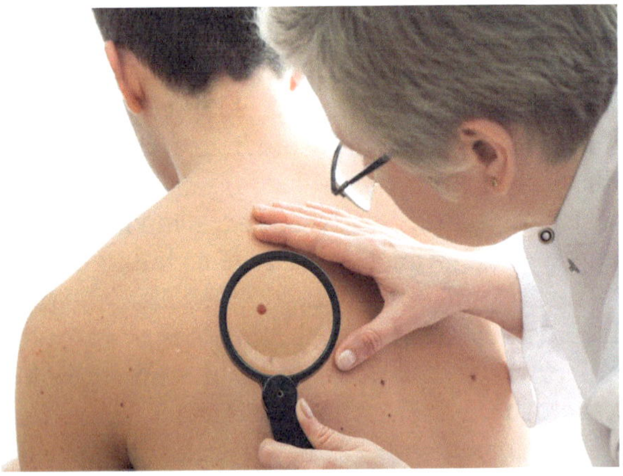

Figure 2.1. Dermatologist examining skin.

Source: U.S. Dermatology Partners. (2016). *GettyImages-158875496* https://www.usdermatologypartners.com//wp-content/uploads/2016/10/GettyImages-158875496-1024x683.jpg.

Following that initial examination, most practitioners resort to dermoscopy—a kind of non-invasive magnifying glass that illuminates details hidden beneath the skin's surface. It does so by revealing tiny vascular structures, pigment networks, and patterns, which give clues about whether or not a lesion is likely to be malignant or benign. This reduces unnecessary biopsies by presenting physicians with a more accurate vision of, for instance, melanoma vs. a benign mole. It also captures early, subtle lesions that may affect a patient's prognosis. Naturally, putting dermoscopy to good use requires the right training, as misreading the images may result in errors.

All this additional insight appreciatively supplements the routine exam, enhancing the whole diagnostic process and, in the end, patient care (Smoller et al., 2021). And then there is the Wood's lamp test—a handy supplement that applies ultraviolet (UV) light to cause specific skin conditions to show themselves. By making the skin glow in unanticipated manners, this test has the ability to bring infections, pigmentation problems, and other abnormalities into clearer focus. For instance, fungal and bacterial infections that may otherwise go unnoticed in normal light suddenly become apparent, and contrasts between lighter or darker regions are more easily discerned. Its rapid, non-invasive quality is an added advantage, albeit that interpretation of the glowing patterns does rely heavily on the clinician's expertise; occasionally normal variations may appear a little pathological when viewed under UV light. Applied in conjunction with other examinations, Wood's lamp effectively refines the entire diagnostic image (Smoller et al., 2021) (Figure 2.1).

2.1.1. Visual Inspection Techniques

When they are diagnosing skin diseases, physicians tend to begin by quite simply looking very hard at the skin. They start with a naked-eye, close examination, looking at lesion size, distribution, and those tiny changes in color or texture that might otherwise pass unnoticed. Even small variations can give a clue as to what test or treatment is the next thing that is required. This is not a cursory look; it is a considered, step-by-step approach that captures both the large picture and the small, palpable details. In general terms, this initial check serves to separate out whether a problem is inflammatory, infectious, or even potentially due to tumors. It demands both keen vision and hands-on practice, and in primary care environments, these early impressions tend to guide the subsequent actions in referrals or management plans (White, 2025). There is more to observing the skin than a mere glance. Frequently, physicians supplement this exercise with additional techniques that refine their vision even more. For instance, equipment such as dermoscopy allows them to zoom out for wider views to capture tiny pigment networks, vascular patterns, or even follicle alterations that would not otherwise be noticed by the unaided eye. Beginning with this close-up skin inspection makes it simpler, in the majority of instances, to select the ideal location for a biopsy ; a decision that can maximize what subsequent tests reveal. Training in these observation protocols, even when occasionally used a little loosely, serves to keep diagnosis generally more consistent; such inconsistency is always a problem with subjective evaluation. Thus, the quaint art of observing hand-in-hand with sophisticated technology fills the gap between a patient's initial visit and more profound, lab-based diagnostics (Lyons & Ousley, 2015; White, 2025). Lighting and patient positioning are also important contributors to what is observed. Natural light or a well-placed artificial source is necessary to capture those subtle colors of pigmentation or faint erythema, and a standard method of placing a patient facilitates easy comparison of symmetric and localized lesions.

Taking a few pictures during the visit—even with a little bit of a careless touch here and there—offers an objective record in which to monitor how a condition changes over time. Such visual examination, careful but unhurried, assists in distinguishing disorders that might otherwise appear nearly indistinguishable; for instance, red, scaly plaques may indicate psoriasis, eczema, or possibly a fungus, each requiring a slightly different response. Ultimately, proficiency with these observation skills is still a foundation skill for dermatologists, paving the way for all the more sophisticated diagnostic work that follows (Lyons & Ousley, 2015; White, 2025).

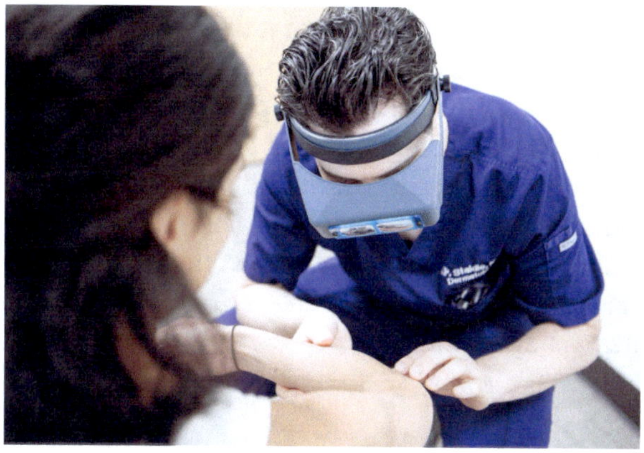

Source: Bend Dermatology Clinic. (2020). *20170906-SDI-Stock-and-Headshots-SDI-0004-1* https://bendderm.com/wp-content/uploads/2020/03/20170906-SDI-Stock-and-Headshots-SDI-0004-1-1024x683-1024x683-1.jpg.

2.1.2. Palpation and Its Significance

Touching skin lesions quite commonly reveals information that a fleeting glance would not. Physicians use their hands to feel variations in texture, hardness, heat, and even the motion of a bump. This simple method, by and large, separates benign marks from those which may require further inspection. Rather than simply depending on a device such as a dermoscope, which shines light to look beneath the surface, palpation makes visible physical signs that may suggest underlying problems. It is particularly useful when checking lumps, patches, or areas that are abnormally hard, where a combination of textures may indicate inflammation or even an early warning of something worse. Briefly, combining a tactile sense with visual information increases the accuracy of a skin examination and informs decisions regarding whether to pursue a biopsy or treatment. Palpation of lymph nodes is also important, especially when staging melanomas or evaluating sentinel nodes, as mentioned in Brazilian melanoma guidelines. A palpation examination that incorporates haptic cues can detect node enlargement indicative of metastasis – information that directly influences prognosis and treatment planning (Castro et al., 2016). Although contemporary imaging has become increasingly adept at detecting node involvement, that initial, non-invasive touch remains a valuable skill. As a rule, it is usually a subtle shift in the feel of adjacent lymph nodes that serves as the first indication that something may be spreading.

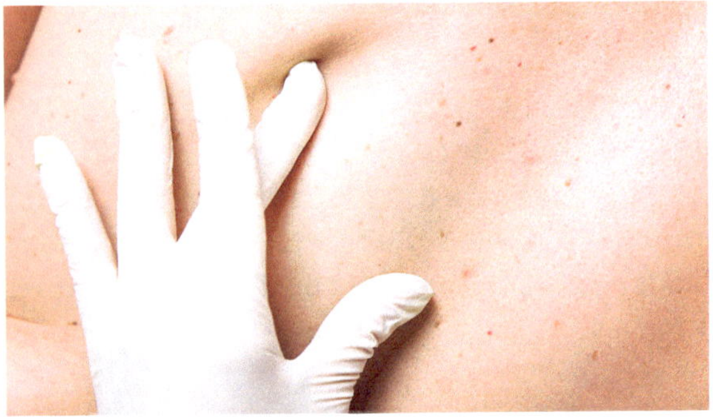

Figure 2.2. Palpation.

Source: Medline. (2019). *Skin Assessment Infographic.* https://www.medline.com/wp-content/uploads/2019/11/STK_SkinAssessment_RGB_840x473.jpg.

A return to touch not only supports the original skin check but also completes a more accurate picture of a patient's skin and overall well-being. Combined with sophisticated methods such as dermoscopy, feeling out lesions remains its own strong skill. While an optical illusion caused by a dermoscope discloses structures underneath the skin, a physical examination can detect variation in firmness or softness that suggests fibrosis, cysts, or even mild inflammatory changes. The doctors can decide which parts to biopsy based on these sensory pointers, thus enhancing the quality of the tissue specimen. And, incidentally, this method can also monitor whether a treatment is succeeding by observing changes in the texture or softness of a lesion—even without using expensive machinery. Combining palpation with other diagnostic modalities provides a more comprehensive assessment, affirming its enduring relevance to contemporary dermatologic practice (Adaskevich, 2016) (Figure 2.2).

2.1.3. Patient History and Its Role in Diagnosis

A good dermatological diagnosis begins long before any physical examination or laboratory test—it begins with the complete patient history. Clinicians ask when the skin problem first cropped up, how long it has been occurring, if and when there have been ups and downs in its course, and what appears to induce or calm it. They also ask what has been tried for treatment and if other body systems are affected. In general, this background information not only serves to limit the range of potential problems but also directs the selection of tests, avoiding unnecessary interventions. For instance, knowledge of a patient's history with systemic or autoimmune conditions generally directs the dermatologist to one specific range of tests such as skin biopsies or other specialist investigations. Without delving deep into an individual's background, even sophisticated instruments like dermoscopy or a Wood's lamp examination can wind up providing ambiguous or even off-base results, highlighting just how pivotal history is to the entire process of diagnosis. Beyond the fundamentals, a complete patient history then becomes crucial when attempting to unravel skin diseases that resemble one another quite closely. Consider hyperkeratotic papules on the palms and soles; these can be a challenge because they look somewhat the same in a group of various conditions. Current evidence tends to imply that although dermoscopy increases clinical awareness, it is not a panacea device by itself but also requires backup histopathology (Chaduvula et al., 2023). For most instances, a meticulous history may offer hints at environmental exposures, occupational dangers, or universal allergens that suggest chronic hand-foot eczema rather than psoriasis or lichen planus. This additional background investigation usually tightens the differential diagnosis, making the cumulative results of dermoscopy and laboratory tests more pertinent to the patient's treatment. Taking it further, an in-depth patient history truly counts when handling complex, immune-mediated dermatoses impacting other systems as well. Psoriasis, for instance, is highly renowned for its genetic and immune origins; in the majority of the instances, the patient's history not only identifies the skin issue but also reveals other issues, such as cardiovascular or even psychiatric problems, for that matter, to the fore (Alessandra-Mădălina et al., 2023). Knowing these additional variables enables the clinician to create a more integrative treatment plan instead of narrowly targeting skin symptoms. Further, an understanding of the patient's response to previous therapy and their daily lifestyle can inform a more tailored intervention plan and enable the prediction of possible side effects. At its core, sitting down to take a thorough patient history is not simply a preliminary gesture—it is an essential component of refining the diagnosis and making sure that the whole care is indeed focused on the individual.

2.2. Dermoscopy

Non-invasive testing practices have truly revolutionized the way skin examinations are conducted these days. New imaging technologies allow us to view areas of the skin that are inaccessible to the naked eye, and dermoscopy has gained popularity because of this. It employs convenient magnifiers and polarized light to bring out concealed layers—getting a close examination of pigmented marks and even vascular patterns so physicians can make better judgments about whether or not something is harmless or maybe risky. This method reduces the number of intrusive procedures, allowing clinicians to make real-time evaluations, which in turn accelerates decisions and enhances results. Those subtle patterns it reveals have a significant role when identifying early melanomas and other severe skin cancers, which, in most cases, can make a significant difference in treatment. Dermoscopy is not only about pigmentation problems, however. It is also helpful for investigating inflammatory and parasitic skin conditions. That is, it provides a non-invasive glimpse into the general appearance of different dermatological conditions, sometimes detecting missed details such as pustules, scales, or abnormal follicular patterns. For instance, when dealing with parasitic infestations such as Demodex mites, this device can detect subtle alterations near hair follicles indicating their presence, thus helping diagnose diseases like rosacea and demodicosis (Chioveanu et al., 2024). Similarly, a dermoscopic assessment can differentiate scabies from other types of scratchy rashes by revealing burrows and small mite bodies, directing clinicians toward a more specific diagnosis without the urge toward invasive sampling (Al J-Dabbagh et al., 2023).

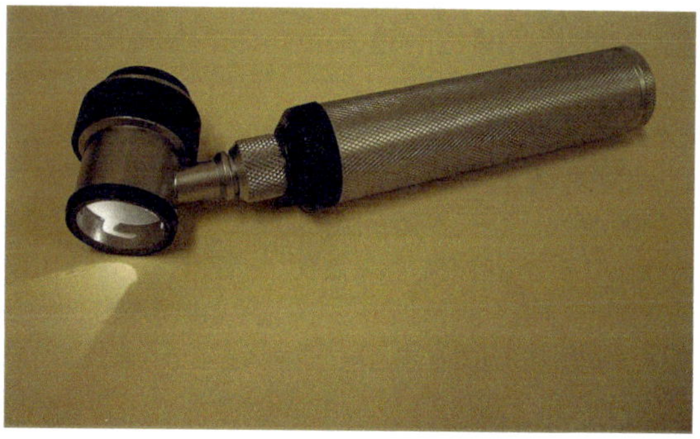

Figure 2.3. Immersion oil dermatoscope.

Source: Wikipedia contributors. (n.d.). *Dermatoscope1*. https://upload.wikimedia.org/wikipedia/commons/thumb/e/e6/Dermatoscope1.JPG/800px-Dermatoscope1.JPG.

Across the majority of instances, this general utility illustrates how dermoscopy is now a definitive component of the diagnostic process for many skin ailments. Of course, becoming proficient at dermoscopy is not precisely easy. It has a high learning curve, and mastering it takes plenty of practice hands-on—because even the smallest misreading will cause errors in diagnosis, especially if the signs are tricky or unusual. While it indeed sharpens clinical judgment, dermoscopy cannot substitute the absolute proof of skin biopsy and histopathology, especially if the lesions appear suspicious or complex., Integrating the results of dermoscopy with clinical information, and sometimes with additional measures such as a Wood's lamp examination or biopsy—provides the most comprehensive view. Thus, dermoscopy must be considered not as an independent fix but as a key component in a larger, multi-step approach to truly maximize patient care (Figure 2.3).

2.2.1. Definition and Purpose of Dermoscopy

Physicians frequently struggle to distinguish innocuous spots on the skin from those that could mean something more serious. Instead of relying on what initially meets the eye, a combination of diagnostic equipment sheds additional information about the skin's appearance and feel. An attractive trick is a dermoscopy, a painless technique (also referred to as epiluminescence microscopy) that allows doctors to magnify surface textures and even look under the skin. This enhanced perspective can reveal small details that are typically not visible to the naked eye, enabling early detection of cancers such as melanoma. It bridges the gap between a routine checkup and those more invasive tests, which, in most instances, can make a significant impact on treatment planning. At its core, dermoscopy works by using optical magnification along with either cross-polarized filters or immersion techniques to cut down on glare, thus exposing hidden pigment networks and tiny blood vessel patterns. By doing so, it makes it easier for doctors to tell apart lesions that come from melanocytic origins versus other kinds. Not only does it play a lead role in detecting melanoma, but it can also identify early manifestations of conditions such as actinic keratoses, which, honestly, can be a hassle to differentiate from benign lesions based on a routine examination alone (Reinehr et al., 2019). This technique of capturing faint morphological clues allows doctors to more accurately determine levels of risk and even reduce the number of unnecessary biopsies, increasing overall confidence in a diagnosis and resulting in better outcomes. In recent years, dermoscopy has been technologically upgraded with some quite sophisticated image analysis software. New computer-aided diagnostics, for instance, use feature discrimination to enhance lesion identification. Lightweight convolutional neural networks (CNNs) have been designed to overcome obstacles such as variations you could experience within a lesion type or the similarities experienced between various ones (Wei et al., 2020). Such breakthroughs are useful for segmenting and classifying dermoscopic lesions without tons of preprocessing, which is particularly useful in clinical laboratories and research environments alike. By marrying the old way with automated examination, the entire diagnostic process somehow becomes less subjective, more efficient, and even accessible in poor regions. This blend of experiential clinical skills and new technology has solidified dermoscopy's essential place in contemporary skin care.

2.2.2. Equipment and Technology Used in Dermoscopy

Dermatology has experienced some nice changes over the years. Consider the dermatoscope, for example—a pen-like device that combines a magnifying lens with polarized or plain light. It allows physicians to see underneath the skin, finding spots of pigment variation, small vascular patterns, and other things that typically remain hidden to plain observation. This device is not only a question of sophisticated optics; it frequently takes pictures that can subsequently be examined or even have sent off for a remote second opinion. In general, this sort of system makes a tremendous difference in eliminating the difference between what you see on a cursory look and what subsequent laboratory tests may validate. And then there is the digital spin on it. Digital dermoscopy goes the extra mile toward high-resolution images with intelligent algorithms that essentially aid in detecting skin lesion changes. These digital devices are utilized by many experts combined with built-in image databases, such that minor changes in the look of a lesion can be followed over a period of time. More often than not, artificial intelligence (AI) is added into the mix as an assisting second set of eyes, analyzing patterns and providing recommendations regarding malignancy risk. It is similar to the equipment marrying human ability with computer knowledge, providing more quantitative in-depth rather than merely a subjective interpretation (Smoller et al., 2021). Another development involves newer methods utilizing videodermatoscopes that project live images onto screens. This real-time glimpse is quite convenient for collaborative commentary, classroom use, or teledermatology consultations, even remote second opinions. Various configurations appear as well: some sensors touch the skin and others maintain a slight distance, each to accommodate patient sensitivities and lesion locations. Polarization capabilities, for instance, reduce glare to expose deeper skin features, providing a further sense of sharpness. These ever-changing tools allow physicians to personalize their approach, coordinating technical advances with day-to-day clinical requirements, and they increasingly support dermoscopy's fundamental role in contemporary skin assessments (Smoller et al., 2021) (Figure 2.4).

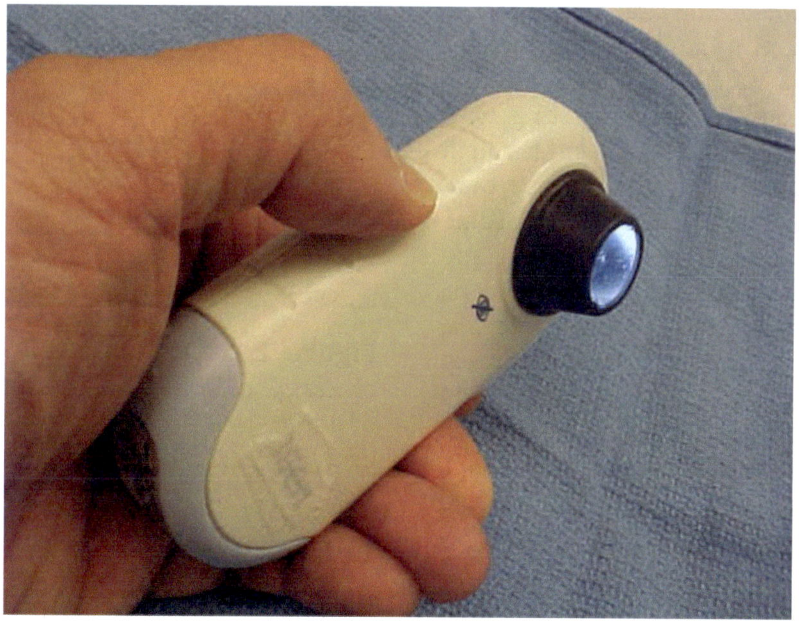

Figure 2.4. Polarized light dermatoscope.

Source: Wikimedia Commons. (n.d.). *Dermatoscope.* https://upload.wikimedia.org/wikipedia/commons/c/c2/Dermatoscope.jpg.

2.2.3. Common Conditions Diagnosed with Dermoscopy

Dermoscopy provides physicians with a means to view areas of skin that normally remain concealed, making it quite useful for determining a variety of skin problems. It allows clinicians to look under the surface to identify information that may not be readily visible to the naked eye. For instance, lesions such as melanocytic nevi and even melanoma are more understandabledetermine whether a growth is benign or otherwise. Inflammatory diseases like psoriasis, eczema, and lichen sclerosus tend to have their own specific patterns; consider lichen sclerosus, for example, which tends to present as chronic, whitish, atrophic lesions in anogenital sites that may be scrutinized under dermoscopy before a biopsy even being contemplated (David et al., 2023). This non-invasive technique contributes a worthwhile addition to a clinician's arsenal, assisting them in making decisions on everything from minor inflammations to potentially fatal malignancies. Recent advancements have really pushed dermoscopy into a new frontier—nowadays, machine learning and AI are competing with conventional techniques. CNNs can sift through images of skin lesions with an accuracy that, more often than not, is virtually on the same level as veteran specialists. This is a game changer for the detection of early skin cancers, such as melanoma and non-melanoma forms, but the accuracy of the results still largely depends on a physician's own experience. The hope of AI platforms is to smooth over such discrepancies and reduce variability, perhaps making them more critical where such advanced dermatologic service is lacking; nonetheless, it remains an issue of implementing such algorithms successfully with every group of patients and all lesions (Liopyris et al., 2022). In other words, great gains are here but still are best left in some way up to the clinician in interpreting dermoscopic results. Dermoscopy is not just for detecting cancers—it shines just as brightly when it comes to diagnosing inflammatory or infectious skin diseases by detecting typical vascular and structural signs. Psoriasis, for instance, usually has a pattern of regularly dotted vessels with white scales, while eczema tends to present yellowish serocrusts with patchy blood vessel patterns. Even in an attempt to distinguish a benign hyperpigmented lesion from a melanoma, the distribution of pigmentation and network pattern can provide essential clues. Minute variations are particularly evident in chronic diseases such as lichen sclerosus, when there is overlapping clinical appearance and it remains uncertain (David et al., 2023). Together, this method not only increases a clinician's confidence in placing a call but also assists in directing treatment and monitoring decisions—frequently eliminating unnecessary biopsies and leading to faster, more targeted treatment (Figure 2.5).

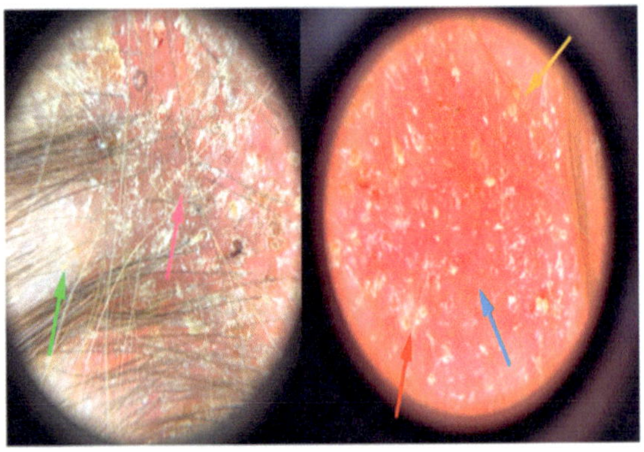

Figure 2.5. The dermoscopic presentation of *Kerion celsi* in an 8-year-old girl on the day of admission. Green arrow—white scales, pink arrow—broken hairs, red arrow—pustules, blue arrow—erythema, orange arrow—yellow crusts.

Source: Putek J, Nowicka D, Jankowska-Konsur A. Dermoscopy and Ultraviolet-Enhanced Fluorescence Dermoscopy (UEFD) Increase the Accuracy of Diagnosis and Are Useful in Assessing the Effectiveness of *Kerion celsi* Treatment. *Journal of Fungi*. 2025; 11(1):52. https://doi.org/10.3390/jof11010052

2.3. Wood's Lamp Examination

Doctors do not always have to use just regular lighting when they are attempting to diagnose skin issues—every now and then, they want a little assist. One well-known trick is to use a Wood's lamp, which is essentially a kind of special UV light that makes subtle details surface. It is an interesting device that reveals minor color variations in the skin, where such things as bacteria, fungus, or pigment changes could be at work. The lamp emits long UVA rays, and most often, this light causes substances like porphyrins (that is what certain bacteria emit) to glow with distinct colors. For example, consider erythrasma, a recalcitrant, superficial bacterial infection that will glow coral-red under the lamp, a handy diagnostic clue. The ease and non-invasive nature of this test is such that it usually gets combined with other examinations such as dermoscopy or even a skin scraping to ascertain what is happening (Jesús et al., 2024). That being said, the advantages of the Wood's lamp extend beyond bacteria. It may also suggest fungal problems or pigment abnormalities in more subtle ways. Fungal structures occasionally exhibit a yellow-green sheen, prompting physicians to think about tinea or candidiasis, whereas areas of vitiligo, due to loss of melanin, can burst forth in white brilliance. By and large, the test needs a darkened room and an observant eye, misreads are possible if creams or contaminants fool the lamp into false alarms. While the concept is simple, getting the glow to translate well requires some good clinical experience, connecting the pieces of evidence presented by the visible signs with a patient's history and exam results.

It is more of an ancillary aid that provides early clues, setting up more definitive testing such as skin scrapings or even a histopathologic examination if necessary (White, 2025). This layered strategy has the effect of refining the overall picture, assisting with a more targeted treatment regimen. In the day-to-day clinic, the value of the Wood's lamp is its fast bedside application and its ability to reduce invasive biopsies.

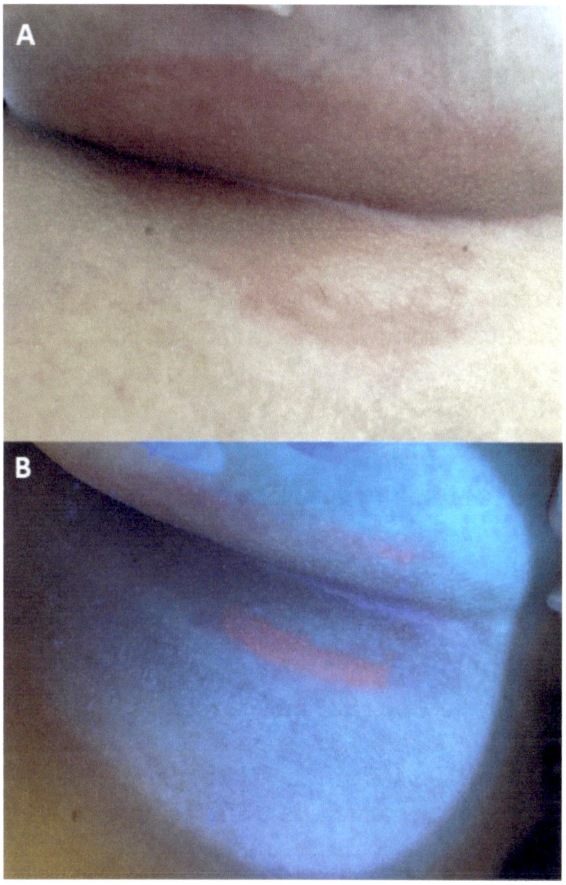

Figure 2.6. Wood's lamp examination revealed a white, partially golden-yellow fluorescence.

Source: Martínez-Ortega J, Franco González S (August 31, 2024) Erythrasma: Pathogenesis and Diagnostic Challenges. Cureus 16(8): e68308. doi:10.7759/cureus.68308

It is convenient because it uncovers telltale fluorescence patterns, sometimes the very cues that indicate a particular microbe or pigment alteration. For instance, catching sight of that coral-red shine in erythrasma will prompt a physician to initiate topical antibiotics immediately, and that typically translates to quicker recovery (Jesús Iván Martínez-Ortega et al., 2024). Additionally, when things become complicated and symptoms compound, this technique provides a second opinion. Nevertheless, one has to bear in mind the lamp's limitations; its sensitivity will depend on the spot of the lesion, the skin type, or even the number of bacteria involved. Everything considered, Wood's lamp examination is most effective as part of a larger picture that encompasses patient history, skin scrapings, a little bit of dermoscopy here and there, and, if it comes to that, histopathological examination (White, 2025). This combination of tests ensures that the ultimate diagnosis is as accurate as can be (Figure 2.6).

2.3.1. Mechanism of Wood's Lamp

Physicians employ specific lights to observe skin problems that would otherwise go unnoticed. Consider the Wood's lamp, for instance, it is not merely a light but one employing UV rays to cause specific skin components to glow suddenly. When skin absorbs this UV light—typically between 320 and 400 nanometers with a peak of around 365 nanometers, chemicals on or in the skin capture that energy and then release it as visible light. This simple process, derived from photoluminescence, allows clinicians to detect various patterns of glowing that suggest different skin issues. The lamp does this by awakening small molecules known as fluorophores that reside in our skin or even on its surface due to microbes.

These small molecules soak up the UV energy and eventually emit light at a longer wavelength, producing specific colors. For instance, in most instances, porphyrins from some bacteria emit a coral-red color, while fungal material may flaunt a yellow-green or blue-white light. Physicians typically perform this test in a dark room—so stray light does not overpower the glow effects (Smoller et al., 2021). In addition to making things shine, the Wood's lamp has a significant function in identifying conditions such as vitiligo, erythrasma, and tinea infections. For the most part, various fluorescence patterns reflect underlying biochemical changes, such as changes in melanin content or the accumulation of bacterial metabolites. For example, vitiligo patches glisten in brilliant blue-white due to melanin loss, while erythrasma-infested areas appear in coral-red as a result of porphyrins. Interpreting such signs improves accuracy in diagnosis and informs effective therapy, thus positioning the Wood's lamp as an invaluable, innocuous asset within clinical dermatology (Smoller et al., 2021).

2.3.2. Conditions Identifiable with Wood's Lamp

Wood's Lamp is an instant favorite in dermatology—it is harmless, fast, and reveals how skin components shine under UV light. You can see infections, pigment anomalies, and other skin peculiarities that would otherwise go unnoticed. For instance, infections by Microsporum species tend to fluoresce a bright green color, which helps physicians pinpoint a diagnosis more easily, particularly in clinical situations when waiting for lab cultures or microscope findings. It also reveals bacterial problems such as erythrasma, which fluoresce coral-red color due to the production of porphyrins; this provides a great punch of specificity without the need for more complex tests (Moskaluk et al., 2022). This rapid differentiation of pathologies significantly reduces the total time taken for decision-making. The lamp is not only for infections—it also has a significant role to play in picking up pigmentary disorders. The long-wave UV light brings out minor alterations in skin color that appear, highlighting patches of either a lack of or an excess of pigment that may be difficult to detect during a standard exam. Consider vitiligo, for example; its depigmented lesions are quite conspicuous under the lamp, making diagnosis and mapping of lesion borders easy. This method is usually less taxing on patients as it spares additional discomfort and simplifies monitoring. Of course, methods such as dermoscopy or spectrometry probe molecular specifics, but Wood's Lamp is still a convenient, inexpensive first-line screening tool for vitiligo and other pigment conditions (Airiss et al., 2023).

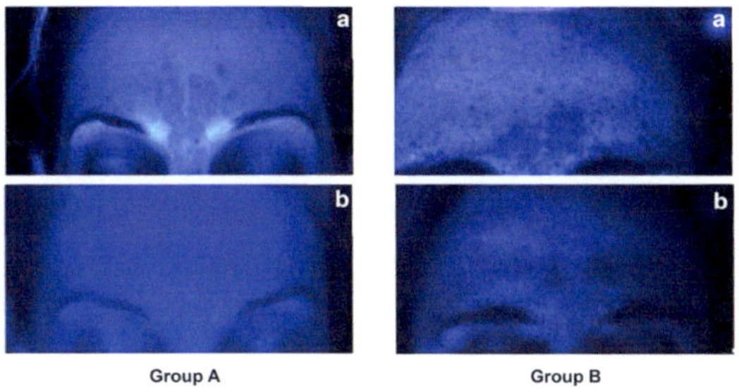

Figure 2.7. Photographs from subjects in the Wood's lamp examination before (a) and on the 60th day after the 1st treatment; and (b) for different treatments: Group A (microneedling and 5% retinoic acid) or Group B (5% retinoic acid only)

Source: Bergmann, C. L. M. da S., Pochmann, D., Bergmann, J., & Dani, C. (2021). Photographs from subjects in the Wood's lamp examination before (a) and on the 60th day after the 1st treatment (b). In The use of retinoic acid in association with microneedling in the treatment of epidermal melasma: Efficacy and oxidative stress parameters. *Archives of Dermatological Research*, *313*(8), 585–592.

In the vast majority of cases, that everyday advantage supports its position in an extended dermatological examination. At times, though, the lamp's true asset is in demystifying a presentation that superficially appears almost indistinguishable from others with definite fluorescent diagnostic signs. For instance, in *Microsporum canis* dermatophytosis, the characteristic fluorescence aids in its differentiation from other non-fluorescent fungal infections or inflammatory conditions, thus leading to a more targeted antifungal therapeutic regimen (Moskaluk et al., 2022). It can also detect alterations in skin flora and metabolic end-products that the naked eye would surely miss. Granted, the level of fluorescence may also differ with the duration a lesion has been present or according to the skin type of a patient, so its results tend to be verified by double-checking with histopathology or culture reports. Despite these imperfections, however, Wood's Lamp is still a quick, inexpensive bedside test that increases dermatological diagnostic efficiency when combined with other tools such as dermoscopy and biopsy (Figure 2.7).

2.3.3. Limitations and Considerations of Wood's Lamp

Although numerous people employ the Wood's lamp, it is not infallible in detecting all types of skin conditions. It greatly depends on having the right glowing chemicals in a patch of skin—something, let us admit, that is not always present. Consider pigment issues such as vitiligo, for instance; the lamp may detect those quite well, but if a condition does not radiate or the changes in the pigment are too subtle to see with UV light, the lamp may easily miss them. Ambient lighting, prior creams applied to the skin, and varying skin types can all interfere with the way bright that glow is going to look, so you essentially need to interpret the results cautiously. Frequently, it is just smarter to employ the Wood's lamp in combination with other tests instead of being the exclusive diagnosis tool—clinicians need always to take into account these characterestics as part of a larger context (Airiss et al., 2023). Another concern is that the lamp is not so particular about infections or inflammation. Okay, sometimes the flash of fluorescence, like that eerie green light from Microsporum species, can provide clues regarding bacterial or fungal microbes, but not all germs emit a similar message. In general, studies on dermatophytes have proven that some species or even some newly emerging fungal strains may not glow very much in Wood's light, so relying on it alone is a bit dangerous (Moskaluk et al., 2022). Furthermore, deciding how active or bad a condition is based on the way it glows turns out to be quite subjective, as there is no objective measurement involved. Thus, although the lamp does lend a helping hand, its diagnostic punch is weak and must be balanced against these subtleties, particularly as pathogens continue to evolve. In addition to that, a host of practical barriers prevent the Wood's lamp from being a go-to in clinics. First, it requires a darkened room and someone who is thoroughly familiar with it, which is not always feasible in all environments due to resource or population variations. There is also the issue of variable device quality: variations in the wavelength of the light, power output, and general construction can result in variable outcomes. And do not forget about skin color; in individuals with a darker complexion, the underlying pigmentation may mask that fluorescence, reducing the lamp's sensitivity. Newer non-invasive imaging techniques and molecular diagnostic tests increasingly have greater sensitivity and specificity for most conditions Wood's lamp would previously be depended on for (Airiss et al., 2023). All in all, if practitioners want to get the best out of this tool, they need to keep these real-world limitations in mind while mixing it with other testing methods.

2.4. Skin Biopsy and Histopathology

Microscopic inspection of skin tissue is usually the actual game-changer in the case of making a diagnosis—it goes significantly beyond an easy, eye-level evaluation. A skin biopsy, a fairly low-key and uncomplicated procedure, provides physicians with a small tissue sample that can be diverted into a histopathological examination. This procedure, in the majority of instances, picks up significant information regarding changes in cells and tissue design. It becomes an essential tool for detecting cancers, inflammation, or infections that may not appear as evident with only noninvasive screening. Dermoscopy, Wood's lamp testing, and other diagnostic techniques usually follow on the heels of these more definitive results. Combining a biopsy with a close examination under the microscope truly flaunts how accurate a dermatologic diagnosis should be. Yes, sophisticated imaging, such as Reflectance Confocal Microscopy (RCM), can almost replicate what you would observe from a complete histopathological analysis, but as a whole, the old-fashioned method still carries immense significance (Pimenta et al., 2020).

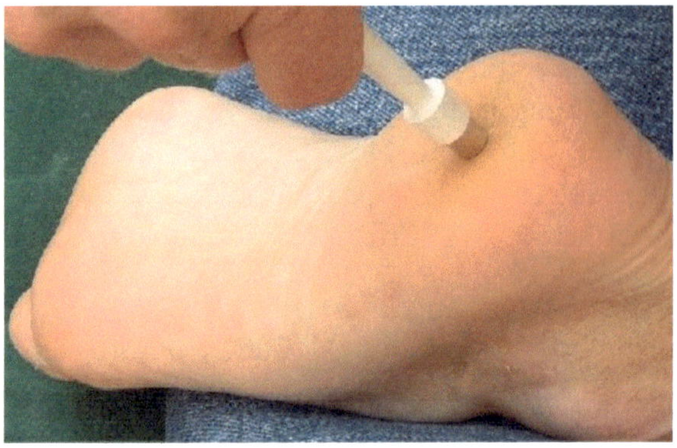

Figure 2.8. Skin biopsy.

Source: By Brimstone - Own work, CC BY-SA 3.0, https://commons.wikimedia.org/w/index.php?curid=19680773

Examining the tissue structure in detail enables distinguishing between benign hits and malignant ones, and it can detect subtle inflammatory anomalies or concealed microbial effects that often go unnoticed by a standard inspection. In most instances, the findings of these biopsies serve as the anchor for the overall clinical impression and guide the treatment course. Despite the more recent noninvasive technologies like Optical Coherence Tomography providing on-the-spot images and even some degree of layer-by-layer examination, nothing compares to the delicate detail of histopathology

(Adabi et al., 2017). The new imaging can enhance the image, but it does not necessarily obviate the necessity of a tissue sample; it is primarily what is on the surface or immediately below. That degree of cellular detail allows dermatologists to fine-tune treatments better, track how a disease progresses, and even estimate how things could turn out down the line. Integrating biopsy results with the microscopic perspective enriches our comprehension of skin conditions, bringing together what we observe in a physical exam and what is occurring at the molecular and cellular level (Figure 2.8).

2.4.1. Types of Skin Biopsies (Excisional, Incisional, Punch)

Obtaining a specific diagnosis for skin lesions is paramount in dermatology, particularly when there is concern for melanoma. Biopsy tends to be the method of choice; sampling tissue for examination, it literally sets the stage for correct diagnosis and appropriate staging. Take excisional biopsy, for example; it cuts out the lesion whole and unbroken, leaving physicians a shot at as good an estimation as possible of tumor depth and other important characteristics. All the same, this is typically a technical procedure and not always feasible when lesions are truly enormous or in unsuitable locations, so clinicians must weigh diagnostic accuracy against what is realistic in the real world (Arjunan et al., 2024; Aslanyan et al., 2022). Incisional biopsies provide an alternative approach by taking a sample of only a part of the lesion. This partial sample can be successful when the lesion is too large to be excised entirely or is in cosmetically or functionally delicate locations. It provides sufficient tissue for a diagnosis in most instances while maintaining low patient morbidity. However, by only obtaining a portion of the lesion, there is always a risk of not sampling malignant tissue in non-uniform tumors. This is the reason incisional biopsies are sometimes employed as a first step or when suspicion for malignancy is relatively low, and although a second excision procedure may be necessary later if cancer is discovered, Aslanyan et al. (2022) remind us. Then there is the punch biopsy, a frequently used, less invasive method. Using this technique, a circular blade is employed to clip out a tiny, cylindrical area of skin containing the epidermis, dermis, and a small amount of subcutaneous tissue.

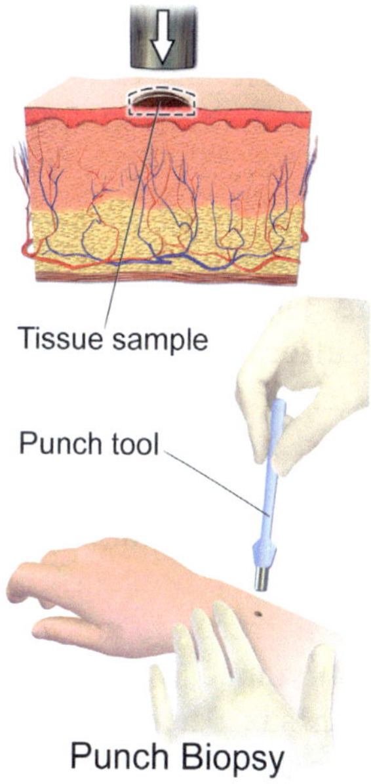

Figure 2.9. Punch biopsy.

Source: By BruceBlaus - Own work, CC BY-SA 4.0, https://commons.wikimedia.org/w/index.php?curid=61404539

This technique is a compromise between ease of procedure, patient comfort, and volume of diagnostic information yielded, which is why it is used with so many dermatologic conditions. Nonetheless, there is evidence that punch biopsies occasionally will underappreciate the depth and extent of the tumor—perhaps leading to underdiagnosis or suboptimal staging. This is especially concerning in pediatric presentations or in atypical melanocytic lesions, in which an incomplete sample can only make things more complicated. Briefly, whereas punch biopsies are certainly valuable, their application in suspected malignancy is weighed cautiously to ensure that the ultimate diagnosis and plan of treatment are maximally accurate (Arjunan et al., 2024; Aslanyan et al., 2022) (Figure 2.9).

2.4.2. Histopathological Analysis and Its Importance

Frequently, determining skin lesions requires more than a passing glance or non-invasive examination. A biopsy that culminates in a microscope examination can reveal cell information and minute alterations not apparent to the naked eye. Histopathological examination gets down to these microscopic aspects, revealing the small structural components and certain alterations in the tissues that even sophisticated imaging may not detect. For instance, although instruments such as dermoscopy or RCM enhance our perception of surface features and somewhat below, tissue examination is still important, particularly if there is even a trace of malignancy. In the majority of instances, examination of the pattern of the tissue is helpful in discriminating inflammatory conditions, infections, tumors, and other dermatoses, guiding practitioners toward therapeutic interventions that enhance patient outcomes (Basra et al., 2024). In pediatric dermatology, histopathological findings carry more significance. Children may present skin issues in unusual ways with symptoms confusingly combined, so a precise diagnosis is difficult. A paper from a tertiary center in southeast Nigeria, for example, noted that nearly half the clinical hypotheses coincided with what they found on biopsy. This discrepancy truly demonstrates that using what is visible upon taking an exam may be insufficient—verification of the diagnosis via tissue examination is usually required.

The same research underscored that neoplasms, skin appendage diseases, and papulosquamous diseases were some of the frequent biopsy results, a testament to how helpful this practice is in distinguishing benign from malignant issues. All this diligence ensures timely treatments and emphasizes the importance of a collaborative effort from dermatologists, pediatricians, and pathologists to provide appropriate care (Ndukwe et al., 2023). It goes beyond just diagnosing, as histopathological examinations also inform what is next in treatment. Consider skin cancers such as basal cell carcinoma (BCC): tissue examination verifies the presence of cancer and also examines aspects such as tumor margins and depth of invasion; information that are vital to surgical planning and ensuring complete excision occurs.

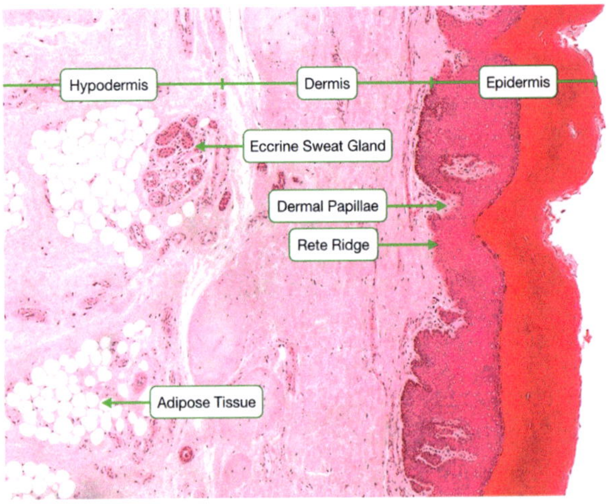

Figure 2.10. Histology of the skin.

Source: Takizawa, P. (2013). Histology of skin layers. *Yale Histology.* https://s3.us-east-2.amazonaws.com/yalehistology/skin/skin_layers.jpg.

While new imaging modalities appear promising as non-invasive alternatives, nothing can quite substitute for the high degree of detail viewed under the microscope when it comes to seeing small cellular changes. By combining what the histopathology indicates with clinical observations and dermoscopic findings, dermatologists are often able to fine-tune their diagnostic precision, modify treatment regimens, and even gain a sense of how the disease may progress. Thus, histopathology occupies the middle ground in dermatologic diagnosis, reconciling recent tech developments with established methods of tissue analysis (Basra et al., 2024) (Figure 2.10).

2.4.3. Interpretation of Biopsy Results

Reading a skin biopsy is not all about finding weird cells. It is more akin to heading directly into the hidden world of the tissue, examining everything from its general structure to how the cells cluster together. The sample literally gives a glimpse into the skin at a microscopic level, which can distinguish harmless marks from those potentially malignant, or even indicate inflammatory or infectious pathology. Good evaluation tends to rely on combining clinical history with additional tests, for example, what you observe with a dermoscopy test or even a Wood's lamp examination. Of late, AI is beginning to fill in, in general, in order to improve accuracy and efficiency in these examinations, possibly reducing man-made errors while maintaining standards constant (Ahmad et al., 2021).

This combination of technology and tradition lays the groundwork for individualized care by correlating what is observed on the slide with clinical and molecular evidence. Histopathology is still at the center of skin diagnoses, although getting every aspect correct really depends on how well the sample was collected. For instance, if a biopsy is inadequately oriented or simply too superficial, it may quite literally miss the point, resulting in potential misreads. For the most part, a pathologist's work is not just to tally up abnormal cells, but to notice subtle clues such as cellular atypia, unlooked-for mitotic outbursts, or groups of immune cells. Emerging imaging technologies, such as photoacoustic imaging, provide an interesting spin by showcasing vascular and structural information that ordinary microscopy could not see (Attia et al., 2019).

Deploying these newer approaches with traditional histopathology can truly cut diagnostic accuracy down to size and, by doing so, lead treatment options in a more in-tune direction for the individual patient's particular case. With all of these technological leaps and bounds, interpreting skin biopsy results always has to be integrated into a larger clinical context. Frequently, pathologists and dermatologists collaborate, juxtaposing microscopic observations against what is happening with the patient, considering additional tests such as patch tests or skin scrapings.

This interaction is rather significant, particularly when tissue slides alone do not provide a crystal-clear diagnosis. And, new AI technologies in surgical pathology are gradually alleviating the burden, allowing experts to concentrate on those difficult, subtle judgments (Ahmad et al., 2021). Finally, combining microscopic vision with contemporary imaging and sound clinical judgment forms the dynamic base of precision dermatology, guiding us toward brighter, more personalized patient care (Figure 2.11).

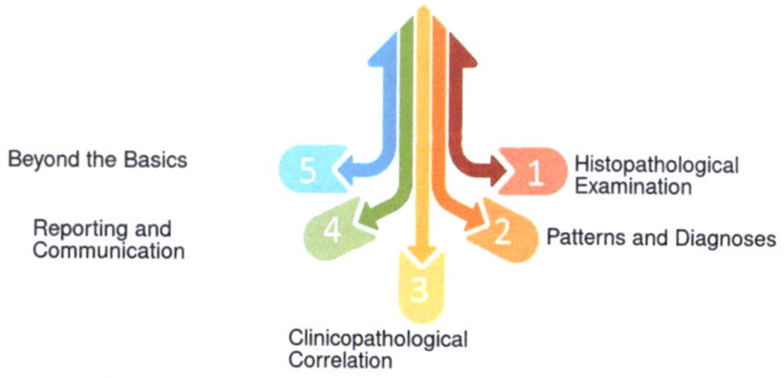

Figure 2.11. Biopsy results interpretation.

Source: FasterCapital. (2025). *Clinical Laboratory Dermatology: Understanding Skin Biopsies – A Guide for Dermatologists*. https://fastercapital.co/i/Clinical-laboratory-dermatology-Understanding-Skin-Biopsies--A-Guide-for-Dermatologists--Interpreting-Skin-Biopsy-Results.webp.

2.5. Patch Testing

Among all the methods of determining skin allergies, determining precisely which substance causes allergic contact dermatitis can be extremely difficult. Patch testing, for instance, involves applying minuscule amounts of suspected allergens on the skin—most often on the back, and then waiting between 48 and 96 hours to observe what occurs. Physicians seek out indicators such as redness, swelling, small bumps, or even small blisters; these signals enable them to determine which allergen could be the culprit. It is a relatively non-invasive technique that, in the majority of cases, differs from other tests that only rely on the appearance of the skin or potential infections. In addition, it complements a patient's history well by presenting concrete proof of sensitivity, which subsequently guides a more individualized treatment strategy. The method of patch testing is based on a number of central concepts. In general, it is really just a matter of employing a standardized panel of allergens, combining them to an appropriate strength, and exposing the skin for a certain length of time in order that the findings can always be relied upon. Our increasing knowledge about the immune system, and specifically how the T cells react over time, has truly influenced this process. In contrast to immediate reaction tests, patch testing requires patients to have precise instructions so they avoid exposing themselves to the likes of topical steroids or excessive sunlight—both of which may dampen the skin's genuine response. The choice of what allergens get often also relies on one's surroundings, occupation, or geographical location one resides in, so the test is highly personalized to each subject. Recent adjustments to the technique even permit more prolonged or repeated testing, which can trap those occasional or delayed responses and assist in guiding not only a diagnosis but lifestyle adjustments as well. Beyond merely coming to a diagnosis, patch testing plays a significant role in how a patient's course of treatment is handled and what the future may hold for them. When the test specifically identifies the individual allergens, dermatologists can then recommend extremely specific avoidance measures—frequently resulting in improved treatment and fewer flare-ups. This is particularly significant for work-related cases, where early identification of a workplace allergen can truly prevent long-term problems and even cause companies to make changes at the workplace. On other occasions, patch testing may be combined with other techniques such as skin biopsies or dermoscopy in order to see the complete picture of what is occurring underneath the surface of the skin. Okay, granted the technique itself is usually deemed to be safe, interpreting the findings can sometimes be an art, an art whereby an experienced eye can distinguish a plain irritant response from an actual allergy. It is therefore why specialized training is necessary. Ultimately, patch testing is a central weapon in the dermatologist's armory, underpinning evidence-based, individualized decision-making within patient management (Elgamal et al., 2023; Muhsin et al., 2024) (Figure 2.12).

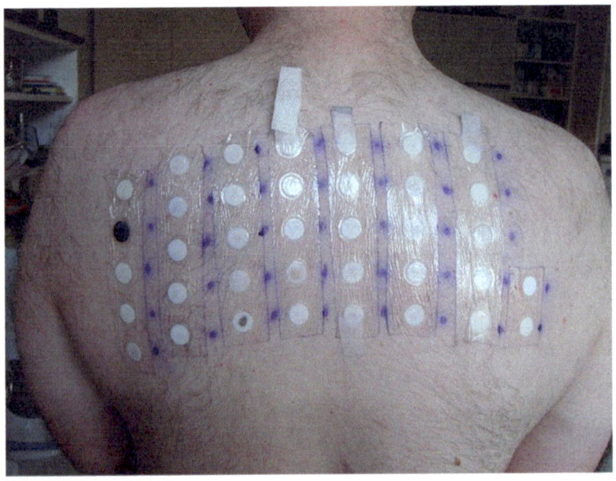

Figure 2.12. Patch test.

Source: Wikimedia Commons. (n.d.). *Epikutanni Test.* https://upload.wikimedia.org/wikipedia/commons/thumb/4/4c/Epikutanni-test.jpg/800px-Epikutanni-test.jpg.

2.5.1. Purpose and Methodology of Patch Testing

Skin diagnostics begin with a sharp emphasis on determining why skin responds the way it does, a consideration that counts a great deal when treating patients. Patch testing is one of those reliable procedures where physicians apply the skin to various possible irritants under laboratory conditions. It is primarily a matter of focusing on those perpetrators that produce negative skin reactions, allowing clinicians to focus on culprits and make informed avoidance maneuvers. In contrast to other tests such as dermoscopy or wood lamp use, with their emphasis on the appearance or fluorescence of items—patch testing explores delayed immune processes, frequently demonstrating type IV hypersensitivity in the form of tiny, localized inflammation. This type of pinpoint precision significantly enhances patient care by catching allergenic pals that may fall through techniques that are based only on vision or lab slides. The procedure itself is quite simple: standardized panels of allergens are applied to the patient's back or another appropriate location, typically with small chambers or discs retained by hypoallergenic tape. After placement, these allergens remain on for about 48 hours while the skin is observed for such indications as redness, swelling, or blistering, indications of a hypersensitive response. Readings are subsequently obtained around 48 hours and again subsequently between 72 to 96 hours so that those delayed immune responses, which are quite typical of allergic contact dermatitis, can be separated from more transient and immediate irritant responses. One of the most important aspects of this regimen is the scoring system, in which the severity and appearance of skin alterations are assessed to make it reproducible and reliable across patients. This systematic yet adaptable approach remains a gold standard for allergy detection in dermatology. Although patch testing has been an established presence for many years, newer advances in drug delivery and non-invasive diagnostics—dissolving microneedles come to mind—appear set to adjust the means of allergen application and the stimulation of immune response (Sartawi et al., 2022). In general, these advances may assist in surmounting challenges such as how well an allergen is absorbed through the skin or coping with variations in skin barriers, leaving room for even more sensitive and effective tests in the future. Nevertheless, the existing method stands its ground in clinical practice, thanks in no small measure to its strength and the simplicity of its results. When integrated into an extensive skin analysis involving features such as biopsies or histopathology, patch testing provides a multi-level approach that enhances the accuracy of dermatitis diagnoses and aids in tailoring treatment plans (Codella et al., 2017).

2.5.2. Common Allergens Tested in Patch Testing

Management of contact dermatitis depends on determining which allergens are responsible. Patch testing is where this comes in – tiny quantities of various allergens are applied to the skin, and local reactions that follow reveal possible culprits. Nickel sulfate, cobalt chloride, and even chromium, for instance, tend to trigger allergic reactions because they are ubiquitous in jewelry, coins, and metal tools you touch every day. Perfume blends, as well as preservatives such as parabens and formaldehyde releasers, are a second group of suspects that appear in most cosmetics and creams. Because these chemicals emerge so much in our environment, they usually end up being added to stock patch test panels to increase diagnostic sensitivity and guide patients toward useful avoidance maneuvers. Looking slightly more in-depth, such as including agents such as neomycin, an antibiotic added to several topical preparations, is important because it will be likely to cause reactions in a significant percentage of cases. Potassium dichromate comes in as well, which occurs in environments involving cement or leather work, so some patients may require a more customized technique in testing. And then there is para-phenylenediamine (PPD), that active ingredient in dyes one finds in hair colorants which usually leads not only to physical distress but also to psychological and social distress. Most often, these multiplicities of allergens—from the routine exposure to those related to occupation or lifestyle— serve to underscore further the benefit that patch testing brings in illuminating the scenario and aiding patient education (Adaskevich, 2016). Emerging trends also continue to redefine how patch testing is done. Scientists have been detecting novel allergens by studying populations epidemiologically, and so the test panels are increasingly comprehensive. Plant perpetrators such as poison ivy, poison oak, and even fragrance components of essential oils now are being recognized for causing delayed hypersensitivity reactions. The entire allergen spectrum continues changing with shifting consumer behavior and manufacturing processes, and so test series have to be constantly revised to capture such new sensitizers. By combining newer allergens with the older ones, dermatologists are able to make more precise diagnoses and recommend improved avoidance strategies, ultimately alleviating the burden of allergic contact dermatitis and enhancing the quality of life (Adaskevich, 2016).

2.5.3. Interpretation of Patch Test Results

Patch test results interpretation is a critical step in identifying allergic contact dermatitis and determining the course of action for further care. Shortly after the patches are placed, the test areas are checked, usually at the 48- and 72-hour points, for indications such as red patches, swelling, small bumps, or even small blisters. Instead of depending on high-sounding jargon, physicians merely grade these reactions from "nothing" up through a couple of levels of positivity, depending on how strong the reaction appears and what shape it takes. A definite reaction typically indicates that the patient is allergic to the allergen, but generally, one has to compare these with what the patient's history and exposure patterns indicate. Misinterpretation of a response could cause either unnecessary avoidance or missed issues, so keen clinical vision is entirely essential. And occasionally, by irritant reactions or even phototoxicity, false positives will be seen, that is to say, the reading is not always as good as it seems on first inspection.

The subtleties at the sites of the test can contribute greatly to what we know of these responses. For example, reading too early can at times equate to missing an early warning, and delayed responses may not be evident on standard readings, suggesting that repeat observations may be necessary. It is also important to distinguish between a simple irritant response, which usually has indistinct boundaries and may resolve quickly, and an actual allergic reaction. Variables like where on the body the test was administered and the subject's individual sensitivity of the skin can change the way the reaction appears. More recent techniques, such as dermoscopy, can cause fine signs of inflammation to become visible, providing a better image than the naked eye would otherwise pick up. For the most part, these varied methods complement more extensive dermatological routines, affirming that increasingly multimodal evaluation increases diagnostic precision (Cheng & Guitera, 2015). Staying current with the continuously evolving discipline of dermatology requires patch test interpretations to be augmented by additional instruments that enhance clinical judgment. For instance, when a skin lesion appears aberrant, performing a histopathological examination will be able to distinguish an allergic reaction from inflammatory or even neoplastic pathology. Patch testing remains the yardstick for revealing contact allergens, but by using it with techniques such as skin biopsies and dermoscopy, one is presented with a complete picture of dermatological problems. Clinicians, in return, must be competent not only at identifying patterns of reactions but also at integrating results from multiple tests to tailor how patients are treated. With practice over time, more experience and training in this field can truly make a person more confident and less prone to making mistakes, ultimately resulting in improved patient care outcomes (Ahnlide, 2015) (Figure 2.13).

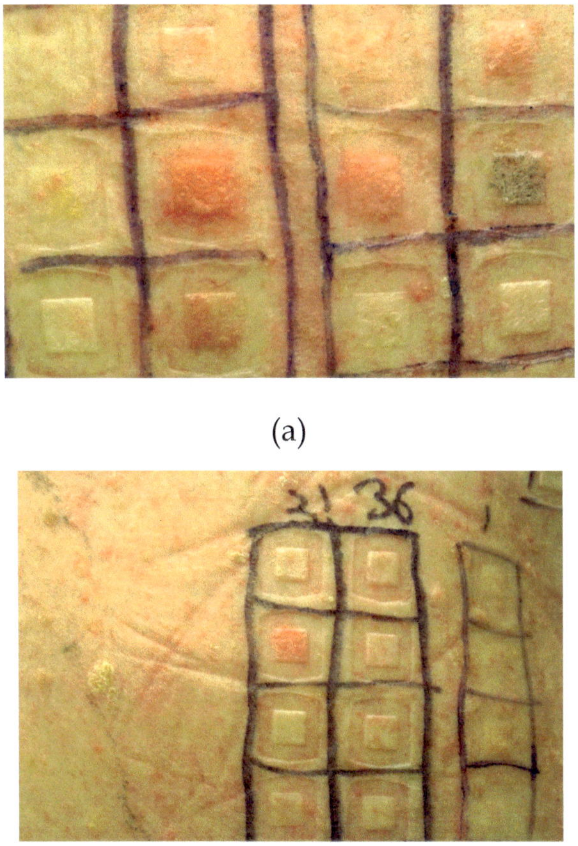

(a)

(b)

Figure 2.13. Interpretation of results.

Source: Wikimedia Commons. (n.d.). *Epikutanni Test.* https://en.wikipedia.org/wiki/Patch_test.

2.6. Skin Scrapings

Microscopic analysis is most important when dealing with skin disease, particularly when you are searching for infection or changes in the tissue. One of the methods used is taking scrapings of the skin, essentially harvesting a sample of what lies on the surface from a lesion—to look for fungal infections such as dermatophytoses. Generally put, after these scrapings have been collected, they are blended with potassium hydroxide (KOH), which breaks down keratin so the fungal components can be observed under the microscope. This technique proves to be a real lifesaver when fungal problems fail to appear conventionally; for example, *Tinea incognito*—a fungal infection distorted by the application of topical steroids—depends on this method to make its concealed signs manifest, thereby preventing misdiagnosis and guiding treatment in the correct direction (Zacharopoulou et al., 2024).

In real-world clinical practice, performing a good skin scraping is not merely a matter of course; it takes a gentle touch and some good knowledge of what lesions are supposed to look like. The key is to scoop up material from the very edge of the lesion where fungal or parasitic debris is most likely to be persisting. Once you get the sample, it is treated with KOH to remove the excess keratin and preserve the diagnostic clues. This method usually differentiates fungal infections from other skin conditions that present with like symptoms, such as eczema or psoriasis—because employing an inappropriate treatment (e.g., corticosteroids on a fungal issue) could make the problem worse by inducing *Tinea incognito*. This is the reason why, in most situations, the skin scraping method continues to be such a vital component of both initial diagnosis and post-diagnosis treatment planning (Zacharopoulou et al., 2024).

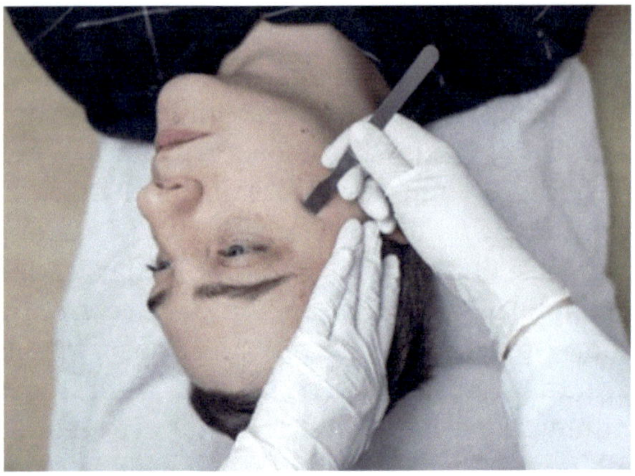

Figure 2.14. A dermatologist takes skin scraping test.

Source: Shutterstock. (n.d.). *Dermatologist Takes Skin Scraping Tests for Demodicosis and Dermatitis.* https://www.shutterstock.com/image-photo/dermatologist-takes-skin-scraping-tests-260nw-2600975265.jpg.

Not only do fungi become swept up this way, but skin scrapings also come into play when investigating parasitic issues such as those of scabies. A rapid microscopic examination may show mites, eggs, or even fecal pellet remnants, all of which corroborate clinical suspicion. The ease and low expense of the procedure make it a convenient choice in most healthcare settings, frequently yielding rapid results that can directly influence treatment plans.

And, too, it well supplements other exams, such as employing a dermoscope or the Wood's lamp—by providing direct microscopic evidence instead of depending on such as fluorescence or the way a lesion merely appears. Naturally, the entire procedure relies on the quality of sample taking and handling as well as the clinician's expertise at identifying features microscopically; these are particularly relevant in environments where high-level testing is not possible (Zacharopoulou et al., 2024) (Figure 2.14).

2.6.1. Technique for Performing Skin Scrapings

Getting an accurate diagnosis in dermatology really all comes down to catching a good sample—just taking the right piece of skin is the name of the game. For infections or infestations on the surface, a skin scraping is generally the move of choice. You use a clean scalpel or something of the sort and gently scrape the infected area to collect skin cells along with any underlying pathogens. Getting a meaningful sample means zeroing in on active spots like vesicles, pustules, or flaky patches so that even the deeper layers of the skin get represented. After you obtain the material, it is usually put on a microscope slide, usually combined with KOK (or an equivalent clearing agent) to facilitate the detection of fungi, parasites, or abnormal cells, all while being careful not to contaminate and keeping the patient as comfortable as possible. Scabies adds a new wrinkle to this procedure. Because the mites are small and are living under the skin, scraping becomes especially necessary. The standard method is looking for intact burrows—those definitive telltale marks, and then gently opening the end of a burrow to capture mites, eggs, or even small pellets of feces. At times, though, scratching or crust may cover over these burrows, and they become difficult to spot. Recently, dermoscopy has been greatly beneficial by magnifying those typical features, such as the so-called "jet with contrail" sign that suggests both the mite and tunnel. The non-invasive method assists clinicians in identifying optimal sites for scraping, particularly where it is difficult in areas such as finger webs and the genitalia, thereby increasing both sample yield and patient satisfaction (Nie et al., 2023). Apart from parasites, also utilized in skin scrapings to identify fungal infections and even certain instances attributed to deeper pathogens like *Leishmania donovani*. In most instances, these conditions necessitate a combination of microscopic analysis and molecular studies since the typical clinical manifestations tend to be rather nonspecific or even overlapping. In essence, skin scrapings constitute a minimally invasive method of obtaining samples that, upon microscopic examination, can demonstrate amastigotes or other forms of the pathogen. Combined with other diagnostic techniques such as biopsy and histopathology, this method tends to increase sensitivity and specificity for the detection of cutaneous leishmaniasis. This entire integrated strategy comes in very handy in areas confronted with endemic disease, where preliminary, proper diagnosis through skin scraping can direct on-time treatment and control interventions (Piyasiri et al., 2023).

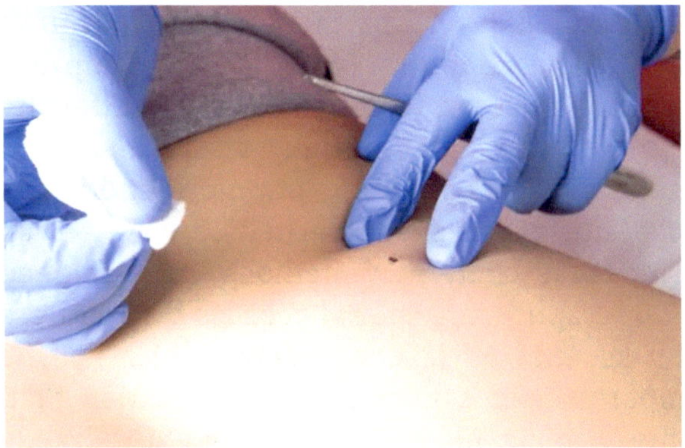

Source: California Dermatology Institute. (2023). *Scraping and Burning Procedure for Skin Lesions.* https://www.calderminstitute.com/wp-content/uploads/2023/09/scraping-and-burning.webp.

2.6.2. Conditions Diagnosed Through Skin Scrapings

Dermatologists tend to rely on less invasive techniques to obtain rapid, trustworthy clues regarding skin problems. A quick skin scraping frequently provides clues to unwanted parasites or small infections. For instance, when scabies is suspected, a microscopic examination can reveal mites, eggs, or even small pieces of fecal material. As a general rule, this method best applies when the scraping is precisely conducted and its results balanced against other clinical information; after all, its sensitivity can vary depending on the context. The 2020 International Alliance for the Control of Scabies (IACS) Consensus Criteria, for example, emphasizes that visual confirmation of the mite alone is insufficient—it is also prudent to look at the general symptoms (Engelman et al., 2020). Although scrapings are a convenient diagnostic tool for parasitic skin infections, they are a useful adjunct, not a sole test. Outside of parasites, scrapings are used to identify fungal infections with diverse appearances that occasionally overlap with other skin conditions. In the instance of dermatophytoses such as ringworm or tinea infections, a basic slide, usually pre-treated with KOH—may reveal fungal hyphae or spores on a microscopic examination. This simple procedure provides quite rapid and economical feedback, which will enable clinicians to separate fungal infections from other conditions such as eczema or even psoriasis. Granted, histopathology provides more detailed information, but skin scrapings are likely to be the initial referral due to preserving the patient's tissue and being on-the-spot. Naturally, the technique's specificity and sensitivity can vary based on the quality of the sample as well as the skill of the examiner, so employing additional diagnostic devices such as dermoscopy is sometimes needed (Engelman et al., 2020). Occasionally, the applicability of scrapings extends into cancer diagnostics as well. In the setting of oncologic assessment, exfoliative cytology, from skin scrapings, can mark basal cell carcinoma (BCC) rapidly, avoiding some of the delay associated with complete biopsy processing. Although skin biopsy and histopathology are still the gold standard because they preserve tissue architecture and provide an absolute diagnosis, cytology from scrapings introduces a noninvasive, expeditious option when BCC is strongly suspected. Research tends to show that cytologic examination from these scrapings provides high sensitivity and specificity for BCC, offering an aid before proceeding to treatments such as radiotherapy (Di Ruffano et al., 2018). For more invasive cancers like squamous cell carcinoma or melanoma, though, the method is lacking in evaluating the entire tissue structure, leaving biopsies firmly at the wheel. In other words, though scrapings can well supplement the overall clinical picture, they never substitute for full histological assessment.

2.6.3. Advantages and Limitations of Skin Scrapings

Physicians attempting to sort out dermatological issues typically combine a physical examination with some laboratory work to double-check whether something odd is afoot, such as unusual cells or unwanted microbes. Skin scrapings, for instance, provide a very handy short cut: by scraping off a small piece of the outer skin, clinicians can rapidly obtain samples to search for things like fungi, parasites, and sometimes bacteria. This small trick is particularly useful for detecting dermatophytes, as these fungi are typically located in keratinized tissue, a place they prefer. It is usually simple and inexpensive, too, avoiding the additional pain a biopsy could inflict on patients. In most clinics, particularly where quick examination must be used to initiate treatment, this procedure is the standard approach (Moskaluk et al., 2022). Nevertheless, even with such benefits, there are definite boundaries to how much skin scrapings can offer. Chief among them is that the test's sensitivity can hang in the balance depending on the clinician's expertise and whether the sample is quality. In the event, for instance, the scraping is shallow or off-target, the test could return a false-negative result, which is especially egregious with deeper or atypical infections. Although scrapings have been effective in capturing surface-level fungi and parasites, they do not always suffice for more complex skin diseases—those that may require an in-depth exploration using histopathological examination to uncover internal cell disorders. More often than not, this implies that physicians must complement scrapings using other techniques in order to get the complete picture (Hulei, 2020). Concurrently, new diagnostic technologies have added layers to the process. Machines like dermoscopy or even a Wood's lamp can occasionally emit visual clues of skin difficulty without ever taking out any tissue, and rapid molecular tests are being put more into action to identify pathogens earlier. However, even with these chilly new methods, old-fashioned skin scrapings are special because they address the keratinized layers directly, which can be important for a microscopic verification that, quite frankly, molecular tests may not exactly duplicate. Combining these tried-and-true scrapings with more modern tools can truly hone precision, but it also points to why using scrapings alone could result in misses in the larger diagnostic picture (Hulei, 2020; Moskaluk et al., 2022).

CLOSER LOOK

Reflectance Confocal Microscopy (RCM)

RCM is an imaging modality that is non-invasive and offers in vivo visualization of skin at near-histologic resolution. It can be employed to facilitate the diagnosis and management of many skin diseases, especially skin cancers such as melanoma and BCC. RCM enables a cellular-level, detailed exploration of the epidermis and superficial dermis, and therefore clinicians can evaluate structures and patterns of the skin.

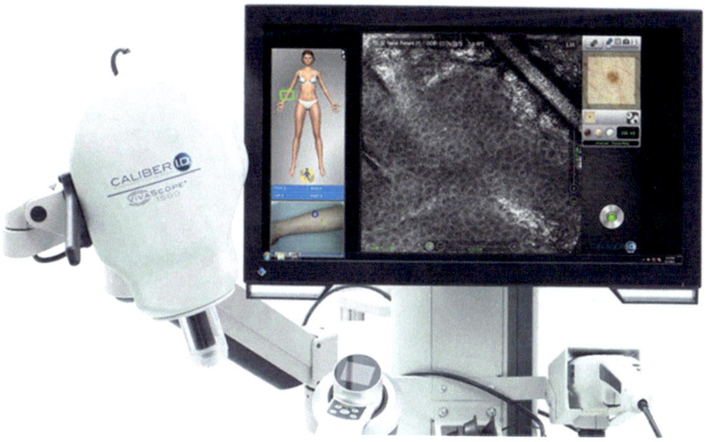

Source: Skin Cancer and Reconstructive Surgery Center. (n.d.). Reflectance Confocal Microscopy for Skin Cancer Diagnosis. https://scarscenter.com/wp-content/uploads/2018/01/Skin-Cancer-Specialists-Skin-Cancer-Diagnosis-Techniques-Reflectance-Confocal-Microscopy-Skin-Cancer-and-Reconstructive-Surgery-Center-Orange-County.jpg.

- **How RCM Works:** RCM employs a confocal microscope to scan the skin surface with a laser beam. The skin's reflected light is then captured and processed to develop a three-dimensional image of tissue. This picture gives a horizontal view of the skin, depicting cellular and subcellular structures.

Key Features and Benefits:

- **Non-Invasive:** RCM is not biopsied or invasive and is thus a comfortable and safe procedure for patients.
- **High Resolution:** RCM delivers near-histologic resolution with the ability to clearly visualize skin patterns and structures.
- ***In Vivo*:** RCM permits real-time imaging of the skin, allowing dynamic observation of temporal changes.
- **Less Need for Biopsies:** RCM can reduce the demand for biopsies, especially for less suspicious or benign lesions.
- **Better Accuracy:** RCM can increase the accuracy of diagnosis over clinical examination and dermoscopy alone.

- **Several Clinical Applications:** RCM is applied for skin cancer diagnosis, evaluation of inflammatory skin diseases, and monitoring of treatment response.

Limitations:

- **Finite Depth:** RCM is mainly informative about the epidermis and superficial dermis, with finite imaging depth.
- **Needs Expertise:** RCM images' interpretation demands certain knowledge of histomorphological characteristics; hence it is not easily available for daily clinical practice.
- **Gray Scale Imag**es: RCM images are grayscale, which may be difficult for some clinicians who are used to dermoscopy's color approach to analysis.

SUMMARY

Skin problem diagnosis has gone a long way since. Sure, the good old skin biopsy and histopathology remain at the top for pinpointing an unmistakable diagnosis—giving a glimpse of the cellular and structural detail—yet newer, less invasive examinations have come into the picture to help out. Dermoscopy and Wood's lamp examinations, for example, assist physicians in identifying subtle pigment and shape alterations without digging too deeply, which can equate to more rapid treatment decisions. Patch tests and skin scrapings sometimes serve their role in revealing allergies or infections, typically in conjunction with the more meticulous visual and microscopic examinations. All these approaches, blended together in a type of holistic stew, lay the foundation for customized treatments and overall improved patient care, and in most instances, they even open the door for next-gen diagnostic technology (Adaskevich, 2016). There is also hype surrounding vibrational spectroscopic methods that could possibly revolutionize things. Essentially, these newer methods allow us to peek into molecular information, sensing even faint biochemical changes that conventional histopathology could possibly miss. In most instances, such methods assist surgeons in improving the delineation of margins of premalignant or malignant lesions during surgery, which hints at better outcomes. Additionally, with its ability to distinguish between different skin problems—some of which are hard to diagnose like vulval disease, with high sensitivity and specificity, vibrational spectroscopy is flaunting its accuracy. Mostly, these techniques provide an accelerated, less invasive, and much more comprehensive peek at what is happening, possibly improving both patient care and overall outcomes (Frost et al., 2020). Looking forward, the trend appears to be towards mixing the new with the old. Classic tests are still vital, but coupling them with modern spectroscopic and imaging instruments can infuse fresh, real-time, and molecular information into day-to-day clinical choices. This combination may not only cut diagnostic accuracy razor-sharp but also facilitate early detection and more personalized treatment protocols. Constant research, and, yes, a dash of trial and error—is truly at the heart of testing and refining such new approaches prior to their going mainstream. As dermatology begins to incorporate this blend, clinicians are more than ever in a position to attack chronic skin disease in a more comprehensive manner, representing a move toward a new diagnostic and treatment-planning era (Adaskevich, 2016; Frost et al., 2020).

Physicians use a combination of instruments to determine skin problems, and each of the varied tests contributes toward improving overall accuracy while maintaining patient outcomes as a priority. Occasionally it begins with a hasty glance and touch—the sort of by-hand examination that identifies rudimentary shapes and textures that indicate some ailments. And then there is dermoscopy, which in effect is like a magnifying glass for the skin; it reveals details invisible to the naked eye and allows it to more easily distinguish between harmless marks and possibly serious ones, particularly where pigment is involved. To this, a Wood's lamp adds the use of UV light to take a sneak peek at pigment changes or even small infections in the outer layer of the skin. Combined, these non-invasive measures construct an initial image that directs physicians toward more extensive testing only when necessary, keeping discomfort minimal and resources concentrated. When a simple test simply will not do, a skin biopsy enters the picture followed by histopathological examination—a process that quite literally functions as the gold standard for a definitive diagnosis. In general, the biopsy could be as minimal as a punch sample or a more excisional type, whereby physicians can examine the cells and their pattern closely. Histopathology provides all-important clues regarding what is happening, whether the problem is inflammatory, cancerous, or infectious. Surprisingly, newer approaches such as vibrational spectroscopic techniques are proving to be promising. They can identify molecular alterations that routine microscopy may miss out on, perhaps eliminating the necessity for some of the more invasive procedures and increasing both diagnostic specificity as well as sensitivity in difficult situations (Adaskevich, 2016). In total, these laboratory examinations, along with clinical examination and imaging, constitute a type of indispensable triad in daily dermatological practice (Frost et al., 2020). Other tests, such as patch testing and skin scrapings—serve critical uses in the identification of allergic and infectious dermatoses. For instance, patch testing entails placing known allergens on the skin to determine whether it will react after a period of time; this can be particularly helpful in diagnosing diseases such as allergic contact dermatitis and assisting patients with knowing what to avoid. Likewise, skin scrapings enable microscopic and culture-based examinations that can uncover parasitic or fungal problems, opening the door to more specific treatments. Although these tests may at times be eclipsed by high-tech imaging and laboratory tests, they remain essential to identifying the more frequent but occasionally confounding skin issues. Effectively bringing together all these multifarious methods depicts a multidisciplinary methodology aspiring for spot-on diagnosis, personalized care, and eventually improved patient care (Adaskevich, 2016; Frost et al., 2020).

KEY TERMS FROM THIS CHAPTER

Benign hypopigmentation	Benign mole	Consultations
Convolutional neural networks	Dermatophytes	Dermoscopy
Fluorophores	Fungi	Histopathology
Leprosy	Lichen sclerosus	Lumps
Melanoma	Microbial fluorescence	Microsporum species
Mites	Palpation	Patches
Patch tests	Photoluminescence	Physicians
Pityriasis alba	Potassium dichromate	Psoriasis
Reflectance confocal microscopy	Skin biopsy	Skin scrapings
Supplements	Teledermatology	Videodermatoscopes
Vitiligo	Wood's lamp tests	

REFERENCES

1. Adabi, S., Clayton, A., Conforto, S., & Daveluy, M., et al. (2017). Universal *in vivo* textural model for human skin based on optical coherence tomograms. *arXiv.* http://arxiv.org/abs/1706.02758 (accessed on 12 May 2025).
2. Adaskevich, V. P. (2016). A-25 Skin Diseases and Sexually Transmitted Infections : handbook / U.P. Adaskevich. – Vitebsk: VSMU, 2016. – 396 p. ISBN 978-985-466-830-7(accessed on 12 May 2025).
3. Ahmad, Z., Rahim, S., Zubair, M., & Abdul-Ghafar, J. (2021). Artificial intelligence (AI) in medicine, current applications and future role with special emphasis on its potential and promise in pathology: Present and future impact, obstacles including costs and acceptance among pathologists, practical and philosophical considerations. A comprehensive review. *Diagnostic Pathology, 16*. https://doi.org/10.1186/s13000-021-01085-4.
4. Ahnlide, I. (2015). *Aspects of skin cancer diagnosis in clinical practice.* [Doctoral Thesis (compilation), Dermatology and Venereology (Lund)]. Department of Clinical Sciences, Lund University. (accessed on 12 May 2025).
5. Al-Dabbagh, J., Younis, R. T., & Sliman, R. (2023). The differential diagnoses and complications of scabies variants. *Portuguese Journal of Dermatology and Venereology, 81*. https://doi.org/10.24875/pjdv.23000062.
6. Al-Dhalimi, M. A., & Mahdi, N. (2024). Onychoscopic evaluation of inflammatory nail disorder and their relationship with disease duration: A clinical descriptive study. *Kufa Medical Journal, 20*, 84–109. https://doi.org/10.36330/kmj.v20i2.15011.
7. Arjunan, A., Wardrop, M., Malek, M. M., Davit, A. J., 3rd, Sargen, M. R., Kirkwood, J. M., Demanelis, K., & Seynnaeve, B. K. N. (2024). Treatment outcomes following partial shave biopsy of atypical and malignant melanocytic tumors in pediatric patients. *Melanoma research, 34*(6), 544–548. https://doi.org/10.1097/CMR.0000000000001002(accessed on 12 May 2025).
8. Pimenta, R., Soares-de-Almeida, L., Arzberger, E., Ferreira, J., Leal-Filipe, P., Bastos, P. M., & Oliveira, A. L. (2020). Reflectance confocal microscopy for the diagnosis of skin infections and infestations. *Dermatology online journal, 26*(3), 13030/qt9qz046f1.
9. Aslanyan, S., Gumeniuk, K., & Lysenko, D. (2022). Modern views on skin biopsy in the diagnostic algorithm of dermatooncological diseases. *Український радіологічний та онкологічний журнал.* https://www.semanticscholar.org/paper/b2e41459a4ca11729078e8c16c1c0bcd0152ffac (accessed on 12 May 2025).
10. Attia, A. B. E., Balasundaram, G., Moothanchery, M., Dinish, U. S., Bi, R., Ntziachristos, V., & Olivo, M. (2019). A review of clinical photoacoustic imaging: Current and future trends. *Photoacoustics, 16*, 100144. https://doi.org/10.1016/j.pacs.2019.100144.
11. Castro, L. G., Bakos, R. M., Duprat Neto, J. P., Bittencourt, F. V., Di Giacomo, T. H., Serpa, S. S., Messina, M. C., Loureiro, W. R., Macarenco, R. S., Stolf, H. O., & Gontijo, G. (2016). Brazilian guidelines for diagnosis, treatment and follow-up of primary cutaneous melanoma - Part II. *Anais brasileiros de dermatologia, 91*(1), 49–58. https://doi.org/10.1590/abd1806-4841.20164715 (accessed on 12 May 2025).
12. Basra, M., Shapiro, L., Patel, H., Payne, C., Brazen, B., & Biglione, A. (2024). Exploring the Utilization of Imaging Modalities in the Diagnosis of Basal Cell Carcinoma: A Scoping

Review. *Cureus, 16*(3), e56047. https://doi.org/10.7759/cureus.56047(accessed on 12 May 2025).

13. Ferrante di Ruffano, L., Dinnes, J., Chuchu, N., Bayliss, S. E., Takwoingi, Y., Davenport, C., Matin, R. N., O'Sullivan, C., Roskell, D., Deeks, J. J., Williams, H. C., & Cochrane Skin Cancer Diagnostic Test Accuracy Group (2018). Exfoliative cytology for diagnosing basal cell carcinoma and other skin cancers in adults. *The Cochrane database of systematic reviews, 12*(12), CD013187. https://doi.org/10.1002/14651858.CD013187 (accessed on 12 May 2025).

14. Engelman, D., Yoshizumi, J., Hay, R. J., Osti, M., Micali, G., Norton, S., Walton, S., Boralevi, F., Bernigaud, C., Bowen, A. C., Chang, A. Y., Chosidow, O., Estrada-Chavez, G., Feldmeier, H., Ishii, N., Lacarrubba, F., Mahé, A., Maurer, T., Mahdi, M. M. A., Murdoch, M. E., ... Fuller, L. C. (2020). The 2020 International Alliance for the Control of Scabies Consensus Criteria for the Diagnosis of Scabies. *The British journal of dermatology, 183*(5), 808–820. https://doi.org/10.1111/bjd.18943 (accessed on 12 May 2025).

15. Chaduvula, J., Chintada, D., Vijayashree, J., Chalamalasetty, S. S., Vudayana, K., & Vaggu, A. (2023). A clinico-epidemiological study of hyperkeratotic palmoplantar lesions and its correlation with dermoscopy and histopathology in a tertiary care center. *Cureus, 15*, e36561. https://doi.org/10.7759/cureus.36561.

16. Chan, A. R., Kooner, A., Farkouh, C., Maibach, H., Anthony, M. R., Abdi, P., & Qureshi, S. (2023). Non-invasive skin measurement methods and diagnostics for vitiligo: A systematic review. *Frontiers in Medicine, 10*, 1200963. https://core.ac.uk/download/573547226.pdf (accessed on 12 May 2025).

17. H.M. Cheng, P. Guitera, Systematic review of optical coherence tomography usage in the diagnosis and management of basal cell carcinoma, *British Journal of Dermatology*, Volume 173, Issue 6, 1 December 2015, Pages 1371–1380, https://doi.org/10.1111/bjd.14042 (accessed on 12 May 2025).

18. Chioveanu, F., Niculeț, E., Torlac, C., Bușilă, C., & Tatu, A. L. (2024). Beyond the surface: Understanding *Demodex* and its link to blepharitis and facial dermatoses. *Clinical Ophthalmology, 18*, 1801–1810. https://doi.org/10.2147/OPTH.S440199.

19. Codella, N., Nguyen, Q. B., Pankanti, S., Gutman, D., Helba, B., Halpern, A. C., & Smith, J. R. (2017). Deep learning ensembles for melanoma recognition in dermoscopy images. *IBM Journal of Research and Development, 61*, 5:1–5:15. https://doi.org/10.1147/JRD.2017.2708299.

20. De Luca, D. A., Papara, C., Vorobyev, A., Staiger, H., Bieber, K., Thaçi, D., & Ludwig, R. J. (2023). Lichen sclerosus: The 2023 update. *Frontiers in Medicine, 10.* https://doi.org/10.3389/fmed.2023.1106318.

21. Elgamal, A. E. M. M., Elfar, N. N., Amer, W. H., & Abdel-Latif, A. M. (2023). Photodynamic therapy in treatment of onychomycoses. *International Journal of Dermatology Venereology and Leprosy Sciences, 6*(2b), 146–151. https://doi.org/10.33545/26649411.2023.v6.i2b.163.

22. Frost, J. (2020). *Vibrational Spectroscopy for The Assessment of Vulval Disease*. https://core.ac.uk/download/305078391.pdf (accessed on 12 May 2025).

23. Hulei, L. O. (2020). Advanced noninvasive diagnostic methods of parasitic skin diseases. *Clinical & Experimental Pathology, 19*. https://doi.org/10.24061/1727-4338.XIX.3.73.2020.24.

24. Liopyris, K., Gregoriou, S., Dias, J., & Stratigos, A. (2022). Artificial intelligence in dermatology: Challenges and perspectives. *Dermatology and Therapy, 12*, 2637–2651. https://doi.org/10.1007/s13555-022-00833-8.

25. Lyons, F., & Ousley, L. (2015). *Dermatology for the Advanced Practice Nurse.* https://hsti.edu.krd/HSTI_Student/images/cars/cars11799992609780826136435.pdf (accessed on 12 May 2025).

26. Man, A. M., Orăsan, M. S., Hoteiuc, O. A., Olănescu-Vaida-Voevod, M. C., & Mocan, T. (2023). Inflammation and psoriasis: A comprehensive review. *International Journal of Molecular Sciences, 24*, 16095. https://doi.org/10.3390/ijms242216095.

27. Martínez-Ortega, J. I., & Franco González, S. (2024). Erythrasma: Pathogenesis and diagnostic challenges. *Cureus, 16*(8), e68308. https://www.cureus.com/articles/285587-erythrasma-pathogenesis-and-diagnostic-challenges.pdf (accessed on 12 May 2025).

28. Moskaluk, A. E. (2022). *Novel Approaches to Characterizing Feline-Associated Dermatophytic Fungi.* https://core.ac.uk/download/553287495.pdf (accessed on 12 May 2025).

29. Moskaluk, A., & VandeWoude, S. (2022). Current topics in dermatophyte classification and clinical diagnosis. *Pathogens, 11*, 957. https://doi.org/10.3390/pathogens11090957.

30. Ndukwe, C., Eziagu, U., Eni, A., Nnamani, C., & Alexander, A. K. (2023). Histopathologic spectrum and clinicopathologic concordance of pediatric skin biopsies: 18-year experience in a tertiary hospital in southeast Nigeria. *Medical Journal of Dr. D.Y. Patil Vidyapeeth.* https://www.semanticscholar.org/paper/9b30d856725a248d1af063d0aa93fc07ee30c546 (accessed on 12 May 2025).

31. Nie, Y., Hong, Y., Xie, X., Fu, G. L., & Zheng, Y. Q. (2023). Dermoscopic features of children scabies. *Frontiers in Medicine, 10.* https://doi.org/10.3389/fmed.2023.1097999.

32. Piyasiri, S. B., Dewasurendra, R., Samaranayake, N., & Karunaweera, N. D. (2023). Diagnostic tools for cutaneous leishmaniasis caused by *Leishmania donovani*: A narrative review. *Diagnostics, 13*, 2989. https://doi.org/10.3390/diagnostics13182989.

33. Reinehr, C. P. H., & Bakos, R. M. (2019). Actinic keratoses: Review of clinical, dermoscopic, and therapeutic aspects. *Anais Brasileiros de Dermatologia, 94*, 637–657. https://doi.org/10.1016/j.abd.2019.10.004.

34. Ari Karmila Sari, Irma D.Roesyanto – Mahadi, Kristo A.Nababan, Remenda Siregar (2019); Diagnostic Analysis of Dermoscopy on Nail Psoriasis; International Journal of Scientific and Research Publications (IJSRP) 9(8) (ISSN: 2250-3153), DOI: http://dx.doi.org/10.29322/IJSRP.9.08.2019.p9206 (accessed on 12 May 2025).

35. Sartawi, Z., Blackshields, C., & Faisal, W. (2022). Dissolving microneedles: Applications and growing therapeutic potential. *Journal of Controlled Release, 348*, 186–205. https://doi.org/10.1016/j.jconrel.2022.05.045.

36. Smoller, B., & Bagherani, N. (2021). *Atlas of Dermatology, Dermatopathology and Venereology.* Springer. https://doi.org/10.1007/978-3-319-45134-3(accessed on 12 May 2025).

37. Thomas, I. N., James, J. J., Bala, A., Mohan, S., Dogiparthi, S., & Shanmugam, N. P. S. (2023). Usage of dermoscopy as an effective diagnostic tool in pityriasis alba: A prospective observational study among children in a suburban hospital in South India. *Cureus, 15*(6), e40271. https://www.cureus.com/articles/157164-usage-of-dermoscopy-as-an-effective-diagnostic-tool-in-pityriasis-alba-a-prospective-observational-study-among-children-in-a-suburban-hospital-in-south-india.pdf (accessed on 12 May 2025).

38. Wei, L., Ding, K., & Hu, H. (2020). Automatic skin cancer detection in dermoscopy images based on ensemble lightweight deep learning network. *IEEE Access, 8*, 99633–99647. https://doi.org/10.1109/ACCESS.2020.2997710.

39. White, S. (2025). *Dermatology: In-House Testing.* https://www.dvm360storage.com/cvc/proceedings/sd/Dermatology/White/White,%20Stephen_Dermatology_inhouse_testing.pdf (accessed on 12 May 2025).

40. Zacharopoulou, A., Tsiogka, A., Tsimpidakis, A., Lamia, A., Koumaki, D., & Gregoriou, S. (2024). *Tinea incognito*: Challenges in diagnosis and management. *Journal of Clinical Medicine, 13*, 3267. https://doi.org/10.3390/jcm13113267.

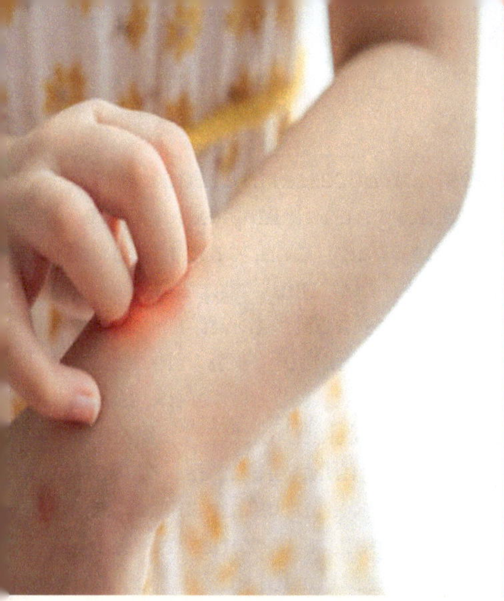

Chapter 3

INFLAMMATORY SKIN DISEASES

Contents

Introduction

Inflammation comes in as the body's mechanism of self-defense against dangers—bacteria, damaged cells, irritants, and although it generally does us a good thing, occasionally it goes awry. When imbalances happen, especially in our skin, this healthy response becomes a complicated ailment known overall as inflammatory skin disease. You may experience everything from a little irritation to all-out, full-body problems, really complicating life for individuals involved and physicians alike. Our skin is a frontline defense; it depends on a mess of immune cells, signaling molecules, and layers of tissue to keep everything under control. When that combination gets disrupted, chronic inflammation kicks in, causing damage to tissues and exacerbating symptoms. In most instances, gaining an understanding of how these mechanisms work is central to developing treatments that assist in restoring the skin's normal sensation and function. Contemporary treatment approaches to these skin afflictions have revolutionized the arena—it is not merely a question of alleviating pain but also reorienting the disease. Consider photodynamic therapy (PDT), for example, this innovative method marries light energy with specific photosensitizing agents to specifically eradicate rogue cells by inducing reactive oxygen species. The method has proven to have real potential, not only for precancerous or actual cancer lesions, but also for disease where viruses are involved. The non-invasive nature of PDT, its selective targeting, and extremely minimal side effects make it a truly desirable choice. Its capacity to modulate local immune responses and reduce viral loads suggests even broader potential in addressing skin inflammation induced by infections, unveiling a new window of opportunity for controlling these difficult challenges (Bartosińska et al., 2025). At the same time, scientists are also focusing on the regulatory systems of the skin itself. The endocannabinoid system, with its receptor network and endogenous ligands, has become an appealing target due to its ubiquitous function in regulating immune responses in the skin itself. Cannabinoids, the substances that bind to the system, have exhibited anti-inflammatory actions in a variety of conditions, including psoriasis and atopic dermatitis (AD), as well as dermatomyositis and systemic sclerosis (SSc). Initial clinical trials are quite promising but further strong, randomized trials are required to validate their safety and efficacy. These findings propose that the incorporation of new biological pathways into therapeutic regimens could perhaps set the stage for improved control of inflammatory skin disorders (Kuzumi et al., 2024).

Definition of Inflammatory Skin Diseases

Inflammatory skin disorders are a broad category of diseases that begin when the immune system gets a little out of control. They frequently result from a misfire of communication between our innate protections and the cells that recall old danger, resulting in a type of persistent or recurrent skin inflammation. Instead of being triggered directly by germs, these issues typically consist of a false or higher reaction that may, but does not necessarily, require an external irritant or allergen. You may experience red patches, swelling, flaky skin, and intense itching – all symptoms that truly impact daily life. In the majority of instances, having a clear view of what is going on beneath the skin is most important since it is not so much a single easy, localized reaction, but a complex web of cell signals and immune messengers in operation. Uncovering a little more depth, how these conditions operate at times reveals that the immune system's confusion is not so much fixed to the skin. These can be brought on by genetic predispositions, environmental stressors, or even an abnormally higher reaction to the microbes that we generally coexist with, all of which makes clinical management harder. Cells such as T lymphocytes, dendritic cells, and macrophages, for instance, continue the inflammation process by producing cytokines and displaying antigens, which further triggers tissue alteration and breaks down the skin's barrier.

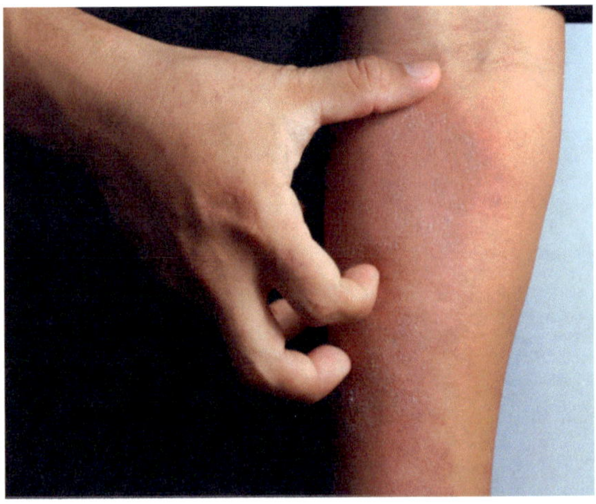

Source: Yuzu. (n.d.). *Study Banner.* https://yuzu-studypages-prod-east.s3.amazonaws.com/study_banners/469076-7b4b746e-b0f7-463c-a8be-077d75fe49e2.jpg.

This constant inflammatory condition disrupts regular tissue architecture, resulting in the types of lesions we tend to find – a scenario that reflects more widespread systemic immune disorders (Christopher et al., 2022). Determining when an individual has one of these disorders is not as straightforward as merely identifying an infection or tumor on the skin. Physicians typically put the puzzle together of the patient's history, a physical examination, and possibly lab work or biopsies to identify inflammation that is not infectious or neoplastic in origin. For the most part, as opposed to simple pain syndromes where the pain is obviously due to nerve or acute trauma problems, these dermatological ailments both have a local immune response and even some central sensitization from chronic inflammation (Kosek et al., 2021). This combination of residual immunological activity, propagation of its influence, and combination of symptoms makes the case for diagnostic criteria that culminate in therapies aimed at minimizing inflammation and preventing irreparable damage.

Importance of Effective Treatment

The nature of inflammatory skin diseases requires careful and multifaceted treatment to avoid chronicity and enhance patient outcomes. Disorders such as AD need management programs not just based on observable signs but also subjective sensations like itch and discomfort that have a direct impact on quality of life. Successful treatment must include both immediate resolution of the lesion and long-term prevention of flare, with incorporation of barrier repair by means of topical hydration and anti-inflammatory drugs. Emerging biologic treatments, with increased cost and possible side effects, have shown encouraging efficacy against underlying immune dysregulation, and precision medicine has become a necessary consideration. In addition, treatment of secondary microbial colonization can prevent exacerbations, highlighting the holistic nature of effective treatment. Unless combined with an integrated, proactive solution, patients experience cyclical relapses that worsen physical symptoms as well as emotional burden, ensuring effective treatment is crucial to modulating disease trajectory and enhancing the quality of life for inflammatory skin disease patients (Wollenberg et al., 2020). Acne vulgaris presents another aspect of inflammatory skin disease in which early and effective intervention is crucial to avoid irreversible damage to the skin and psychosocial damage. The pilosebaceous inflammation present in moderate to severe acne usually results in scarring, which can significantly reduce self-esteem as well as play a role in psychological distress, especially in young people. Oral isotretinoin, known to be the only therapeutic agent that can produce long-term remission or cure for severe acne, exerts multifactorial mechanisms such as sebaceous gland inhibition and immunomodulation. Its effectiveness exceeds that of topical and antibiotic combination regimens, placing in bold relief the central importance of aggressive early treatment in modifying disease course. Although the drug requires careful monitoring because of possible side effects, the gains in preventing chronic lesions and enhancing psychosocial outcomes verify the indispensable role of therapeutic modalities in inflammatory cutaneous diseases. Beyond symptomatic control, the significance of successful treatment of inflammatory skin diseases carries over into wider health and social spheres, a testament to its holistic effect. Visibly apparent skin lesions and chronic inflammation routinely engender social stigmatization and lowered mental well-being, underscoring the demand for treatments that spur healing and minimize relapse. Adjuvant treatments including phototherapy and patient education induce long-term disease control and enable patients to become active participants in trigger management and treatment compliance. Further, individualized approaches based on patient age, severity of disease, and associated comorbidities maximize therapeutic efficacy and reduce the risk of adverse effects. In this respect, treatment goes beyond symptom suppression, aiming at enhanced function and quality of life. Hence, investment in evidence-based and personalized interventions continues to be crucial for reducing the substantial burden caused by inflammatory skin conditions (Wollenberg et al., 2020).

Overview of Treatment Options

Chronic inflammatory dermatoses require a multidimensional strategy that reconciles symptom control with the normalization of pathologic processes. Recent developments point toward the power of biological therapies directed against immune dysregulation and inflammatory cascades specifically. For example, mesenchymal stem cell-derived exosomes represent a promising cell-free therapeutic option. These exosomes help to re-establish the epidermal barrier by enhancing the ceramide and dihydroceramide synthesis, which is crucial for skin hydration and integrity. This strategy also minimizes pro-inflammatory cytokines like IL-4 and TNF-α, which are key players in inflammatory signaling. The capacity of these exosomes to restore the stratum corneum and regulate gene expression associated with lipid metabolism and immune response highlights their therapeutic potential for diseases such as AD, where barrier dysfunction is central to disease pathogenesis (Kyong-Shin et al., 2020). In addition to biologics, anti-inflammatory pharmacologic agents continue to be a mainstay of inflammatory dermatoses treatment. Artemisinin, a classical antimalarial drug, has been recently repurposed to take advantage of its anti-angiogenic and anti-inflammatory activities against rosacea, an inflammatory skin disease. Its therapeutic benefit was proven by reducing redness of the skin and inhibiting the expression of pro-inflammatory cytokines such as IL-1β and IL-6. Artemisinin also regulates immune cell infiltration and suppresses chemokines participating in immune cell trafficking, which plays a critical role in managing inflammation. The mechanism of the drug consists of NF-kB signaling pathway inhibition, which is a crucial mediator of inflammation, and diminishment of pathogenic angiogenesis through restraint on endothelial migration. The bimodal efficacy treats both dysregulation of the immune process and vascular disease inherent to rosacea with an integrated therapeutic strategy (Yuan et al., 2019). Apart from novel biological and pharmacologic treatment options, conventional therapies like topical corticosteroids, immunomodulators, and phototherapy remain elementary. Such drugs are designed to dampen acute inflammation and block exacerbations of disease while facilitating the repair of the skin barrier. The chronicity of inflammatory skin disorders, however, often curtails prolonged corticosteroid therapy because of toxicity, so there is a need for new therapies with improved safety and efficacy profiles. The incorporation of cutting-edge molecular therapies, such as stem cell-derived products and targeted anti-inflammatory medications, into practice has the potential to change paradigms by tackling disease mechanisms directly instead of just symptom relief. Optimizing therapy for inflammatory skin diseases, therefore, calls for a strategic synergy between conventional and new modalities fashioned to patient profiles.

3.1. Types of Inflammatory Skin Diseases

Inflammatory skin conditions are a broad assortment of disorders that appear to arise from a variety of immune messes and manifest themselves in all sorts of ways. Psoriasis is one example, a chronic autoimmune condition in which skin cells grow too quickly and immune cells pour in to form thick, scaly patches. Atopic dermatitis (AD) is another case entirely – it usually stems from a jumbled mix of genetics, environment, and immune triggers that mess up the skin's barrier and drive a Th2-skewed inflammation. Then there are disorders linked to mast cell overactivity: these disorders see mast cells go into overdrive and pile up, setting off inflammatory symptoms without the telltale signs of classic allergies or *clonal mastocytosis*. In such cases, mediators such as histamine and prostaglandin D2 are released, driving inflammation that may persist locally or travel more peripherally (Valent et al., 2012). Generally speaking, pinning down these various etiologies is important if we are to target treatments that truly hit the spot. Macrophages, for instance, are center stage in orchestrating skin inflammation – they are no one-trick ponies, either. When skin is injured or infected, these cells typically switch into a proinflammatory gear, revving up responses predominantly through Toll-like receptor signals. This surge of activity clears infections, but if it gets out of control, it may contribute to doing more harm to tissues. Eventually, as the wounds begin to heal, these same cells generally switch again to send out signals that dampen the inflammation and aid in repair. And if that flip does not occur just so, the process can drag on as chronic inflammation or even result in fibrosis, because macrophages sometimes begin nudging fibroblasts to lay down more extracellular matrix. This sort of adaptive flexibility – sometimes crazy, sometimes reparative – illustrates just how macrophage heterogeneity can control both flare and resolution phases in inflammatory dermatoses (Weidenbusch & Anders, 2012). The other skin diseases in this category occur when the immune system gets it wrong with its own signals, either by presenting antigens in unusual ways or by releasing too many inflammatory mediators from a variety of cell types. Consider contact dermatitis, for instance; in this case, allergens induce a delayed hypersensitivity reaction that ultimately injures local tissues and attracts lymphocytes. Meanwhile, systemic autoimmune disease such as lupus erythematosus typically stimulates lesions in the skin via immune complex deposits and activation of the complement system, causing distinctly different varieties of lesions. There is chronic urticaria, of course, a disorder based on mast cell behaviors that create transient wheals due to bursts of transient mediators; strangely enough, it shares a few common properties with mast cell activation found with other conditions. For the most part, wrapping our minds around these idiosyncratic inflammatory pathways – and how mast cells and macrophages, in their own capricious manner, initiate and ultimately bring the inflammation to a stop – is vital for making proper diagnoses and crafting customized therapies (Valent et al., 2012; Weidenbusch & Anders, 2012).

3.1.1. Psoriasis

Grasping inflammatory skin diseases involves combining molecular and genetic information to clarify shared control loops and pathways. Scientists have been charting gene co-expression networks and protein connectivity networks, sometimes in surprising fashion—to understand the complex interplay between disparate maladies, psoriasis included. They even identified approximately 55 genes that continue to appear on the scene in immune functions, quietly emphasizing just how complicated immune regulation can be. It is noteworthy that certain network analyses identify regulators such as IKZF1, which in most instances proves to be a critical switch responsible for the problems encountered in psoriasis, AD, and other inflammatory skin ailments.

Identifying these proteins not only enhances our molecular understanding of psoriasis but also suggests exciting targets for therapies that may one day make a dent in the disease's burden (Mishra et al., 2023). By and large, this approach represents a departure from conventional transcript-based procedures towards the nascent discipline of precision dermatology. Psoriasis has made considerable progress, albeit its chronicity and heterogeneity continue to present a few challenges. Biologic agents that target tumor necrosis factor-alpha

(TNFα) are a popular go-to nowadays, but interestingly enough, sometimes these therapies cause psoriasis themselves, particularly in those living with inflammatory bowel disease (IBD) on anti-TNFα treatment regimens.

This unexpected twist makes decision-making more difficult; physicians then find themselves balancing whether to maintain the anti-TNF treatment to cover both skin and gut diseases or to change direction completely. Recent multicenter trials indicate that if the psoriasis induced by the drug is minor, it may be okay to continue with the therapy, while the more severe cases may do well by switching to alternatives like Ustekinumab. Such a strategy appears to alleviate skin lesions without significantly raising the risk of IBD flare-ups, highlighting the fact that treatment truly needs to be individualized (Segura et al., 2023). Even though biologics have revolutionized how we manage psoriasis, a lot of patients continue struggling with incomplete management and sporadic side effects—leading us to search for newer therapeutic options. Identifying frequent master regulators between several inflammatory diseases of the skin now presents an opportunity to build medicines that target the molecular faulty firing responsible for psoriasis. By fusing transcriptomic information with multi-omics data, scientists have established a modular system that probes more deeply than solitary gene expression; it records the constantly shifting ballet of immune signals and keratinocyte responses. This strategy, with its emphasis on central networks and high-impact protein targets, may just accelerate the development of combination therapies matched to individual profiles. In the majority of instances, to progress psoriasis treatment demands not just new clinical concepts but also steady, systems-wide investigation of the disease's complex biological design (Mishra et al., 2023) (Figures 3.1 and 3.2).

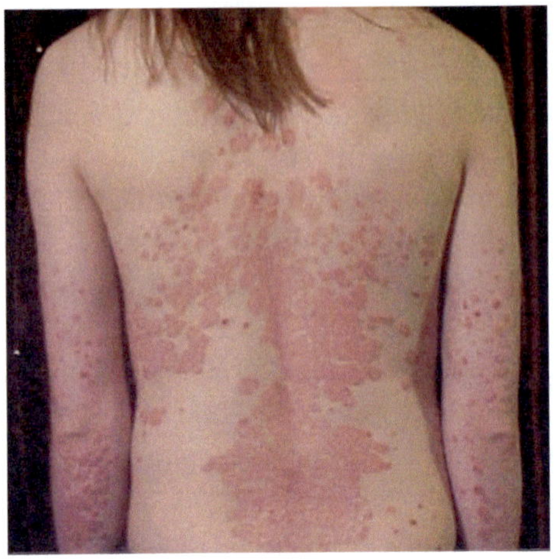

Figure 3.1. Psoriasis of the back.

Source: Wikimedia Commons. (n.d.). *Psoriasis on Back.* https://upload.wikimedia.org/wikipedia/commons/f/f5/Psoriasis_on_back1.jpg.

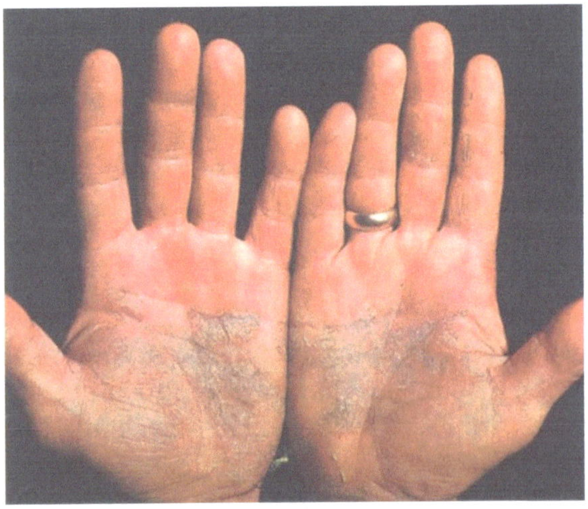

Figure 3.2. Psoriasis of the palms/

Source: Wikimedia Commons. (n.d.). *Psoriasis of the Palms.* https://upload.wikimedia.org/wikipedia/commons/8/88/Psoriasis_of_the_palms.jpg.

3.1.2. Eczema (Atopic Dermatitis [AD])

AD demonstrates how nasty inflammatory skin diseases can be. It appears as a chronic, relapsing condition that is becoming increasingly widespread worldwide – particularly in developed regions. Genes, an overresponsive immune system, and routine environmental stress all combine, so to speak, to trigger the condition. You usually see it as red, itching lesions that quite literally wreak havoc on day-to-day existence. Even though AD itself is not an infection, it occasionally lays the groundwork for other atopic conditions such as asthma, suggesting that its influence extends beyond the skin itself. Ongoing investigation, examining both where it originates and how it functions, indicates that a more intimate knowledge of such underlying causes is critical to orchestrating intelligent treatments that address both the skin barrier and immune characterestics (Szewczyk et al., 2024).

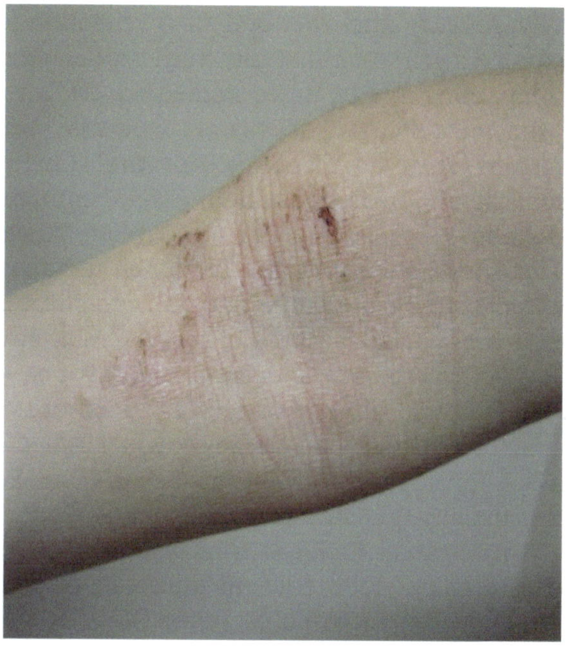

Figure 3.3. Atopic dermatitis (AD).

Source: By James Heilman, MD - Own work, CC BY-SA 3.0, https://commons.wikimedia.org/w/index.php?curid=10429479

New treatment methods for AD include repairing the protective barrier of the skin and decreasing the immune system's overreaction to maintain low levels of inflammation. The standard initial steps include applying generous amounts of emollients and topical corticosteroids to manage the flare-ups, although chronic steroid use can generate its own problems.

3.1.3. Contact Dermatitis

Our skin is a frontline defense against everything in our world, but it is surprisingly susceptible to irritation when it comes into contact with different substances. At times this irritation erupts as contact dermatitis, where the natural barrier of the skin is disrupted and the immune system suddenly intervenes. You may notice redness, itching, or even some scaling, all signs that allergens or irritants have disrupted the equilibrium. Children are particularly vulnerable; their skin simply is not geared to protect itself, so they react more intensely and over larger body surfaces. Doctors in most instances attempt to reduce the exposure to these triggers and concentrate on repairing that barrier. Often, a combination of topical anti-inflammatory hormones with barrier-assisting agents like ceramides is pure magic for young patients, accelerating recovery (Soboleva, 2024). More recently, studies have thrown some new light on the small, molecular specifics of inflammatory skin disease, highlighting epigenetics as a major player in both how they begin and how we can address them. In general terms, contact dermatitis takes its place within a spectrum of long-standing skin afflictions that draw on a messy mixture of genetic messages and epigenetic adjustments. As an example, histone modifications—those small chemical stickers that assist in deciding whether genes are either on or off—can contribute significantly to both the inflammation mechanism and the repair system of the skin. In the majority of instances, adjusting such marks presents an opportunity to target the precise pathways that are causing harm without halting the immune system. Thus, through examining such histone modifications, we not only uncover more about how contact dermatitis works but also unlock new avenues for therapies that could be more effective and have fewer adverse effects (Zhang et al., 2024). Managing contact dermatitis is a twofold process: immediate relief of annoying symptoms and a long-term strategy to keep flare-ups at bay. Treatment is never one-size-fits-all and typically begins with topical corticosteroids—especially prevalent in children, where the inflammation can be recalcitrant and diffuse. Certain recent case studies even indicate that employing methylprednisolone acetonate in combination with ceramide-packed creams soothes the inflammation and at the same time patches up the barrier of the skin, thus reducing side affects you would normally get from using steroids alone. Such a two-pronged strategy enables the skin to return to its balanced state and avoids chronic conditions by maintaining that all-important lipid layer.

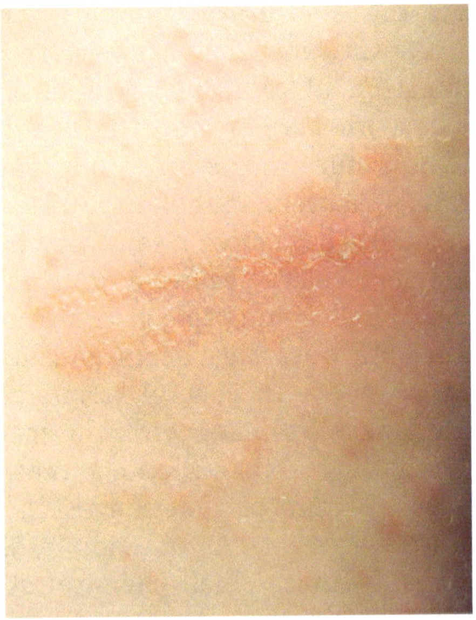

Figure 3.4. Contact dermatitis around a healing rugburn.

Source: Digitalgadget. (2007). Contact dermatitis around a healing rugburn. *Wikimedia Commons.* https://upload.wikimedia.org/wikipedia/commons/a/a8/Contact_dermatitis_around_wound.jpg.

Concurrently, instructing patients in the identification and avoidance of triggers and adherence to a proper skin care regimen really supports the therapy as a whole. Combining these practical techniques with new perspectives from epigenetic studies could well result in more sophisticated, individualized therapies for contact dermatitis and other inflammatory skin disorders (Soboleva, 2024; Zhang et al., 2024) (Figure 3.4).

3.2. Causes and Triggers

Inflammatory skin diseases appear to come from a sort of mishmash of factors—genes, environment, and the body's own immune responses all combine as both underlying explanations and at times immediate triggers. If you look at a tissue sample, you may see patterns such as thickening of the skin in psoriasis or peculiar accumulations of immune cells that suggest what is happening. These structural changes are not static, either; they will shift around over time, and that complicates matters as far as giving a diagnosis. At times, you even witness a spectrum of reactions—going from sponge-like engorging to abnormal behavior of the blood vessels, which reflects how unpredictable reactions can be of the skin. Usually, physicians have to equate what they observe in a patient with what the slides indicate, since a lot of the time the actual trouble is not limited to the skin itself (Khachikyan et al., 2025). Such layered thinking opens the door to investigating what particular stimulus may trigger flare-ups. Most often, environmental factors such as catalysts jump in, sometimes nudging or even aggravating these inflammatory skin conditions; usually, they partner with genetic predispositions to determine how severe the condition turns out to be. Daily perps may range from a harsh knock against the skin, infections, everyday allergens, or even excessive

UV exposure—all of which can compromise the skin's barrier and trigger local immune reactions. The effects of such triggers can be incredibly variable from individual to individual, which might be one reason that patients so often present with such disparate symptoms. Added to this, certain genetic research suggests that disorders such as AD could have underlying associations with more generalized autoimmune issues (such as IgA nephropathy), suggesting a more profound, entwined immunogenetic association (Li et al., 2024). Briefly, the identification of both external influences and one's inherent vulnerabilities is essential to truly understanding the complete range of these precipitating factors. Concurrently, immune system malfunctions are firmly at the center of both the development and continuation of such skin issues. In essence, once cytokines, such as interleukins and TNF-alpha, and T-cell responses become out of kilter, not only do they ignite the initial lesions but also continue to cause the inflammation to return over time. That immune-mediated process is the reason why treatments that target those unpredictable pathways tend to be so successful, providing cause-specific strategies for management. It should also be mentioned here that the associations of chronic skin inflammation with other body disorders highlight the point that the skin functions as an active immunologic organ, and not as a passive barrier (Li et al., 2024). It would appear that the triggers of these conditions go far beyond their presentation as local skin conditions, intertwining systemic immune imbalance with genetic susceptibility (Figure 3.5).

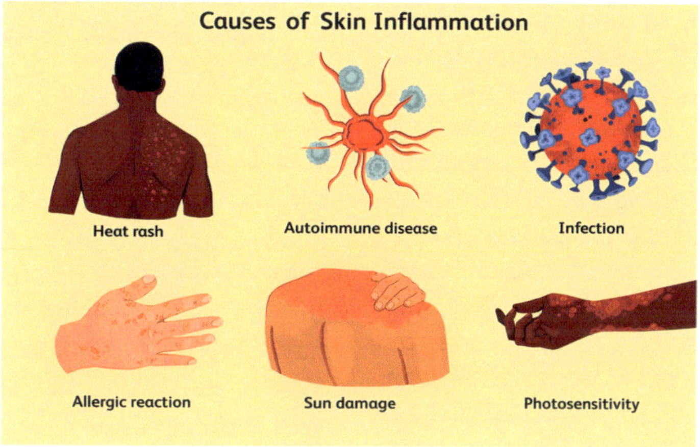

Figure 3.5. Causes of skin Inflammation.

Source: Hansen, Z. (2025). *Pimply Rash on Buttocks.*

3.2.1. Genetic Predisposition

Inflammatory dermatoses arise through a mishmash of factors—environmental ones combine with our internal mechanisms, and genetics appears to be a large component of that equation. It seems that differences in our genes most frequently affect how our skin is held together and how our immune system responds. Certain gene variations can fine-tune everything from cytokine signals to who is present at the scene, and even to the very small proteins that make our skin work. This gene variation does not only influence how the disease looks; it can also influence how well one responds to treatments. Recent advances in genomics have highlighted a handful of significant DNA areas associated with conditions such as psoriasis and AD, suggesting hereditary patterns that provide an argument for treatments shaped by one's individual genetic plan. Genetic influences are, in the majority of circumstances, quite important when it comes to why these skin conditions persist or recur. Family research and even twin studies have suggested greater similarity among relatives, highlighting the fact that hereditary influences play a significant role—often in unforeseen manners. For instance, mutations or minor alterations in genes related to the immune system, such as those associated with interleukins or tumor necrosis factor, are associated with more intense inflammatory responses. There is a kind of give-and-take between these genetic characterestics and environmental stimuli that could trigger flare-ups in a person who already has a weakness. Even with all the progress, the varying expression of so many gene variants still represents a complicated challenge to researchers attempting to develop predictive models and identify targeted therapies. Pharmacogenomics, where treatments are individualized according to genetic composition, holds the potential for increasing efficacy while reducing side effects (Pinckney, 2017). Recently, new treatment modalities have relied on our improving knowledge of genetic tendencies to assist patients in managing inflammatory skin conditions more effectively. Techniques such as employing nanotech-based drug delivery or microneedle patches are being developed as methods to deliver treatments directly where they are needed, to counteract how genetic differences can change responses. Some existing clinical trials are evaluating therapies designed to modulate the molecular pathways influenced by these genetic alterations, such as those in cytokine signaling. Although the specific causes of certain chronic, fibrotic skin diseases are still somewhat unclear, the notion that genetics provides a substantial cornerstone for such diseases is difficult to dismiss. This revelation leads scientists to consider the larger picture, combining genetic, immune, and environmental factors in an effort to potentially chisel out more promising treatments in the future (Pinckney, 2017).

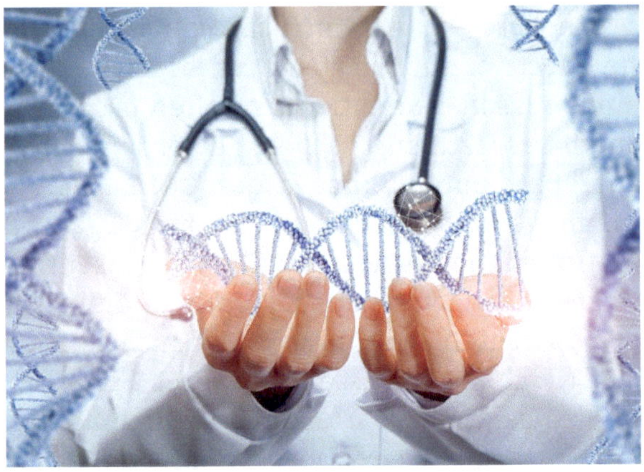

Source: Center for Family Medicine. (2021). *What Does it Mean to Have a Genetic Predisposition? Family History and Your Health.* https://centerforfamilymedicine.com/wp-content/uploads/2021/02/center-for-family-medicine-What-Does-It-Mean-To-Have-A-Genetic-Predisposition-Family-History-And-Your-Health.jpg.

3.2.2. Environmental Factors

The human body's interaction with the environment truly comes into play when we consider why inflammatory skin diseases occur. Genes permitting, daily exposures to microbes have the potential to modify our immune system in a way that can ultimately trigger skin flare-ups. The skin and gut contain active microbial communities that at times interact with our defenses – and these interactions have the potential to stimulate, or even exacerbate, inflammation. Small changes in these resident microbes can tip over the immune balance, potentially initiating chronic conditions such as psoriasis or AD. Recently, scientists have been exploring how these host-microbe interactions contribute, in general, and it appears that microbial imbalance could be an important external factor guiding disease development. This combination of factors, both the internal programming and external triggers explains why we must consider environmental cues with genetics in order to truly comprehend and treat these disorders (Castelino et al., 2014). Add lifestyle habits like diet, smoking, and even stress, and you have a whole additional level of complexity. Small daily routines such as what we eat or how stressed we are can re-model the gut microbiota, which then gives the body's immune systems a push and manifests on the skin. For instance, when the gut flora is off balance (or dysbiosis occurs), the inflammation that is caused tends to increase, illustrating the gut-skin relationship in fairly obvious terms. Outside pressures also disrupt the system out of balance, both by undermining the barrier of the skin and enhancing the synthesis of inflammation-producing chemicals. For the majority, these results emphasize that inflammation of the skin is not straightforward—it is the consequence of an complex knot of environmental contacts and our own immune reactions, indicating that fighting these external influences could contribute to better managing the disease (D'Amelio et al., 2016). Getting a clear picture of inflammatory skin conditions means combining insights from microbial ecology with everyday lifestyle and immune factors. Since different microbial communities across our body, along with stressors from our daily lives, have a say in how our immune system handles inflammation, personalized approaches seem pretty necessary. Altering what we eat, quitting smoking, or simply coping with stress could be nudging the microbial blend in a healthy direction, reducing the severity and speed of these ailments. Ongoing research into how our genes interact with our microbes is starting to reveal new biomarkers and potential therapeutic targets – hints that could make the prediction and treatment of these diseases slightly more specific. Awareness of these environmental factors provides a pathway to a more integrative type of care and invites new notions for treatments specific to the complex nature of inflammatory skin conditions (Castelino et al., 2014; D'Amelio et al., 2016).

3.2.3. Immune System Dysfunction

Our skin health mostly relies on a sensitive balance of our immune system—if it tips off, even a minor glitch could trigger an entire cascade of problems. Occasionally, immune cells become overly enthusiastic or uncharacteristically calm, and that can result in ongoing inflammation and tissue damage in skin disease. This imbalance can be brought on by things within us such as genetic characterestics or external irritants that we encounter daily. Interestingly, mitochondria, those small powerhouses within our cells, do not simply produce energy; they also impact the generation of reactive oxygen compounds that dial the inflammation up. When these tiny motors shift with age or respond to environmental signals, they may exacerbate the current immune dysregulation in chronic skin disease, forcing disorders to persist and making it more difficult for the body to restore equilibrium (Haas , 2019). It is a complicated dance that suggests potential targets for soothingly adjusting our immune reactions back to equilibrium. Modern lifestyles and shifting environments seem to play a huge part too. There is this idea of "biome depletion" which, generally speaking, argues that we are losing a lot of the diverse microbes and symbiotic species once common in our everyday lives, especially given the push of industrialized living. When this microbial diversity disappears, the natural dialogue between our immune system and its beneficial microbial friends becomes confused, tending to initiate overly extreme responses and even autoimmune reactions. That is, the evolutionary distance between our ancient environment and present conditions can make our skin more susceptible to irritation and allergic outbursts. Some scientists propose that by attempting to revitalize this eliminated microbial diversity, , or what they term biome reconstitution, we can potentially unlock new avenues to help alleviate inflammatory skin issues (Parker & Ollerton, 2013). And then there is the genetic component, which delicately interplays with all of this. Some gene variations, for instance, may set a person up for an overactive immune response by altering how antigens are presented, modulating levels of cytokines, or influencing important proteins that maintain our skin's seal. Next thing you know, even a typically benign stimulus will cause a full-fledged inflammatory response. When the skin environment becomes stuck in a loop of ongoing immune stimulation, it effectively devours itself by attracting still more inflammatory cells—a vicious feedback loop that merely continues. As a whole, this complicated situation illustrates that immune dysfunction is not solely a matter of a single stimulus; it is a combination of internal messages and external pressures that accumulate over time. As scientists integrate findings from molecular immunology with more general ecological and evolutionary perspectives, they aim to identify more specific means of unraveling these intermingling causes and assist in reestablishing a healthier balance.

3.3. Symptoms and Diagnosis

Inflammatory skin disorders present themselves in all manner of ways that can completely confuse a diagnosis. Patients may struggle with red areas, scaling skin, and that distracting itch, with the occasional additional, body-wide signs included. Consider dermatomyositis, for example—this is not merely a matter of overt skin manifestations; it frequently presents with muscle weakness and other systemic complications, so physicians are left with taking a broad-based approach to things, including a thorough patient history, physical examination, and occasionally laboratory work or imaging. Too often, treatment becomes activated to alleviate the outward symptoms even before the actual inflammatory issue is identified, and this delay in a final diagnosis complicates the entire process (Kielhorn et al., 2023). The variety and severity of these symptoms truly emphasize why getting them early is important, particularly in disorders such as AD that affect so many children and adolescents. You acquire chronic, recurring itchy lesions that are merely part of the issue, patients may also endure stress or even slight depressive moods which, in most situations, only provide another level of complexity. Socioeconomic and lifestyle determinants also like to guide these mental health issues, a reminder that a wider, more general examination of a patient can be critical. These non-skin findings, in combination with the classic lesions, enable physicians' interventions to come earlier, alleviating the physical as well as the psychological strains of the disease (Park et al., 2023). In clinical practice on a daily basis, the diagnosis of these inflammatory dermatoses requires a combination of simple observation and precise testing. In a condition such as myopathic dermatomyositis, physicians must observe not only the cutaneous findings but remain vigilant for complications such as interstitial lung distress or even gastroesophageal reflux that may arise subsequently and alter prognosis. It is not uncommon, in most instances, to initiate immunosuppressive treatments early because the symptoms are obdurately ongoing. In general, the high complication rate after diagnosis indicates that we still need to optimize our early detection and diagnostic prowess, which, for the most part, would more effectively inform treatment and reduce risks (Kielhorn et al., 2023).

3.3.1. Common Symptoms Associated with Inflammatory Skin Diseases

Inflammatory skin conditions are accompanied by a combination of vexing symptoms that can truly upend someone's daily routine. You may notice those patches of redness—kind of like a blush on the skin—because additional blood flows into the area, and that usually accompanies small bumps such as papules or pustules, which are essentially small, raised bumps filled with inflammatory cells. Another regular visitor is swelling, which sometimes tends to make the face slightly uneven, and itching or burning is not a stranger either, making any scratch further irritation. Many individuals also have a tough time emotionally, as the outward signs can burden the mind; for example, rosacea is famous for inducing waves of fear and depression along with its physical manifestations (Furgalska-Kud et al., 2024). And, of course, the severity of these problems can fluctuate up or down based on what is happening inside the body and out in the world.

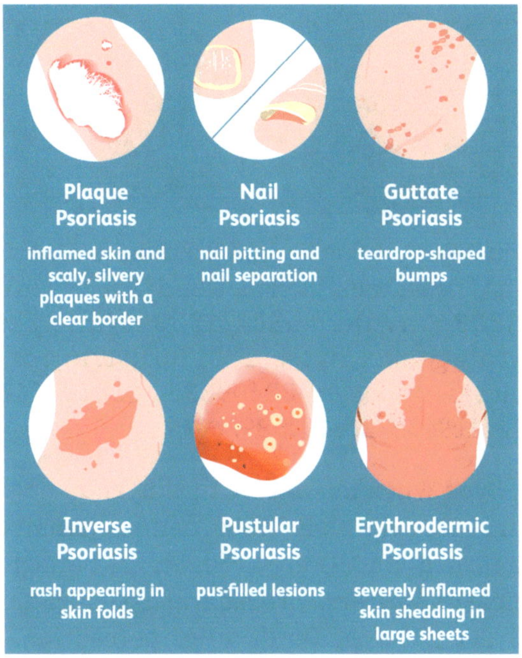

Figure 3.6. Psoriasis: Symptoms by type.

Source: Verywell Health. (n.d.). *Psoriasis Symptoms.* https://www.verywellhealth.com/thmb/dbWoPrhHl42JBqu6mM5ekHlKe4g=/1500x0/filters:no_upscale():max_bytes(150000):strip_icc()/psoriasis-symptoms-5b6880af46e0fb002538c5ad.png.

That persistent itch, usually called pruritus in the medical community, is another huge piece of the puzzle in these skin conditions. It is particularly an issue in diseases such as AD, which strikes children and adolescents particularly hard. The almost constant need to scratch not only exacerbates the damage to the skin but can also invite secondary infections, complicating treatment further. Persistent itch can take a toll on one's emotional health, even driving individuals to depressive states. There have been studies that also highlighted the presence of a strong correlation between such skin problems and mental health issues, particularly among youths who suffer from AD, where depression and stress appear to go hand in hand (Park et al., 2023). It turns out to reveal that these conditions are all about much more than superficial discomfort. Beyond what you can feel or see on the outside, inflammatory skin disorders tend to give messages that the body is way off. Individuals occasionally report a burning or stinging feeling—an indication that nerves may be caught up in the inflammation brood. More importantly, the lesions can give rise to dry, scaly lesions that compromise the barrier function of the skin, making it more susceptible to environmental irritants and even pesky microorganisms. Consider rosacea, for instance; this skittish disorder can even play havoc with your eyes, causing drying or red, inflamed appearance, which suggests that the problem is not merely skin-deep (Furgalska-Kud et al., 2024). These diverse symptoms in many instances require clinicians to take a detailed, thorough examination to differentiate the subtype and adjust treatment accordingly. Determining the numerous aspects of these conditions assists clinicians in developing care plans that treat both the physical pain and the emotional stress that patients quite often experience (Figure 3.6).

3.3.2. Diagnostic Methods Used by Healthcare Professionals

Technology has truly disrupted the manner in which physicians view inflammatory skin diseases. In most instances, it is not merely what appears during an examination or what a patient recollects of their past. These days, equipment such as dermoscopy, skin biopsies, and advanced imaging are integrated into everyday practice, diverting the process from the conventional routine.

Machine learning has also found its niche, particularly when it comes to problems such as psoriasis. Through the process of winnowing through enormous sets of skin images and clinical records, techniques such as convolutional neural networks and support vector machines identify subtle details that may otherwise be missed by even the most experienced clinicians. These automated methods tend to assist in improving diagnostic precision while reducing valuable time, ultimately making patient management and resource allocation easier. Adding these new gadgets and algorithms into the equation promises to deliver quicker, more personalized treatment plans for inflammatory skin diseases (Raut et al., 2024). It is not merely machines, however; how physicians and patients collaborate also plays a significant role. Usually, an integrated process has dermatologists, immunologists, rheumatologists, and primary care providers all chipping in, each with a piece of their own expertise. With this blend of viewpoints, what results is that assessments tend to address everything from verifying symptoms to conducting lab work and adding in clinical scoring for ailments such as eczema or psoriasis.

Patient involvement, where open communication and joint decisions come into play, can, in the majority of instances, ensure that treatment regimens are adhered to and the proper actions are taken on time. Nevertheless, these interprofessional practices encounter some bumps along the way; variations in how content various medical providers are and the uneven implementation of such models among areas sometimes impacts the uniformity of diagnoses (Van Den Steen et al., 2024). A consistent, uniform method for diagnosing these conditions continues to be one of the large objectives of the discipline. Since dermatoses can present themselves in so many ways, physicians require tools that range from a mere observation of the skin to more sophisticated histopathological and immunological examinations.

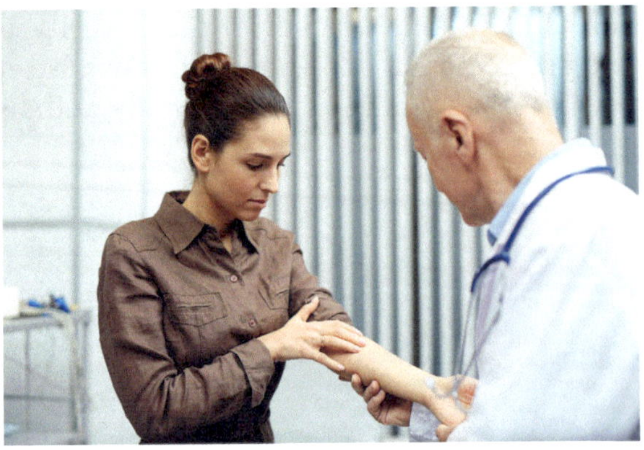

Source: Getty Images. (n.d.). *Psoriasis on Hand.* https://www.health.com/thmb/ZhCk9nTqW3YZA8Q3u3nVGR2dmEc=/1500x0/filters:no_upscale():max_bytes(150000):strip_icc()/Health-GettyImages-886098366-5a2b34568cc04e26ac9e1e72ce19c589.jpg.

Even when laboratory testing and imaging improve, relatively few comprehensively established models are available that integrate clinical indicators, procedural specifications, and even the patient's own perception. In most instances, having a full set of outcome measures would be a more systematic method for evaluating how well diagnosis is delivered; combining hard clinical statistics with advice from patients and professionals. This wider, more whole-picture perspective has the potential to highlight where things are going wrong, aid agreement on best practices, and guide quality improvements. Finally, the development of these diagnostic techniques through continued research and collaboration will support the transition to more accurate, patient-centered care for complicated inflammatory skin diseases (Raut et al., 2024; Van den Steen et al., 2024).

3.3.3. Importance of Early Diagnosis

Skin inflammatory issues have surprises in store—what we observe on the surface may not be everything. Conditions that appear to be mere skin issues at times are accompanied by deeper, body-wide issues that present themselves as mild pain or stiffness, such as a mild neck or backache that some may simply brush apart. Capturing these early is quite significant; in most instances, grabbing the signs before they have a chance to fully bloom means treatments can get started sooner and may even prevent a worse outcome, like disabling later on. Consider psoriatic arthritis, for example—it is frequently married to psoriasis and includes those hardly perceptible axial symptoms. Studies indicate that the identification of early inflammatory back pain and other such symptoms in psoriasis patients can be the difference-maker, in establishing the proper treatment regimen before the onset of permanent damage to joints (Pereverzina et al., 2024). Briefly, early detection is far from simply managing symptoms—it becomes part of overall treatment. Occasionally, skin problems hint at something larger occurring internally. Inflammatory diseases are not skin-deep; they may be initial cues of more systemic issues such as IBD. Skin signs, in general, may appear even before gastrointestinal signs come into the limelight. Such characteristic marks, though superficial, tend to have significant messages behind them, alerting us to possible flare-ups that necessitate an instant adjustment in treatment strategies (Antonelli et al., 2021).

Physicians can utilize these additional skin manifestations as part of a larger puzzle, enabling them to intervene earlier to prevent further complications, and in most situations, maintain a higher quality of life. That intimate relationship between skin and widespread inflammation truly emphasizes the importance of keeping a watchful eye out for even the smallest hints. Pre-emptive diagnosis is not merely a matter of avoiding physical backsliding—it also has a significant impact in reducing the social and psychological burdens that usually accompany chronic skin conditions. Individuals suffering from these conditions feel uncomfortable not only because of visible lesions or pain but also because of the ever-present fear of misdiagnosis or uncertainty.

By catching problems early, physicians can intervene with treatments that can alleviate symptoms, retard the progression of the disease, and reduce the likelihood of long-term disability. In most instances, even detecting subtle axial signs in psoriatic arthritis can save a person from severe functional loss through more focused treatment. This interactive method calms both the body's pain and the mind's tension—kind of decreasing anxiety and alleviating social isolation. Early diagnosis remakes patient care, restoring physical health and mental well-being as one, and demonstrating just how vital early detection is (Pereverzina et al., 2024).

3.4. Conventional Treatments

Treatment of inflammatory dermatoses typically starts with long-standing systemic treatments that have been in use for many decades, a testament to a background of clinical experience and extensive research. Even older drugs like methotrexate, cyclosporine, and retinoids are still the cornerstones due to their anti-inflammatory and immunosuppressive effects. Methotrexate, for instance, is a prodrug, which requires metabolic activation before it can bring about its action, and is generally administered subcutaneously to maximize its bioavailability and safety. Cyclosporine, similarly, is utilized for its quick action but its administration requires vigilant monitoring because of the threat of nephrotoxicity and hypertension. Retinoids, while effective, call for strict precautions because of teratogenicity and long-term hazards of toxicity. The clinical use of these traditional therapies requires balancing therapeutic effects and side effects, highlighting the need for personalized patient evaluation and regular assessment of disease severity and quality of life measures to inform therapeutic decisions (Nast et al., 2021). A significant point of consideration within traditional therapies is their effect upon certain presentations of inflammatory skin diseases, like psoriasis of the nails, that, although a relatively small anatomy, severely undermine patient quality of life. Of clinical concern is the differentiation from concomitant conditions, i.e., psoriatic change of the nail versus onychomycosis, since antifungal and immunosuppressive therapy, which is frequently utilized in psoriasis—can enhance fungal infection in the case of undiagnosed onychomycosis. Traditional systemic treatments such as steroids, methotrexate, and cyclosporine are effective in controlling nail psoriasis but tend to be encumbered by cumulative organ toxicities in the long term. This complicates the need for diagnostic alertness and full clinical assessment before treatment initiation, with fungal infection exclusion to avoid possible exacerbation by immunosuppression. The interaction between efficacy, safety, and diagnostic clarity sets the traditional therapeutic strategy for nails with inflammatory disease (Ventura et al., 2017). In spite of these, traditional treatments remain worth considering within integrated management plans. The toxicities and safety profiles have limited the use to more specific applications with combinations or as bridging treatments awaiting the start of biologics or new oral small molecules. Focus on regular monitoring such as laboratory tests and patient-reported outcomes such as the Dermatology Life Quality Index (DLQI) allows for early detection of adverse events and informs dose adjustments. Also, education of patients regarding risks like teratogenicity, drug-drug interactions, and lifestyle changes, such as alcohol abstinence with methotrexate treatment—increases compliance and reduces complications. The changing paradigm in the management of inflammatory skin disease is complemented by these well-established systemic therapies, supporting their position as mainstays in the therapeutic arsenal when used judiciously and in the context of patient-specific factors and disease severity (Nast et al., 2021).

3.4.1. Topical Corticosteroids

Management of inflammatory skin conditions frequently depends on the attainment of symptomatic improvement with minimal adverse effects, especially in chronic diseases. Among topical drugs, corticosteroids have continued to play a pivotal position because of their strong anti-inflammatory action, which suppresses immune reactions and decreases epidermal hyperproliferation. Their therapeutic efficacy cuts across a wide range of dermatoses, and hence they are considered a first-line treatment for diseases like psoriasis, eczema, and AD. However, the long-term use of topical corticosteroids is of concern with regard to cutaneous atrophy, telangiectasias, and possible systemic absorption causing suppression of the hypothalamic-pituitary-adrenal axis. These risks demand careful dosing and meticulous patient education about application time and strength choice. Even with these drawbacks, corticosteroids' quick onset and widespread clinical use still favor their use, pointing to the continued need for the assessment of safety profiles in combination with therapeutic effects (Gooderham, 2024). Recent developments in topical therapy have aimed to overcome the tolerability and safety constraints inherent in corticosteroids by searching for other immunomodulatory drugs. Calcineurin inhibitors pimecrolimus and tacrolimus have presented themselves as steroid-sparing alternatives with mechanism-based T-cell activation inhibition without the thinning of the skin that is seen with corticosteroids. However, their therapeutic efficacy can be hampered by physicochemical limitations, such as inadequate dermal penetration by virtue of their large molecular size and lipophilicity. This pharmacokinetic barrier tends to lead to inadequate dosing and localized irritation in the form of stinging or burning, which compromises patient compliance. Additionally, new drug delivery systems like nanocarriers are being explored to maximize drug bioavailability and reduce side effects. These advancements are a crucial milestone in the development of topical therapy for inflammatory skin conditions, substituting or otherwise diminishing the need for corticosteroids. Even with the introduction of newer topical immunomodulators, corticosteroids continue to be invaluable due to their immediacy of action and flexibility. Therapeutic strategies now routinely involve the use of corticosteroids as an adjunct to other drugs to optimize treatment while restricting side effects.

For example, corticosteroid intermittent therapy with follow-up maintenance therapy on calcineurin inhibitors can maintain disease control and decrease damage due to corticosteroids. Besides, corticosteroid potency stratification based on disease severity and anatomical location facilitates more accurate management. Concomitantly, molecular mechanisms of inflammation and disruption of the skin barrier are continually under investigation in order to guide the future development of therapeutic agents, specifically to produce molecules that retain the action of corticosteroids without their safety liabilities. Finally, the inclusion of corticosteroids as part of a larger, multimodal therapeutic strategy reflects both their enduring utility and the changing environment for inflammatory skin disease treatments (Gooderham, 2024) (Figure 3.7).

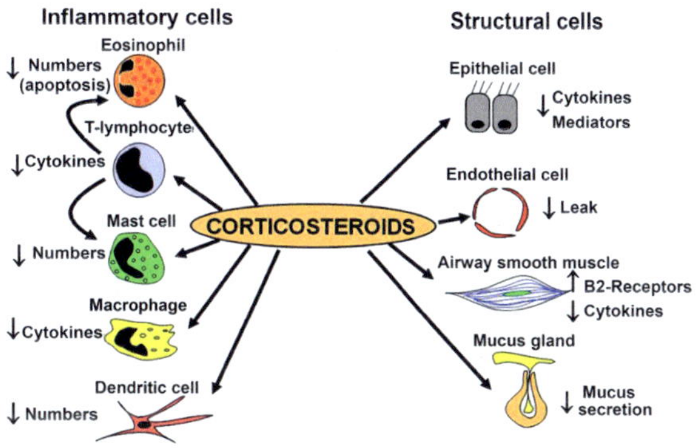

Figure 3.7. Corticosteroids.

Source: Maringer, K., Saheb, E., & Bush, J. (2014). Vesicular trafficking defects, developmental abnormalities, and alterations in the cellular death process occur in cell lines that over-express Dictyostelium GTPase, Rab2, and Rab2 mutants. *Biology, 3*(3), 514–535.

3.4.2. Systemic Medications

The pathophysiology of inflammatory skin diseases usually requires therapeutic intervention that transcends the use of topical agents, particularly in cases that are moderate to severe. Systemic therapy offers a way to treat the pathophysiologic immune dysregulation underlying these conditions, which target pathways that drive chronic inflammation and tissue injury. Among newer systemic therapies, cannabinoids have been recognized because of their anti-inflammatory effects and the localization of cannabinoid receptors to the endocannabinoid system of the skin. This complex system regulates inflammatory reactions and skin homeostasis, implicating cannabinoid potential to mitigate the symptoms of disease in psoriasis, AD, and systemic sclerosis (SSc). Preclinical and initial clinical data look promising, yet evidence to date depends mostly on restricted and diverse research. Broad, randomized controlled trials are crucial to determine efficacy, dosing, and safety profiles before being able to include cannabinoids in regular systemic treatment of inflammatory dermatoses confidently. Apart from cannabinoids, systemic therapy typically includes modulation of lipid metabolism, which has increasingly been recognized to play a role in inflammatory skin pathogenesis. Dyslipidemia is commonly seen in inflammatory dermatoses like psoriasis and AD, and this emphasizes a potentially causative link between lipid derangements and skin inflammation. Mendelian randomization analyses in recent years show that genetic inhibition of the major lipid-regulating proteins, including PCSK9, is associated with decreased risks of psoriasis and AD. This causal evidence places PCSK9 inhibitors as potential systemic drugs that may modulate both lipid profiles and inflammatory processes, and hence a dual therapeutic advantage. In contrast, HMGCR inhibitors, better known as statins, have more nuanced effects, potentially improving conditions such as seborrheic dermatitis but worsening others such as rosacea and allergic urticaria. Therefore, detailed knowledge of lipid-targeted systemic agents can inform individualized treatment decisions in inflammatory skin diseases. Systemic therapy with drugs involves cautious weighing of efficacy about safety and tolerability since side effects may affect patient compliance and outcome. Although conventional systemic treatments, such as corticosteroids and immunosuppressants, are still the basis, new agents like cannabinoids and lipid modulators enhance therapeutic options. Clinical choice increasingly involves genetic and molecular information that can forecast response to treatment and disease course, allowing more specific interventions. However, the heterogeneity of inflammatory skin diseases requires strict clinical trials for individual subtypes and patient groups to confirm these new systemic treatments. Ongoing investigation into effects on mechanisms of action and long-term consequences is necessary to incorporate these systemic drugs into multidisciplinary management approaches to enhance quality of life and control of disease (Figure 3.8).

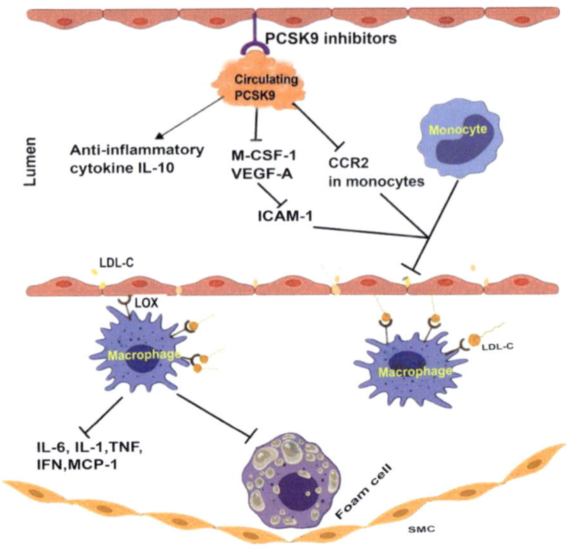

Figure 3.8. The effect of PCSK9 inhibition on vascular inflammation.

Source: Wu N-Q, Shi H-W and Li J-J (2022) Proprotein Convertase Subtilisin/Kexin Type 9 and Inflammation: An Updated Review. Front. Cardiovasc. Med. 9:763516. doi: 10.3389/fcvm.2022.763516

3.4.3. Phototherapy

Breakthroughs in dermatologic therapy have substantially increased the range of options for individuals with inflammatory skin conditions, with phototherapy proving to be especially significant. It involves the use of certain wavelengths of ultraviolet (UV) light that affect areas of involvement, thus decreasing inflammation and controlling the immune response in the skin. Conventional cabinet phototherapy, although effective, carries high operating costs and has to be operated by trained individuals, thereby reducing its availability and utilitarian value in certain contexts. New technologies like the 308-nm excimer pulsed light have overcome these drawbacks by enabling focused treatment of localized lesions with reduced sessions and improved patient compliance. Interestingly, research has shown that excimer pulsed light can provide significant clearance in severe cases that are refractory to traditional treatments, improving clinical outcomes and quality of life without adverse effects (Mohammed et al., 2024). These advancements highlight its new role as an individualized, effective treatment for problematic skin diseases. Given the potential of phototherapy, its use will need to be cautiously weighed against the larger picture of inflammatory skin disease treatment, particularly when adverse effects from other drugs are involved. As an example, in children with IBD treated with tumor necrosis factor α inhibitors, psoriasiform rashes are a frequent side effect that presents clinical management problems. In such cases, phototherapy is usually an adjunct or alternative to systemic medications, particularly when topical steroids are not enough. Treatment compliance can be complicated, though: about one-third of involved pediatric patients needed discontinuation of the initial biologic therapy because of refractory cutaneous eruptions. Phototherapy, in combination with methotrexate and acitretin, has been shown to be crucial for the management of recalcitrant lesions, underscoring the role of a multidisciplinary care system that incorporates phototherapy to achieve maximum benefits with retention of underlying disease control. Such complexity underscores the role of phototherapy in subtle clinical decision-making. The safety and efficacy profile of phototherapy establishes it as a useful option, especially for patients with inflammatory skin diseases who are refractory to other forms of therapy.

Results show that targeted excimer pulsed light therapy is associated with high rates of rapid lesion clearance and significant patient-reported improvements in quality-of-life measures, including the DLQI. Notably, the chance of serious adverse effects is low, with localized burns occurring in a minority of patients and no serious complications reported in most. The decrease in a number of treatment sessions needed relative to conventional phototherapy regimens increases patient convenience and possibly decreases healthcare system loads. However, additional rigorous, large-scale randomized controlled trials are needed to standardize dosing regimens and evaluate long-term benefits. Ongoing research will determine phototherapy's definitive role in treatment algorithms for inflammatory skin diseases, affirming its potential as a powerful, patient-friendly therapeutic modality (Mohammed et al., 2024) (Figure 3.9).

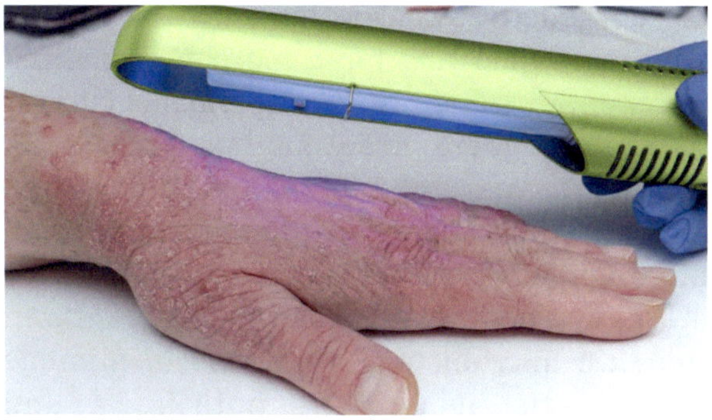

Figure 3.9. Phototherapy treatment psoriasis.

Source: Medical News Today. (2021). *Phototherapy Treatment for Psoriasis.* https://i0.wp.com/post.medicalnewstoday.com/wp-content/uploads/sites/3/2021/09/Phototherapy-Treatment-psoriasis-1296x728-header-1024x575.jpg?w=1155&h=1528.

3.5. Alternative and Complementary Therapies

The intricacy of inflammatory cutaneous diseases, like psoriasis, has made clinicians and scientists venture into treatments other than mainstream pharmacotherapy. Although traditional therapy is primarily immune-focused, treatments sometimes fail to treat the comprehensive aspect of the disease. Complementary and alternative treatments provide pathways that can enhance or complement mainstream therapies by adjusting underlying biological pathways. For example, some approaches target vascular modulation, given the involvement of vascular endothelial growth factor-A (VEGF-A)-mediated angiogenesis in the maintenance of inflammation in psoriatic plaques. Anti-angiogenic therapy targeting VEGF-A has been promising in experimental models, and based on clinical experience, patient administration of VEGF-A inhibitors has been indicated to alleviate symptoms. These therapies may be especially useful for patient subsets genetically at risk for increased VEGF-A expression, allowing for a more personalized therapeutic strategy that complements current immune-targeted treatments. Outside of vascular targets, the bidirectional interaction between the immune system and the skin microbiome represents another fertile area for alternative and complementary interventions. The skin microbiota plays a role in immune homeostasis, modulating both local and systemic inflammatory responses. Dysbiosis or imbalances in this microbial community may worsen inflammatory skin diseases, and restoring microbial homeostasis may improve the severity of disease. New evidence highlights the need to modulate host-microbiome interactions, possibly by prebiotics, probiotics, or directed microbial therapies. These treatments can re-tune immune responses by supporting healthy microbial communities, thus supporting conventional immunomodulatory therapies, and treating disease mechanisms at a fundamental level (Zheng et al., 2020). Incorporation of alternative and complementary therapies into the treatment model for inflammatory skin diseases necessitates stringent evaluation of efficacy and safety across diverse patient populations. Disease heterogeneity and underlying immune profiles necessitate individualized treatment regimens that take into account genetic, microbial, and environmental determinants. As the available data indicate, a combination of anti-angiogenic and microbiome-directed therapies with standard immune-suppressive or biologic agents may maximize therapeutic benefits while reducing adverse effects. In addition, this integrative paradigm recognizes the limitations of single-modality treatments, encouraging a multidisciplinary approach more in keeping with the multifactorial pathophysiology of inflammatory skin diseases. Ongoing research into these complementary modalities promises to further define patient-tailored care and broaden the therapeutic armamentarium against chronic dermatoses (Zheng et al., 2020).

3.5.1. Herbal Remedies

The search for safer and more potent treatments for inflammatory cutaneous disorders has generated renewed interest in natural therapeutic agents, and notably, herbal remedies. These therapies utilize the complex bioactive molecules present in plants, which tend to show anti-inflammatory, antioxidant, and antimicrobial activities crucial to repairing the skin and controlling symptoms. In contrast to synthetic drugs, most herbal remedies have fewer side effects, holding great promise as an alternative or adjunctive therapy for patients with chronic skin diseases. Their capacity to target multiple pathways in inflammation and tissue repair maximizes their therapeutic effectiveness. New technologies developed in biomedical research have opened the possibility of incorporating herbal extracts in new delivery systems, such as nanofibers, maximizing their bioavailability and potency. This new method not only allows for extended release but also promotes wound healing mechanisms, suggesting an advanced refinement of conventional medicine in contemporary dermatology. The addition of certain plant remedy interventions has proven to be quite effective in terms of managing the complexities involved with inflammatory skin conditions. For instance, specific herbs contain agents that modulate immune function, inhibit oxidative stress, and suppress microbial adhesion, all important components in diseases such as eczema and psoriasis. In addition, most herbal extracts play a part in scalpel-like exactness of tissue healing by stimulating the synthesis of collagen and reducing scar formation. Clinical experience and preclinical research have proven that such natural substances are able to hasten healing while improving symptoms like redness, swelling, and itching. Such therapeutic pliability raises the profile of herbal remedies from mere symptomatic treatment to agents with the ability to affect subclinical pathological processes. Such data highlights the capability of phytomedicine to bridge gaps left by traditional remedies, particularly in long-term care and reduce recurrence (Varsha et al., 2024). Furthermore, including herbal medicine into dermatology needs strict scientific authentication and standardization to prove safety and reproducibility.

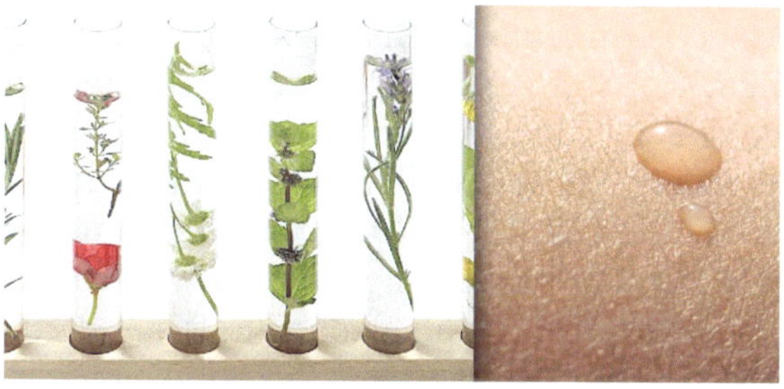

Figure 3.10. Herbal anti-inflammatory agents for skin.

Source: Skin Therapy Letter. (2000). *Herbal Anti-Inflammatory Agents for Skin Disorders.* https://www.skintherapyletter.com/wp-content/uploads/2000/04/herbal-anti-inflammatory-agents-skin.jpg.

The bioactivity of plant molecules can also differ significantly based on extraction techniques, formulation, and concentration. Research activities must thus aim to clarify pharmacodynamics and pharmacokinetics, as well as the interaction of these substances with human skin at molecular levels. Advances such as electrospun nanofiber matrices loaded with herbal extracts represent advances towards standardized delivery and controlled release, achieving maximum therapeutic effect while limiting systemic exposure. Extensive clinical trials and mechanistic investigations are needed to rationalize dosing regimens and clarify possible synergistic interactions with traditional drugs. Such a systemic strategy opens the door for herbal medicines to be adopted as key elements of evidence-based treatment regimens for inflammatory skin disorders (Figure 3.10).

3.5.2. Dietary Modifications

Inflammatory dermatoses, like psoriasis and AD, encompass multifactorial etiopathogenesis including immune dysregulation and environmental influences. New evidence indicates that dietary interventions can significantly impact the disease by modulating systemic inflammation and immunity. The gut microbiota, closely associated with immune system function via the microbiota-gut-brain axis, is the key player in this process. Dietary fibers and resistant starches fermented into short-chain fatty acids (SCFAs) by gut bacteria have anti-inflammatory actions that could translate to clinical benefits for skin health. SCFA production maintains immune homeostasis by modulating neuro-immunoendocrine circuits and potentially lessening the severity of inflammatory skin disease. Combining dietary strategies aimed at increasing beneficial microbial metabolites is a promising adjunctive method in the treatment of chronic skin inflammation. In addition, the interplay between nutrition, gut microbiota, and systemic inflammation highlights the therapeutic benefit of dietary interventions in inflammatory dermatoses. Changes in the composition of gut microbiota, in accordance with dietary habits, have been associated with abnormal immune signaling pathways in skin inflammation. Certain nutrients like omega-3 fatty acids, antioxidants, and prebiotic fibers correct microbial diversity and decrease pro-inflammatory cytokines. Early life influences such as diet have the ability to influence long-term microbiota profiles and confer susceptibility to inflammatory disease. Similarly, stress and aging, which converge to regulate the microbiota-gut-brain axis, can worsen skin pathology by disrupting immune homeostasis. Hence, precision dietary interventions designed to preserve microbial diversity and increase anti-inflammatory metabolites present a new path to preventing the inflammatory manifestation of skin disease (Olbryś & Cyran, 2025). In clinical practice, patient-specific dietary regimens that focus on whole foods high in fiber, vitamins, and anti-inflammatory substances show positive impacts on inflammatory skin disease progression. Prohibition of pro-inflammatory foods like processed sugars and saturated fats can decrease systemic oxidative stress and inflammation, enhancing therapeutic results.

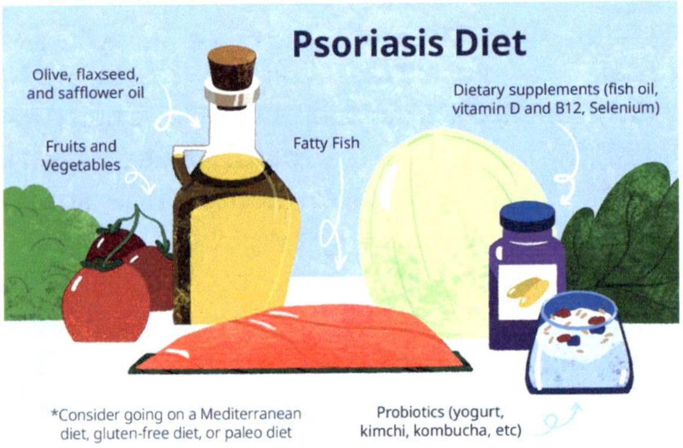

Figure 3.11. Psoriasis diet.

Source: Porter, L. (n.d.). *Psoriasis Diet: Foods to Eat and Avoid.* https://www.verywellhealth.com/thmb/103EaPD5dsDkdo5eM28rYXobaFw=/1500x0/filters:no_upscale():max_bytes(150000):strip_icc()/VWH-LauraPorter-PsoriasisDiet-Standard-c37bfc3b4ae14f2488568b3009b9a544.jpg.

Furthermore, interventions aimed at gut microbiota through probiotics and prebiotics have proven to be effective in modulating immune responses pertinent to skin disease. However, the heterogeneity of the response highlights the necessity of additional research defining particular dietary constituents and their mechanistic effects on inflammation of the skin. Probing an understanding of the microbiota-gut-skin axis will support the development of integrative treatment paradigms that include dietary interventions and thus optimize the management of disease and the quality of life of patients (Figure 3.11).

3.5.3. Stress Management Techniques

Chronic stress has also been identified as a critical determinant of worsening inflammatory dermatoses, with an impact on the severity and course of disorders like SSc and psoriasis. The pathophysiological cascade initiated by stress increases inflammatory mediators and upsets immune homeostasis, thus worsening cutaneous manifestations. Therefore, utilizing effective stress management strategies can become an adjunct therapy in managing such disorders. Practices such as mindfulness meditation, cognitive behavior modification, and regulated deep breathing have shown promise in regulating the hypothalamic-pituitary-adrenal axis with the resultant reduction in inflammatory processes. Additionally, the reduction of stress can potentially counteract increased plasma proteins such as Heat shock protein 90 that is associated with the degree of skin involvement and severity of inflammation in SSc patients. By acting on the neuroendocrine-immunological mechanisms, these methods not only enhance psychological well-being but also affect the outcome of disease by suppressing systemic inflammation. In addition to psychological advantages, stress management plays an essential role in the physiological homeostasis necessary for inflammatory skin disease management. Chronic stress triggers peripheral and central nervous system mechanisms that sustain inflammation, as observed in complex pain syndromes associated with skin and soft tissue inflammation. Methods that induce parasympathetic activation, like vagal nerve stimulation or relaxation training, can break the cycle by limiting proinflammatory cytokine release. This biochemical change creates an anti-inflammatory milieu, enhancing skin barrier function and lessening lesions. In addition, stress management enhances patient compliance with dermatologic treatment by strengthening coping skills and decreasing symptom-related distress. Therefore, the incorporation of structured stress-reducing interventions into dermatological disease management models is a necessary step towards comprehensive disease management, highlighting the interdependence of somatic and mental health in inflammatory skin pathology.

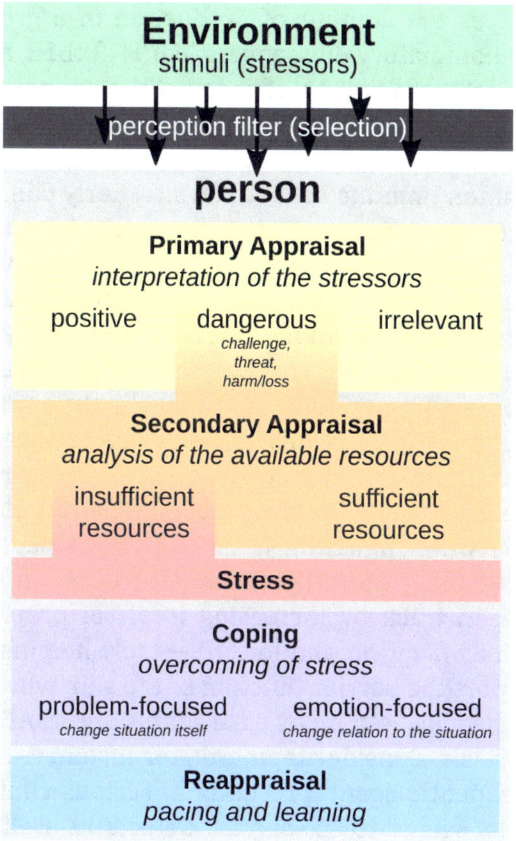

Figure 3.12. Stress management.

Source: By Philipp Guttmann - Own work, CC BY-SA 4.0, https://commons.wikimedia.org/w/index.php?curid=45616588

Clinically, the addition of individualized stress management routines supplements pharmacological interventions by acknowledging the multidimensional dimensions of inflammatory skin disease. With the heterogeneity in the patient response to stress and its immunological outcomes, individualized strategies based on biofeedback, yoga, or hypnosis can produce better results. Moreover, the view of stress as a modifiable risk factor comports with progressive therapeutic frameworks promoting patient-centered care. This facilitates resilience against stimuli that induce skin flare-ups, subsequently decreasing the frequency and severity of inflammatory episodes. Studies of biomarkers such as Hsp90 emphasize the biological viability of modulation of stress to influence disease progression, with objective criteria for measuring therapy efficacy. In conclusion, stress management strategies are an essential, evidence-supported element of multi-component treatment programs designed to enhance quality of life and prognosis in individuals with inflammatory skin disorders (Figure 3.12).

3.6. Current Research and Advances

Recent advances at unraveling the numerous molecular pathways to inflammatory skin disease have placed the aryl hydrocarbon receptor (AHR) in a surprising forefront position—no longer is it all about detoxing environmental pollutants. Instead, AHR now appears intimately connected with how keratinocytes mature, whether the skin's protective barrier remains intact, and even how inflammatory messages get modulated. Dysregulation of this signaling pathway has been implicated in diseases such as psoriasis and AD, where immune missteps and barrier failings take center stage. Recent research with certain AHR modulators, in the majority of instances, suggests treatments that could be more effective and have fewer side effects than the traditional approaches. This new emphasis on AHR reflects a wider trend toward precision medicine in dermatology, a model that seeks to leverage the body's own regulatory sleights of hand to reinstate skin wellness (Michał et al., 2024). In the meantime, new research into the immune repertoire (IR) is expanding our understanding of the adaptive immune system's role in inflammation of the skin. By unearthing the B-cell and T-cell receptor sequences, scientists are finding leads on what antigens are causing issues and in what ways immune regulation goes awry in autoimmune and inflammatory diseases. While full-scale IR profiling in skin disease is still in its infancy, preliminary hints indicate that certain prevalent antigen-binding motifs might be associated with particular presentation and course of disease. These findings, in general, unveil promising avenues for the development of targeted immunotherapies that can assist in rebalancing immune tolerance and reducing pathological autoimmunity in conditions such as lupus erythematosus and vitiligo (Terhaar et al., 2024). Adding another layer, newer technologies that integrate genomic, transcriptomic, and proteomic analyses are refining our capacity to identify the subtleties of inflammatory skin diseases. These integrative strategies uncover new biomarkers and surprising pathogenetic routes, which in turn enable researchers to classify patients according to their specific molecular "fingerprints." Rather than using broad immunosuppressants, such strategies open the door to treatments specific to the individual disease mechanism. And on top of that, developments in bioinformatics and machine learning—though with a few bumps along the way—are accelerating the analysis of complicated datasets, so that responses to treatment can be monitored in real-time and possible side effects identified earlier. Together, these advances represent a revolutionary era in dermatology, unscrambling the intricacies of skin inflammation and guiding us toward more personalized and effective management strategies.

3.6.1. New Therapies and Medications in Development

Improvements in our understanding of inflammation have prompted some new ideas about the treatment of skin diseases, particularly by targeting the very molecular stimuli themselves. Nuclear transport checkpoint inhibitors (NTCIs) are one such promising new option. They do this by inhibiting the travel of the major inflammation leaders such as NF-κB and STAT3 from entering the nucleus. This, in turn, reduces the amount of production of a group of inflammatory messengers like TNF, IL1B, and IL6. In the majority of instances, this method not only reduces the overall inflammatory peak but also lowers the number of chemokines that summon immune cells to the site. Early clinical trials even suggest that these medications will dampen gene expression associated with diseases such as AD, showing a new route to manage inflammation driven by keratinocytes (Liu et al., 2024). On another front, there is also increasing talk about arylhydrocarbon receptor (AhR) agonists. These are viewed as an organized means to enhance skin barrier stability while calibrating the immune response. AhR/ARNT signaling is an important part of maintaining the differentiation process in the skin on track by increasing levels of proteins such as filaggrin and loricrin—truly helping to support the barrier function of the skin when it has been beaten up by such conditions as AD or psoriasis. Consider tapinarof, for instance. This therapeutic agent, presently in serious clinical trials, seems to fix barrier defects as well as modulate immune circuits (including Th17/22 and T regulatory cells) to cause significant clinical improvement. It is a two-part mechanism that, if it pans out, may nicely address both the immune and structural deficits in inflammatory skin disorders (Aoki et al., 2023).

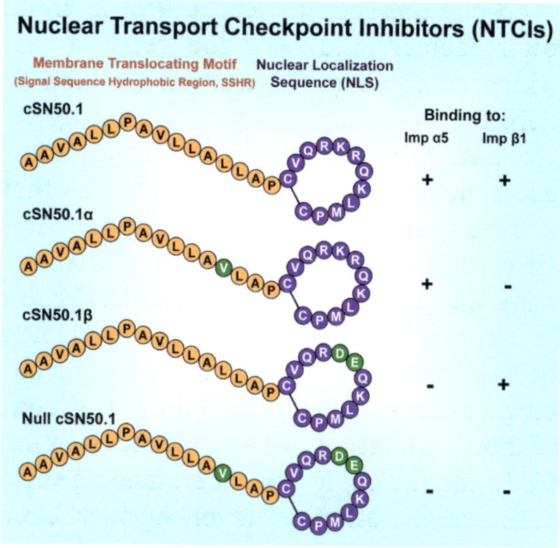

Figure 3.13. Nuclear transport checkpoint inhibitors (NTCIs).

Source: Nong, J., Glassman, P. M., Shuvaev, V. V., Reyes-Esteves, S., Descamps, H. C., Kiseleva, R. Y., et al. (2024). Targeting lipid nanoparticles to the blood-brain barrier to ameliorate acute ischemic stroke. *Molecular Therapy, 32*(4), 857–871.

Concurrently, therapeutic approaches to inflamed skin are changing to encompass targeted small molecules and biologics that specifically inhibit cytokine signaling pathways. This shifts away from broad, blanket immunosuppression toward precision therapies appears to hold greater promise for safety and longer duration of control. For example, therapy focused on modulating the IL-23/IL-17 pathway in psoriasis and the judicious inhibition of Th2 cytokines in AD highlight the utility of these cytokine-specific agents. At the same time, treatments such as NTCIs and AhR agonists are being tested in phase 3 trials, implying that they will soon join our arsenal. In summary, these advancements promise a future where the treatment of chronic inflammatory skin diseases not only becomes more individualized but also more efficacious in enhancing daily life and long-term outcomes (Aoki et al., 2023; Liu et al., 2024) (Figure 3.13).

3.6.2. Role of Biotechnology in Treatment

More recently, biotech has transformed the way we treat inflammatory skin conditions. Rather than simply covering up symptoms like older methods tend to do, newer methods get at the actual, messy biology of chronic inflammation and compromised skin barriers. Individuals now employ such things as organ-on-a-chip systems, which replicate human skin behavior in the lab—to develop a more realistic sandbox for drug testing and disease modeling. These microfluidic systems encapsulate the give-and-take between cells and the immune system, and scientists can test out new treatments that feel much more like real life. Most times, this advance is a game-changer compared to animal models that usually get it wrong when they predict what happens in humans (Donald, 2022). Consider wound healing in inflammatory skin disorders—a messy web of cells and molecules working endlessly to restore the integrity of the skin, but chronic inflammation can really make things difficult. Normal wound healing is one thing, but once inflammation gets out of control, healing is slowed down and tissues fail to recover as they should. Biotechnology comes in here by designing novel solutions such as engineered scaffolds, growth factors, and bioactive molecules, all of which combine to create a more healing atmosphere. By combining genetically engineered cells and targeted molecular therapies, researchers believe that the inflammation process will be made less painful while promoting faster wound closure; this in turn can reduce scarring and mitigate recurring issues. In sum, these bioengineered interventions deviate from the traditional one-size-fits-all methods by providing a better-tuned cure that may even reduce hospitalization durations (Tottoli et al., 2020). In the future, it also appears evident that biotech's contribution to overcoming inflammatory skin ailments is moving in the direction of personalized medicine as well as regenerative treatments. All things considered, in general, with a reliance on advances in genetic engineering, molecular biology, and tissue engineering, researchers are attempting to customize therapies based on the individual patient's own inflammatory fingerprint and genetic characteristics. Consider the case of using organ chips as a kind of "living avatars" to observe therapy responses in real time—this might make it possible to make adjustments in real-time to enhance safety and efficacy. Despite the continued challenges, such as adapting these methods for day-to-day application and securing appropriate regulatory approvals, the convergence of biotech and dermatologic treatment is an auspicious age; one where inflammatory dermatosis could not only be controlled more efficiently but even possibly turned around with precision medicine therapies (Tottoli et al., 2020; Donald, 2022).

3.6.3. Future Directions in Inflammatory Skin Disease Research

Skin microbes have been in the spotlight of late—they contribute more to our immune system than most of us ever guessed. New research indicates that when the skin's natural cocktail of microbes gets out of control; what some refer to as dysbiosis—it can readily worsen problems like eczema and psoriasis by interrupting local immune messages and damaging the skin's defense. Individuals are starting to see these microbial hiccup fits not merely as an afterthought but as possible hints at new diagnostic markers and tailored treatments. Probiotic treatments and even microbial transplants, for example, are proving promising as a means of shifting the balance back in the direction of a more healthful skin environment. In most instances, this increasing understanding suggests that individual therapies involving microbiome altering may soon alleviate chronic inflammation and rebalance (Fritts et al., 2025). Beyond the microbial universe, molecules like lactate are getting new interest. Previously brushed apart as mere metabolic waste products, lactate is now viewed as a vital participant in skin biology. It seems that, through binding to some receptors, lactate can modulate how cells handle inflammation and tissue repair, an observation that was rather surprising. Current research into genes and pathways for lactate has even made it possible to attack a variety of skin conditions, ranging from persistent inflammation and hair loss to skin tumors. By examining these metabolic indicators alongside microbial components, researchers hope to identify new targets for future therapies (Ruan et al., 2025). Combining knowledge from skin microbes and metabolic indicators may be the next giant leap in tackling inflammatory skin diseases. Precision medicine, which studies each individual's distinct combination of molecular, microbial, and metabolic characteristics, is likely to transform the way we diagnose and treat these diseases. A dual strategy—applying techniques to restore the microbial balance with approaches that modulate metabolic pathways—may well provide a synergistic increase in dampening inflammation and promoting skin repair. Long-term studies, despite a few setbacks here and there, will be important to verify the safety and efficacy of these novel treatments. As scientists push more into high-tech biotech and systems biology (with all its built-in eccentricities), the dream of genuinely personalized, mechanism-based treatments for skin disease comes closer and closer (Smith et al., 2020).

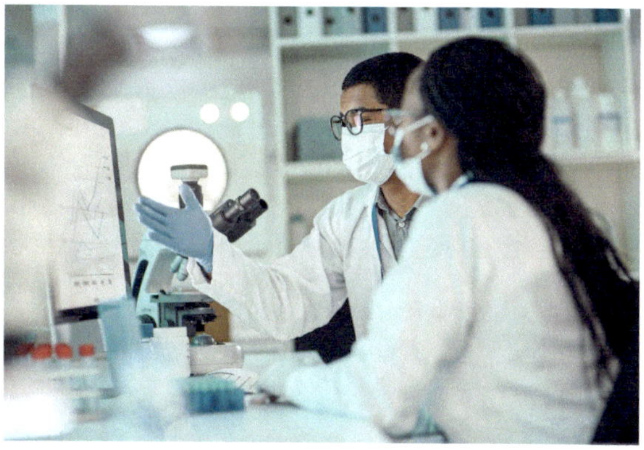

Source: British Association of Dermatologists. (2022). *Research Journals Landing Page Main Image.* https://cdn.bad.org.uk/uploads/2022/02/29200027/Research-Journals_Landing-Page_Main-Image.jpg.

CLOSER LOOK

Photodynamic Therapy (PDT)

PDT is a non-surgical therapy that employs a light source along with a photosensitizer to kill pathological cells, more so in the case of skin disorders such as precancerous lesions and certain skin cancers. The photosensitizer is brought in contact with the skin and subsequently exposed to a certain wavelength of light that leads to a reaction between the photosensitizer and oxygen, generating reactive oxygen species that result in the killing of target cells.

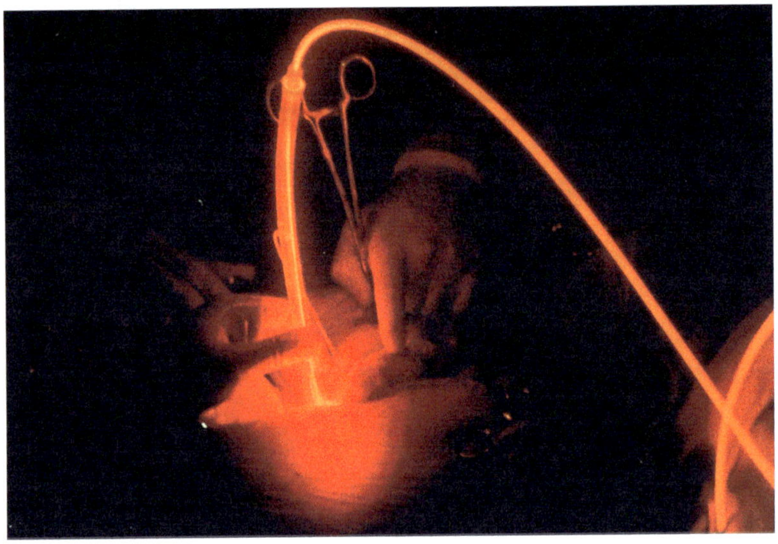

Source: By John Crawford (Photographer) - This image was released by the National Cancer Institute, an agency part of the National Institutes of Health, with the ID 2267 (image) (next)., Public Domain, https://commons.wikimedia.org/w/index.php?curid=24059596

- How it Works:
  - **Photosensitizer:** A compound that is selectively absorbed by the diseased cells and is not toxic to the normal cells until it is triggered by light.
  - **Light Source:** A light source or laser used to cause the photosensitizer to become active by producing reactive oxygen species.
  - **Reactive Oxygen Species:** Cell-damaging molecules that destroy the target cells.
- **Common Applications:**
  - **Skin Cancer:** PDT is utilized to treat multiple skin cancers, such as BCC, squamous cell carcinoma, and actinic keratosis, based on the National Institutes of Health (NIH) (nih.gov).
  - **Precancerous Lesions:** PDT is also applied in the treatment of precancerous lesions such as Bowen's disease and actinic keratosis.

- **Acne and Other Skin Issues:** PDT is becoming more common for acne, sun damage, and other types of skin imperfections, according to Skin Care Doctors.
- **Aesthetic Dermatology:** PDT is also applied for skin rejuvenation and other aesthetic reasons.

- **Advantages of PDT:**
    - **Non-invasive:** PDT is a non-invasive treatment that is not performed through surgery or other invasive treatments.
    - **Targeted Treatment:** PDT specifically targets the disease cell but spares healthy tissues.
    - **Effective:** PDT has had positive outcomes in the management of most skin diseases, such as skin cancer, precancerous lesions, and acne.
    - **Reduced Recurrence Rates:** PDT can reduce recurrence rates of skin cancer lesions, according to Cancer Research UK.

SUMMARY

Inflammatory skin diseases are difficult to nail down since a mix of factors, genes, environmental factors, and even the small microbes that live on our skin, have a role. Our resident microbe, *Cutibacterium acnes*, is normally harmless, but under specific circumstances, it can trigger inflammation. It is surprising that abscesses associated with this bacterium are quite uncommon even in individuals who have very good immune systems, so we tend to require molecular tests to distinguish a genuine infection from a small amount of contamination. This pressure towards clearer diagnosis aligns with the general trend of individualizing medicine according to differences—acknowledging that how diseases present can truly differ. In concluding the discussion of inflammatory skin conditions, it is vital to highlight the delicate equilibrium between the body and its microbes, and there is much more to learn as to why some bacteria switch from being good neighbors to bad troublemakers (Angèle et al., 2024). This is an important mindset when creating therapies that try to repair the issue without destroying the skin's natural ecosystem. Skin breakouts, though, are not merely a skin-deep melodrama; they can be signs of greater distress within the body. For example, advanced glycation end-products (AGEs) are apt to accumulate and trigger a cascade of inflammatory processes, which not only fuel cutaneous inflammation but also vascular aging. Noninvasive methods such as skin autofluorescence (SAF) provide a glimpse into these internal mechanisms through the assessment of AGE deposits, which tend to correlate with many of the risk factors for heart disease and metabolic disease. This association of what occurs on the skin with what occurs within the body serves as a reminder that the skin is not simply a barrier—it tends to reflect overall health. By integrating SAF into routine check-ups, clinicians may be able to detect early warning signs of other health problems that persist with chronic inflammatory diseases (Du et al., 2023). The combination of systemic and skin-specific inflammation truly necessitates a more expansive, holistic approach to patient care. In conclusion, treating inflammatory skin diseases requires a combination of knowledge from microbial behavior, systemic inflammation pathways, and individualized diagnostic tools. The evolving landscape of dermatological research is exposing both challenges and new opportunities in addressing these diseases. Methods such as single-locus sequence typing inform us about how bacteria fuel the inflammatory blaze, while noninvasive markers such as SAF uncover the broader consequences of chronic skin disease. Ultimately, these breakthroughs are propelling us toward a multidisciplinary framework, one that brings dermatology, microbiology, and internal medicine together—to more effectively care for patients. Work ahead must home in on the particular virulence factors and inflammatory mediators advancing disease and open the door to treatments that strike the correct note. In this manner, we can largely alleviate the onerous burden of inflammatory skin disorders and elevate patients' living standards (Du et al., 2023; Angèle et al., 2024).

Inflammatory skin conditions are a broad category of problems, all caused by the immune system attacking tissue and leading to challenging symptoms in general. Psoriatic arthritis, or PsA, is a prime example; it does not merely confine itself to the skin but also likes to infiltrate joints and even organs. Over the past few years, there have been newer treatment options available that appear to make the patient feel better, but there is still much to be explored. For example, there not being enough direct, head-to-head clinical trials and real-world data makes it more difficult to create firm, overall guidelines. Balancing treatments that relieve joint pain without sacrificing soothing skin issues and other associated health concerns is something physicians truly need to consider. All of this drives us toward more adaptable, patient-specific plans and reminds us that a combination of various specialties and studies that keep the patient at the center is essential (Stephanie et al., 2024). Occasionally, boundaries between inflammatory skin conditions and systemic autoimmune diseases overlap in unexpected manners. Consider neuropsychiatric lupus, for instance, it not only accompanies neurological problems but may also exhibit unusual skin manifestations such as erythema multiforme. It is not always easy to determine whether a rash represents an adverse effect of drugs such as hydroxychloroquine or whether it represents part of the underlying process of lupus. Neuropsychiatric symptoms can further complicate the picture, blurring into symptoms of other brain disorders. Imaging devices such as MRI in most instances clarify things by identifying definite inflammatory changes from other etiologies, which then dictates treatment options. A consistent combination of supportive therapy and immunosuppressive medications usually manages these difficult symptoms, emphasizing the importance of meticulous clinical screening and collaboration among experts (Ravindran et al., 2024). Inflammatory dermatoses are a very heterogeneous group that demands adaptive strategies for both local and systemic problems. Increased knowledge of the functioning of these diseases and improved diagnostic techniques have sharpened the treatment programs, but gaps remain when it comes to total, evidence-based guidelines. The knotty correlation between skin findings and general inflammation makes physicians attentive to atypical symptoms and drug effects that can influence treatment options. In broad terms, persistent study of tailormade therapy—along with monitoring patients throughout their course—holds the key to overcoming them. Ultimately, educating clinicians on just how complex these disorders may be can lead the way toward care that does not feel so rigidly box-like and instead is more responsive to the unique, ever-changing needs of each patient (Harrison et al., 2024; Ravindran et al., 2024).

KEY TERMS FROM THIS CHAPTER

Ailment	Atopic dermatitis	Bacteria
Calendula officinalis	Curcuma longa	Damaged cells
Dendritic cells	Dermatomyositis	Endocannabinoid system
Immune dysregulation	Immunomodulation	Inflammatory bowel disease
Inflammatory skin disease	Irritants	Light energy
Localized reaction	Macrophages	Photodynamic therapy
Sebaceous gland	Self-esteem	Systemic sclerosis
T lymphocytes	Tumor necrosis factor-alpha	Ustekinumab

REFERENCES

1. Parker, W., & Ollerton, J. (2013). Evolutionary biology and anthropology suggest biome reconstitution as a necessary approach toward dealing with immune disorders. *Evolution, medicine, and public health, 2013*(1), 89–103. https://doi.org/10.1093/emph/eot008 (accessed on 12 May 2025).
2. Valent, P., Akin, C., Arock, M., Brockow, K., Butterfield, J. H., Carter, M. C., Castells, M., Escribano, L., Hartmann, K., Lieberman, P., Nedoszytko, B., Orfao, A., Schwartz, L. B., Sotlar, K., Sperr, W. R., Triggiani, M., Valenta, R., Horny, H. P., & Metcalfe, D. D. (2012). Definitions, criteria and global classification of mast cell disorders with special reference to mast cell activation syndromes: a consensus proposal. *International archives of allergy and immunology, 157*(3), 215–225. https://doi.org/10.1159/000328760
3. Aoki, V., & Orfali, R. L. (2023). Aryl-hydrocarbon receptor agonist: A novel topical therapeutic approach for inflammatory skin diseases. *Journal of the European Academy of Dermatology and Venereology, 37*, 1093–1094. https://www.semanticscholar.org/paper/e8cbccf85f529fb4cc75ac317da307efbb0a1673 (accessed on 12 May 2025).
4. Castelino, M., Eyre, S., Upton, M., Ho, P., & Barton, A. (2014). The bacterial skin microbiome in psoriatic arthritis, an unexplored link in pathogenesis: challenges and opportunities offered by recent technological advances. *Rheumatology (Oxford, England), 53*(5), 777–784. https://doi.org/10.1093/rheumatology/ket319
5. Bartosińska, J., Kowalczuk, D., Szczepanik-Kułak, P., Kwaśny, M., & Krasowska, D. (2025). A review of photodynamic therapy for the treatment of viral skin diseases. *Antiviral Therapy, 30*(2), 13596535251331728. https://www.semanticscholar.org/paper/c29cf09237fa2962c52874888addfaada7624e25 (accessed on 12 May 2025).
6. Groshek, J., Basil, M., Guo, L., Parker Ward, S., Farraye, F. A., & Reich, J. (2017). Media Consumption and Creation in Attitudes Toward and Knowledge of Inflammatory Bowel Disease: Web-Based Survey. *Journal of medical Internet research, 19*(12), e403. https://doi.org/10.2196/jmir.7624 (accessed on 12 May 2025).
7. Smith, M. P., Ly, K., Thibodeaux, Q., Bhutani, T., Liao, W., & Beck, K. M. (2019). Acrodermatitis continua of Hallopeau: clinical perspectives. *Psoriasis (Auckland, N.Z.), 9*, 65–72. https://doi.org/10.2147/PTT.S180608
8. Cano, A., Espina, M., García, M. L., Muñoz, J., et al. (2021). Psoriasis: From pathogenesis to pharmacological and nano-technological-based therapeutics. *International Journal of Molecular Sciences, 22*, 4983. https://core.ac.uk/download/428286014.pdf (accessed on 12 May 2025).
9. Cryan, J. F., O'Riordan, K. J., Cowan, C. S. M., Sandhu, K. V., Bastiaanssen, T. F. S., Boehme, M., Codagnone, M. G., et al. (2019). The microbiota-gut-brain axis. *Physiological Reviews, 99*, 1877–2013. https://doi.org/10.1152/physrev.00018.2018.
10. OLBRYŚ, Julia and CYRAN, Piotr. Stress-Coping Strategies in Healthy Individuals and Patients with Atopic Dermatitis – Literature Review. *Journal of Education, Health and Sport.* Online. 3 March 2025. Vol. 79, p. 58328. [Accessed 12 June 2025]. DOI 10.12775/JEHS.2025.79.58328.
11. D'Amelio, R., Laganà, B., Rosado, M. M., Picchianti Diamanti, A., et al. (2016). Microbiota and chronic inflammatory arthritis: An interwoven link. *Journal of Translational Medicine, 14*, 233. https://core.ac.uk/download/54535728.pdf (accessed on 12 May 2025).

12. Dec, M., & Arasiewicz, H. (2024). Aryl hydrocarbon receptor role in chronic inflammatory skin diseases: A narrative review. *Advances in Dermatology and Allergology/Postępy Dermatologii i Alergologii, 41*, 9–19. https://www.semanticscholar.org/paper/e0a3ffbe06760a569cd4260e90d7d96789959947 (accessed on 12 May 2025).

13. Du, T., Brandl, B., Hauner, H., & Skurk, T. (2023). Skin autofluorescence mirrors surrogate parameters of vascular aging: An Enable study. *Nutrients, 15*. https://www.semanticscholar.org/paper/27db3679c499d02628eb09a08f8a28ab51ff2cbd (accessed on 12 May 2025).

14. Fritts, H., Frasier, K., Herrick, G., Li, V., & Sebastiao, E. (2025). Unravelling the role of the skin microbiome in immunodermatological diseases: implications for therapeutic interventions . *International Journal of Research in Dermatology, 11*(2), 190–198. https://doi.org/10.18203/issn.2455-4529.IntJResDermatol20250442(accessed on 12 May 2025).

15. Furgalska-Kudła, J., Suława, A., Targoński, O., Targońska, M., Fedorowicz, S., Basiak, A., Ptasiński, A., et al. (2024). Association between rosacea and risk factors: A literature review. *Quality in Sport*. https://www.semanticscholar.org/paper/aba7d8884c6ac394d1990a80aad264363a141804 (accessed on 12 May 2025).

16. Solimani, F., Meier, K., & Ghoreschi, K. (2019). Emerging Topical and Systemic JAK Inhibitors in Dermatology. *Frontiers in immunology, 10*, 2847. https://doi.org/10.3389/fimmu.2019.02847 (accessed on 12 May 2025).

17. Gooderham M. Exploring Newer Topical Therapies for Inflammatory Skin Diseases: A Guide for Rheumatologists. Can Rheumatol Today [Internet]. 2024 Sep. 17 [cited 2025 Jun. 12];1(2):18–22. Available from: https://canadianrheumatologytoday.com/article/view/1-2-Gooderham(accessed on 12 May 2025).

18. Grine, L., Hofbauer, G. F. L., Lambert, J., Lapeere, H., et al. (2020). Comparison of personality traits among patients with psoriasis, atopic dermatitis, and stress: A pilot study. *Dermatology, 236*(4), 324–328. https://doi.org/10.1159/000505543.

19. Haas R. H. (2019). Mitochondrial Dysfunction in Aging and Diseases of Aging. *Biology, 8*(2), 48. https://doi.org/10.3390/biology8020048

20. Harrison, S. R., Aung Din, B. N. R., Marzo-Ortega, H., & Helliwell, P. S. (2024). Recent advances in the management of psoriatic arthritis: practical considerations. *Polish archives of internal medicine, 134*(1), 16639. https://doi.org/10.20452/pamw.16639 (accessed on 12 May 2025).

21. Hop, I., Kołodziejczyk, K., Branewska, J., Ostrowska, B., Olszanicka, A., Niemiec, R., Galas, A., et al. (2023). The most common dermatological manifestations of inflammatory bowel diseases. *Journal of Education, Health and Sport*. https://www.semanticscholar.org/paper/5cb47352b191a8594eba938d34f4d86cad8352bf Antonelli, E., Bassotti, G., Tramontana, M., Hansel, K., Stingeni, L., Ardizzone, S., Genovese, G., Marzano, A. V., & Maconi, G. (2021). Dermatological Manifestations in Inflammatory Bowel Diseases. *Journal of clinical medicine, 10*(2), 364. https://doi.org/10.3390/jcm10020364(accessed on 12 May 2025).

22. Ingber, D. E. (2022). Human organs-on-chips for disease modelling, drug development and personalized medicine. *Nature Reviews Genetics, 23*(8), 467–491. https://doi.org/10.1038/s41576-022-00466-9.

23. Iraji, F., Zolfaghari, B., Mousavi, A., & Mousavi, F. (2024). Efficacy of a herbal cream formulation incorporating *Calendula officinalis*, *Glycyrrhiza glabra*, *Curcuma longa*, and *Fumaria parviflora* versus topical mometasone in the management of atopic dermatitis. *Journal of Skin and Stem*

Cell. https://www.semanticscholar.org/paper/2c496fd4eedaafdf2a598e14cb64254b1fb334e3 (accessed on 12 May 2025).

24. Jiang, W., Wang, X., Duan, X., Li, S., Li, N., & Dou, J. (2024). Review of the relationship between mental stress and inflammatory skin diseases. *International Journal of Social Sciences and Public Administration.* https://www.semanticscholar.org/paper/ab9ceb47362ddd40415a6e76fd4ddce1ae71bda8 (accessed on 12 May 2025).

25. Kanatoula, D., Bodner, E., Ghoreschi, K., Meier, K., & Solimani, F. (2024). Non-biologic immunosuppressive drugs for inflammatory and autoimmune skin diseases. *JDDG: Journal der Deutschen Dermatologischen Gesellschaft, 22*, 400–421. https://www.semanticscholar.org/paper/178cd796ad75300948eae1645ea75bff5cfc9e0d (accessed on 12 May 2025).

26. Khachikyan KhM, Michenko AV, Topchyan AP. Main pathohistological reactions of inflammatory skin diseases, dermoscopic patters and their correlation (essay). Russian Journal of Clinical Dermatology and Venereology. 2025;24(1):102-110. (In Russ.)

27. https://doi.org/10.17116/klinderma202524011102(accessed on 12 May 2025).

28. AB1458 TREATMENT UTILIZATION, SYMPTOMS, AND COMORBIDITIES IN DERMATOMYOSITIS: AN ANALYSIS OF ELECTRONIC MEDICAL RECORDS IN THE UNITED STATES

29. Smith, M. L., Farkas, D. K., Sumner, J. A., Jiang, T., Lash, T. L., Galea, S., Sørensen, H. T., & Gradus, J. L. (2020). Associations between adjustment disorder and hospital-based infections in the Danish population. *Journal of psychosomatic research, 132*, 109976. https://doi.org/10.1016/j.jpsychores.2020.109976

30. Kosek, E., Clauw, D. J., Nijs, J., Baron, R., Gilron, I., Harris, R. E., Micó, J. A., et al. (2021). Chronic nociplastic pain affecting the musculoskeletal system: Clinical criteria and grading system. *Pain, 162*(11), 2629–2634. https://doi.org/10.1097/j.pain.0000000000002324.

31. Kuzumi, A., Yamashita, T., Fukasawa, T., Yoshizaki-Ogawa, A., Sato, S., & Yoshizaki, A. (2024). Cannabinoids for the treatment of autoimmune and inflammatory skin diseases: A systematic review. *Experimental Dermatology, 33*, 1–12. https://www.semanticscholar.org/paper/807e885f55b08d376da93959fe9a37f97e77fa1a (accessed on 12 May 2025).

32. Lemarcq, L., Reynaert, V., Van den Steen, E., Evers-Lebrun, C., Marinović, B., De Cock, D., & Gutermuth, J. (2025). Outcome Measures for Interdisciplinary Care in Immune-mediated Inflammatory Skin Diseases (skIMIDs): A Scoping Review. *The British journal of dermatology*, ljaf153. Advance online publication. https://doi.org/10.1093/bjd/ljaf153(accessed on 12 May 2025).

33. Li, C., Wang, B., Han, T., Xu, Y., & Li, X. (2024). Causal relationship between inflammatory skin diseases and immunoglobulin A nephropathy: A Mendelian randomization and enrichment analysis study. *Skin Research and Technology, 30.* https://www.semanticscholar.org/paper/addc000eb80ff0acd17383cfad4faa66d51eb2a9 (accessed on 12 May 2025).

34. Yajia Li, Ziqin Cao, Jianhuang Wu, Identifying novel risk targets in inflammatory skin diseases by comprehensive proteome-wide Mendelian randomization study, *Postgraduate Medical Journal*, 2025;, qgaf032, https://doi.org/10.1093/postmj/qgaf032(accessed on 12 May 2025).

35. Liu, Y., Qiao, H., Zienkiewicz, J., & Hawiger, J. (2024). Anti-inflammatory control of human skin keratinocytes by targeting nuclear transport checkpoint. *Skin health and disease, 4*(3), e356. https://doi.org/10.1002/ski2.356(accessed on 12 May 2025).

36. Mishra, B., Gou, Y., Tan, Z. *et al.* Integrative systems biology framework discovers common gene regulatory signatures in mechanistically distinct inflammatory skin diseases. *npj Syst Biol Appl* **11**, 21 (2025). https://doi.org/10.1038/s41540-025-00498-x(accessed on 12 May 2025).

37. Haya Mohammed, Victoria Vilenchik, Alexandra Banner, Daniel Keith, PD13 A UK single-centre prospective audit and clinical experience of developing an ultraviolet B phototherapy service using 308-nm excimer pulsed light for inflammatory skin disease, *British Journal of Dermatology*, Volume 191, Issue Supplement_1, July 2024, Page i87, https://doi.org/10.1093/bjd/ljae090.177(accessed on 12 May 2025).

38. Monaenkova M.K., Abalukhova E.D., Zlobin D.E., Molochkov A.V., Gureeva M.A., Karzanov O.V., Molochkova Y.V. Worsening of the skin diseases' severity during SARS-CoV-2 pandemic is confirmed irrespective of the leading immune response pattern // Almanac of Clinical Medicine. - 2024. - Vol. 52. - N. 8. - P. 437-445. doi: 10.18786/2072-0505-2024-52-042(accessed on 12 May 2025).

39. Murray, C. J. L., Ikuta, K. S., Sharara, F., Swetschinski, L. R., Robles Aguilar, G., Gray, A. P., Han, C., et al. (2022). Global burden of bacterial antimicrobial resistance in 2019: A systematic analysis. *The Lancet, 399*, 629–655. https://doi.org/10.1016/s0140-6736(21)02724-0.

40. Nagre, V. S., Dhole, Y. R., & Deshmukh, S. P. (2024). The power of herbs: Effective treatment for skin diseases. *GSC Advanced Research and Reviews.* GSC Advanced Research and Reviews, 2024, 21(03), 293-298.

41. Article DOI: 10.30574/gscarr.2024.21.3.0494(accessed on 12 May 2025).

42. Nast, A., Altenburg, A., Augustin, M., Boehncke, W. H., Härle, P., Klaus, J., Koza, J., et al. (2021). German S3-guideline on the treatment of psoriasis vulgaris, adapted from EuroGuiDerm–Part 1: Treatment goals and treatment recommendations. *JDDG Journal der Deutschen Dermatologischen Gesellschaft, 19*, 934–150. https://doi.org/10.1111/ddg.14508.

43. Park, J. H., Prochnow, T., Chang, J., & Kim, S. J. (2023). Health-related behaviors and psychological status of adolescent patients with atopic dermatitis: The 2019 Korea Youth Risk Behavior Web-Based Survey. *Patient Preference and Adherence, 17*, 739–747. https://www.semanticscholar.org/paper/f4f5b19de9eb95cd5976dff908ccca9894eea41f (accessed on 12 May 2025).

44. Pereverzina N.O., Kruglova L.S., Korotaeva T.V. Prevalence and clinical signs of inflammatory back pain in patients with skin psoriasis and axial involvement // Russian Journal of Skin and Venereal Diseases. - 2024. - Vol. 27. - N. 1. - P. 69-82. doi: 10.17816/dv624169(accessed on 12 May 2025).

45. Pinckney, Leah C., "Dupuytren's Disease" (2017). *Student Publications.* 534. https://cupola.gettysburg.edu/student_scholarship/534(accessed on 12 May 2025).

46. Raut, R. D., Zade, A., & Gaikwad, A. (2024). Implementation paper on dermatological psoriasis and other skin diseases diagnosis using machine learning. *International Journal for Research in Applied Science and Engineering Technology.* ISSN: 2321-9653. (accessed on 12 May 2025).

47. Ravindran, Y., Mahmood, A., & Erb, N. (2024). P48 Lupus with a neurological twist: from skin rash to sudden confusion and a diagnosis of posterior reversible encephalopathy syndrome. *Rheumatology Advances in Practice, 8*(Suppl 1), rkae117.079. https://doi.org/10.1093/rap/rkae117.079(accessed on 12 May 2025).

48. Roudeau, A., Corvec, S., Heym, B., d'Epenoux, L. R., Lidove, O., & Zeller, V. (2024). Unusual *Cutibacterium acnes* splenic abscess with bacteremia in an immunocompetent man: Phylotyping and clonal complex analysis. *BMC Infectious Diseases, 24.* https://www.semanticscholar.org/paper/e362d01a16a574e4f676d92f3be5a53487bb886d (accessed on 12 May 2025).

49. Ruan, D., Hu, T., Yang, X., Mo, X., & Ju, Q. (2025). Lactate in skin homeostasis: Metabolism, skin barrier, and immunomodulation. *Frontiers in Immunology, 16.* https://www.semanticscholar.org/paper/bc75e5a685843498869350c6a9929c5a32058ab6 (accessed on 12 May 2025).

50. P Sanz Segura, F Gomollón, S García García, M Vela, A Fernández-Clotet, R Muñoz, I García de la Filia, M García Prada, J A Ferrer Rosique, M J García, R de Francisco, L Arias, J Barrio, I Guerra, A Ponferrada Diaz, J P Gisbert, M Carrillo-Palau, X Calvet, L Márquez-Mosquera, B Gros, F Cañete, D Monfort, R E Madrigal, O Roncero, V Laredo, M Montoro, C Muñoz, B López-Cauce, R Lorente, A Fuentes, P Vega, D Martín, J Nerín de la Puerta, P Varela, D Casas-Deza, P Martínez, R Pajares, A J Lucendo, E Domènech, S García-López, on behalf of the ENEIDA project of GETECCU, P643 Psoriasis induced by anti-TNF therapy in Inflammatory Bowel Disease: analysis of therapeutic management and evolution of both diseases in a nationwide cohort study, *Journal of Crohn's and Colitis*, Volume 17, Issue Supplement_1, February 2023, Pages i774–i775, https://doi.org/10.1093/ecco-jcc/jjac190.0773(accessed on 12 May 2025).

51. Scholar, M. D., & Nevagi, K. (2024). Traditional Ayurvedic practices in the management of Vicharchika w.s.r. eczema: A case report. *AYUSCRIPT.* https://www.semanticscholar.org/paper/d9213672de49110624cf6a858458115bb9cc9629 (accessed on 12 May 2025).

52. Shin, K. O., Ha, D. H., Kim, J. O., Crumrine, D., Meyer, J. M., Wakefield, J. S., Lee, Y., et al. (2020). Exosomes from human adipose tissue-derived mesenchymal stem cells promote epidermal barrier repair by inducing de novo synthesis of ceramides in atopic dermatitis. *Cells, 9*(3), 680. https://doi.org/10.3390/cells9030680.

53. Soboleva VA. The effectiveness of topical anti-inflammatory hormonal therapy in irritant contact dermatitis management in toddlers. *Meditsinskiy sovet = Medical Council.* 2024;(11):107–112. (In Russ.) https://doi.org/10.21518/ms2024-237(accessed on 12 May 2025).

54. Su, X., Ou, Y., Ruan, S. F., Lv, X., Qin, K., Mao, J., & Ji, C. (2025). Risk of serious infection with JAK inhibitors in immune-mediated inflammatory skin diseases: A meta-analysis of randomized clinical trials. *The Journal of Dermatological Treatment, 36*(1), 2474507. https://www.semanticscholar.org/paper/cdadac571abbfb3602f5d21b47d175a5656471ae (accessed on 12 May 2025).

55. SZEWCZYK, Kamila, SZEWCZYK, Bartlomiej, PYTEL, Paulina, KRZESŁOWSKA, Wiktoria Julia, HOŁOWNIA, Weronika and WIŚNIEWSKI, Szymon. Understanding and Managing Atopic Dermatitis: Insights into Pathogenesis and Treatment Strategies. *Quality in Sport.* Online. 30 September 2024. Vol. 22, p. 55014. [Accessed 12 June 2025]. DOI 10.12775/QS.2024.22.55014. (accessed on 12 May 2025).

56. Terhaar, H., Jiminez, V., Grant, E., Collins, C., Khass, M., & Yusuf, N. (2024). Immune repertoires in various dermatologic and autoimmune diseases. *Genes, 15.* https://www.semanticscholar.org/paper/71a7a727de4606326a1604ebd7f095a5435d1f57 (accessed on 12 May 2025).

57. Tottoli, E. M., Dorati, R., Genta, I., Chiesa, E., Pisani, S., & Conti, B. (2020). Skin wound healing process and new emerging technologies for skin wound care and regeneration. *Pharmaceutics, 12*, 735. https://doi.org/10.3390/pharmaceutics12080735.

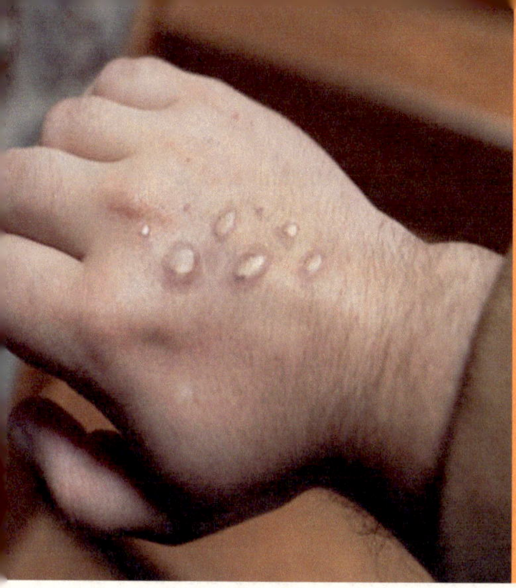

Chapter 4

INFECTIOUS SKIN DISEASES

Contents

Introduction

Human skin is not merely a protective barrier; it is the body's primary face to the world, and it is always hanging out with thousands of microbes. Most of the time, the skin's ecosystem, commonly referred to as the microbiota, has a gigantic role in keeping things copacetic by assisting the immune system and keeping unwanted microbes at bay. More often than not, when this small community is disrupted—a situation usually referred to as dysbiosis—it appears to manifest in tandem with several skin ailments that can be quite frustrating to deal with in the clinical environment. In general terms, understanding the confused interactions between our skin's natural condition and these tiny roommates is sort of the key to understanding how infectious skin issues begin and, consequently, developing improved treatments (Anderska et al., 2025). In the real world, nature itself can agitate more havoc. Climate change, say, appears to play havoc with nearly everything—temperature, humidity, and even air pollution, and all told, it ends up leaving our skin more vulnerable to infection. Global warming and declining ozone leave us exposed to more UV radiation, which, given time, can thin out the skin's immune defenses and allow pathogens to move in more readily. And daily pollutants at times bring about inflammatory responses that weaken our skin's protective barriers even further. These changing circumstances obviously suggest more conscious and responsive public health policies in combating skin infections (Anderska et al., 2025). And then there is the role of the way we live our lives. Exercises involving a lot of skin-to-skin contact, such as wrestling and gymnastics, tend to result in small tears in the skin layer and even faster germ spread. It seriously illustrates how our everyday routines are able to increase the risk of infections, entwining with those minuscule microbial partners we just discussed. Not to mention, the skin also produces its own antimicrobial peptides—little warriors, essentially—that attempt to ward off the bad stuff. Our natural defenses and healthy practices aid in reducing the progress of infections, directing the treatment choice and prevention steps in the long term (Mennitti et al., 2025).

Definition of Infectious Skin Diseases

Skin and mucosal surfaces usually signify that point where our bodies and the rest of the world come together—they are at once a rugged barrier and an active immune area. Daily, these areas come under attack from all sorts of environmental debris, including the microbe invaders that could be a problem. Essentially, when our built-in defenses' balance against the invading microbes fails, skin infections can establish themselves. One nice aspect of our skin's first line of defense is its arsenal of sensors, commonly referred to as PRRs, which detect special molecular markers, referred to as PAMPs, found only on bad guys. When these sensors are activated, they trigger an immune attack designed to neutralize or boot out the baddies. Concurrently, our body recruits adaptive immune power from lymphoid tissues to maintain things under control and ward off additional invasions. In a majority of situations, the sophisticated, dynamic dance between what our body performs and the environmental microbials forms the basis of these infectious diseases (Oscar and Pearay, 2019). There are so many different infections of the skin out there - from those ignited by bacteria, viruses, fungus, and even parasites that infiltrate or colonize the skin - and they can appear almost anywhere and in pretty much any variety. The specific manner in which an infection occurs typically indicates not only which microbe is the culprit, but also how our body's defense system responds. Fundamentally, the defining characteristic of these diseases is how dangerous microbes get into skin layers and begin to multiply, frequently causing explosions of inflammation. You may experience this with red patches, rashes, lesions, or even ulcers which indicate that something is seriously wrong. That is, to grasp these infections, you must observe how the pathogens get around our defenses and cause subsequent immune reactions. It turns out that, apart from just being a covering, the skin plays a critical role in our overall immune system, and that is why it is both vulnerable to attack and so important system-wide (Oscar and Pearay, 2019). Consider, for instance, dermatological conditions such as cutaneous tuberculosis—this type of case sheds light on just how challenging it can be to identify and treat such infections, particularly when individuals are already vulnerable. Tuberculosis, which is Mycobacterium tuberculosis, sometimes presents in the skin with a vast range of symptoms that bewilder conventional diagnostic tools. While some would maintain that relying on symptom-based diagnosis can be quite sound if strict clinical criteria are employed (especially in low-resource environments), no one can deny it gets complicated. For example, the host's immune status can have a tremendous influence on how the disease manifests and whether we can get the diagnosis nailed down, demonstrating that such infections are far from simple. By and large, these diagnostic challenges underscore how critical it is to combine clinical wisdom with a thorough understanding of immune responses to truly address skin infections properly.

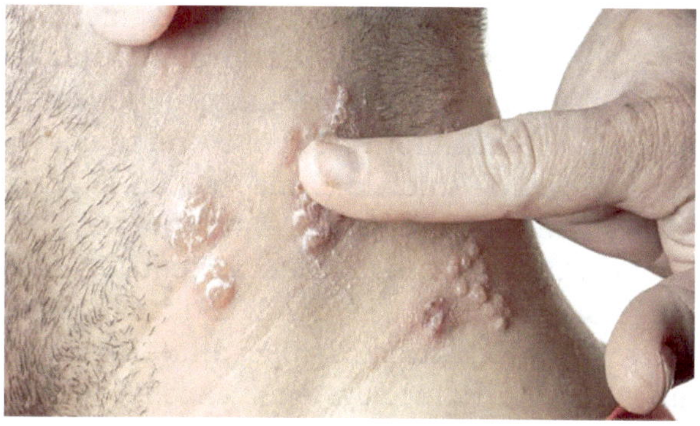

Source: RVO Health. (2025). *Slide 4: Skin Infections.* https://media.post.rvohealth.io/wp-content/uploads/2025/02/642x361_Slide_4_Skin_Infections.jpg.

Importance of Studying Skin Infections

In most of the globe, infectious diseases continue to be a big problem, particularly where medical care is not available. Skin infections, for example, usually do not receive attention despite appearing all the time and can develop difficult complications when left untreated. Scientists have observed that these skin problems if left untreated, can provide insight into why bacteria continue to become more resistant to medications. Resistant microbes continue to emerge, and overall, we require more comprehensive data to inform more effective treatment strategies and public health guidelines. Obtaining a glimpse of how prevalent skin insects resist not only informs focused initiatives to diminish sickness and mortality but also necessitates combining clinical observations with larger patterns of antimicrobial resistance (Christopher et al., 2022). In the practice of medicine, being able to precisely identify why a skin infection begins, how it is transmitted, and what its signs and symptoms are is crucial for speedy and correct diagnosis—this, in turn, is a big help for the patient. Occasionally, such infections start out as trivial superficial lesions and can suddenly develop into serious, even life-threatening cases that necessitate immediate attention. It becomes even more complex when there are issues like diabetes, weakened immune systems, and even discrepancies in age or sex involved; these factors dictate who is most at risk and how the infection manifests. I find myself regularly noticing that it is truly valuable to know all these details, even if I repeat them once or twice to drive the point home, when it comes to establishing treatment regimens that are as individualized as the patient's situation. This improved clinical profile, in the majority of instances, improves responses to treatment, reduces hospital admissions, and is able to decrease total healthcare expenditures by preventing infections from becoming systemic issues (Valent et al., 2012). In addition to direct patient management, research on skin infections also has an important role in public health planning and education. Normally, these conditions are all indicative of larger problems, such as daily hygiene habits and whether individuals easily have access to medical facilities. By examining trends and observing how patterns of resistance emerge, health officials can create preventive measures that address the underlying causes and reduce the likelihood of further spread. In addition to that, constant research calls for the discovery of new antibiotics, vaccines, and control schemes specially formulated to combat resistant strains that most adversely impact vulnerable populations. Such a broad perspective not only assists in preventing future outbreaks but also maintains health systems agile enough to cope with unforeseen challenges. Finally, cutaneous infections reflect how closely medical care, microbiology, and public health correlate in our fight against infectious illness worldwide (Valent et al., 2012).

Importance of Treatment

Successful control of infectious skin conditions depends on early and effective treatment to avoid complications and contain the spread of pathogens. Infections can break down the skin's protective barrier function, leading to tissue integrity disruption and enhanced microbial invasion. Therapies that are judiciously chosen not only kill the causative microorganisms but also aid in restoring the skin barrier. For instance, the application of topical antiseptics such as chlorhexidine gluconate (CHG) provides considerable antimicrobial advantage, as evidenced by its capacity to significantly decrease bacterial load when properly applied. However, concentrations beyond certain levels have the potential to harm the skin's protective properties, highlighting the need to strike a balance between antimicrobial activity and avoiding injury to skin cells. These results emphasize the essential importance of tailoring treatment protocols to both cure infection and maintain skin integrity, highlighting the greater role of treatment in the management of infectious skin infections while protecting the body's natural defenses (Matsuda et al., 2025). In addition to antimicrobial use, prompt diagnosis and treatment of infectious skin diseases are necessary to the prevention of their development and resultant systemic complications. The complex ecosystem of microorganisms and keratinocytes in the skin works together to suppress pathogenic colonization, but these defenses can be breached if not addressed immediately. Timely and precise diagnosis enables clinicians to institute specific therapies that minimize the infectious load and avert the establishment of chronic lesions or secondary infections. Furthermore, technological advancements, such as artificial intelligence (AI), have greatly improved diagnostic precision and treatment approaches for skin infections. This advancement allows for more targeted and efficient care plans, which are invaluable in light of the heterogeneity of pathogens involved and variability in patient immune responses. The significance of treatment, therefore, goes beyond curing the infection—it also entails intervention strategies that maximize skin healing, lower healthcare expenses, and enhance patient quality of life (Han et al., 2024). In addition, proper management of infectious skin conditions is also a critical element in the fight against more general public health issues like antimicrobial resistance. Dependence on systemic antibiotics for the treatment of superficial skin infections may encourage the development of resistant bacterial strains that will make subsequent treatment difficult. Therefore, therapeutic models increasingly opt for local treatments, like diluted topical antiseptics, to reduce systemic exposure while still offering antimicrobial efficacy. As studies show, local CHG at moderate concentrations may safely decrease bacterial numbers without compromising the skin barrier functions and thus represent a potential alternative to systemic medications. This subtle insight underpins rational decision-making concerning infection control alongside reducing resistance potential. Thus, the value of therapy for infectious cutaneous diseases extends beyond the care of individual patients and affects approaches to the management of microbial resistance at a population level, demonstrating the essential interaction of clinical practice with public health principles.

4.1. Types of Infectious Skin Diseases

Skin infections may take a lot of different forms and may be quite difficult to identify. Different germs—bacteria, viruses, fungi, and even parasites—are commonly responsible for them. Bacteria, for example, are responsible for things like impetigo, cellulitis, or erysipelas; these typically appear as red, swollen spots that sometimes have pus oozing from them. There are also viral causes, like herpes simplex or varicella-zoster, which cause small clusters of blisters on the skin. Fungus microbes, such as those responsible for ringworm or candidiasis, typically cause scaling, redness, and itching, either just on the surface or deeper. And do not forget parasites; consider scabies from mites, for instance, notorious for intense itching and those characteristic burrow tracks. In most instances, the symptoms may overlap, so it is crucial that doctors pin down precisely what germ is responsible. This combination truly illustrates the necessity of careful testing in the treatment of these conditions. Occasionally, the body's own immune system can introduce an added level of complexity. When skin infections occur, mast cells tend to get involved—though we typically associate them with mastocytosis, and this can cause additional symptoms such as itching, flushing, or even hives. This response is commonly referred to as mast cell activation syndrome (MCAS), a type of cascade that increases the skin problems beyond what the infection would naturally induce.

All in all, identifying these immune side effects is important, as it could indicate that other treatments in addition to antibiotics or other anti-microbial regimens are required. How MCAS is diagnosed, by examining mediator release and the way symptoms resolve when those mediators are inhibited, gives physicians some helpful tools to unravel complicated cases (Valent et al., 2012). Briefly, monitoring these immune signals can truly enhance treatment results and care in general. Other skin infections also extend into larger public health issues, particularly when they intersect with body-wide infections or strike vulnerable populations severely. Consider skin tuberculosis, for example. While not the most prevalent type, it can be a significant problem and is sometimes found in individuals such as refugees or immunocompromised children. Epidemiological information generally reveals foreign-born children to be at greater risk for TB, so physicians may have to conduct rigorous screening , through examinations such as the old tuberculin skin test or the interferon-gamma release assay, to find latent infections.

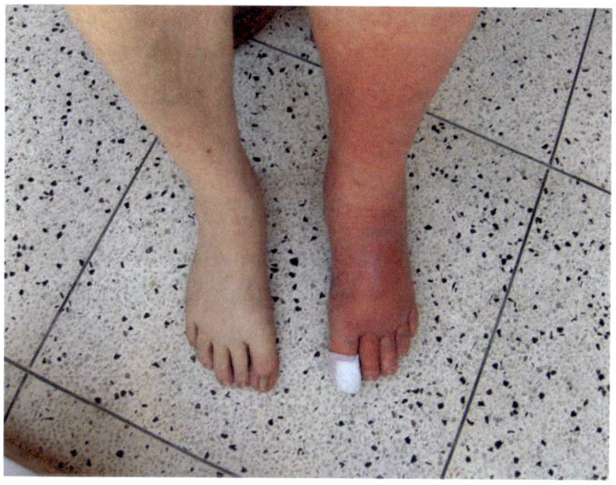

Figure 4.1. Skin infection.

Source: CC BY-SA 3.0, https://commons.wikimedia.org/w/index.php?curid=1517111

These are not all the same; interferon-gamma release assays, for instance, tend to reduce false positives in individuals vaccinated with BCG. TB that involves the skin requires a combination of prompt diagnosis, the appropriate type of antimicrobial treatment, and other public health efforts to assist populations that have been displaced in an effort to suppress transmission (Lamb , 2019). All this serves to illustrate how certain skin infections have a close connection with broader social and health problems (Figure 4.1).

4.1.1. Bacterial Infections

Bacterial infections of the skin are a serious concern, particularly when people find themselves in close proximity. Take contact sports, for instance – players collide with each other throughout the game and exchange equipment that can easily transfer microbes such as methicillin-resistant *Staphylococcus aureus* (MRSA). Oftentimes, these germs create red areas on the skin, small abscesses, or even frank cellulitis – and if you allow them to run wild, the issue can spread all over the body. As a general rule, the fix is to identify the problem ahead of time, practice good hygiene, and follow sound cleaning habits. Both coaches and athletes must be taught the early warning signs and adhere to fastidious cleanliness; not only does this reduce infection rates but also keeps teams from experiencing unnecessary downtime (Kucharczyk et al., 2025). Consider, for example, how some bacteria function—this is a twist in treating skin infections. *Streptococcus pyogenes*, a Gram-positive microbe, is an example. It is said to be responsible for a range of complaints from an uncomplicated sore throat to severe skin infections such as impetigo and cellulitis. Reports tend to observe its seasonal highs and lows and the way that it has a pronounced effect on children in schools and daycare. A timely antibiotic treatment, particularly penicillin, is often effective in most cases since the microbe tends to retain its sensitivity. However, if left untreated, things can suddenly turn into complications, which truly speaks to the necessity of vigilant monitoring and quick action. Public health surveillance of these infections, in essence, is still paramount to avoiding bigger outbreaks and alleviating the overall disease burden of the community (Maris et al., 2024).

Management and prevention of such infections require a combination of approaches to respond to the various ways bacteria present and circulate. Both systemic and topical antibiotics frequently comprise our first line of weaponry, chosen depending on severity and the microbe's resistance pattern. But here is the catch—increasing antibiotic resistance requires us to use these drugs carefully and even investigate additional prevention strategies such as vaccines where it is appropriate. Apart from medications, basic changes in behavior like enhanced personal cleanliness, not sharing personal items, and proper wound care can pay dividends. In high-risk areas such as contact sports, regular screening and even quarantine of infected patients can serve to keep the spread under control. Combining medical treatment with preventive proactive measures is often seen to have better results and mitigate the disruptions brought about by these diseases (Kucharczyk et al., 2025) (Figure 4.2).

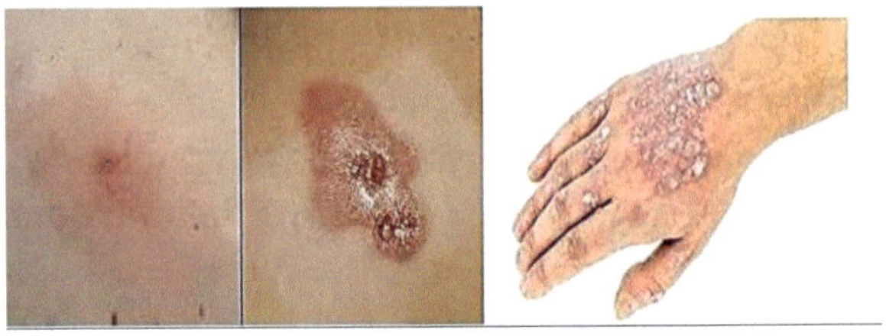

Figure 4.2. Spread of bacterial infection.

Source: Aljamali, N. M., Alzubaidy, Z. H., & Enad, A. H. (2021). Spread of bacterial infection. In Bacterial infection and common bacterial diseases: A Review. *Trends in Pharmaceuticals and Nanotechnology, 3*(2), 13–22.

4.1.2. Viral Infections

Coping with infections is not merely a case of fighting bacteria or fungi –; viruses that infect the skin add another kink in the works. These annoying viral problems have a nasty habit of occurring in all manner of ways, from dense groups of blisters to rashes that break out in unexpected patterns, which tends to make it quite difficult to work out what is happening. In environments such as sports communities, where bodily contact is the standard, these viruses jump from person to person before you can say Jack Robinson; focused preventive action becomes essential. Vaccinations, in general terms, have a large role to play here as well: inoculations against influenza, whooping cough, and even meningitis reduce contagion in communal settings. It is not just an individual protective shield – these steps prevent populations like athletic teams or school communities from getting hurt in general. Ultimately, managing these infections entails combining good hygiene habits, prophylactic medications, and immunizations together with each other in one versatile, layered regimen (Luke & d'Hemecourt, 2007). The interaction between our immune systems and the environment determines the frequency and severity with which these viral skin afflictions strike. Although numerous studies have investigated how viruses act in human populations, the same research on organic livestock – whose health can influence disease transmission to humans – is much rarer. Organic farming, with all its offbeat ecological and immune-related considerations, may alter the extent to which susceptible animals are affected by these viral pests or even modify how skin disease arises. Since organic operations tend to bypass the customary antibiotics and chemical solutions, they may be more vulnerable, so exploring further this aspect of things is certainly justified. Investigating why various breeds react and the influence of environmental stressors may offer some insight as to why such viral skin diseases erupt or deteriorate, and ultimately contribute toward the development of larger-scale initiatives to contain zoonotic viruses that could become bothersome for human skin wellness (Luke & d'Hemecourt, 2007). Fresh viral threats keep putting holes into the set scripts for the avoidance and management of skin infections. Because viruses are continually in motion, perpetually changing, there is indeed a call to study new antiviral drugs and immune-enhancing vaccines that honor both clinical necessities and ecological realities. Particularly in organic environments where genetically modified vaccines may conflict with fundamental principles, discovering alternative methods of vaccination is critical in order to keep these pests in check without undermining organic principles. And it does not end there – public health campaigns need to ensure that individuals receive uncomplicated, no-nonsense information regarding how viruses are transmitted and why good hygiene counts, especially where infections spread quickly in certain areas. Combining the findings of vets, medical professionals, and environmental scientists might be the way to unlock better, more flexible strategies for managing these cunning skin viruses. This kind of comprehensive game strategy could lead to more effective prevention, treatment, and containment efforts in the future (Luke & d'Hemecourt, 2007) (Figure 4.3).

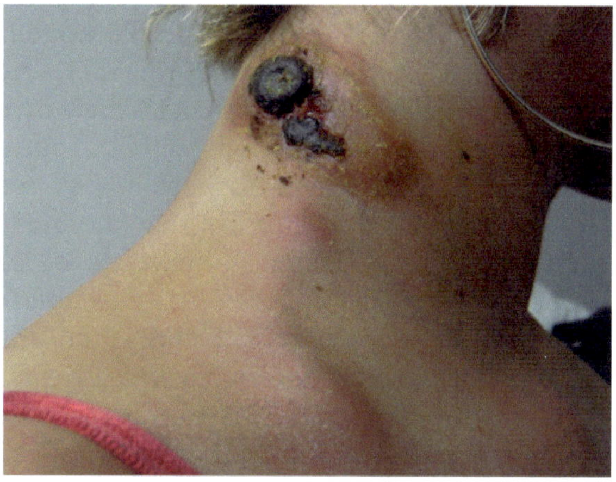

Figure 4.3. Necrotic lesion and lymphangitis due to cowpox virus infection.

Source: Wollenberg, A., Vogel, S., Sárdy, M., Glos, K., Prkno, A., Hoffmann, D., et al. (2012). Necrotic lesion and lymphangitis due to cowpox virus infection (patient 1). In The Munich outbreak of cutaneous cowpox infection: Transmission by infected pet rats. *Acta Dermato-Venereologica, 92*(1), 126–131.

4.1.3. Fungal Infections

Infectious skin problems are a medical doctor's worst nightmare since they originate from a variety of causes and appear in so many different forms. Fungal infections, for instance, appear to thrive particularly well in warm, moist areas—that is why football players in collision sports tend to get them. These fungi, particularly those dermatophytes which are fond of keratin (which is present on our skin, hair, and nails), like to persist in areas where cleanliness tends to fall short. They spread directly from skin-to-skin contact or indirectly when equipment and surfaces are not cleaned well enough. All of this makes it rather obvious that understanding what you are working with—how it presents and how it travels—is the key to keeping outbreaks under control and making sure training or games are not disrupted (Kucharczyk et al., 2025). If you examine dermatophytosis more closely, it is clear why identifying the specific fungus is so important. Pathogens such as *Microsporum canis*, *M. gypseum*, and Trichophyton mentagrophytes cause their own distinct inflammatory reactions. Think about it this way: you notice hair loss, scaling, or red areas at times, punctuated by that annoying itch. Because these manifestations can be so nonspecific, physicians most often must piece together what they observe in the exam with some lab work to truly determine which fungus is causing the problem. This is not only for selecting the proper antifungal cream or tablet, but it also sets up how to prevent further spread, particularly when animals are involved, such as with skin infections in dogs. The treatments can be as simple as applying a topical agent or as serious as systemic therapy, so it definitely pays to customize the therapy for each instance (Elânia et al., 2024). Prevention, however, is where much of the war against fungal skin infections is fought and won. In situations such as group living or group sports, where infection can take off quickly, enlightening competitors regarding proper hygiene, disinfecting shared equipment aggressively, and identifying skin problems early on make a significant impact. , keeping anyone infected relatively segregated and making sure that wounds get attended to properly can significantly reduce the risk of transmission. Because fungal infections strike from many sides, it requires an effort from all members of the team—from coaches to medical professionals to the athletes themselves—to implement plans that work and target specifically. And, by and large, staying current on research about more accurate diagnostics and more potent antifungal medications is important if we want to cut down on infections in both humans and animals (Elânia et al., 2024; Kucharczyk et al., 2025) (Figure 4.4).

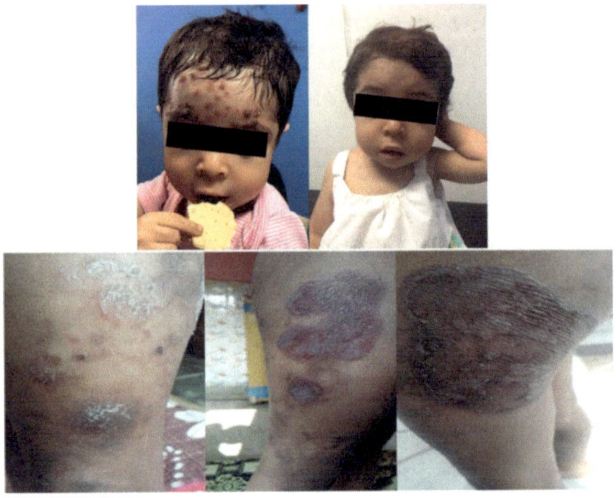

Figure 4.4. Pictures of fungal skin lesions in two girls with STAT1-GOF. Upper panel: Cutaneous fungal infection resembling cryptococcosis in patient 1, before (left), and after antifungal treatment. Lower panel: Verrucous *Tinea corporis* on the thighs of patient (With authorization from the patients' mother).

Source: Staines-Boone, A. T., Vignesh, P., Tsumura, M., Lugo-Reyes, S. O., & others. (2023). Pictures of fungal skin lesions in two girls with STAT1-GOF. In Fatal COVID-19 infection in two children with STAT1 gain-of-function. *Journal of Clinical Immunology, 43(6)*, 1112–1120.

4.2. Common Bacterial Skin Infections

Bacterial skin infections continue to appear increasingly frequently these days, and they quite literally leave both healthcare professionals and patients in a bind. Impetigo, cellulitis, and folliculitis come to mind for most individuals here. Impetigo predominantly affects children and appears as red, infectious patches that tend to have their roots in microbes such as *Staphylococcus aureus* or *Streptococcus pyogenes*. When an infection penetrates deeper (consider cellulitis), it can result in swelling, redness, and even fever, making things considerably more serious—as if the infection had decided to settle in for the long term. And then there is folliculitis, a hair follicle irritation that frequently results in those pesky, pus-filled bumps and overall discomfort. Although antibiotics typically take care of these problems, the misuse, and even overuse—of broad-spectrum antibiotics since penicillin was first isolated back in 1928 has created resistant strains, diminished the effectiveness of routine treatments, and increased the chances of complications (Lillestolen , 2018). Clearly, prudent antibiotic use is not optional—it is mandatory. There is also an interesting connection between these human medical issues and animal husbandry practices. Organic farming practices, guided by global standards such as the IFOAM standards and even EU regulation 2092/91 (Eijck et al., 2006), do their best to restrict drug usage while maximizing the welfare of the animals. For most instances, these practices work to keep zoonotic bacteria—those that can leap from animals to humans and infect them similarly on the skin—at bay. Organic farming allows animals to act naturally and does not stress them out, which naturally strengthens immunity, many think, and decreases infection rates, so fewer antibiotics are needed. Some infections remain, though, even despite these efforts, and employing fewer of the traditional antibiotics may at times allow certain bacteria to stay in livestock a bit too long, with a potential to spread to humans. This complicated interplay of farming practices and infection control demonstrates how many elements go into managing infectious diseases. Diagnosing and treating these bacterial skin infections requires a blended approach—mating street-level clinical intuition with new perspectives from both medicine and agriculture disciplines. As long as we rely on antibiotics, stewardship is crucial in managing resistance; at the same time, other therapies are still in the process of being discovered, especially in practice such as organic livestock production where usual drug consumption is minimal (Eijck et al., 2006). Clinicians must monitor arising resistant strains and modify treatment accordingly to achieve optimum outcomes for patients. In addition to that, emphasizing good hygiene practices, early intervention, and continuous education can facilitate the alleviation of such infections. Antibiotic resistance, therefore, becomes a multidisciplinary problem cutting across human medicine, veterinary medicine, and agricultural policies (Lillestolen , 2018). In the vast majority of cases, additional study and wise investment in novel antimicrobial approaches and preventive measures hold the key to alleviating the burden of bacterial skin infections and maintaining our therapies effective in the long term.

4.2.1. Impetigo

Our skin is really good at keeping germs away, but even a small cut or a pesky bug bite can compromise that barrier and invite unwanted microbes in – sometimes initiating conditions such as impetigo. It begins as red, swollen spots that suddenly become tiny pus-filled bumps topped with a honey-colored crust. Children most often get struck first, although adults are not entirely exempt. *Staphylococcus aureus* and *Streptococcus pyogenes* are the most common culprits, taking advantage of any opening in the skin to establish a localized infection. Because it is very contagious, however, impetigo becomes a genuine public health concern when individuals are close together or when there is not proper cleanliness. The issue is not only bacteria growth; there is also an acute inflammation that really forms the appearance of the condition. Treating it, in general, involves balancing firm antimicrobial activity with increasing worries about antibiotic resistance, which in turn generates interest in other treatment and prevention concepts (Tang et al., 2025). Getting a little deeper into the story shows just how complicated things can become between our body's defenses and the underhanded tactics of these microbes. Recent research, for instance, indicates that how our antibodies respond may alter the trajectory and severity of skin infections, occasionally exacerbating them or even providing some protection. Despite the fact that impetigo is typically a short, localized episode, the entire back-and-forth between pathogens and immunity reinforces why obtaining an accurate diagnosis and treatment designed specifically for the patient is so critical. Scientists with some very sophisticated genetics and immunological techniques , such as genome-wide association studies – continue to discover how infections trigger and sustain inflammation in the skin. These observations are important not just for a disease such as impetigo but also for other chronic inflammatory skin diseases, where microbial influences appear to have a large, sometimes surprising, influence on how much of a problem the condition can become (Li et al., 2024).

With antibiotic resistance spreading, alternative treatments are attracting increasing interest on the global skin infections scene. Consider moxibustion, for example – an ancient technique from traditional Chinese medicine that employs heat and the special properties of burning moxa. Anciently, it has been used to treat many skin ailments, and while its place in the treatment of infections such as impetigo is still being sorted out, initial indications are sort of promising. Its complex set of biological effects may be able to modify local immune reactions and enhance tissue repair, which may reduce our reliance on traditional antibiotics and minimize resistance threats. Of course, more stringent clinical trials, and some precise, mechanistic investigations—are required to truly establish its safety and efficacy. Merging such traditional methods with contemporary standards of medicine may well provide a multi-faceted approach to the treatment of impetigo and other such infections, perfectly accommodating the trends and demands in infectious disease studies today (Tang et al., 2025) (Figure 4.5).

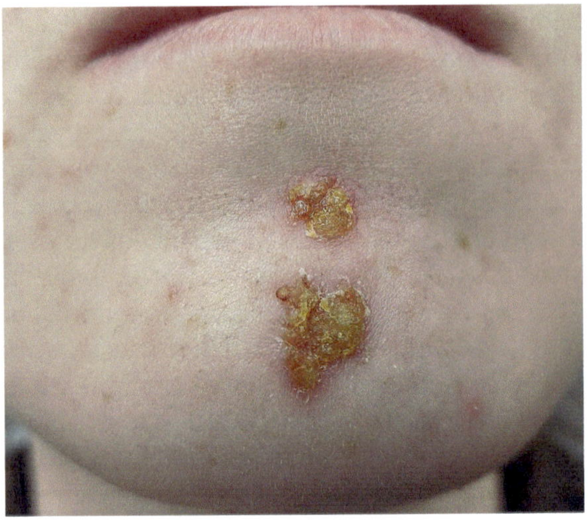

Figure 4.5. A case of impetigo on the chin.

Source: Heilman, J. (2000). Impetigo. *Wikimedia Commons.*

4.2.2. Cellulitis

Our skin generally does a fairly good job of keeping the unwanted microbes out, but even a small cut or scratch can allow bacteria to sneak in. Cellulitis, for instance, is an everyday but potentially serious infection that makes the deeper layers of the skin swell suddenly. Usually, bacteria such as *Streptococcus pyogenes* or *Staphylococcus aureus* capitalize on even small ruptures in the skin, sometimes from minor cuts or even ulcerations—to initiate an infection. You may see red areas that are warm and tender with some swelling, and in most cases, a fever or that overall feeling of being "under the weather.." Unless the diagnosis is made early, the infection can accelerate its process, and one can develop complications such as abscess or even a dissemination throughout the body. Treatment, in general, consists of administering the appropriate antibiotics depending on the causative germ, with additional care for controlling pain and swelling. Determining how and why cellulitis occurs is the most important way to keep it in check (Eric et al., 2019). It does not make it easier that each patient may have a slightly different presentation, and other conditions such as deep vein thrombosis, stasis dermatitis, or contact dermatitis can look very similar to cellulitis and frequently lead physicians down the wrong path if they are not vigilant. In certain cases, chronic edema from lymphedema or diabetes, which disrupts the local immune response—can result in recurring episodes of cellulitis. While newer imaging and laboratory methods have enhanced the ability to distinguish cellulitis from other dermatologic disorders, much of diagnosis continues to depend on clinical acumen. And then there is the issue of MRSA, a type that is becoming all too prevalent in certain areas, leading clinicians to cover these resistant organisms at times from the get-go. In the majority of instances, a tailored strategy that considers both the patient's unique findings and local patterns is the best bet (Eric et al., 2019). In terms of treatment, the idea will be to hit the antibiotics as early as possible while also adhering to the principles of symptom relief in the meantime. Physicians tend to begin treatment in a fashion that targets both Streptococcus and Staphylococcus, and then refine the strategy if culture reports provide more direction. For the less severe cases, oral antibiotics such as cephalexin or dicloxacillin are typically sufficient, but where there is a more severe infection or the overall state of the patient is poor, intravenous antibiotics take over. In addition to the medication, as little as elevation of the infected limb, pain control, and adequate amounts of fluids can make a big difference in decreasing the inflammation. It also cannot hurt to emphasize preventive care, such as simple skin hygiene, treating any persisting fungal infections (e.g., tinea), and attempting to avoid even small skin traumas—as these measures can forestall subsequent episodes. Even with enhanced medical treatments, cellulitis remains a formidable foe in healthcare. A managed protocol across primary care, dermatology, and infectious diseases usually produces improved results, particularly with complex or recurrent cases (Eric et al., 2019) (Figure 4.6).

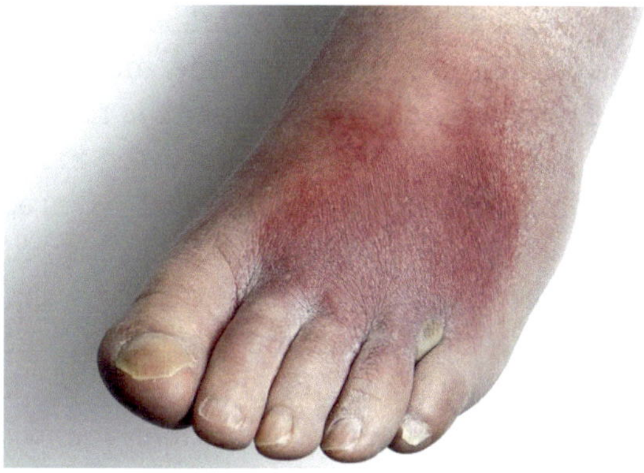

Figure 4.6. Cellulitis.

Source: Science Photo Library. (n.d.). Cellulitis of the foot. *NHS.*

4.2.3. Folliculitis

Sometimes microbes infiltrate by way of the smallest skin scratches and initiate a domino effect that culminates in disease, and folliculitis is one such process. Hair follicles can become colonized, typically with *Staphylococcus aureus*, and that colonization induces a localized episode of inflammation that cannot be ignored. It is fascinating how the architecture of a follicle itself becomes a snug little haven for these germs, particularly when the skin's natural barriers are low or local immunity is out of control. You may see red, pimple-like bumps that are painful or itchy, and really, this illustrates how the battle between microbial mayhem and our own defenses is more nuanced than it appears. In the majority of instances, fundamental hygiene and environmental conditions also affect whether or not these germs become established, highlighting the difficulty of controlling skin infections effectively. Diagnosing these follicular eruptions is not always easy, primarily since they may resemble a great deal of other skin conditions like acne or dermatitis. Usually, physicians need to dig deeper—performing cultures or even a biopsy—to determine precisely which microbe is causing the problem (Talapko et al., 2021). At other times, fungal perpetrators such as specific varieties of Candida come into play, particularly when the immune system is somewhat compromised. For the most part, treatment is individualized to both the microbe and the patient: mild infections may be helped by a cream or topical antibacterial, whereas more resistant or diffuse infections may call for systemic antibiotics. In addition to that, steps to reduce the itch and prevent further complications are significant aspects of the complete plan, repeating suggestions found in guidelines for chronic itch management (Wei et al., 2019).

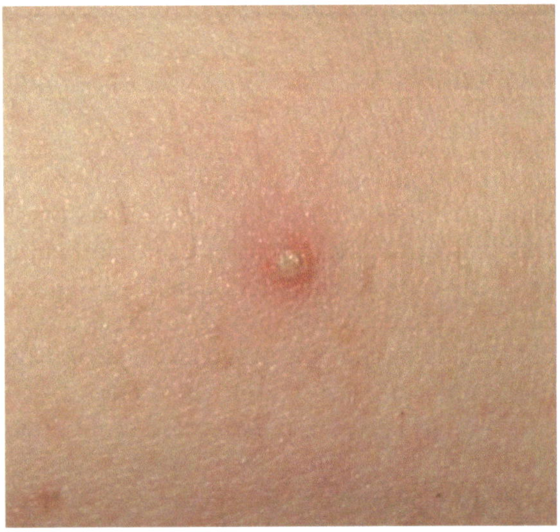

Figure 4.7. Folliculitis, single lesion.

Source: Jmarchn. (2015). Isolated folliculitis. *Wikimedia Commons.*

Maintaining the skin's barrier is paramount to preventing folliculitis. Normal activities, such as proper wound care, good hygiene, and even less tight or occlusive clothing—can all assist in reducing the risk of infection. Those with compromised immune systems or existing skin problems must be vigilant, as what begins as minor irritation sometimes can quickly become a bigger issue. With antibiotic-resistant pests becoming more prevalent today, clinicians are looking more and more for alternative antimicrobial agents and new therapies. Public health measures and patient education also contribute significantly to preventing these infections from recurring. Folliculitis not only appears regularly in clinical practice but also serves as a reminder of the larger issues of dealing with infectious skin disease (Figure 4.7).

4.3. Common Viral Skin Infections

Viral skin infections appear quite a lot when individuals spend time in close proximity. You might even see that outbreaks tend to spread rapidly in situations such as sports, where skin-to-skin contact is involved and there is the added factor of shared equipment. HSV , the herpes simplex virus , is a common pathogen. It usually causes painful blisters around the mouth or genitals in most instances, but among athletes, it sometimes manifests as "herpes gladiatorum" in such areas as the face, head, and arms from contact during competition. Early diagnosis, rapid isolation, and proper antiviral treatment are usually important for mitigating the spread, while frequent cleaning of communal equipment and proper personal hygiene also avoid outbreaks (Kucharczyk et al., 2025). Our skin provides a first line of defense, but it is not infallible, particularly under the physical stress of sports activities. Ongoing sweating, rubbing, and small abrasions can compromise this natural defense, allowing viruses to penetrate. It is because of this that you may notice conditions such as molluscum contagiosum or HPV, usually presenting as small bumps or warts—persisting if not treated early. Add to that contact with challenging surfaces further increasing the risk; regular dermatologist visits can go a long way towards identifying these issues before they have long-term complications (Szot et al., 2024). As for treatment, a combination of treatments and clever precautions is the answer. In addition to taking antiviral drugs, it is also very helpful to follow good hygiene habits and not share personal belongings, particularly for those who are at greater risk such as athletes. Washing hands thoroughly and drying them well, and treating cuts and scrapes immediately, reduces viral entry points. Coaches and medical professionals, by keeping an eye out for early indications, can isolate cases earlier and prevent wider outbreaks. For the most part, a little more study about how these viruses is transmitted and streamlining prevention strategies will better equip us to manage these skin conditions in tight living settings (Szot et al., 2024; Kucharczyk et al., 2025).

4.3.1. Herpes Simplex Virus

Skin infections take a variety of forms, and of those some of the viral ones just make life difficult, particularly in full clinics or in cases involving athletes. HSV is unique; it is primarily transmitted through actual skin contact, which is why contact sports can increase the risk. You usually find it in the form of painful blisters on parts such as the face or hands, and outbreaks can not only be uncomfortable but also tamper with individuals' capacity to engage in regular activities. In close-knit communities, an outbreak can easily go viral, so getting it figured out quickly and managing it properly is crucial. Unlike a fungal or bacterial problem, this virus requires a different approach, so it is a particularly difficult microbe to handle (Kucharczyk et al., 2025). Sometimes HSV is more than your average cold sore. At times and in most cases, it can become a serious skin issue such as Kaposi Varicelliform Eruptions—a more commonly known eczema herpeticum. This situation tends to crop up when the skin is already compromised in some way, like with long-term dermatitis or in individuals whose immune response is out of control , resulting in generalized and excruciating blistering with other bodily symptoms. It becomes a bit of an emergency situation where immediate, antiviral therapy (acyclovir, for instance) is needed to prevent things from becoming worse. In totality, tight surveillance and accommodative treatment scheme come a long way when dealing with these advanced manifestations of HSV (El-Masry et al., 2024). Prevention of HSV from establishing in teams, particularly within sports personnel, relies critically on intelligent protection and sound learning.

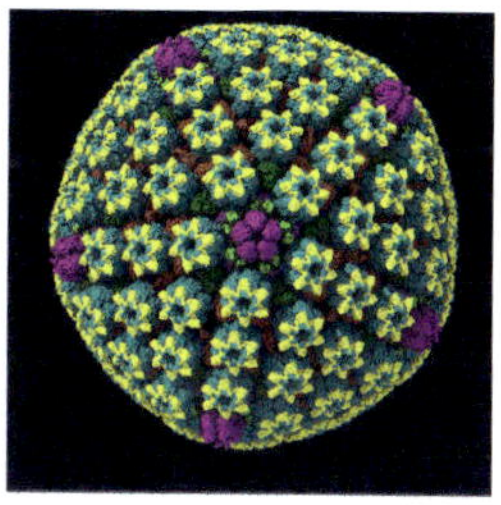

Figure 4.8. Herpes simplex virus.

Source: By Victoramuse - Own work, CC BY-SA 4.0, https://commons.wikimedia.org/w/index.php?curid=83926203

As the disease is contracted through direct transmission and even from off surfaces or athletic equipment, clean wounds and thoroughly sanitized apparatus must be the policy. It also pays if people with evident signs of infection are avoided from group activity until they are cleared to return—a strategy given some credibility when coaches and players remain vigilant. Since HSV tends to re-emerge and lay low in the body, these measures should not be a temporary measure but part of a broader public health initiative. Briefly put, combining early diagnosis, successful treatment, and continued prevention can reduce the burden of HSV in community as well as sports environments (Kucharczyk et al., 2025) (Figure 4.8).

4.3.2. Human Papillomavirus (HPV)

Infections involving skin lesions arise in a variety of unexpected manners, so their diagnosis and prevention is a bit of a tricky business. HPV, or Human papillomavirus (HPV), is a good example—there are more than 200 different types of this virus, each having its own peculiar way of interfacing with our tissues. It can infect both skin and mucosal surfaces and just hang around, which in general terms accounts for its ubiquitous prevalence. Its genetic material, a double helix of DNA wrapped in a protein shell, not only enables it to copy itself but even pushes cells to abnormal actions at times. You may have heard that types 16 and 18 tend to be associated with cancerous change, which is to say that the virus does more than result in slight skin issues. It is largely transmitted by skin-to-skin contact—typically in sexual situations, and a large number of the infections go undetected without symptoms, which makes controlling it even more difficult (Ireti et al., 2024). Even though HPV is long regarded as a sexually transmitted microbe, new evidence is obscuring that line. In most instances, non-sexual channels such as direct skin-to-skin contact can also initiate its spread, and evidence suggests it may be particularly so for women. Certain individuals, such as those who share needles in intravenous drug use, may experience additional risks, expanding the generally underappreciated range of transmission. Recognizing these varied pathways pushes us to look beyond the standard sexual health advice and broaden our efforts—this means rethinking surveillance and adjusting vaccine strategies to capture the full picture (Kawssan et al., 2024). Dealing with skin infections tied to HPV calls for a mixed approach. Vaccination, early testing, and treatments that match an individual's needs all come into play. Introduction of vaccines for the riskiest types of HPV was a true breakthrough, cutting incidence of cervical and other cancers associated with HPV in half. Around the same time, technologies such as HPV DNA testing have become more adept at detecting early warnings of danger, allowing physicians to intervene before it gets bad. Combined, these new instruments imply that we are moving towards a more specific method of addressing infectious skin ailments. However, initiating widespread vaccination is still a hard nut to crack, with issues of public education and equitable access even now. There are also rumors about future concepts, such as therapeutic vaccines, that may be used to treat active infections and mitigate the long-term impact of the virus (Ireti et al., 2024) (Figure 4.9).

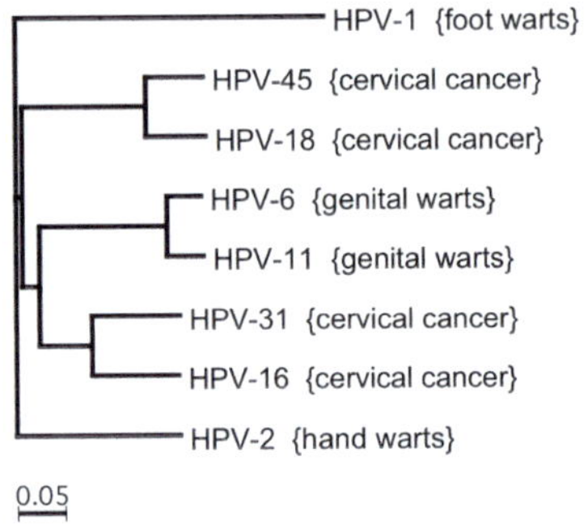

Figure 4.9. Human papillomavirus (HPV).

Source: By Remember the dot at English Wikipedia - Transferred from en.wikipedia to Commons by Premeditated Chaos using CommonsHelper., Public Domain, https://commons.wikimedia.org/w/index.php?curid=18827304

4.3.3. Varicella-Zoster Virus (Chickenpox)

Infectious skin conditions often start when a virus infiltrates, then goes into hiding again, only to emerge again unexpectedly. Consider VZV as an example, first appearing in children, it causes chickenpox with its complete rash and all those on-and-off symptoms such as fever and overall feeling of illness. Typically, once the first episode occurs, the virus simply remains dormant in the nerve groupings, as if in waiting for the time when it will erupt again. Despite most of the time this quiet period going by without too much fanfare, there are instances, particularly with individuals who are immunocompromised, pregnant, or neonatal—where the situation can become quite serious, which is part of why determining VZV's behavior is such a big deal (Gershon et al., 2018). Vaccination programs targeting chickenpox have genuinely reduced how frequently and severely the illness appears, which brings prevention into the spotlight. Years, and sometimes decades, later, things can change. The virus can re-emerge in a more agonizing manner, usually unsettling older persons, or those with compromised defenses with an ailment called shingles. This type of reemergence often strikes with a one-sided pain-and-blisters situation that follows a predictable nerve pattern, kind of like an aching ribbon along the skin. In most instances, the pain does not remain at the surface; it has the ability to cause neurological problems as well. Most individuals find themselves struggling with postherpetic neuralgia, a chronic aching that refuses to go away. And more dangerous options like encephalitis, localized muscle weakness (segmental motor paresis), or even vasculitis, sometimes requiring a combination of antiviral medications and steroids, exist. Even if that initial infection is a minor one, the likelihood of those subsequent complications brings us back to the realization that the virus will bite harder than anticipated (Gershon et al., 2018). Considering the bigger picture, how VZV unfolds in its course reveals a great deal about general public health issues. Chickenpox is primarily a childhood illness, while shingles is more likely to afflict the old—posing an image of the virus affecting different age brackets in widely differing ways. For most, live vaccines that utilize weakened forms of the virus have been implemented to maintain both chickenpox and shingles at bay; several developed nations now make these inoculations part of regular immunizations. Not only do these vaccines reduce the incidence of chickenpox, but they also lighten the heavy burden that shingles puts on older individuals. As more and more communities meet higher vaccination levels, monitoring disease patterns and how effective the vaccines are remains an important part of controlling these difficult skin infections (Pace , 2008) (Figure 4.10).

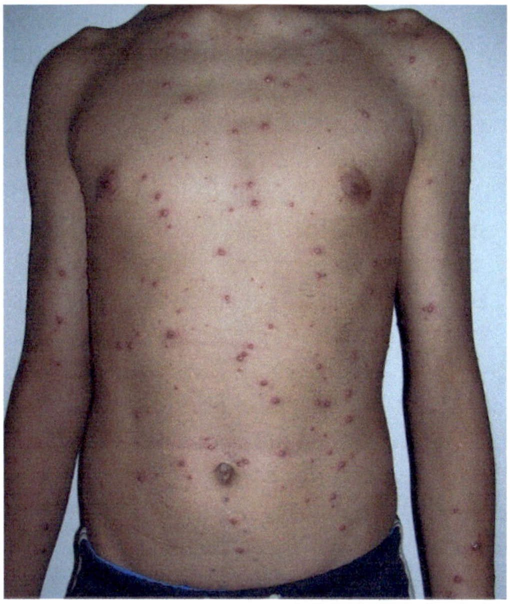

Figure 4.10. A patient presenting with the characteristic blisters of chickenpox.

Source: Aranzales, C. (2010). Varicela. *Wikimedia Commons.*

4.4. Common Fungal Skin Infections

Fungal infections of the skin are fairly prevalent and are apt to occur where individuals, well, stick close together or congregate—think locker rooms, group showers, or even dense sports facilities. These settings begin when fungi enter the outermost layers of skin, typically when defenses are weakened or when there is a tiny breach in the skin barrier. As a general rule, a cluster of organisms called dermatophytes consisting of forms such as Trichophyton, Microsporum, and Epidermophyton is responsible for infections such as *Tinea corporis*, tinea pedis, and tinea capitis. Most often, particularly in contact sports where ongoing skin-to-skin contact makes clean habits a bit of a challenge, these fungi flourish, at times causing a great deal of discomfort and even halting activity. Having good personal hygiene and an eye out for early signs, however, is really the bottom line to maintaining control over an outbreak and decreasing risk among high-risk individuals (Kucharczyk et al., 2025). These fungal infections manifest in the patient in somewhat unpredictable ways. One time, you might mildly itch and red areas that it is easy to overlook; at other times, you will get worse scaling and crusting and really cannot miss it. Tinea pedis—commonly called athlete's foot—often makes itself known with soggy, cracked skin between the toes, especially when occlusive shoes trap moisture. On the flip side, *Tinea corporis* tends to show up as ring-like, clearly outlined spots with a clearer center, which can easily be mistaken for eczema or psoriasis. Although checking under a microscope or culturing a fungal infection continues to be the first choice for a final diagnosis, new technology in the form of dermoscopy now provides noninvasive clues in most instances. Treatment typically begins with topical creams that have antifungal compounds such as azoles or allylamines, and only if they become desperately widespread or recalcitrant do physicians' resort to systemic therapy. Others even resort to natural alternatives like tea tree oil, but more standardized procedures are required before we can ascertain for sure just how safe and effective these are (Daud et al., 2024). Preventing these infections is not only about being clean or treating them fast—it also involves considering the larger picture. Shared equipment, from athletic equipment to shower and locker room surfaces, function as small hubs for fungal spores to propagate, accelerating their dissemination among those who are at risk. Wherever possible, disinfectants effective against such spores, along with education programs to instruct athletes in good hygiene, can work wonders. There is also work being done on alternative medicines, such as antifungal plant oils, that promises new methods of augmenting standard treatments—though, yes, stringent clinical trials remain to be conducted to lock down the optimal dosages and formulations. In general, adopting a strategy that includes clinicians, trainers, and public health professionals collectively is usually the best option to minimize the effect of fungal skin infections in high-density or high-contact environments (Daud et al., 2024; Kucharczyk et al., 2025).

4.4.1. Tinea (Ringworm)

Skin infections may appear in a crazy array of shapes, depending on everything from our environment and habits to small microbes. In tropical and subtropical regions, for instance, some skin-friendly fungi that thrive on keratin can get a foothold. You may see a red, well-defined, circular, or oval area, usually on the trunk—that appears as an indication of something amiss. Individuals who have active lifestyles (and perspire excessively) provide the foundation for fungal development. In general, fungi in the Trichophyton class take hold in the top layers of skin and cause an inflammatory response leading to these characteristic lesions. In most instances, recognizing these patterns is the foundation for receiving proper diagnosis and treatment (Susanto et al., 2022). The scalp has another story to tell. With its high hair follicle density and endogenous oil secretion, it provides a tight, humid place where fungi, such as those of tinea capitis, find it easy to multiply. Fungal transmission commonly occurs via everyday objects—grasp a comb, cap, or styling implement, and you are in danger; occasionally, some self-transmission (autoinoculation) is mixed into the pot. It is difficult because the symptoms, like inflammation, scaling, and some itchiness (pruritus)—can cross over with other scalp issues. So, narrowing down the culprit with precise diagnosis is fairly essential to selecting the right antifungal treatment (Grimalt et al., 2007). Treatment-wise, there is not a one-fits-all solution. For lesser, more contained instances, topical ointments such as clotrimazole, ketoconazole, or terbinafine may suffice. But if the infection is widespread or recalcitrant, oral antifungal drugs like itraconazole or griseofulvin typically enter the picture. Prompt treatment not only accelerates healing but also avoids complications such as resistance, spread, or recurrence. And, educating patients regarding good hygiene and the dangers of sharing items makes a big difference. Ultimately, combining solid diagnosis, judiciously chosen medications, and intelligent preventive practices is key to controlling *Tinea corporis* and capitis efficiently (Susanto et al., 2022) (Figure 4.11).

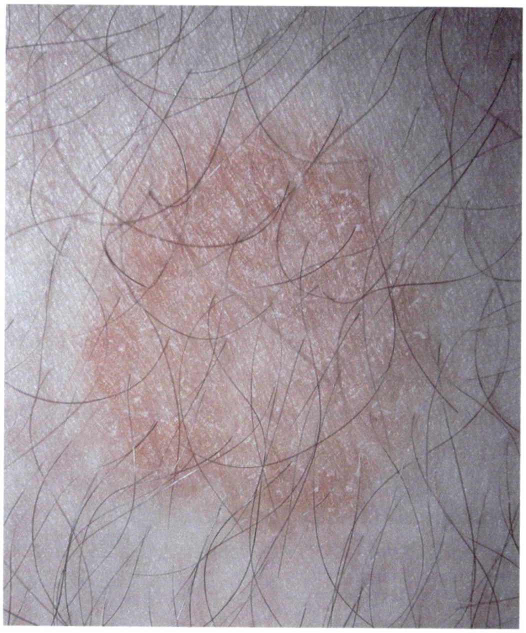

Figure 4.11. Ringworm.

Source: By James Heilman, MD - Own work, CC BY-SA 3.0, https://commons.wikimedia.org/w/index.php?curid=19051050

4.4.2. Candidiasis

Our skin is our initial line of defense, but it is not always perfect, particularly if our immune system is not quite working at full capacity. Candida, being a fungus infamous for taking any opportunity it can get, can take hold on the skin and cause candidiasis. It prefers to grow in warm, moist areas such as skin folds where sweat and friction blend to form the ideal environment. Individuals with compromised immunity—those suffering from HIV/AIDS, diabetes, or undergoing immunosuppressive therapy—are more prone to encounter this hassle. The fungus also possesses this peculiar ability to change its phase from the yeast type to a more penetrating hyphal form, upping its ante significantly. For the most part, understanding these changing dynamics is central to diagnosis and treatment of the infection, as its manifestations can readily be confused with other skin conditions (King et al., 2017). Cutaneous candidiasis, for example, comes in numerous guises—alternately just a faint red rash, alternately as deep, eroded lesions. You tend to feel manifestations such as itching, burning, and that nagging discomfort. In the immunocompromised individual, however, the infection can strike harder sometimes and even suggest issues far beyond the skin itself. More or less by the nature of the work, physicians rely quite heavily on what they see on clinical examination and then back it up with laboratory work like direct microscopy and culture. Early detection is particularly important in HIV-positive patients because these skin alterations may indicate underlying immune compromise and trigger more rapid therapy. In a sense, the skin is a window to our general immune status, providing critical information for monitoring disease progression (Hosseinabad & Abdolhazadeh, 2017). Treating candidiasis successfully involves not only attacking the fungus but also correcting the conditions that predispose us. Topical antifungals are typically the first line of treatment for infections limited to a localized area; however, in more widespread or recalcitrant infections, systemic treatment may be required. It also is crucial to address the things you can, such as limiting moisture, maintaining proper hygiene, and addressing immune problems, in order to avoid a recurrence. Most recent research, overall, highlights the importance of an integrated strategy for those with compromised defenses, pointing out that early detection and rapid treatment usually result in improved results. The manner cutaneous candidiasis is associated with more extensive systemic disorders clearly demonstrates how a multidisciplinary approach can reduce overall sickness and improve quality of life (Hosseinabad & Abdolhazadeh, 2017; King et al., 2017) (Figure 4.12).

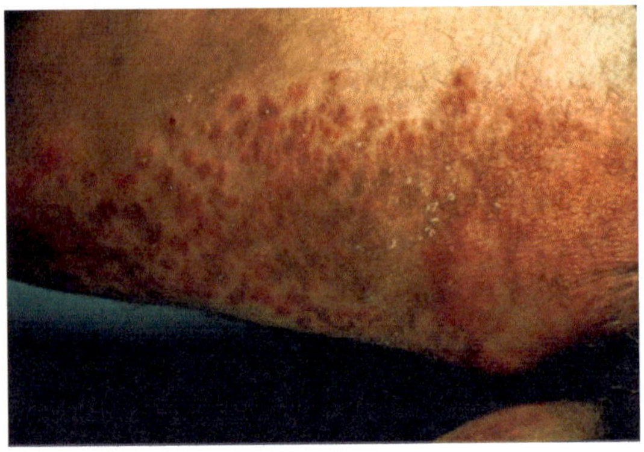

Figure 4.12. Skin candidiasis.

Source: By U.S. Department of Veterans Affairs - http://www.hiv.va.gov/provider/image-library/dermatological.asp?post=1&slide=202, Public Domain, https://commons.wikimedia.org/w/index.php?curid=52313076

4.4.3. Athlete's Foot

Physically active individuals occasionally encounter skin problems due to where they train and how they conduct themselves. Contact sports athletes or those who strike public gyms are most likely to encounter nagging fungal infections, such as athletes' foot. You see, when the feet are rolled up for too long, sweat accumulates and the skin comes into contact with infected surfaces, which allows fungus to grow readily. Most times, receiving an accurate diagnosis and a complete treatment plan is essential, particularly as returning too soon can exacerbate the condition or infect teammates (Luke & d'Hemecourt., 2007). All things considered, combining good hygiene practices with treatment protocols appears rather important to reduce personal discomfort and broader health risks within sports environments. If you think about it, things such as wetness and humidity can be a big contributor to how athlete's foot begins in the beginning. Swimmers and other water-logging wet surroundings struggle with their own skin issues, courtesy of constant wetness, chemicals such as chlorine, and even certain physical trauma to the skin barrier. This combination of excess moist skin, chlorine irritation, and minor equipment injuries increases the risk of fungal infection, essentially tinea pedis or what is commonly referred to as athlete's foot. Accepting these points, by and large, makes it simpler to design solutions. For instance, moisture-wicking equipment and rigorous after-exercise skin cleansing practices ensure that fungus is kept at bay without undermining performance, (Łazicka et al., 2025) whereas overall strategy that weaves together diagnosis, prevention, and treatment ultimately proves vital in sports. Treating athlete's foot is far more than just applying some medicine. It entails staying ahead through prevention education and cleanliness in the environment as well. Simple things, like washing and drying feet well and using antifungal creams or powders, can really lower repeat cases. Meanwhile locker rooms and communal showers need regular cleaning to keep fungal spores from hanging around. Plus, it is important athletes get a heads-up on choosing the right shoes that do not keep too much moisture – and, well, not sharing personal items can make a big difference too. The professionals are usually charged with balancing sound treatment with the need to return athletes to action ASAP, a task that some days is challenging. All of these tactics, mixed in with a little awareness of vaccines and overall prevention tactics, create an effective front for fighting infectious skin conditions (Luke & d'Hemecourt, 2007). With studies continuing to progress, combining novel antifungal therapy with wiser changes in behavior is promising to deliver improved results for those afflicted by athletes' foot (Figure 4.13).

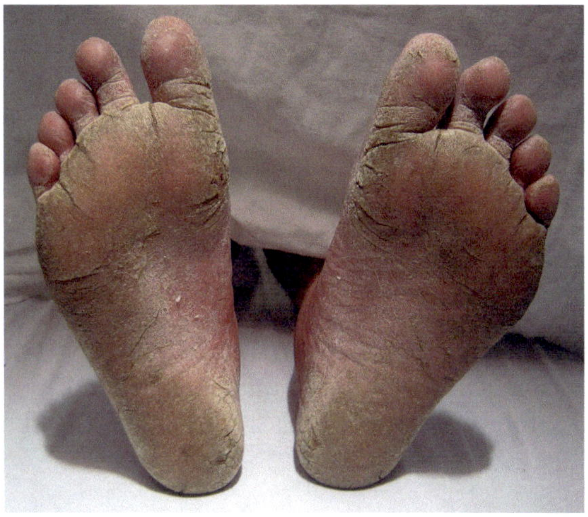

Figure 4.13. Athlete's foot.

Source: By James Heilman, MD - Own work, CC BY-SA 3.0, https://commons.wikimedia.org/w/index.php?curid=17770316

4.5. Risk Factors for Infectious Skin Diseases

A combination of internal factors and external forces can increase the likelihood of developing skin infections. Consider it: diseases like diabetes tend to render the skin's natural defense weaker, allowing germs to penetrate more easily. In most instances, if a person's immune system is already under way – i.e., HIV/AIDS or due to therapies such as chemotherapy or post-organ transplant – the body's protective mechanisms are even weaker. Dwelling in crowded or challenging areas, making transmission of pathogens more probable, merely contributes to the problem. And if the skin is broken by a cut, an insect bite, or even a long-term problem such as eczema, it merely offers an open door to opportunistic insects. All of these factors, when combined, result in doctors tending to have to take account of a patient's history and environment in quite a general sense. Day-to-day routines and cultural traditions have their voice heard as well. Individuals who bathe rarely or who may be apt to forget to wash hands properly—ahem, those tiny things—can predispose the spread and survival of infectious agents. Group situations, such as with team sports or other shared environments, add another element by facilitating direct contact with someone's own stuff or mere contact of the skin that elevates transmission. Occupational aspects come into play as well; the person working in industries such as healthcare, agriculture, or manufacturing can collide with germs or chemical irritants that compromise the strength of their skin. Naturally, wearing protective equipment can be of assistance, suggesting that minor behavioral changes could decrease these risks. Age and where an infection could hit come into play as well. Newborns and elderly, for example, are generally more at risk because their immune systems are still developing or in the process of diminishing, and their skin is typically thinner and more susceptible. Some areas on the body, such as those warm folds where moisture accumulates, provide miniature environments that lend themselves to bacterial growth. There are instances where site-related conditions, for example, diabetic foot ulcers, create an enormous risk. There is some evidence that even the eye region may be targeted by viral infections , and occasionally a systemic problem such as an infection of the urinary tract may set the stage for an ensuing skin infection (Valent et al., 2012). Age, particular site of the body, and general health all correlate in the majority of instances to determine how probable an individual is to contract skin infections.

4.5.1. Age and Immune Status

Getting older can really change how the body defends itself, and these shifts hit the skin in surprising ways. Aging brings on what is often called immunosenescence, meaning the immune system slowly loses some of its punch; fewer new T cells appear and even the cells that "remember" past infections just are not as effective as before. This loss makes it harder for the skin to fight off invading germs, and thus bacteria, viruses, and fungi cause more havoc than before. At the same time, the skin itself changes—its layers become thinner, and its barrier weaker, making it less capable of resisting microbes. When both structural and cellular defense collapse, older adults will experience more severe and more frequent skin infections (Vos et al., 2017). It is not just that our immune system will slow down; there is a larger context when you take a look at global disease patterns. As individuals live longer and mortality declines, more elderly will be struggling with chronic or persistent infections. For instance, the Global Burden of Diseases study indicates that disabling but not fatal conditions—long-standing infections and sequelae skin conditions—tend to increase with age, bulging the number of years spent with disability. With an immune system failing to clear infections as rapidly as previously, recurrent skin troubles become an everyday bane, contributing to total health ailments. This combination of an aging body, waning defenses, and increasing infections unequivocally calls for prevention and treatment plans that target older populations (Hosseinabad & Abdolhazadeh, 2017).

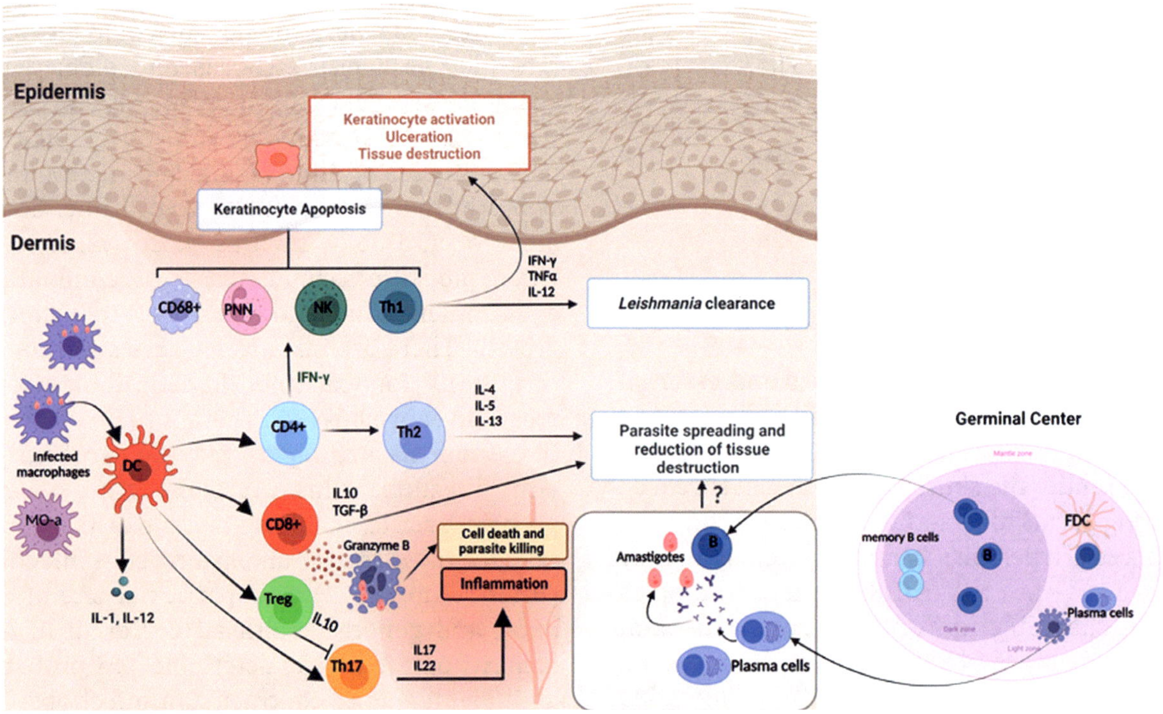

Figure 4.14. Immune responses and skin cytokine profile during cutaneous leishmaniasis infection.

Source: Saidi, N., Blaizot, R., Prévot, G., & Pied, S. (2023). Immune responses and skin cytokine profile during cutaneous leishmaniasis infection]. In Clinical and immunological spectra of human cutaneous leishmaniasis in North Africa and French Guiana. *Frontiers in Immunology*.

In addition to immunological changes, other ailments and daily situations complicate matters further for elderly individuals. Diabetes and other conditions are fairly prevalent among this age group and disrupt both the body's rapid, instinctive defenses and the slower, acquired reactions. High blood sugar and decreased circulation impair healing and compromise the protective layer of the skin, making it easier for opportunistic germs to find a home. Even treatments that benefit other age-related conditions can at times lower the guard further; nutritional deficiencies, reduced mobility, and communal living arrangements all contribute to the hassle by changing general immune resilience. All these complex factors indicate that there should be a holistic, integrated approach towards the management of skin infections among the elderly (Vos et al., 2017) (Figure 4.14).

4.5.2. Environmental Factors

Environmental factors count with skin infections—temperature, humidity, rain, all the tiny weather characterestics are able to fine-tune the way these nagging pathogens act. Consider skin parasites, for example; they tend to have susceptible stages dependent on the climate, which modifies how well they thrive and infect, for the most part. Scientists have even correlated these changes with disease transmission using some rather sophisticated math modeling. In the case of large parasites in diseases, seasonal variation, particularly timing, appears to drive infection patterns, suggesting local public health strategies need to take particular note of the weather (Remais , 2010). Alternatively, however, it is not only the microbes that feel the strain of environmental fluctuations; our skin barrier also takes a blow. Research on such conditions as AD reveals that a combination of environmental stressors and our own genetic predispositions can make our skin's natural barriers more vulnerable. You may notice how when environmental irritants (such as pollutants or extreme weather fluctuations) kick off cytokine-induced inflammation, essentially a cascade reaction that leaves our door wide open for infections. The interaction between the environmental exposures and genetics remains to some extent still a mystery, but in a majority of the instances, this understanding in advance could lay down the path towards better prevention programs (Martyna, 2013). Living in cities makes it an interesting mix yet. In the tightly packed settlements that have low sanitary conditions and inadequate clean water resources, infections among the skin more easily spread. Environmental degradation—habitat modification, pollution—can indirectly reduce our resistance by altering our immune responses or exposing us to novel germs. In general, the fight against these skin diseases is not merely a matter of medicines; it is a matter of examining our living environments and daily habits as well. This more holistic view could result in interventions that cure not only patients but also the environments that allow these diseases to flourish, eventually improving global skin health.

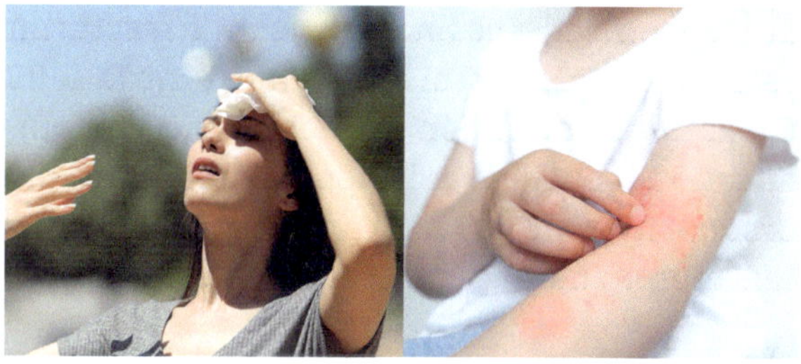

Source: Clocip. (2024). *Scratches Drying Sweat.* https://www.clocip.com/blogs/wp-content/uploads/2024/04/Scratches-drying-sweat.jpg.

4.5.3. Personal Hygiene Practices

Strict personal hygiene is a big concern for warding off skin infections—even if it may appear to be simply getting clean. Using a good many of the following tactics daily can prevent germ spread where lots of individuals converge, such as on sports teams or crowded halls in hospitals. Consider athletes, for instance, they are close and intimate throughout practice and games, so they should frequently wash hands, avoid using other people's personal items, and take care of any cuts or skin conditions immediately to prevent germs from entering (Luke & d'Hemecourt, 2007). Good hygiene is not only a first line of defense; it also serves to maintain your skin's natural barrier strong, as a broken barrier makes you more susceptible to infections. Plainly, if everyone abides by these habits, outbreaks can decline precipitously. In medical environments, proper use of protective gear and adherence to rigorous hygiene practices cannot be overstressed. Current research tends to highlight that despite training, errors during the donning or doffing of PPE can result in self-contamination, which ultimately increases infection risk for the workers themselves (Kwon et al., 2017). At times, even under supervision, these little mistakes occur—demonstrating just how difficult it is to do everything perfectly in a high-pressure clinical environment. Enhancing proper procedures and incorporating brief refreshers in using equipment, with the regular washing of hands beforehand and afterwards patient contact, becomes critical in fracturing the link of transmission. In most situations, an excess of attention to detail and ongoing education are what set it right. Simple everyday personal hygiene has its payoff carry far further than merely halting immediate infection.

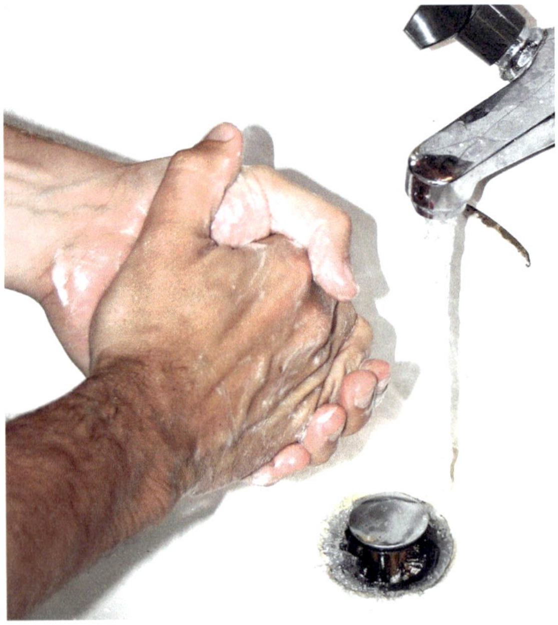

Figure 4.15. Personal hygiene.

Source: By Lars Klintwall Malmqvist (Larsklintwallmalmqvist) - Own work, Public Domain, https://commons.wikimedia.org/w/index.php?curid=4112060

Daily bathing, good hand washing with good cleansers, and even the mere habit of getting your clothes clean all make an environment such that troublesome microbes have difficulty getting a foothold. Particularly in populous areas or areas where there are vaccination gaps, hygiene can collaborate with vaccines and even antimicrobial interventions to reduce disease risks (Luke & d'Hemecourt, 2007). When individuals, especially the more at-risk, learn about the value of these routines, it encourages the initiation of habits that facilitate skin health over the long term—albeit sounding redundant, the little daily things work out. Personal hygiene is an essential public health measure by reducing opportunity exposure and maintaining our natural protective defenses strong (Figure 4.15).

4.6. Diagnosis and Treatment

Accurate diagnosis is critical in the treatment of infectious skin conditions; it determines the treatment used and can prevent complications from occurring in the first place. Physicians typically assemble information from a patient's history, conduct physical examinations, and employ an array of precise tests to determine what is happening. For instance, parasitic conditions (such as those due to fleas or *Sarcoptes scabiei*) tend to get confirmed by skin scrapings followed by a microscopic examination, whereas fungal infections like ringworm usually require either a culture or a direct microscopic examination to identify the fungi. Occasionally, when an allergic reaction complicates the picture, a few additional immunologic studies clarify whether the problem is infectious or not. Most of the time this combination of methods assists in individualizing treatment to both the microbe and the body's response, usually improving results and reducing the likelihood of things returning (Schacht et al., 2008). Treatment for infectious skin conditions can be quite varied based on both the instigator and how bad the infection is. Most surface infections are addressed with topical antimicrobials or antiparasitic medications, which have the advantage of attacking the affected area directly without excessive systemic absorption. In more challenging situations where the infection is deeper or more extensive in the area—systemic medications such as antibiotics, antifungals, or antiparasitics may be required to bring things under control. Doctors even incorporate corticosteroids in the mix at times to soothe inflammation, particularly when troublesome allergic reactions are involved. Maintenance of cleanliness through an emphasis on environmental hygiene and avoidance of additional exposure also becomes a major component of the overall recovery plan, promoting the minimization of transmission risks within affected populations (Schacht et al., 2008). Special attention is required in communities where there is regular physical contact, such as in athletes who regularly have to manage small cuts and share equipment. Rapid diagnosis in these cases is crucial because early detection of an infection can avoid long-term illness and prevent it from spreading to teammates. Treatment programs may even be adjusted a little to accommodate their busy lifestyle—getting them back to activity quickly enough without compromising on healing. A little more guidance on hygiene and protective measures can go a long way as well, reducing the rate of recurrences. In total, the combination of timely, correct diagnosis with tailor-made treatment and active prophylaxis truly demonstrates the importance of a multidisciplinary strategy in the management of infectious skin conditions in these specialist populations.

4.6.1. Diagnostic Methods

Occasionally, skin infections are not so straightforward to diagnose. You begin by seeing the skin—spots, rashes, and sores stand out, but these can all appear strange enough to be confused with other issues. So, physicians add in some lab tests, allowing bacteria, fungi, or viruses to grow from samples to determine what is present. This interactive test not only identifies the sneaky culprit but also aids in shaping treatments so that patients are not dosed with heavy-duty antibiotics when a lighter touch would suffice. Recently, some immune assays , such as tuberculin skin tests and interferon-gamma release assays , have moved in to detect infections that lie low or act strangely, such as that sneaky latent tuberculosis in individuals with less robust defenses. All these checks, operating fairly in concert with one another, provide a fuller picture in the majority of clinical contexts (Miller et al., 2024). Following a bout of virus, matters can become more complicated further. A virus like SARS-CoV-2 may acutely knock you off your feet, but its shadow tends to persist, exciting dermatological pathology that feels nascent or disturbingly chronic. It is not rare for old foes such as herpesvirus to stir, or for chronic skin irritations to flare, suggesting an immune system still a tad out of sorts. Conventional tests sometimes overlook these quieter, persistent changes. Consequently, some doctors today add immunophenotyping and molecular studies in addition to their routine check-ups—a double-check, as it were—to further grasp these viral skin enigmas (Miller et al., 2024). Combining these diagnostic approaches can truly become a game-saver, particularly for individuals living with other chronic issues. Take a person with diabetes; their immune system can be in disarray, leaving the way open for infections that ultimately present themselves with evident skin indicators. In these situations, combining a good clinical risk assessment with investigations such as the tuberculin skin test, and even interferon-gamma assays in certain instances—can identify the problem and indicate when closer observation is necessary. Even when swank, high-tech tests are available, more affordable methods still hold their ground in resource-tight settings. Essentially, adapting the testing plan to fit both the individual's needs and the local conditions is crucial for getting the best outcomes (Miller et al., 2024) (Figure 4.16).

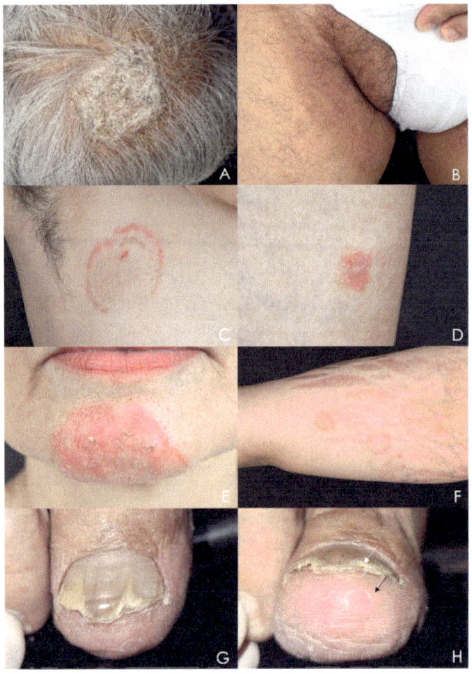

Figure 4.16. Clinical presentations of cutaneous fungal infection. (A) Tinea capitis; (B) Tinea cruris; (C) *Tinea incognit*; (D) *Tinea corporis*; (E) *Tinea faciei*; (F) *Tinea corporis*; and (G) Dorsal view of the right big toenail.

Source: Chanyachailert P, Leeyaphan C, Bunyaratavej S. Cutaneous Fungal Infections Caused by Dermatophytes and Non-Dermatophytes: An Updated Comprehensive Review of Epidemiology, Clinical Presentations, and Diagnostic Testing. *Journal of Fungi*. 2023; 9(6):669. https://doi.org/10.3390/jof9060669

4.6.2. Treatment Options

Skin infections are a pain – they persist on tenaciously and do not always react in the usual way to our usual remedies. For centuries, antibiotics were the default choice for bacterial infections, but as resistance continues to rise, long-term use, particularly for chronic diseases—has the effect of blunting their potency and accompanied by additional side effects. This has encouraged practitioners to seek alternative strategies, such as traditional treatments like moxibustion. Burning moxa releases heat, light, and even some chemical properties that may soothe inflammation and hasten healing. Although these older methods hold promise, strict high-quality randomized controlled trials are still required to fully establish their safety and efficacy in skin infections (Tang et al., 2025). Selecting the best treatment today is knowing that things are rapidly evolving, especially when newly emerging germs and complicated cases arise unexpectedly. Consider, for instance, SARS-CoV-2. Most cases in children only manifest mild cutaneous manifestations, yet there are some cases of full-blown systemic involvement that require highly specific interventions.

Even systematic reviews, by and large—perhaps especially systematic reviews—emphasize the importance of stratifying patients by risk factors, like age, baseline health conditions, and severity of the disease, such that treatments should be individualized for each (Zachary et al., 2024). This patient-specific strategy steps away from a one-size-fits-all philosophy toward safe and effective treatment for diverse patient populations. In the future, combining customary practices with tested, evidence-based medicine may help us break through the barriers of existing treatments. Certain infections that resist conventional antibiotics might be helped by adjunctive therapies such as moxibustion, which appears to stimulate multiple body mechanisms to enhance skin repair and immunity. Nevertheless, since skin infections are so diverse, well-planned clinical studies must be conducted to pin down precisely where these additional steps best fit. New developments in molecular diagnostics and personalized medicine will also help refine our capacity to hone in on particular infections and individual patient requirements. Ultimately, an integrated approach—combining drugs, alternative strategies, and preventive measures all guided by continuous research—will likely be the basis for enhancing outcomes, reducing resistance, and assuring long-term sustainability in controlling infectious skin diseases (Tang et al., 2025; Zachary et al., 2024) (Figure 4.17).

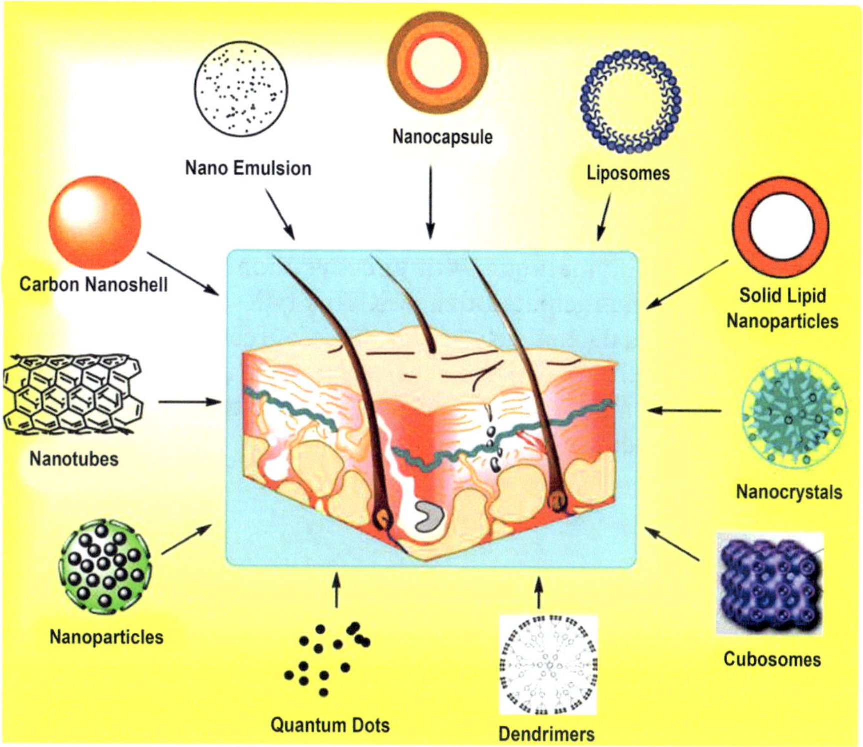

Figure 4.17. Various novel carriers in the treatment of skin fungal infections.

Source: Keshwania, P., Kaur, N., Chauhan, J., Sharma, G., Afzal, O., Altamimi, A. S. A., et al. (2023). Superficial dermatophytosis across the world's populations: Potential benefits from nanocarrier-based therapies and rising challenges. *ACS Omega, 8*(35), 31575–31599.

4.6.3. Importance of Early Intervention

It is important to catch skin infections early—it prevents a minor localized problem from mushrooming into one that involves the entire body. Skin is supposed to be our body's first defense against germs, but once it is injured, bacteria, viruses, or fungi can enter and very easily make things worse if they are not detected soon enough. In the majority of instances, moving quickly means that treatments can be implemented prior to the infection spreading or causing additional inflammation. A rapid clinical response also assists in lowering the chances of these germs transmitting to others, particularly when the illness is very contagious, and keeps outbreaks contained, minimizing public health risks. Recently, some research has highlighted that employing novel diagnostic equipment, such as artificial intelligence (AI), enhances a physician's capacity to identify skin lesions correctly and in a timely manner, thus simplifying intervention measures and overall outcomes (Han et al., 2024). Matters become even more complicated when resistant strains appear. Consider, for instance, Mycobacterium tuberculosis, which sometimes presents with symptoms on the skin. This microbe, increasingly multidrug-resistant, complicates treatment and requires rapid, accurate testing to determine which drugs will be most effective. In general, early identification of these resilient strains is a huge factor in being able to customize treatments and prevent the disease from spreading among vulnerable individuals. In countries such as India, this requirement becomes particularly evident; robust public health infrastructures that adopt early action through education at the community level, convenient access to diagnostic services, and treatment programs sensitive to cultural variations are crucial in reducing both the burden of disease and the development of resistance (Gamon et al., 2013). Implementing early intervention measures earlier than usual does more than simply improve the prognosis of one particular patient; it breaks the transmission chain in the community. Early diagnosis and equally early treatment can stop infections dead in their tracks, preventing not only short-term issues such as abscesses or frank systemic dissemination but also longer-term complications such as scarring or chronic inflammation. By combining sophisticated diagnostic methods with effective monitoring, health systems are more ready to handle outbreaks and unanticipated dangers. This type of multidisciplinary emphasis on rapid, decisive treatment becomes particularly critical in resource-constrained communities where even a momentary delay can result in far more severe consequences. In the majority of instances, early intervention is not only a clinical advantage—it is one of the main pillars of general public health care management (Miller et al., 2024).

CLOSER LOOK

Methicillin-Resistant Staphylococcus aureus (MRSA)

MRSA, or MRSA, is a strain of staph bacteria that is resistant to numerous standard antibiotics. It can result in skin infections in the form of red, painful, swollen bumps that may have pus in them. These infections may spread to other areas of the body and lead to more serious disease.

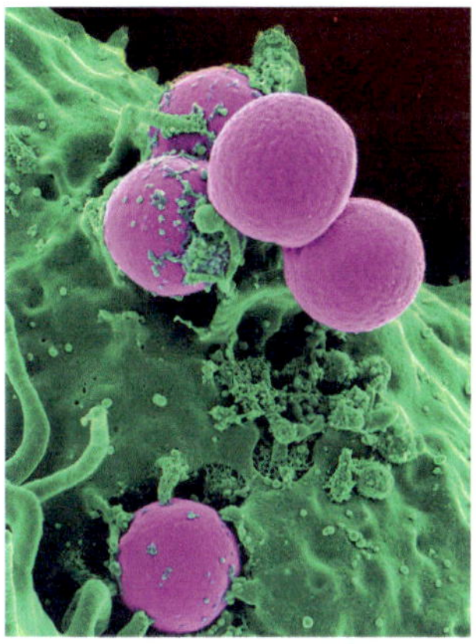

Source: By National Institutes of Health (NIH) - National Institutes of Health (NIH), Public Domain, https://commons.wikimedia.org/w/index.php?curid=29540596

- Signs and Symptoms:
  - **Skin Infections:** MRSA skin infections tend to begin as a bump, pimple, or spider bite-like lesion that can be red, swollen, painful, warm to the touch, and possibly filled with pus.
  - **Development:** The infection may spread and worsen, with the region becoming increasingly tender, red, and swollen.
  - **Other Symptoms:** In certain instances, there may be a fever or tiredness accompanying the skin infection.
  - **Systemic Infections:** When the infection occurs in the blood, it can cause more serious diseases such as pneumonia, endocarditis (infection of the heart valves), or osteomyelitis (bone infection).
- **Important Considerations:**
  - **CA-MRSA (Community-Acquired MRSA):** MRSA infection can occur outside of the hospital or healthcare environment.
  - **Early Detection and Treatment:** Getting immediate medical attention is the key in order to avoid the spread and the forming of more complicated infections.
  - **Infection Control**: Frequent hand washing and not sharing personal items such as towels and razors are some of the hygiene practices that prevent the transmission of MRSA.

SUMMARY

Breakthroughs in delivering drugs far into the skin have essentially revolutionized the way we fight infections today. Nanoparticles, liposomes, and microemulsions—these types of carriers have emerged to provide medicine an added kick in penetrating the skin's hard outer layer. They achieve this by releasing drugs in a slow and controlled manner so that the treatment arrives at the target without inundating the entire system, reducing unpleasant side effects. On top of that, the new approaches also appear to perform better against more recalcitrant microbes like MRSA, which is kind of exciting if you look at the limitations of previous treatments (Ayyüce et al., 2022). This entire targeted, controlled delivery concept has changed the philosophy of topical therapy, holding the promise of greater outcomes and even the possibility to stem the increase in resistant microbes. Although high-tech solutions are dominating the spotlight, it is worth remembering the broader context surrounding skin conditions. Research indicates that a lot of people who have skin issues also have mental health problems—psoriasis and AD, say, tend to co-exist with depression. In the majority of instances, although parasitic infections are not particularly prevalent among psychiatric inpatients, the integration between skin issues and mental health necessitates treatment that is not necessarily unilateral (Mavrogiorgou et al., 2020). Early diagnosis and interdisciplinary treatment that addresses physical and emotional areas can work wonders, even if it may seem a little complicated initially. It is about combining pioneering pharmaceutical technology with a focus on total patient care. The potential of these new drug delivery technologies is thrilling—they could be our best defense against resistant pathogens. Simultaneously, physicians and caregivers must not forget that skin conditions often carry an emotional burden, so it is also about pairing technical advancements with a patient-centered approach. Looking to the future, studies should be moving in the direction of creating treatment plans as individualized as they are innovative, combining new concepts from pharmacology with treatment that speaks to every aspect of a patient's life (Ayyüce et al., 2022; Mavrogiorgou et al., 2020).

Skin infections manifest in so many different ways – they can be bacterial, viral, fungal, or even parasitic. Getting the correct diagnosis often hinges on having a clue as to what tests to order and just how to process the samples. The laboratory chimes in with hard facts that assist in making treatment decisions, which, for the most part, can be the difference-maker. Since these infections also have their own unique twists, tests need to focus on particular culprits, and a slight mishandling of a specimen can complicate the results. Usually, when physicians and lab teams collaborate, additional tests get trimmed out and treatment is initiated earlier, reducing costs and saving patient's further discomfort. Briefly speaking, incorporating lab findings into day-to-day clinical practice is paramount for remaining current with skin infections, and remaining current with new methods of diagnosis is still essential (Miller et al., 2024). Our immune system does not consistently respond the same way, and particularly so with skin infections. New research indicates that hormones , androgens, specifically , influence the way our skin reacts, which could be the reason why severity and even cell types responding to the infection vary between men and women. For instance, androgens appear to silence type 2 innate lymphoid cells (ILC2s), the dendritic cells' supporting cells that are important for initiating an all-out adaptive immune response. This decline in dendritic cells, which commonly occurs in men, results in a significantly more subdued immune response compared to females. Essentially, these hormone-controlled adjustments in the immune system have a significant role in the way our skin protects itself, and understanding these differences is an important move towards creating more individualized treatments (Chi et al., 2024). In summary, fighting infections of the skin requires a combination of wise testing and a sense of how our bodies respond. It is not merely a matter of selecting the proper test and treating a sample gently—the lab's involvement is vital. Concurrently, biological sex is one of those things that subtly changes the behavior of immune cells through the effects of hormones (that androgen–ILC2–dendritic cell connection, for example), so one size truly does not fit all. These findings pave the way for more targeted treatments tailored to an individual's own immune configuration and to more easily clear out infections. Moving ahead on both the front of enhanced tests and a better understanding of immune functions sets up a solid ground for improved, more tailored patient care (Chi et al., 2024; Miller et al., 2024).

KEY TERMS FROM THIS CHAPTER

Active immune
Antimicrobial activity
Candidiasis
Climate change
Erysipelas
Herpes simplex
Impetigo
Lymphoid tissues
Ozone
Pollutants
Screening
Temperature
Tuberculosis
Viruses
Air pollution
Athletic teams
Cellulitis
Dysbiosis
Fungus
Humidity
Jack robinson
Microbes
Parasites
Rashes
Skin insects
Tissue integrity
Vaccines
Vulnerable populations
Antibiotics
Bacteria
Chlorhexidine gluconate
Environmental debris
Global warming
Immune systems
Keratin
Molecular markers
Penicillin
Ringworm
Streptococcus pyogenes
Topical antiseptics
Varicella-zoster

REFERENCES

1. Shakeri Hosseinabad, M. A. & Abdolhazadeh, F., (2017). Cutaneous symptoms and rashes in patients with HIV-positive infections: A review article. Asian Journal of Pharmaceutical Research and Health Care Vol 8(S1), 72-78, 2016(accessed on 12 May 2025).
2. Abdul-Ghani, R., Al-Awadi, A. H., Al-aghbari, N., Al-Mikhlafy, A. A., Abdulmoghni, S. S., Al-dobai, S. S., & Nauman, N. F. (2024). Latent tuberculosis infection and diagnostic performance of the tuberculin skin test among type 2 diabetics in Sana'a city, Yemen. *BMC Infectious Diseases, 24*. https://www.semanticscholar.org/paper/20e61cd2f4dc4dc20be3d45399d3a3744c2b025f (accessed on 12 May 2025).
3. Ajisafe, I. B., Afariogu, D. A., Owa, S., Ndako, J. A., Adekeye, A., Oguntimehin, O., & Owolabi, A. (2024). A review on current trends of human papillomavirus: Need for prompt action. "A Review on Current Trends of Human Papillomavirus: Need for Prompt Action," *2024 International Conference on Science, Engineering and Business for Driving Sustainable Development Goals (SEB4SDG)*, Omu-Aran, Nigeria, 2024, pp. 1-6, doi: 10.1109/SEB4SDG60871.2024.10629835. (accessed on 12 May 2025).
4. Valent, P., Akin, C., Arock, M., Brockow, K., Butterfield, J. H., Carter, M. C., Castells, M., Escribano, L., Hartmann, K., Lieberman, P., Nedoszytko, B., Orfao, A., Schwartz, L. B., Sotlar, K., Sperr, W. R., Triggiani, M., Valenta, R., Horny, H. P., & Metcalfe, D. D. (2012). Definitions, criteria and global classification of mast cell disorders with special reference to mast cell activation syndromes: a consensus proposal. *International archives of allergy and immunology, 157*(3), 215–225. https://doi.org/10.1159/000328760(accessed on 12 May 2025).
5. Jakubczak, Z., Zimniak, M., Miłkowski, P., Głąbień, M., Kusiak, K., Aleksandrowicz, D., ... Śliwiak, P. (2024). Dermatoses among athletes. *Quality in Sport, 23*, 54564. https://doi.org/10.12775/QS.2024.23.54564 (accessed on 12 May 2025).
6. Anderska, A., Osuch, D., Opala, D., Staszczyk, I., Drabik, A., Szczotka, D., Błachnio, K., et al. (2025). The impact of climate changes on skin diseases: A narrative review of the literature. *Przeglad Epidemiologiczny, 78*(4), 400–407. https://www.semanticscholar.org/paper/162f70969ae94d79a5a5eede81af84362350696a (accessed on 12 May 2025).
7. Anger, J. T., Lee, U., Ackerman, A. L., Chou, R., Chughtai, B., Clemens, J. Q., Hickling, D., et al. (2019). Recurrent uncomplicated urinary tract infections in women: AUA/CUA/SUFU guideline. *The Journal of Urology, 202*, 282–289. https://doi.org/10.1097/ju.0000000000000296.
8. Kwon, J. H., Burnham, C. D., Reske, K. A., Liang, S. Y., Hink, T., Wallace, M. A., Shupe, A., Seiler, S., Cass, C., Fraser, V. J., & Dubberke, E. R. (2017). Assessment of Healthcare Worker Protocol Deviations and Self-Contamination During Personal Protective Equipment Donning and Doffing. *Infection control and hospital epidemiology, 38*(9), 1077–1083. https://doi.org/10.1017/ice.2017.121 (accessed on 12 May 2025).
9. Chi, L., Liu, C., Gribonika, I., Gschwend, J., Corral, D., Han, S. J., Lim, A. I., et al. (2024). Sexual dimorphism in skin immunity is mediated by an androgen-ILC2-dendritic cell axis. *Science, 384*. https://www.semanticscholar.org/paper/6ff7d4cc44b6a582fec11598cc814f2f421f14dd (accessed on 12 May 2025).
10. Colavita, F., Lapa, D., Carletti, F., Lalle, E., Bordi, L., Marsella, P., Nicastri, E., et al. (2020). SARS-CoV-2 isolation from ocular secretions of a patient with COVID-19 in Italy with prolonged

viral RNA detection. *Annals of Internal Medicine, 173*, 242–243. https://doi.org/10.7326/m20-1176.

11. Mohd Daud, N. I., Ahmad Raus, R. ., & Mohd Radzuan, H. . (2024). A Scoping Review: Topical Treatment of Infectious Skin Diseases with Remedial Plant Oils. *Borneo Journal of Medical Sciences (BJMS)*, *19*(1), 26–39. https://doi.org/10.51200/bjms.v19i1.5585(accessed on 12 May 2025).
12. d'Hemecourt, P., & Luke, A. (2007). Prevention of infectious diseases in athletes. https://core.ac.uk/download/323072758.pdf Luke, A., & d'Hemecourt, P. (2007). Prevention of infectious diseases in athletes. *Clinics in sports medicine*, *26*(3), 321–344. https://doi.org/10.1016/j.csm.2007.04.006 (accessed on 12 May 2025).
13. Dobrynina, M., Zurochka, A., & Zurochka, V. (2024). Clinical and immunological characteristics of post-COVID patients with infectious immunopathology syndrome. *Russian Journal of Immunology*. https://www.semanticscholar.org/paper/b1a191f30db8c8dfc844d6211c9fdd9895be4858 (accessed on 12 May 2025).
14. Docherty, A. B., Harrison, E. M., Green, C., Hardwick, H., Pius, R., Norman, L., Holden, K., et al. (2020). Features of 20,133 UK patients in hospital with COVID-19 using the ISARIC WHO Clinical Characterisation Protocol: Prospective observational cohort study. *BMJ*. https://doi.org/10.1136/bmj.m1985.
15. Eijck, I., & Kijlstra, A. (2006). Animal health in organic livestock systems: A review. https://core.ac.uk/download/10924572.pdf (accessed on 12 May 2025).
16. Eijck, I., Groot, M., Kasteel, D., Kijlstra, et al. (2003). Analysis of black holes in our knowledge concerning animal health in the organic food production chain. https://core.ac.uk/download/10919416.pdf (accessed on 12 May 2025).
17. El-Masry, H., Gaber, H., Shaheen, N., Abdelbary, A., Sayed, N. M., & Omar, S. (2024). Kaposi varicelliform eruption: An unusual presentation caused by varicella zoster virus in a healthy adult patient–A case report. *BMC Infectious Diseases, 24*. https://www.semanticscholar.org/paper/c7ffb2775ffe3e04f077bf07a23b4e48d3f700bb (accessed on 12 May 2025).
18. Gamon, M. (2013). Multidrug-resistant tuberculosis in India: Solving a problem by reconstructing the public health infrastructure. https://core.ac.uk/download/67755957.pdf (accessed on 12 May 2025).
19. Gershon, A. A., & Kennedy, P. G. E. (2018). Clinical features of varicella-zoster virus infection. https://core.ac.uk/download/161770843.pdf (accessed on 12 May 2025).
20. Gómez-Duarte, O. G., & Ogra, P. L. (2019). Development of mucosal immunity: Functional interactions with mucosal microbiome in health and disease. *Current Immunology Reviews, 15*, 154–165. https://www.semanticscholar.org/paper/13da0b9b1156c3e9d1352714b5d9d2ce36e1326c (accessed on 12 May 2025).
21. Gonçalves da Silva, E., Gomes de Barros, I., Ferreira da Costa, A. C. M. S., Moreira, M. B. P., Martins Cahú, A. K., Romeiro, E. T., Cavalcanti, R. L. P., et al. (2024). Canine infectious fungal dermatopathy: A silent zoonosis in humans. *Caderno Pedagógico*. https://www.semanticscholar.org/paper/f711fc7cb4bb189e93f6bbce4ebb06f7e910e7bc (accessed on 12 May 2025).
22. Grimalt, R. (2007). A practical guide to scalp disorders. *Journal of Investigative Dermatology Symposium Proceedings, 12*(2), 10–14. https://doi.org/10.1038/sj.jidsymp.5650048.

23. Han, R., Fan, X., Ren, S., & Niu, X. (2024). Artificial intelligence in assisting pathogenic microorganism diagnosis and treatment: A review of infectious skin diseases. *Frontiers in Microbiology, 15*. https://www.semanticscholar.org/paper/9d965c4bb57eac5c22224e47468f2aff72ec7a3d (accessed on 12 May 2025).

24. Han, R., Fan, X., Ren, S., & Niu, X. (2024). Artificial intelligence in assisting pathogenic microorganism diagnosis and treatment: a review of infectious skin diseases. *Frontiers in microbiology*, *15*, 1467113. https://doi.org/10.3389/fmicb.2024.1467113 (accessed on 12 May 2025).

25. Łazicka, P., Jakubowska, E., & Tarnowska, J. (2025). Approaches to the diagnosis of Cutaneous Diseases Among Swimmers: Causes, Symptoms, Prevention, Treatment. *Quality in Sport, 37*, 56586. https://doi.org/10.12775/QS.2025.37.56586

26. Johnson, E. K., Vogel, J. D., Cowan, M. L., Feingold, D. L., & Steele, S. R. (2019). The American Society of Colon and Rectal Surgeons' clinical practice guidelines for the management of pilonidal disease. *Diseases of the Colon & Rectum, 62*, 146–157. https://doi.org/10.1097/dcr.0000000000001237.

27. Kawssan, A., Chawiche, C., Shamas, Z., & Hamdar, H. (2024). Non-sexual transmission of sexually transmitted diseases in women. *Journal of Medical Research and Reviews*. JOURNAL OF 2024; 17-22. 10.5455/JMRR.20240702073007(accessed on 12 May 2025).

28. King, J., Pana, Z. D., Lehrnbecher, T., Steinbach, W. J., & Warris, A. (2017). Recognition and Clinical Presentation of Invasive Fungal Disease in Neonates and Children. *Journal of the Pediatric Infectious Diseases Society*, *6*(suppl_1), S12–S21. https://doi.org/10.1093/jpids/pix053 (accessed on 12 May 2025).

29. Lamb, Gabriella S., "Epidemiology Of Tuberculosis In Internationally Displaced Children Resettling In Harris County" (2019). *Dissertations & Theses (Open Access)*. 64. https://digitalcommons.library.tmc.edu/uthsph_dissertsopen/64 (accessed on 12 May 2025).

30. Li, X., Chen, S., Wu, Y., Qiu, G., Cheng, S., Lan, H., Yan, Z., et al. (2024). Antibody immune responses and causal relationships in four immune skin diseases: Evidence from Mendelian randomization and Bayesian weighting (Antibody Responses in Skin Diseases: MR & Bayesian). *Skin Research and Technology, 30*. https://www.semanticscholar.org/paper/ba1a0fc0ca37c7c0ae061550ae13efa4c863834a (accessed on 12 May 2025).

31. Lillestolen, Derek, "Infections Not Fought: Antibiotic Resistance in Underserved Communities" (2018). *Senior Honors Theses*. 741. https://digitalcommons.liberty.edu/honors/741 (accessed on 12 May 2025).

32. Marais, B., Gie, R., Hesseling, A., Schaaf, H. S., Lombard, C., Enarson, D., & Beyers, N. (2006). A refined symptom-based approach to diagnose pulmonary tuberculosis in children. *Pediatrics, 118*, e1350–e1359. https://www.semanticscholar.org/paper/931b6f74736f5f67aa1ce32b0daca512882faa09 (accessed on 12 May 2025).

33. Maris, S., Stošić, M., Šaponjić, V., Giljača, S., Risimović, V., & Tanasijević, Z. (2024). Surveillance of infectious diseases caused by *Streptococcus pyogenes* in the territory of the city of Belgrade. *Glasnik javnog zdravlja*. 2024, vol. 98, iss. 2, pp. 159-170https://www.semanticscholar.org/paper/f19401185c6cc6a6c919bdd2a30d431175bee1f4 (accessed on 12 May 2025).

34. Matsuda, A., Nakamura, Y., Itoi, T., Arai, K., Kutara, K., Sugimoto, K., & Maeta, N. (2025). Daily topical application of chlorhexidine gluconate to the skin in dogs and its impact on skin

barriers and cytotoxicity. *The Journal of Veterinary Medical Science, 87*, 257–262. https://www.semanticscholar.org/paper/146a041fdaf4ebb52ac7e21359d000d2e02a48f9 (accessed on 12 May 2025).

35. Mavrogiorgou, P., Mersmann, C., Gerlach, G., Herpertz, S., & Juckel, G. (2020). Skin diseases in patients with primary psychiatric disorders. *Psychiatry Investigation, 17*, 157–162. https://www.semanticscholar.org/paper/b6f82176d48e4e546fb384b06a0e06439e7a0130 (accessed on 12 May 2025).

36. Mennitti C, Calvanese M, Gentile A, Vastola A, Romano P, Ingenito L, Gentile L, Veneruso I, Scarano C, La Monica I, et al. Skin Microbiome Overview: How Physical Activity Influences Bacteria. *Microorganisms*. 2025; 13(4):868. https://doi.org/10.3390/microorganisms13040868(accessed on 12 May 2025).

37. Miller, J. M., Binnicker, M. J., Campbell, S., Carroll, K. C., Chapin, K. C., Gonzalez, M. D., Harrington, A., Jerris, R. C., Kehl, S. C., Leal, S. M., Jr, Patel, R., Pritt, B. S., Richter, S. S., Robinson-Dunn, B., Snyder, J. W., Telford, S., 3rd, Theel, E. S., Thomson, R. B., Jr, Weinstein, M. P., & Yao, J. D. (2024). Guide to Utilization of the Microbiology Laboratory for Diagnosis of Infectious Diseases: 2024 Update by the Infectious Diseases Society of America (IDSA) and the American Society for Microbiology (ASM). *Clinical infectious diseases : an official publication of the Infectious Diseases Society of America*, ciae104. Advance online publication. https://doi.org/10.1093/cid/ciae104(accessed on 12 May 2025).

38. Murray, C. J. L., Ikuta, K. S., Sharara, F., Swetschinski, L. R., Robles Aguilar, G., Gray, A. P., Han, C., et al. (2022). Global burden of bacterial antimicrobial resistance in 2019: A systematic analysis. *The Lancet, 399*, 629–655. https://doi.org/10.1016/s0140-6736(21)02724-0.

39. Pace, D. (2008). Review of varicella zoster virus: From epidemiology to prevention. Malta Medical Journal Volume 20 Issue 03 September 2008. https://core.ac.uk/download/46602191.pdf (accessed on 12 May 2025).

40. Remais J. (2010). Modelling environmentally-mediated infectious diseases of humans: transmission dynamics of schistosomiasis in China. *Advances in experimental medicine and biology, 673*, 79–98. https://doi.org/10.1007/978-1-4419-6064-1_6 (accessed on 12 May 2025).

41. Saavedra-Lozano, J., Falup-Pecurariu, O., Faust, S. N., Girschick, H., Hartwig, N., Kaplan, S. L., Lorrot, M., et al. (2017). Bone and joint infections. *The Pediatric Infectious Disease Journal, 36*, 788–799. https://doi.org/10.1097/inf.0000000000001635.

42. Schacht, J. (2008). Smittsamma hudsjukdomar hos hund. https://core.ac.uk/download/211578519.pdf (accessed on 12 May 2025).

43. Susanto, I. K. (2022). *Tinea corporis Therapy*. https://core.ac.uk/download/543014253.pdf (accessed on 12 May 2025).

44. Szot, A., Kmak, B., & Górska, M. (2024). The most common dermatoses of athletes. *Journal of Education, Health and Sport*. https://www.semanticscholar.org/paper/938fedcd1b1ab1088067868bc0deb3755b52b72f (accessed on 12 May 2025).

45. Talapko, J., Juzbašić, M., Matijević, T., Pustijanac, E., Bekić, S., Kotris, I., & Škrlec, I. (2021). *Candida albicans*—The virulence factors and clinical manifestations of infection. *Journal of Fungi, 7*(2), 79–79. https://doi.org/10.3390/jof7020079.

46. Tang B, Yuan H, Ji J, Lin P, Pei L. The application of moxibustion in infectious skin diseases. Infect Dis Res. 2025;6(1):5. doi: 10.53388/IDR2025005. (accessed on 12 May 2025).

47. Türkmen, A., İmren Esentürk-Güzel, and B. A. Kara. "INNOVATIVE DRUG DELIVERY SYSTEMS FOR INFECTIOUS DISEASES OF THE SKIN". *Universal Journal of Pharmaceutical Research*, vol. 7, no. 4, Sept. 2022, doi:10.22270/ujpr.v7i4.815.(accessed on 12 May 2025).

48. Vos, T., Abajobir, A. A., Abate, K. H., Abbafati, C., Abbas, K., Abd-Allah, F., Abdulkader, R. S., et al. (2017). Global, regional, and national incidence, prevalence, and years lived with disability for 328 diseases and injuries for 195 countries, 1990–2016: A systematic analysis for the Global Burden of Disease Study 2016. *The Lancet, 390*, 1211–1259. https://doi.org/10.1016/s0140-6736(17)32154-2.

49. Vos, T., Allen, C. A., Arora, M., Barber, R. M., Bhutta, Z. A., Brown, A., Carter, A., et al. (2016). Global, regional, and national incidence, prevalence, and years lived with disability for 310 diseases and injuries, 1990–2015: A systematic analysis for the Global Burden of Disease Study 2015. *The Lancet, 388*, 1545–1602. https://doi.org/10.1016/s0140-6736(16)31678-6.

50. Weißhaar, E., Szepietowski, J. C., Dalgard, F., Garcovich, S., Gieler, U., Giménez-Arnau, A. M., Lambert, J., et al. (2019). European S2k guideline on chronic pruritus. *Acta Dermato-Venereologica, 99*, 469–506. https://doi.org/10.2340/00015555-3164.

51. Wesserlking, M. (2013). Role of genetic aspect in pathogenesis of atopic dermatitis. *Acta Universitatis Lodziensis. Folia Biologica Et Oecologica, 9*, 1–8. https://doi.org/10.2478/fobio-2013-0005 (accessed on 12 May 2025).

52. Willis, Z. I., Oliveira, C. R., Abzug, M. J., Anosike, B. I., Ardura, M. I., Bio, L. L., Boguniewicz, J., Chiotos, K., Downes, K., Grapentine, S. P., Hersh, A. L., Heston, S. M., Hijano, D. R., Huskins, W. C., James, S. H., Jones, S., Lockowitz, C. R., Lloyd, E. C., MacBrayne, C., Maron, G. M., ... Wolf, J. (2024). Guidance for prevention and management of COVID-19 in children and adolescents: A consensus statement from the Pediatric Infectious Diseases Society Pediatric COVID-19 Therapies Taskforce. *Journal of the Pediatric Infectious Diseases Society, 13*(3), 159–185. https://doi.org/10.1093/jpids/piad116 (accessed on 12 May 2025).

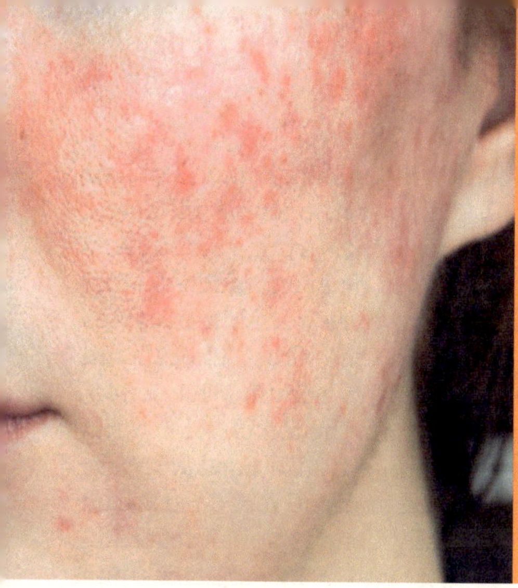

Chapter 5

ACNE AND ROSACEA

Contents

Introduction

Skin diseases strike far beyond what you observe on the outside—they can alter both our physical wellbeing and mood. Acne and rosacea, for example, are both inflammatory conditions but appear in totally different manners. Acne likes to make an appearance in those adolescent years, whereas rosacea tends to appear later in life. Each has its own problems and its own set of symptoms, so it is sort of vital that we recognize these differences early on if we are going to address them in the right way. It is not physical treatment alone either; these conditions tend to play havoc with a person's self-esteem and daily life. That is why methods that combine patient education with a shared decision-making feel are so important (Drug and Bulletin, 2013). In the end, it turns out that balancing the clinical facts with a personal touch really helps in addressing the broad impact of these dermatological concerns. Digging a little deeper, the onset of acne and rosacea comes down to several overlapping factors like inflammation, changes in blood vessel behavior, and shifts in immune response. Acne vulgaris typically takes over when hair follicles become plugged with excess oil, dead skin accumulation, and bacteria making themselves at home, whereas rosacea is more of an enduring inflammation taking place in the facial blood vessels and skin. What this really means is that acne tends to present itself with such manifestations as blackheads, pimples, or pustules, while rosacea hangs in there with a chronic flush and those small, spider-looking veins, , or telangiectasia, you can spot. In general, being aware of these differences aids in establishing the proper game plan. Some treatments may include straightforward topical creams or even lifestyle adjustments, whereas others require more systemic treatment. All that confusion really serves to emphasize just how critical personalized treatment plans, considering severity, particular subtypes, and individual considerations—are. And truly, when patients are included in the decision-making process, the likelihood of improved outcomes increases (Drug and Bulletin, 2013). Broadly speaking, the healthcare landscape of today is trending towards engaging patients in all aspects of chronic disease management such as these. Similar to trends with other long-term health conditions, dermatology is beginning to reap obvious benefits from a more collaborative process. When physicians transfer decision aids and provide individualized counseling, patients are able to make decisions that are more suitable for their lives, which is a significant assistant considering how tenaciously acne and rosacea can return. In most instances, these types of patient-centered approaches not only improve adherence but also render treatment more effective in general. Dermatology practitioners are tuning in to this change, combining a little old-school clinical practice with wider, more individualized conversation. This is reflecting what is occurring in so many other areas of medicine, progressing steadily toward care as unique as it is value-based, which can raise the quality of life for those going through these skin disorders.

Definition of Acne

Acne is not purely a surface issue – it erupts from a combination of bodily functions and the bacteria that reside on our skin. Follicles of hair and adjacent oil glands can become inflamed, and you may notice spots from comedowns and papules to pustules or even nodules. Most times, this will occur where our skin becomes oiled up, such as on the face, chest, and back. In general, excessive sebum production, abnormal shedding within the follicles, bacterial colonization (predominantly by *Cutibacterium acnes*), and an agitated immune response are all part of the mix. Briefly, acne is a manifestation of problems not just with what appears upon the surface of the skin, but also with the small ecosystem that inhabits it. Getting a little more up close (and messy) with the skin microbiome reveals more. This group usually has skin under control, but if it gets out of kilter – i.e., if there is an unexpected derangement – inflammation could become more intense and vicious bacteria could more than normally amplify. For example, even a little change in this microbial system can kick-start lesion formation. Recent research, in the majority of instances, has indicated that therapies to restore this balance—through the use of such as probiotics and prebiotics—can enhance the barrier function of the skin. In doing so, acne management frequently extends beyond the mere use of topical ointments or antibiotics, relying instead on approaches that correct a root microbial imbalance (Al-Smadi et al., 2023). Occasionally, the distinction between acne and rosacea becomes a bit blurred. While they are categorized differently, both diseases could be associated with comparable follicular inflammation.

Peculiarly, Demodex mites – those pesky little insects that typically congregate innocently on our bodies – can occur in abnormal densities in patients who have facial dermatoses, either rosacea or acne-like skin diseases. Their proliferation appears to induce additional inflammation and can even interfere with immune reactions, correlating microbial and parasitic forces in a quite unexpected manner.

There is evidence to indicate that Demodex blooms are associated with both eye and skin symptoms of rosacea, which at times overlap with what we see in acne. Identifying this subtle transition in otherwise harmless skin inhabitants is central to designing treatment strategies that address both the microbial perpetrators and the inflammatory mechanisms (Chioveanu et al., 2024) (Figure 5.1).

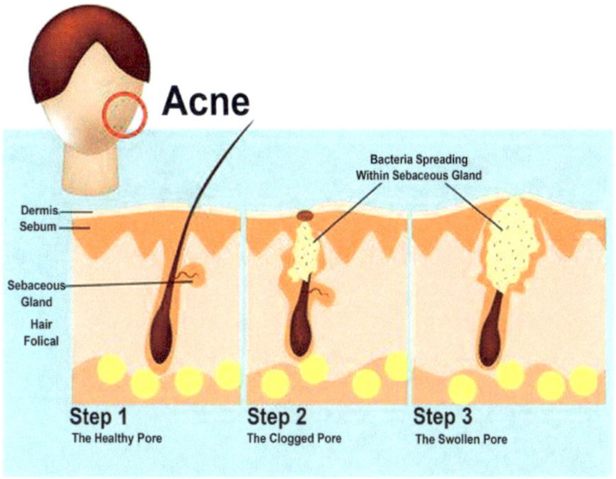

Figure 5.1. Acne.

Source: Unknown. (n.d.). *Businessman Drawing cloud Network Diagram.* https://t3.ftcdn.net/jpg/01/01/64/70/360_F_101647089_wTOSog8D59Xo75rOHdzU43RQ11j9lwyX.jpg.

Definition of Rosacea

Chronic skin conditions with constant inflammation have a way of blurring diagnosis lines—they all have so many similar signs and are caused by a mix of things. Consider rosacea, for instance; it usually appears with constant flushing on the face, a matrix of seen-through blood vessels, and those weird little bumps that appear primarily in the middle. Acne vulgaris, however, tends to come with plugged pores and strikes individuals of all ages, whereas rosacea appears to accompany adults and comes with these bursts of activity that catch you by surprise due to environmental or bodily sparks. Its persistent inflammation suggests a complex combination of immune system snafus and nerve-controlled blood flow problems, creating a scenario that is far from straightforward. Too often, because it is confused with other skin ailments, the actual prevalence of rosacea falls through the cracks—so clear-cut guidelines to distinguish it from acne and other ails are darn near necessary. Attempting to gain some control over rosacea necessitates a look beyond the surface. More recent studies tend to invoke a gut-skin relationship, where alterations in gut bacteria and even in intestinal permeability could push the skin toward inflammation (Mántó et al., 2019). That concept, more often than not, implies an out-of-control gut ecosystem that may be driving the immune system into hyperdrive, with the results manifested as rosacea flare-ups. There is even speculation that support measures, such as experimenting with probiotics—could ease overall inflammation, suggesting that this affliction goes beyond what is apparent. In some sense, these observations lead us to consider rosacea as being more of an overall body complaint than simply an irritation at the surface.

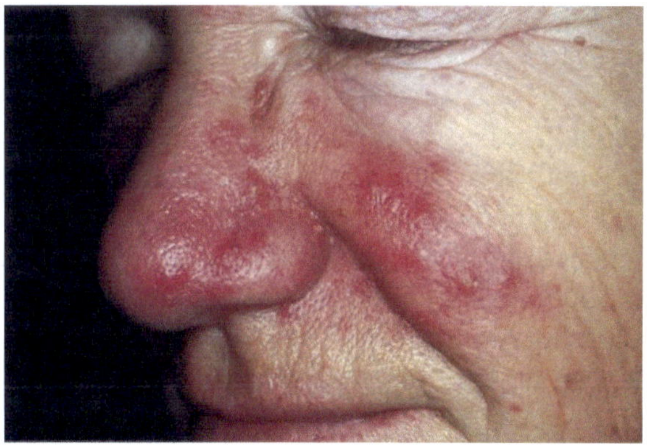

Figure 5.2. Rosacea.

Source: By Michael Sand, Daniel Sand, Christina Thrandorf, Volker Paech, Peter Altmeyer, Falk G Bechara - https://www.ncbi.nlm.nih.gov/pmc/articles/PMC2903548/, CC BY 2.5, https://commons.wikimedia.org/w/index.php?curid=74055900

Even the eyes become pulled into this challenging scenario on occasion. A few patients experience problems such as blepharitis, conjunctivitis, or even dry-eye syndrome, which may occur preceding or concurrent with the typical facial symptoms. These eye problems can literally take a toll on daily life and may even ruin results in eye surgeries (Christopher et al., 2019). Due to this, it is now apparent that a single-track skin check is no longer sufficient—incorporating eye check-ups is the way to go for handling the condition effectively. On the whole, this combined method reminds us rosacea is not all about facial redness; it is a complex disorder that requires an approach treating the skin as well as other associated systems (Figure 5.2).

Importance of Understanding Both Conditions

Skin diseases are not quite as black and white as they may appear to be. Rosacea and acne, for instance, can exhibit symptoms such as facial redness and inflammation but have different causations. Often, the triggers and the underlying problems are not a good match even when the surface indications may be similar, and that can result in treatment strategies that fall short, or even cause harm if the diagnosis is not an exact fit. Many individuals have beliefs regarding diet and skin care that simply do not align with fact, and studies reflect that the majority of people feel nutrition has a great deal to do with healthy skin (Jan et al., 2024). This type of fundamental knowledge seriously raises the bar, relieving both the physical and emotional costs resulting from diagnostic and treatment errors. Measuring how effective treatments are, particularly for something as chronic as the redness of rosacea, requires sharp, trusted measures.

For example, taking baseline photos and then comparing those over time can do a lot to check how effective a treatment is (Eichenfield et al., 2019). In general, employing these sorts of standard measures reduces bias and facilitates doctors in choosing the correct avenue forward. It is not only about achieving solid research results—this type of close monitoring allows clinicians to adjust treatment plans in the moment, which can improve patient satisfaction and result in improved long-term control over both rosacea and acne.

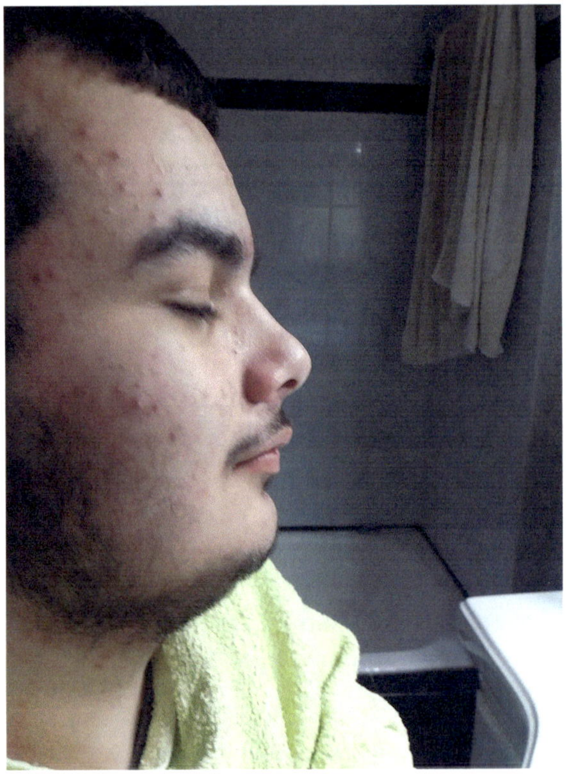

Figure 5.3. Teenager with acne.

Source: Likomitros, N. (2020). *Teenager with Acne. Wikimedia Commons*. https://upload.wikimedia.org/wikipedia/commons/thumb/d/d6/Teenager_with_acne.jpg/800px-Teenager_with_acne.jpg.

It is also important to recall that understanding acne and rosacea involves seeing beyond symptoms. Individuals tend to encounter mixed messages, particularly on the internet, where sound advice becomes submerged in an ocean of opinion and sometimes opposing information (Jan et al., 2024). When physicians take a moment to describe how these conditions are different—not just what you see but also what causes them and how they react to various methods—it empowers patients to make better decisions and even modify their lifestyles slightly. Furthermore, the recognition that such skin problems come close to matters of emotional well-being fosters a more supportive care culture. In most situations, when patients and healthcare workers have a definite, rounded picture of these problems, it translates into better treatment, less flaring, and a generally better quality of life (Figure 5.3).

5.1. Causes of Acne

Acne is more than skin deep – imagine it as a clammy combination of what is going on within our skin, where hormones and immune messages are having an ongoing conversation. The pilosebaceous unit, which combines the hair follicle with its sebaceous gland, is not just hanging around; it produces and fine-tunes hormones like a mini endocrine system. Most of the time, this "in-house" hormone activity operates on a system similar to the hypothalamus-pituitary-adrenal (HPA)-similar axis, which, to be frank, responds to stress and triggers inflammation in the skin. Sex hormones and stress can accelerate the gland's activity, releasing more sebum that, in turn, tends to worsen acne. This mixed-up hormonal waltz leads to thickening of the follicle's lining and inflammation that sets the stage for long-standing acne lesions (Clark et al., 2020). In short, acne is inextricably entangled with our skin's nerve and hormone habits, mixing up both local and body wide issues into one complicated picture. The inflammation we observe in acne vulgaris usually starts with folliculitis – i.e., the hair follicle is inflamed by several stimuli, ranging from internal causes to external causes. Oftentimes, acne vulgaris is classified as folliculitis because its clinical presentation is a mix of other follicular conditions, and therefore it is a puzzle to some degree. It begins with overly active keratinocytes plugging up the follicle's opening, resulting in the development of comedones. Next, when *Cutibacterium acnes* (once known as *Propionibacterium acnes*) enters the picture, the immune system of the skin is stirred into action, fueling the flames of inflammation and exacerbating the lesions. And it is not even acne vulgaris – other inflammatory breakouts such as rosacea also target pilosebaceous units, illustrating the fact that this region is surprisingly susceptible to all sorts of inflammatory issues (Alper & Aksoy, 2017).

Examining these overlapping mechanisms provides a fairly good understanding of why the causes of acne are so complex. Our genetic configuration combined with day-to-day environmental factors puts another spin on the origins of acne. Individuals who have an inherited sensitivity to androgen hormones tend to have larger and more active sebaceous glands that can trigger more aggressive acne outbreaks. Normal, everyday things like diet, climate, hygiene routines, and even the cosmetics we apply can nudge skin conditions and the microbial balance – sometimes improving the situation, sometimes making it worse. And then There is psychological stress, which is always lurking and ready to emerge when you least expect it, amplifying the skin's stress response and releasing additional proinflammatory substances that make the breakouts worse. More broadly, acne must be regarded as a systemic condition rather than as a mere localized cutaneous disease. Its etiology is rooted in an complex interplay of hormonal, microbial, genetic, and environmental influences – an appreciation that demands therapeutic strategies to confront not just the microbes and inflammation but also the underlying hormone dynamics and lifestyle factors (Alper & Aksoy, 2017; Saric-Bosanac et al., 2020) (Figure 5.4).

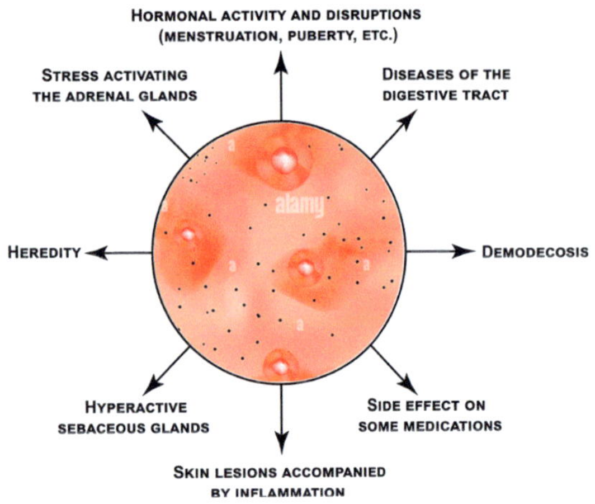

Figure 5.4. Causes of acne.

Source: Timonina, I. (n.d.). *Causes of Acne: Pustules, Papules, Comedones, Blackheads.* https://c8.alamy.com/comp/2A6PBYD/causes-of-acne-pustules-papules-comedones-blackheads-acne-on-the-skin-infographics-vector-illustration-on-isolated-background-2A6PBYD.jpg.

5.1.1. Hormonal Changes

Our skin is not only protective against the outside world—it also plays games with hormones in a way that greatly complicates things like acne and rosacea. Down deep in those pilosebaceous units, which both disorders feature to a large degree, steroid hormones (including the ones linked with stress and sex) get produced and locally metabolized. Interestingly, the skin has its own version of a HPA axis that, in most instances, gets activated during stressful situations by adjusting hormone production. Changes in hormone levels can affect oil gland activity, which then, very predictably, triggers off inflammation and abnormal skin cell accumulation that we so commonly observe in acne. Concurrently, this type of localized endocrine activity also appears to be connected with the inflammatory outbursts in rosacea, bringing entire hormonal fluctuations into visualization with observable skin problems. In a sense, coming to terms with this rather complicated neuroendocrine connection is essential for the development of targeted therapies (Saric-Bosanac et al., 2020). Hormonal fluctuations—during those sleepless teenage years all the way through to adulthood—have a deep influence on the behavior of the skin, and androgens (such as testosterone, although these hormones are not unique to one sex) dominate in the cause of acne. These high androgens stimulate the manufacture of sebum, creating an oil-laden environment of the skin that is susceptible to plugged pores and bacterial accumulation, which stimulates inflammation. Although rosacea's origins are a little more involved and less explicitly linked to hormones, new data typically suggests that hormonal changes could even exacerbate vascular and inflammatory reactions. As an illustration, when stress triggers a torrent of hormone release, it can activate the skin's inflammatory pathways, adding to red patches and minuscule perceptible vessels characterizing rosacea. In most instances, it appears that hormone management might have a helpful application in the management of such skin conditions, particularly when one looks at the common inflammatory and pilosebaceous processes (Saric-Bosanac et al., 2020). In terms of treatments, scientists are emphasizing the strategies that tackle both the hormonal and inflammatory foundations of rosacea and acne by fine-tuning the central biochemical pathways. Certain antibiotic therapies, such as certain tetracycline derivatives—achieve clinical benefit not only by attacking bacteria but also by suppressing inflammation that fluctuating hormones are prone to stimulate; these agents interfere with cytokine signaling, the activity of specific matrix enzymes, and oxidative stress as well. Since the hormonal responses of the skin so frequently involve overlap with inflammatory mechanisms, treatments that reduce both of these effects simultaneously hold great promise. Future research to more clearly define which hormone fluctuations initiate these inflammatory cascades, and precisely how they interact—

will most likely refine treatment approaches. A holistic approach that balances hormones in conjunction with immune regulation appears to be increasingly indicated (Figure 5.5).

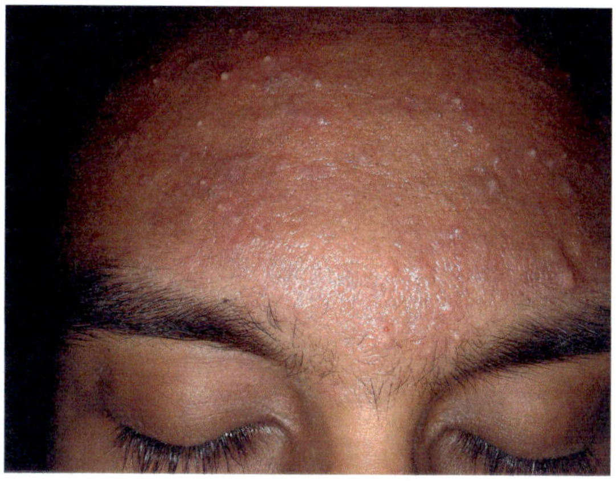

Figure 5.5. Signs of adult hormonal acne.

Source: By Roshu Bangal - Own work, CC BY-SA 4.0, https://commons.wikimedia.org/w/index.php?curid=47832556

5.1.2. Bacterial Growth

Knowledge of bacteria on our skin is important—a big deal, particularly when addressing problems such as acne and rosacea. The skin has a diverse community of bacteria, and at times, some of them will grow too much, disrupting the natural order. When that occurs, these microbes engage with our immune system, usually provoking inflammation seen in skin diseases. For example, a sudden outburst of some bacteria can initiate a cascade that drives inflammation and accentuates symptoms. Furthermore, conditions like sebum production and moisture determine how these microbes reproduce; any interruption here may cause bacterial dysbiosis, which several researchers view as an instigator behind inflammatory skin disorders (Korting & Schöllmann, 2009). Rosacea, however, tends to be more complicated in most instances because it appears that microbes as well as the immune system both lose their typical brakes. The whole picture is not fully sorted out yet, but more recent research tends to suggest overall that inflammatory pathways—involving inciting bacterial antigens—play a primary role in the development of the disease. At other times, bacteria associated with Demodex folliculorum mites may increase levels of matrix metalloproteinases and cytokines, a process that ultimately amplifies inflammation and tissue damage. Therapy such as tetracycline derivatives, for instance, has the tendency to not only inhibit bacterial growth but also to reduce inflammatory responses. This implies that reducing bacterial proliferation may well mollify the general rosacea symptoms (Korting & Schöllmann, 2009). In the case of acne vulgaris, once more, bacteria have an important role.

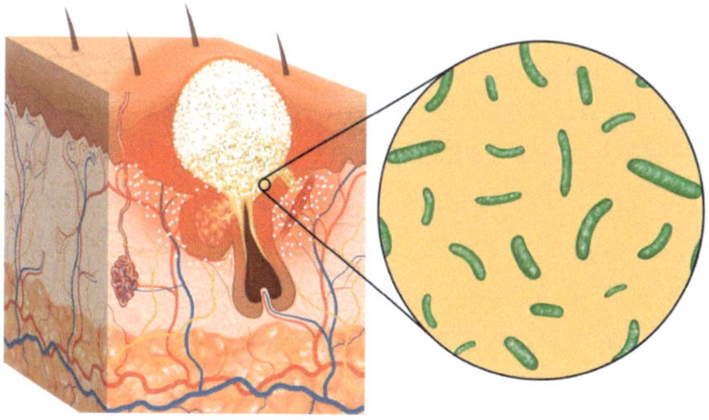

Figure 5.6. The role of bacteria in acne.

Source: Acne.org. (2021). *The Role of Bacteria in Acne.* https://www.acne.org/wp-content/uploads/2021/12/The-Role-of-Bacteria-in-Acne.jpg.

Propionibacterium acnes, the predominant microbe of oily skin follicles, is able to stimulate immune reactions leading to inflammation of the hair follicles. Its continued growth aids in triggering granuloma formation and release of proinflammatory mediators, thereby exacerbating acne. Notably, the communication between the skin and even the gut microbiomes appear to affect systemic immune responses; a sign that issues in one spot may reverberate elsewhere. In most instances, employing antibiotics or even microbiome rebalancing seems to be an effective means of soothing both bacterial proliferation and the resulting inflammation (De Pessemier et al., 2021) (Figure 5.6).

5.1.3. Environmental Factors

Skin problems like rosacea and acne are not just genetically born – what occurs outside is a big contributor as well. We are realizing now that a mix of things, including changing weather, challenging city air, and strong sunlight, seriously disrupts our skin. These factors appear to break the natural barrier of the skin and fine-tune its immune system, at times activating inflammatory mechanisms that increase the intensity of the disease. Even latest research indicates that our skin is not merely a cover; it is an active interface between the external world and our internal processes. And do not forget the skin microbiome, which itself changes in response to these environmental fluctuations, further complicating the picture. All of this goes some way to explaining why some individuals get flare-ups more often – a suggestion that specific preventive measures may one day really pay off (De Pessemier et al., 2021). Another dimension to add is the gut-and-skin axis, where an imbalanced equilibrium between microorganisms is key. When the normally helpful bacteria get out of balance, a condition researchers refer to as dysbiosis, the immune system's equilibrium is disrupted, usually triggering inflammation that exacerbates skin disease. External factors, be they pollutants or even food, can disrupt this subtle microbial blend, compromising the skin's built-in defenses against nasty microbes. This imbalance could even initiate a vicious cycle in which the body's own defense mechanisms turn back on it, making symptoms worse. There is increasing evidence that attempts at resetting this balance of microbes may be central to treating such disorders, highlighting just how interdependent our environment, our microbes, and our immune system are (De Pessemier et al., 2021). There is also the concept of the exposome, which essentially ties together all environmental exposures an individual encounters over their lifetime. This method brings in considerations such as UV rays, chemical exposure, daily life practices, and persistent pollution, to sketch a more complete picture of their combined effect on our skin. While the idea did not gain traction in dermatology initially, more recent studies in exposomics are slowly uncovering how cumulative outside forces could engage with our innate genetic code to cause or exacerbate conditions such as acne and rosacea. By charting these exposures, scientists hope to pinpoint moments for intervention, opening up possibilities for more personal treatment plans. This broader view promises to steer us toward prevention strategies that address both environmental triggers and our individual vulnerabilities (Granger et al., 2023).

5.2. Causes of Rosacea

Rosacea appears to arise from a chaotic mix of external things occurring outside the body and internal characterestics that, together, ignite persistent inflammation. Externally, factors such as ultraviolet (UV) light, heat, and other microbes are involved, while our skin's own nerve and blood vessel impulses, and even its immune responses—add to the mix to keep things perpetually irritated. Consider the pilosebaceous unit: far from being purely a structural component, it is also sort of like a mini endocrine gland, spewing out and metabolizing steroid hormones that fuel the fire of inflammation. In most instances, this hormonal activity in the skin reproduces a HPA process, regulating stress responses that inadvertently perpetuate the condition (Saric-Bosanac et al., 2020). Grasping these mechanisms, is the foundation of how one would develop treatments that address both hormonal pressures and immune malfunctions at play. Another turn in rosacea is how some small creatures, such as Demodex mites, become too friendly with hair follicles and oil glands, or else induce a strange immune reaction to themselves. In other cases, their intrusive presence elicits a chronic inflammation and follicular damage that manifests as the classic lesions we talk about with the condition. Fascinating how this dance, with mites causing an inflammatory response (and sometimes bacterial particles join in), renders rosacea look so much like acne-like breakouts in some areas, even when acne vulgaris typically boils down to bacteria and sebum. In general, what this implies is that although the two conditions have some overlap, rosacea is more of an aberrant immune reaction to these mites and their antigens (Alper & Aksoy, 2017). This subtlety, when combined with clinical and microscopic examinations, generally serves to distinguish rosacea from other disorders with some similarity. Family history and excessive vascular response introduce yet another degree of complexity. Those who have had rosacea usually look even more sensitive to stuff that makes the redness occur, suggesting that there is an inheritable factor behind how the nerves and blood vessels are managed. Abnormalities in the neuropeptides as well as even channels like the TRP channels on the sensory nerves will have you breaking into uninduced episodes of vasodilation—so that repeated instances of the constant redness and swelling arise. Furthermore, the subsequent oxidative stress of these neurovascular hiccups can translate to the inflammation just not residing, and it causes additional tissue pain. When you combine this inborn vascular mismatch with the skin's endocrine characterestics and microbial effects, a vicious cycle follows that progresses the condition over time (Saric-Bosanac et al., 2020). In most cases, recognizing how genetics and vascular factors play into things is essential for moving toward more personalized treatments (Figure 5.7).

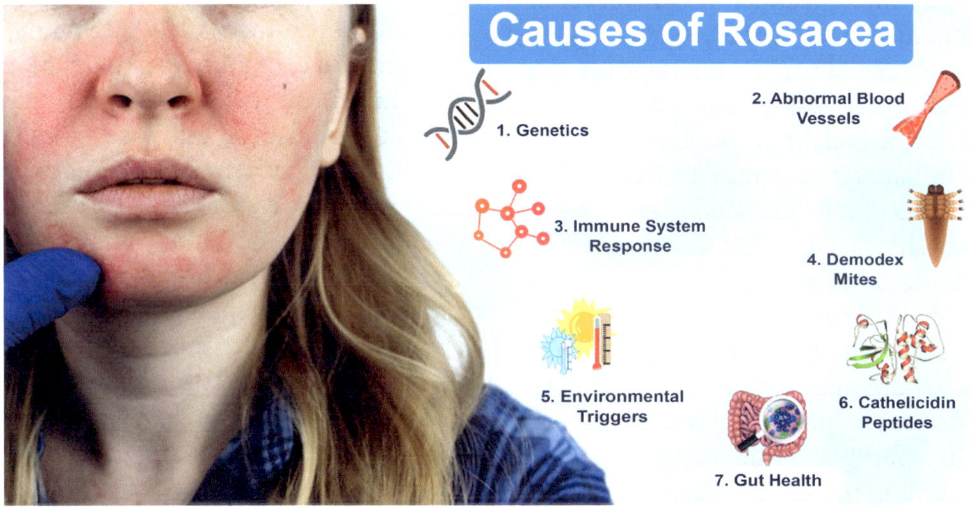

Figure 5.7. Causes of rosacea.

Source: OngoCare. (2023). *Causes of Rosacea.* https://ongocare.com/wp-content/uploads/2023/08/Causes-of-Rosacea.png.

5.2.1. Genetic Predisposition

Acne and rosacea appear due to a combination of factors—your surroundings, how your immune system functions, and what you inherit from your parents. Family studies indicate that if a close relative has these conditions, it increases your risk, and this implies that heredity is a greater factor than we might often attribute to it. Your genes can adjust how your body responds to irritants, keep your skin barrier intact, and even trigger inflammation in surprising manners. But these inherited characterestics never act alone; they mix with external stimuli such as daily microbes or stress, which can alter how severe symptoms may become and how they end up presenting. Exploring these genetic influences provides us with a genuine, if sometimes chaotic, understanding of why these conditions may be so varied and persistent over time. When researchers look into what triggers rosacea at the molecular level, they tend to discover that some genetic pieces pave the way for that combination of inflammation and blood vessel alterations. In general terms, an aberrant innate immune response (affected by family history) can overreact to everyday skin microbes, resulting in the chronic redness, bumps, and sometimes pus-filled lesions we observe in patients (Fortuna et al., 2016). Certain gene mutations also appear to interfere with the functioning of blood vessels and how our oil glands respond, which may be the basis for the chronic inflammation characteristic of the disorder. It seems that focusing on these genetic pathways may allow us to refine treatments that alleviate symptoms associated with inherited characteristics. These hints contribute to a better understanding of rosacea's many forms, pushing us toward more individualized care plans. Acne rosacea joining forces with eye issues truly puts the spotlight on the contribution of genetics to guiding the entire disease process. Evidence is directed at inherited factors that could modify how glands surrounding the eyes operate and adjust immune reactions, with anywhere from 30–70% of rosacea patients also experiencing ocular symptoms (Dogan et al., 2017). Not only do these genetic factors mold skin manifestations, but they can also turn up the volume and duration of eye problems—making a team-based treatment strategy nearly necessary. Understanding more about these genetic contributions assists practitioners in being able to make better educated guesses about how the condition is going to progress and develop long-term plans that take into account both inflammation and troublesome microbes. Ultimately, family history becomes a significant protagonist behind both the skin and eye sides of acne rosacea, and this serves as a reminder of why exploring genetics is of such importance when providing improved patient care.

5.2.2. Triggers and Flare-Ups

Acne and rosacea tend to arise due to a mixture of causes that act in combination—both from outside and inside our bodies. Sunlight, pollution, and even changes in the weather can trigger inflammation in the skin, worsening these conditions. Meanwhile, hormonal fluctuations at puberty, around the time of menstruation, or when stress strikes can shift levels of sebum and adjust immunity responses, sometimes resulting in bumps or outbreaks. What you do daily, such as what you consume, your alcohol use, or even your facial routine, can turn the skin's defense and the minuscule universe of microbes that inhabit it. Digital twin technology now brings all these variables together, typically assisting in identifying individual triggers and paving the way for a form of precision medicine that can at times anticipate and soothe future flares (Haykal, 2025). In most instances, this type of information assists physicians in molding treatments that alleviate pain and improve long-term results. Blinking back in time, to see the inside story on flare-ups, you will observe a complex web of inflammatory reactions at play—initiated by microbes lodging in and the body's immune machinery going awry. Consider *Cutibacterium acnes* (formerly *Propionibacterium acnes*), for example; it is fairly central in igniting up follicular inflammation within acne. With rosacea, it is somewhat the same: disruption of the skin's microbial balance and overactive blood vessels are typically responsible, with microbes like Demodex mites sometimes throwing fuel on the fire. Drugs like clindamycin do their job by fighting these microbes while also calming inflammation, thus decreasing both lesions and redness (Maria et al., 2024). That being said, overusing antibiotics can result in resistance, so caution is necessary in prescribing them. In general, gaining an understanding of these microbial actions and how they contribute to the initiation of inflammation is crucial for developing treatment regimens that are both effective and sustainable. Occasionally, stress and intense emotions also have a large role in causing acne or rosacea flares. Cortisol, the stress hormone, tends to disrupt the balance of the immune system and allow inflammation to get out of control.

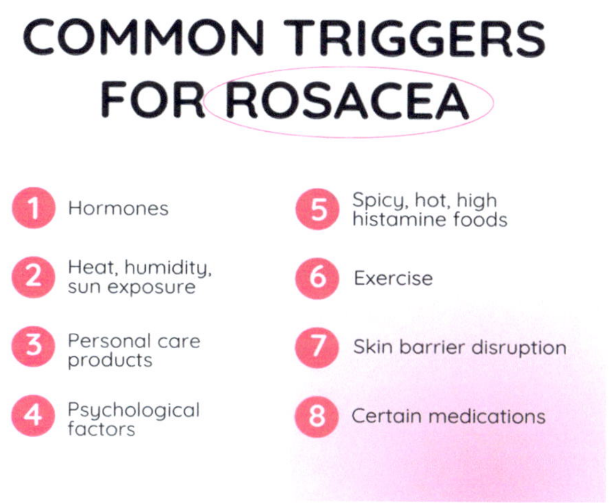

Figure 5.8. Common triggers for rosacea.

Source: Brighten, J. (2023). *Rosacea on Face Triggers.* https://cdn.drbrighten.com/drbrighten/20230809085054/Rosacea-on-Face-Triggers-1024x1024.png.

Additionally, normal skincare products, cosmetics, or even environmental factors could weaken the skin barrier or initiate allergic-like responses, again triggering symptoms. As the causes can be so numerous, monitoring one's own conditions becomes fairly critical. New methods such as digital twins collect data from wearable sensors and patient history to identify moments when the skin could be at risk and recommend initial actions (Haykal, 2025). In most instances, such precision instruments might transform the way patients deal with their conditions, enabling them to comprehend and avoid their individual triggers, and – ultimately – contribute to overall quality of life and disease management (Figure 5.8).

5.2.3. Vascular Abnormalities

Vascular concerns with acne and rosacea do count—even if they never command the center stage. Vessels in the skin behave somewhat erratically, emitting more signals such as redness and flushing; occasionally, a leaky vessel or spontaneous dilation just fuels on-going inflammation in a loop that may be difficult to escape. Sunlight, fluctuating temperatures, or even a case of bacteria can push these vessels into overdrive, so it makes some sense that fundamental anti-inflammatory Band-Aids would not always reach the target. For the majority of patients, targeting treatments straight at those vessels appears to be the missing component for managing persistent redness and those pesky, problematic little broken vessels. When you look more broadly, you can see that what is occurring within your body also influences these vascular characterestics. Your neighborhood skin—the composition of microbes on your skin and in your intestines—feeds into the way your immune system reacts. And when that gets out of control, the vessels get a little rebellious, making inflammation more deep-seated that may occur with rosacea. For the most part, what you see on the skin might be only one symptom of a bigger, challenging interaction between our immune systems and microbial communities. So, approaches that attempt to balance these microbial communities and soothe the immune system might simply reduce the vessel problems indirectly, suggesting that a more integrated approach is necessary (Pessemier et al., 2021).

Tech is not far behind. Today, methods such as machine learning and computerized drug screens are accelerating the pursuit of chemicals capable of dampening abnormal vessel response without introducing yet more issues. Scientists can now simulate how the blood vessels are likely to respond at a molecular level, which, to be real, reduces way down on treatment development time. This cross of cutting-edge tech and precision medicine is opening the doors to treating directly irritated vessels in cases of acne and rosacea. In the majority of instances, as these devices improve, they have the potential to unlock new methods to repair the underlying vessel problem and change patient outcomes for the positive (Carracedo-Reboredo et al., 2021).

5.3. Symptoms of Acne

Acne is a mixed bag, to say the least. It begins when small hair follicles become plugged—those small bumps we refer to as comedowns, or better known as blackheads and whiteheads—packed with excess sebum and dead skin cells. Occasionally these small pimples take a turn; in no time at all, they become red, puffy bumps such as papules and pustules that are easily inflamed. Sometimes you will develop deeper, more sore lesions—cysts or nodules—that not only are painful but will scar.

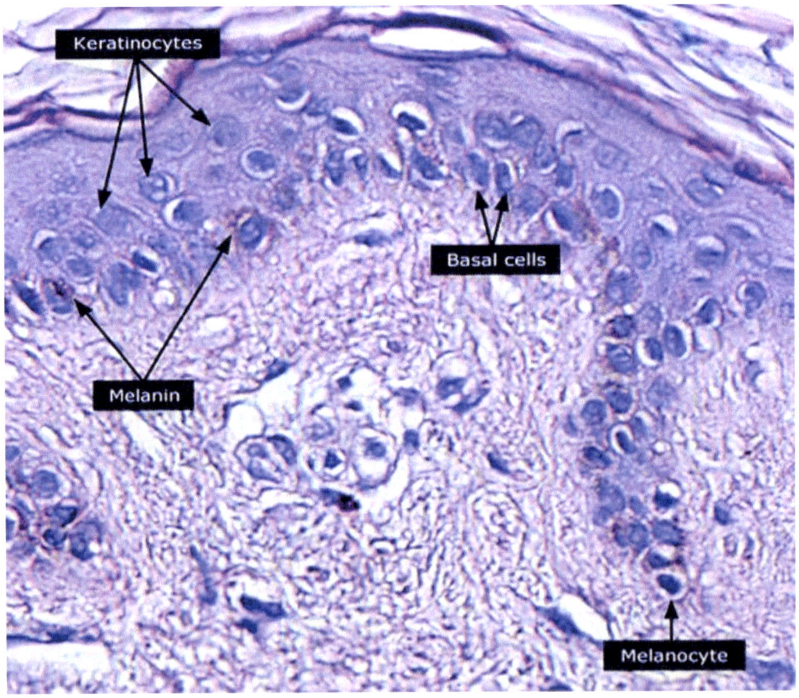

Figure 5.9. Acne symptoms.

Source: By James Heilman, MD - Derivative work of File:Cysticacne.JPG, CC BY-SA 3.0, https://commons.wikimedia.org/w/index.php?curid=125339269

The inflammation is not superficial, either; it can penetrate down to the cellular level, causing both physical distress and emotional tension. Acknowledging all of these symptoms illuminates why customized treatment is truly necessary. Inflammation in general takes a big hand in the way that acne appears, and it rings a lot of changes similar to what occurs in rosacea. Both diseases follow very similar inflammatory pathways, consider the engagement of cytokines and matrix metalloproteinases—to stimulate redness, swelling, and lesion formation. Your immune system and even bacteria such as *Cutibacterium acnes* essentially get into this sloppy game in a manner, contributing to the fire. The intensity of this inflammation generally corresponds to the extent of the lesions, directing treatment strategies in turn. Interestingly, therapies like tetracycline derivatives, have been found to alleviate such inflammatory reactions by reducing cytokine production and inhibiting reactive oxygen species, which really underscores the way the treatments for acne tend to parallel those for rosacea (Korting & Schöllmann, 2009). Apart from what you just see on the skin, acne usually appears with other health problems that may complicate treatment even further. New research generally indicates that skin ailments such as acneiform disorders often coincide with systemic disorders—fibromyalgia, for example—still impacting an individual's way of life. This is not merely about marks on the surface; it implies that the inflammation we observe may also be one among broader body upsets. Although the precise pathways through which acne are connected to these conditions are not as yet completely outlined, the fact that inflammation of the skin can reflect larger physiological changes reminds us how complex acne truly is, and it prompts a more integrated examination of treatment (D'Onghia et al., 2024) (Figure 5.9).

By Setijanti H.B., Rusmawati E., Fitria R., Erlina T., Adriany R., Murtiningsih - Chapter: Setijanti H.B., Rusmawati E., Fitria R., Erlina T., Adriany R., Murtiningsih (2019) Development the Technique for the Preparation and Characterization of Reconstructed Human Epidermis (RHE)Book: Kojima H., Seidle T., Spielmann H. Alternatives to Animal Testing, Springer, Singapore DOI: 10.1007/978-981-13-2447-5_3. ISBN: 978-981-13-2446-8.License: Creative Commons Attribution 4.0 International License, CC BY 4.0, https://commons.wikimedia.org/w/index.php?curid=82095836

5.3.1. Types of Lesions

Acne lesions appear in numerous varieties, and being aware of these distinctions is important in order to receive the proper diagnosis and treatment protocol. For example, the initial presentation tends to appear as comedones—those plugged pores we refer to as blackheads when open or whiteheads when closed off. Then inflammatory subtypes such as papules and pustules will develop as your body responds to bacterial accumulation and broken follicles; nodules and cysts, in contrast, typically indicate more serious, more internal inflammation. Practitioners, most of the time, discover that replicating these findings allows them to not only measure severity, but also determine what treatments may be most effective—even if appearance occasionally appears a bit erratic.

Rosacea, though, has a different story to tell. It typically presents with persistent flush and redness over the mid-face, with inflammatory papules and pustules, but without comedones of acne – something which aids the differential diagnosis quite a bit. You may also see small vascular spots (telangiectasia), and in some cases, even phymatous changes that indicate tissue thickening. Subdividing rosacea into subtypes, like the papulopustular subtype characterized by those red, inflamed bumps, seems to direct treatment and follow-up very well (Alegre et al., 2019).

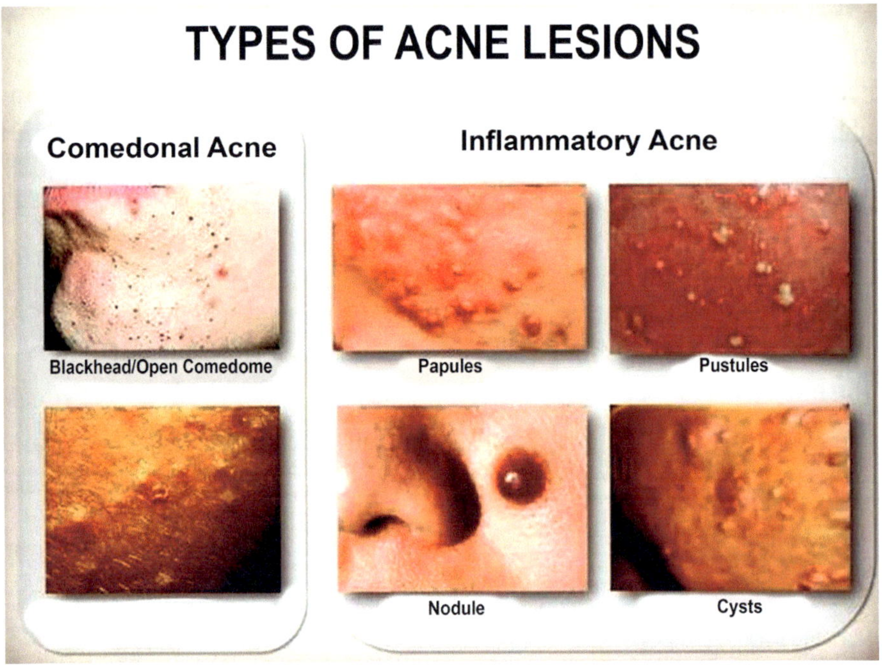

Figure 5.10. Types of acne lesions.

Source: Unknown. (n.d.). *Medical illustration.* https://cdn.medizzy.com/I2Qn_oIMM_O7kYgG-T6NVeGJoXE=/680x510/img/posts/3506e84a-38a9-4a92-86e8-4a38a9fa9297.

Both have prompted scientists to investigate new avenues of treatment with the goal of removing lesions and avoiding scarring. There is early evidence, as a whole, that botulinum toxin may have advantages in treating inflammation, decreasing sebum production, and even regulating inflammatory cytokines, enhancing lesion appearance in those particularly recalcitrant cases. Again, these results are early, and more rigorous clinical trials will have to sort out such issues as optimal dosing and long-term effects. To some extent, the complex information behind every lesion features a pivotal impact in advancing therapeutics and thereby improving the quality of a patient's life (Chmiel et al., 2025) (Figure 5.10).

5.3.2. Severity Levels

Inflammatory skin diseases such as rosacea and acne appear in all sorts of ways, and how they appear makes a difference when deciding on treatment. You may notice something as straightforward as a few comedones and the occasional red spot in mild acne, whereas more serious cases can erupt into widespread nodules, cysts, and ultimately scarring. Rosacea, also, may simply be an episode of brief redness or flushing one day, only to become chronic erythema, papules, pustules, and even tissue hypertrophy down the road.

Hormonal changes, immune reactions, even environmental factors all combine to create this image. In the majority of instances, even the mechanisms behind, such as the activity of an HPA-like axis of a skin and the metabolism of hormones locally—differ between the milder and more severe forms (Saric-Bosanac et al., 2020). This, in most cases, necessitates a very personalized approach when treating these conditions. Inflammation is not merely an afterthought in these skin conditions—it drives the disease forward. Take, for example, antimicrobial peptides (AMPs); as intended to eliminate the pathogen, they will interfere with our signal for immune reactions, sometime worsen the inflammation. With aggressive flares, there may result an higher AMP reaction causing perpetual inflammation, destruction of the follicle, and ultimate scarring resulting in forms of acne seen on phymatous rosacea (Matanic et al., 2012).

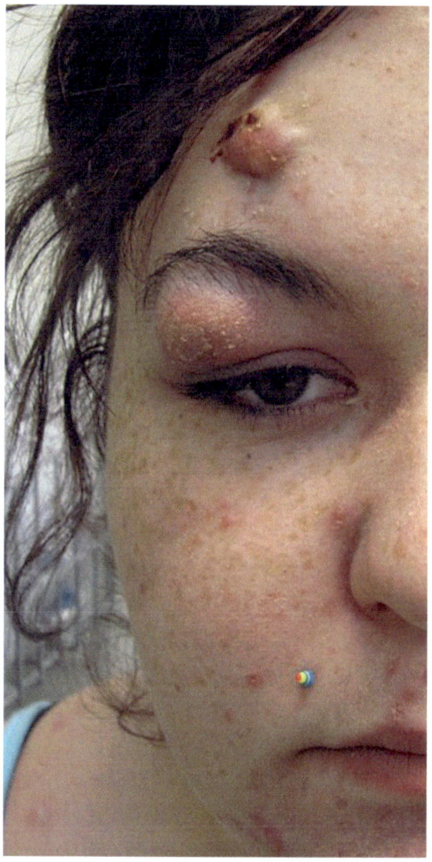

Figure 5.11. A severe case of nodular acne.

Source: Heilman, J. (2010). *Closeup Photo of a Severe Case of Cystic Acne.*

It is a little ironic how the body's own defenses could become part of the problem, and this dynamic truly highlights why it is so important to get these immune factors right in order to get the full picture of disease severity. Acne and rosacea become even more problematic due to their chronic, sometimes changing nature. Hormonal changes, particularly those associated with stress or sex steroids—can trigger flare-ups, and that indicates how far the skin's own glandular, pilosebaceous unit can dance with inflammatory pathways. For rosacea, a chronically unstable vascular system and a form of immune imbalance can cause redness and inflammatory lesions to persist, at times culminating in tissues becoming permanently altered if not maintained under tight control. Assessing the severity of these conditions, therefore, is not merely a matter of what you can see on the surface; it is also a matter of the underlying molecular and hormonal signals (Matanic et al., 2012; Saric-Bosonac et al., 2020). This more integrated, holistic perspective is more likely to direct treatments that are more naturally suited to a patient's individual biological configuration, ultimately leading to better outcomes and quality of life (Figure 5.11).

5.3.3. Psychological Impact

Skin diseases that you can easily see ultimately burden more than just the body—these tend to screw with one's head too. Individuals suffering from acne or rosacea usually feel abnormally self-conscious and anxious in social situations; sometimes these emotions can even go on to make them withdraw from friends or work and lower their self-esteem. Continuous skin problems can have a person always in fear of their look, creating an unfavorable attitude about themselves that merely contributes to their stress. Most of the time, this weighing emotional burden may also cause additional skin breakouts since stress itself has the capability to bring on both acne and rosacea. It is an entangled mess, —a dead giveaway that taking care of someone's mind in addition to their skin might add up to a lot of difference in total care. Entangled with all of this is the subtle dance between stress and conditions such as rosacea and acne. Stress tends to function as a kind of primer, exacerbating symptoms and triggering outbreaks more frequently. In addition to the clear signs on the skin, stress will drive individuals away from enjoyable or necessary activities, and this fueling of isolation and inner distress stokes. At times, these very strong, negative emotions, such as shame or even embarrassment—begin to build and build and build to more difficult concerns like anxiety or depression. This ping-pong between mood and skin condition truly illustrates the reason why a balanced strategy that calms body and mind alike is necessary to reduce flare-ups and stay on course with treatment (Chmiel et al., 2025). Even with all the latest developments in skin therapies, the psychological aspect of coping with acne and rosacea sometimes falls by the wayside. New research into treatments such as mindfulness-based stress reduction (MBSR) is suggesting a promising solution to reducing the anxiety and low moods that usually accompany these chronic conditions. By providing individuals with valuable tools for coping with stress, MBSR can provide emotional resilience, prevent patients from dropping out of treatment, and ultimately result in improved overall outcomes. While more work is certainly necessary to pin this down, preliminary evidence indicates that combining some mental health care with the standard treatment for rosacea and acne may enhance both mood and skin health—toward a more integrated approach to managing these ubiquitous skin ailments (Chmiel et al., 2025).

5.4. Symptoms of Rosacea

Rosacea is a tenacious skin disease that appears as a chronic flush of redness on the face. Individuals find that they first notice it most on the cheeks, nose, forehead, and chin, and the severity can fluctuate wildly. Small, nearly spider-like capillaries occasionally appear too, suggesting that all is not well beneath the surface. This is not merely superficial; that chronic redness typically indicates a induced immune system and persistent inflammation—much as occurs in other long-term diseases in which persistent provocation eventually does tissue damage (Rahman et al., 2021). It serves as a reminder that these vascular markings typically accompany other symptoms, making both comfort on a daily basis and appropriate treatment difficult. There is then the additional inconvenience of acne-like pimples. They may appear as papules or pustules, but you will not see blackheads or clogged pores as you would with normal acne. Rather, they are accompanied by a burning or stinging sensation, leaving the skin even more sensitive. Although they share certain similarities with acne, their spread and development are quite different, leaving one to question what the actual culprit is. This additional irritation appears connected to localized skin immunity and an upset microbiome (Pessemier et al., 2021)—a combination that only serves to highlight the way multiple factors, ranging from blood vessel characterestics to immune miscalculations, can accumulate in rosacea. Others experience problems even deeper than the skin's surface. Many, for example, experience angry, dry, and red eyes—a condition commonly referred to as ocular rosacea that, if left unaddressed, could even impact vision. With time, constant inflammation can gradually thicken the skin around the nose, a transformation called rhinophyma (more common in men) that probably results from excessive inflammatory signals causing excess oil production and even fibrosis. Treatment in general attempts to quiet this internal tempest by addressing the inflammation and sometimes even restoring the skin and gut microbiome (Pessemier et al., 2021; Rahman et al., 2021). All in all, the range of symptoms—from a flushed face to uneasy bumps and eye issues—paints a picture of a complex condition where immune, vascular, and microbial factors all have a hand in the mix (Figure 5.12).

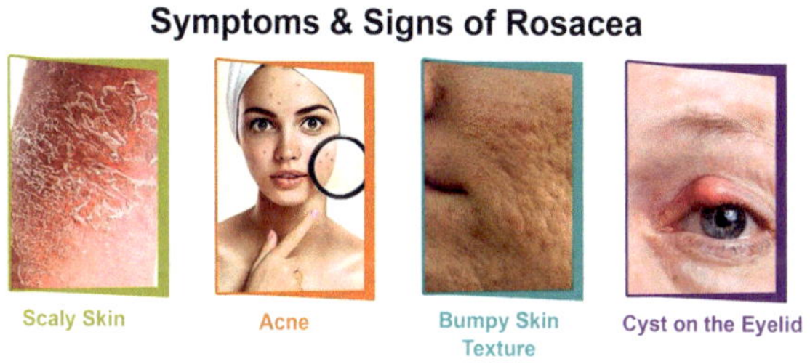

Figure 5.12. Symptoms and signs-of rosacea.

Source: Medindia. (n.d.). *Symptoms and Signs of Rosacea.* https://www.medindia.net/images/common/patientinfo/950_400/symptoms-and-signs-of-rosacea.jpg.

5.4.1. Skin Redness and Flushing

Redness and flushing appear as obvious indicators in most inflammatory skin conditions such as rosacea and acne. You notice the blood vessels opening up and allowing more blood circulation on the face, not simply a temporary flush due to heat or rapid emotion—it indicates something different is happening. When the red persists, it tends to indicate deeper, long-term inflammation, with nerves and immune cells sort of married to a state of chronic inflammation (Manjula & Kumar, 2024). Constant redness indicates that the skin is under ongoing stress, which in turn feeds into both the physical irritation and the emotional distress that individuals tend to experience. Addressing these changes in blood flow can aid in reducing the noticeable appearance and even simplify some of the daily discomfort associated with it. Rosacea, specifically, will often begin with that telltale red flush, sometimes before the occurrence of bumps, pustules, or small dilated blood vessels. Most commonly, the central face becomes red and then, at random, additional flushes are added to the equation, sometimes heat, stress, or even a skincare product that simply does not get along with the skin. Rosacea patients tend to have reactive, sensitive skin that requires special attention: imagine gentle cleansers and products that restore its natural barrier.

This type of tender treatment, typically combined with medical therapies, can genuinely alleviate both redness and pain, although the skin's activity fluctuates unpredictably between flare-up and quiescent moments (Chmiel et al., 2025). In a majority of instances, individualizing therapies to stabilize these vascular reactions while calming the overall sensitivity is the best way to encourage more wholesome, resistant skin. New treatment concepts are also on the horizon to treat the blood vessel alterations responsible for the redness of acne and rosacea.

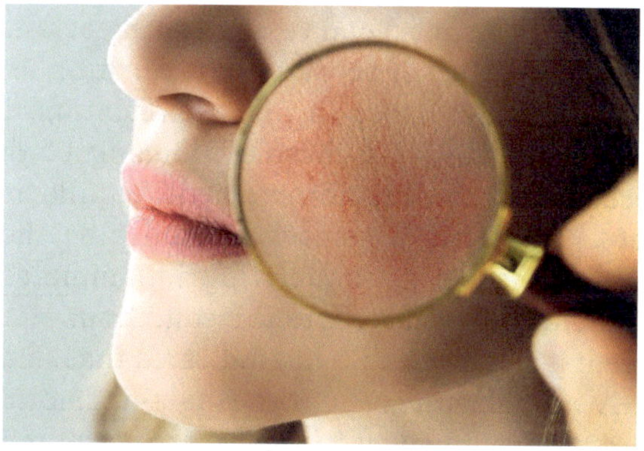

Figure 5.13. Skin redness.

Source: CosmeticsDesign-Europe. (n.d.). *Image of Cosmetic Packaging.* https://www.cosmeticsdesign-europe.com/resizer/v2/NHCORD7DJ5O3VOL2JJ3RTTNIJM.jpg?auth=8ffb562d94bc794c45519dca7b1c77ab0a5db8bf55188cd81dca4b87fd32923a.

For instance, botulinum toxin therapy has garnered some interest since it may reduce the chronic flush. Initial research suggests that this toxin can disrupt neurovascular signaling, essentially changing the way nerves talk to blood vessels to cut down on the sudden dilation and related inflammatory rush. While those initial results are promising, additional large-scale studies are necessary to pin down the optimal dosing and safety for regular use in the management of skin redness (Chmiel et al., 2025). In the majority of instances, investigating these novel approaches appears to be an exciting path forward to not only address the inflammatory lesions but also address the apparent vascular effects, which could contribute to enhanced patient comfort and self-confidence (Figure 5.13).

5.4.2. Visible Blood Vessels

Genes and the air around us can combine in subtle ways to lay the groundwork for difficult skin issues, particularly when it has to do with vessels appearing in unusual locations. Rosacea, for instance, tends to appear with those clear, visible blood vessels (telangiectasia) that are a result of constant inflammation and a disheveled balance in blood circulation. In most instances, this chronic widening of the vessel and the resultant brittle capillaries not only bother a person aesthetically; they also develop more underlying inflammatory problems that exacerbate the condition. More recent genetic research has indicated that small DNA adjustments, such as single-nucleotide alterations and some HLA markers—may tend to enhance an individual's susceptibility to develop rosacea, correlating naturally with greater inflammation in the vicinity of the blood vessels in the skin. Exploring these molecular drivers also accounts for why those sensitive vessels tend to make themselves noticeable and become even more sensitive, which in most instances sets the stage for treatments targeted both at the blood vessel characterestics and the inflammation (Chang et al., 2015). Rosacea generally announces itself with a persistent flush of redness and those conspicuous blood vessels that both patients and practitioners notice fairly early in the disease. The look of these vessels appears to be the result of a combination of persistent skin inflammation and a peculiar vascular reaction—small capillaries expand and draw attention throughout the cheeks and nose.

But it is not merely a matter of a change in appearance; these visible vessels are also an indication of deeper errors in the way nerve impulses and immune reactions are regulated. Current clinical practice guidelines typically recommend addressing these vascular findings not only to reassure cosmetic concerns but also to assist in inhibiting the exacerbations of inflammation and preventing the condition from developing into more dangerous forms. In essence, the red, obvious vessels serve as a double-barreled clue both for diagnosis and as an aim for therapeutic interventions, indicating their place within a complete spectrum of patient care (Del Rosso, 2016). In terms of dealing with visible blood vessels in acne and rosacea, the method is quite diverse—a combination of genetic understanding and practical clinical approaches. Acne primarily appears with plugged pores and bacterial accumulation and does not tend to put these vascular problems on center stage, whereas rosacea is characteristically defined by vessel abnormalities that contribute to its tenacity. Rosacea treatments usually include drugs that, in a sense, pinch the blood supply or inhibit vessel growth, nicely complementing anti-inflammatory choices. In general, catching these vessel changes early and treating them head-on can prevent further enlargement and the tissue changes that tend to make what you see on the skin worse.

Synthesizing our growing knowledge of vascular genetics with new, emerging clinical guidance provides a promising path toward more individualized care, one that, in the end, should improve outcomes and overall quality of life for patients (Chang et al., 2015; Del Rosso, 2016).

5.4.3. Eye Involvement

Eye problems in rosacea can be a nuisance, frequently confusing both diagnosis and treatment. Patients may present with hardly discernible eye symptoms that may appear before any skin manifestations or even independently, which can quite commonly result in the condition being missed. The severity bounces around a little – beginning with mild dryness or irritation and possibly progressing to problems such as chalazion, blepharitis, or conjunctivitis. The symptoms are chronic and just keep returning, seriously disrupting daily life. Also, in the absence of one sure test for ocular rosacea, misdiagnosis or delayed treatment is frequent, particularly when eyelid inflammation appears stubborn or when eye discomfort just does not calculate. In general, identifying the connection between rosacea and eye symptoms is critical for early treatment, which further slows down the progression of the disease and reduces permanent eye damage (Han et al., 2024). Treating eye issues in rosacea associated with acne requires additional caution since the skin around the eyes is sensitive and can quickly flare up with improper treatment. Common approaches are maintaining the eyelids clean, the warm compresses, and counting on anti-inflammatory treatments to soothe the irritation. Systemic and topical antibiotics are at work here, such as the case with doxycycline, which has been found to reduce surface inflammation and prevent chalazions from reoccurring too often. If these conservative measures just are not sufficient, systemic antibiotics can step in by altering the fundamental inflammatory process. All that being said, it is important to exercise care when choosing the appropriate treatment; females of childbearing age are particularly cautious because medications like isotretinoin are teratogenic. That is, safer topical treatments, such as clindamycin, which tends to exhibit little phototoxicity—are usually more commonly selected, considering also that exposure to UV light is found to exacerbate rosacea (Mildzikhova et al., 2024). Associating systemic rosacea with its ocular symptoms quite dramatically emphasizes the necessity of a multidisciplinary approach among specialists. Both ophthalmologists and dermatologists, in the majority of instances, have to collaborate with each other to address both the skin and the ocular components, eventually enhancing patient outcomes.

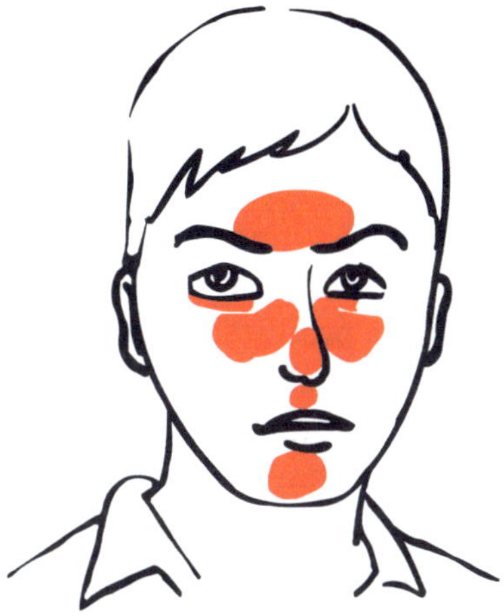

Figure 5.14. Ocular rosacea.

Source: By PNG: Jean-no SVG: Karl Udo Gerth - Rasacee_couperose_zones.png, FAL, https://commons.wikimedia.org/w/index.php?curid=8697877

Rosacea's chronic eye inflammation may manifest in different forms, whether it is through repeated chalazions, chronic dryness, or even blepharitis, and each form requires its own treatment protocol. Though surgery may at times be the solution for the extraction of a chalazion, it many times fails when the underlying inflammation is not addressed, allowing opportunity for problems to recur. Combined therapy—combing systemic antibiotics with anti-inflammatory therapy—very often enhances outcome after surgery. In addition, clinicians should also discuss with patient's simple lifestyle adjustments, such as sun protection and good skin care, to minimize flare-ups. Knowing the early signs of ocular rosacea and recognizing them is imperative in averting permanent eye damage (Han et al., 2024; Mildzikhova et al., 2024) (Figure 5.14).

5.5. Treatment Options for Acne

Acne treatment has evolved significantly over the years. Physicians now take into account how bad the breakouts are and tailor their treatment to suit each individual's case. Mild-to-moderate breakouts in most cases tend to respond well to simple topical therapy—retinoids, benzoyl peroxide, and even a splash of antibiotics. Recently, there has been hubbub over azelaic acid, which individuals such as for its numerous tricks, ranging from soothing inflammation to combating microbes and mollifying skin accumulations. Azelaic acid, frequently applied singly or in combination with oral antibiotics to avoid resistance issues, is regarded as a good bet—even in pregnant patients. Treatment typically takes the form of anywhere from six to eight weeks, on average, which most professionals agree appears to be the therapeutic sweet spot (Uddin & Yesmin). New treatments are emerging as well and they do not adhere to a rigid formula. There are new retinoid formulas promised to be gentler, though, on the skin and new topical or systemic treatments that target adjusting sebum production and the entire inflammatory process. Combination treatments are becoming more popular precisely because acne is not one-dimensional; it requires a multi-angled approach. And then there is a trend towards laser and light-based methods, which sometimes act as additional tools, particularly when normal treatments are not doing enough or when a person's skin type requires special attention. As we continue to discover what drives acne on a cellular level, more specific treatments are being developed, promising a truly dynamic practice of care (Dursun et al., 2019).

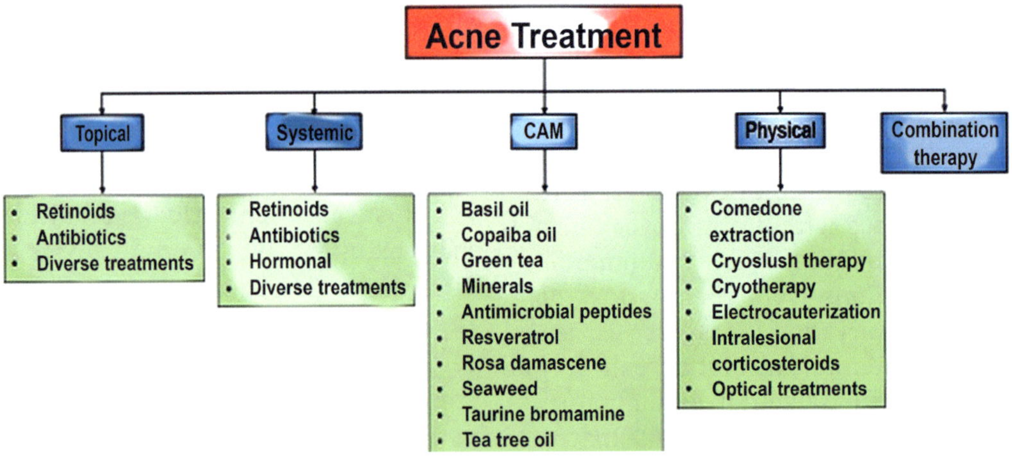

Figure 5.15. Acne treatment.

Source: Kalia, Y., & Muñoz-Torrero, D. (2016). Treatment modalities for acne. *Molecules, 21*(8), 1063.

Ultimately, following through on a treatment regimen and tailoring it is most important. Dermatologists tend to point out that any regimen ought to be complementary in terms of conditions such as skin sensitivity, even conditions such as rosacea which may ride alongside and confuse, and lesion types. Azelaic acid stands out then because not only does it tackle the lesions but also does work on residual marks after inflammation. And, of course, patients receive guidance on good skin care and even a bit of lifestyle adjustments that complement the medications in the long term. Finding the best balance of how well something does work, is safe, and what the patient likes still is the essence of successful acne management (Dursun et al., 2019; Uddin & Yesmin) (Figure 5.15).

5.5.1. Topical Treatments

Treating skin problems is not always a matter of one-size-fits-all solutions. Sometimes you require a specific solution to soothe inflammation and the overgrowth of microbes on your skin. Topical treatments are helpful in such situations because they address the area directly, reducing those undesirable side effects elsewhere. You may discover that products such as retinoids, antibiotics, and anti-inflammatory creams combine to reduce bumps, redness, and inflammation and make the skin smoother. Acne treatment, for instance, now addresses both the current breakouts and the residual marks left behind, such as scars or dark spots. A small clinical trial even discovered that a new cream reduced both scars and discoloration with virtually no side effects (Bruce et al., 2025). This type of double-duty treatment illustrates, in general, how our knowledge of acne continues to advance. Retinoids are not merely about unclogging pores—they also reduce inflammation. Consider trifarotene, a fourth-generation retinoid that is formulated specifically for your skin. Its targeted application is not something you need to be as concerned about with the medicine floating around in your system and irritating things. Some new research combining trifarotene with oral antibiotics indicates promising news for moderate to severe acne, reducing the numbers of lesions dramatically and increasing clinical check-up scores (Uddin & Yesmin, 2024). Together, these treatments slow the propagation of Propionibacterium acnes while calming excessive skin cell proliferation. This combination not only boosts treatment efficacy but also makes patients nicer and more inclined to comply with their regimens. Trifarotene's clever design works well in most cases for different skin types, and it is especially helpful for refractory truncal acne that tends to disregard more conventional creams. Treatment of rosacea borrows some concepts from acne care but takes a different turn. Rather than having a single-track approach, creams for rosacea directly address soothing inflammation and alleviating those blood vessel concerns that create the typical redness and papulopustular pustules.

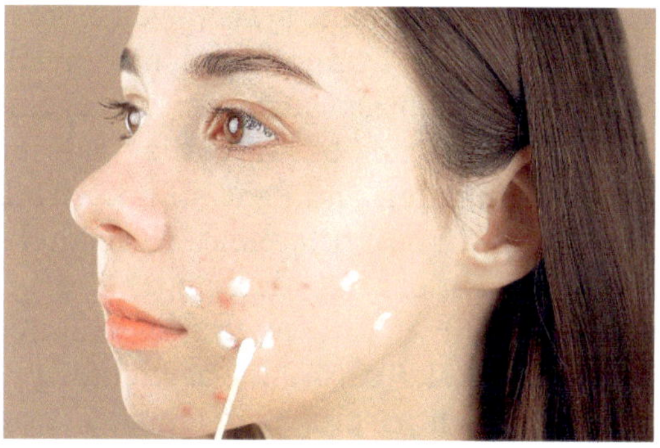

Figure 5.16. Using retinoids for acne.

Source: Minimalist. (n.d.). *Cover Image for Article on Skincare.* https://beminimalist.co/cdn/shop/articles/cover_image_1_8feddbc1-6612-4f12-8f61-06408f155a58.jpg?v=1612849156.

Although rosacea and acne both have red, inflamed areas, their causes are different enough that treatment is as well. Typical choices, such as metronidazole, azelaic acid, and ivermectin—attack the microbes and inflammatory cycles that cause rosacea outbreaks. Layering topical treatments not only calms the redness but can also address any persisting cosmetic effects, which is important because undiagnosed rosacea could leave skin appearing to be forever red or mottled. Finding the balance between how potent a cream is and how comfortable it feels is finicky, something common to acne treatment as well. In general, dermatology is trending toward more personalized, effective, and tolerable treatments that allow each patient's individual skin narrative to shine through (Figure 5.16).

5.5.2. Oral Medications

Occasionally, stubborn skin problems require more than a mere cream on the surface. Chronic conditions tend to drive us to treatments that are bodywide, not just in one location. For example, when daily topicals simply do not work for acne or rosacea, many physicians turn to oral medications that attempt to quiet hormone imbalances, out-of-control bacteria, and an overactive immune system—all elements that fuel those chronic blemishes. Rather frequently, antibiotics such as tetracyclines become the solution because they not only reduce inflammation and fight off bacteria but provide an all-in-one treatment. Nevertheless, it is not always easy to determine the ideal oral medication; it is a matter of balancing benefits and risks carefully, particularly for populations such as pregnant females, where even minute risks to the fetus must not be taken lightly (Kaptanoglu & Mullaaziz, 2017). In most instances, this complicated picture highlights why treatment must be individualized to achieve the proper balance between good outcomes and few side effects. Sorting out rosacea and acne with pills involves adopting a blended approach that aligns each drug's effect with what the patient is experiencing. Retinoids, for instance, act powerfully to even out skin cell turnover but have severe risks of causing birth defects, which restricts the usage to certain individuals. Hormonal solutions can smother the overproduction of oil, particularly significant for most women—but these also need careful use. Patient reactions are unpredictable, and because these conditions tend to persist for years, regular check-ups and even mixing therapies at times become required in order to maintain the skin in a clear state and enhance the quality of life. Clinicians generally find themselves balancing options between antibiotics, retinoids, and hormone-related agents, attempting to cause more good than bad while working through each patient's individual case (Nojek et al., 2024). Pregnancy, though, adds another wrinkle to the situation. In the case of treating acne or rosacea in pregnant women, the typical systemic treatments might not be safe due to possible harm to fetal development, and frequently the safety information just is not robust enough. Physicians then tend to rely on non-teratogenic, or safer—treatments and more conservative options that will alleviate symptoms without harming mom or baby. Hormonal changes and a little immune suppression during pregnancy also tend to confuse the picture further, and hence, close, and cautious monitoring becomes imperative. Being precise about these challenges prevents aggravation of skin conditions, prevents secondary infections, and even alleviates some of the psychological distress during such a sensitive period (Kaptanoglu & Mullaaziz, 2017). This sensitive scenario really calls for a cautious, evidence-based approach that respects the need for individualized care.

5.5.3. Lifestyle Modifications

Skin microbes play a larger part in maintaining our healthy skin than we once thought. Recent research indicates that maintaining these tiny animals in balance may be the ticket when addressing such problems as acne and rosacea. What we do every day—what we put in our mouths, how we cleanse, and even where we hang out—has the power to push this microbial blend in one direction or another, either relieving or exacerbating skin issues. For instance, gentle washing and the avoidance of very harsh products can prevent the disruption of the skin's natural crowd, keeping it resistant to unwanted invaders. Environmental factors like heavy pollution or excessive UV light also hang over the head and must be carefully managed. Observing how our selections engage with this mini environment presents us with useful, occasionally complementary, methods to address skin issues that transcend mere dependence on medications (Kortekaas et al., 2024). Mental well-being and diet also contribute heavily to skin issues such as acne and rosacea. Stress, by triggering inflammation, can tip the balance and cause flare-ups; therefore, interventions such as mindfulness or cognitive-behavioral therapy are often advocated in the general treatment regimen. Diet may be as powerful—reducing sugary foods and some dairy foods, for example, may reduce acne conditions. There is also increasing hype surrounding probiotics, which may assist in modulating both local and systemic immune responses, slowly restoring the micro balance to a healthier position while reducing inflammation. Essentially, addressing these lifestyle factors in addition to conventional treatments not only assists with the physical symptoms but may also improve overall quality of life, allowing individuals to feel better about managing a chronic skin condition (Sieradocha, 2024).

Treating acne and rosacea requires an individualized solution and not a one-size-fits-all solution. Following skincare regimens appropriate for your own skin type can generally preclude flare-ups and maintain the integrity of the skin barrier. It should also be noted that lifestyle advice should emphasize avoiding known culprits, excessive sun, excessive alcohol, and temperature extremes tend to induce rosacea specifically. When patients understand how their everyday decisions affect their skin, they tend to engage more with their own care, which can lead to better, longer-lasting results. This type of comprehensive, multi-faceted plan, blends lifestyle adjustments with appropriate medical treatment, emphasizes a biopsychosocial perspective in dermatology and places a high premium on combining varied approaches to alleviate the burdens of acne and rosacea while helping maintain general skin well-being (Kortekaas et al., 2024; Sieradocha, 2024).

5.6. Treatment Options for Rosacea

Rosacea is not a simple puzzle to solve because its symptoms appear in so many different ways and we still do not entirely understand why it occurs. Physicians tend to end up combining various strategies, one-part creams, one-part pills—to customize treatment for each individual. For instance, a newer variation has been microencapsulated benzoyl peroxide, which now finds application specifically for papulopustular rosacea despite being long a first choice for acne. Most practitioners are loathe to dive in with it due to concerns about irritation and an unclear understanding of precisely how it impacts rosacea lesions; however, newer incarnations attempt to minimize side effects while providing actual benefits in reducing inflammation. In general, this option provides another avenue for clinicians attempting to home in on the inflammatory bad aspect of the condition (Rosso et al., 2024). When creams fall a little short in handling more challenging cases, systemic treatments take center stage as an encouraging alternative. Consider minocycline foam in a 1.5% strength; it provides anti-inflammatory action right where it is needed while reducing the risks commonly associated with oral antibiotics. The design of the foam results in the medicine remaining primarily where you put it, resulting in less opportunity for common systemic side effects you might get with conventional tetracyclines. Since rosacea is likely to be a chronic condition, treatment regimens simply must trend toward safety and convenience over the long term. With the release of minocycline foam, practitioners now stand in an improved position to treat those erythematous papules and pustules without subjecting patients to the traditional systemic risks (Rosso et al., 2024). Several of those topical remedies formerly in favor of acne therapy have also revealed benefits for rosacea, and fittingly, that is perhaps because the two disorders have pieces of the same inflammatory processes. Azelaic acid, which was first used to treat acne and even hyperpigmentation, is now gaining traction as a sound option for soothing inflammatory rosacea. It acts in a number of ways, being an antimicrobial, calming inflammation, and even aiding in the shedding of dead skin; all of this with a safety profile that usually accommodates even very sensitive skin. Physicians tend to prescribe azelaic acid on its own or combine it with other treatments, allowing them to make targeted adjustments to alleviate general concerns such as redness and bumps. Its versatility makes it become a go-to in the clinician's cabinet for addressing rosacea flare-ups.

5.6.1. Topical Therapies

When addressing acne and rosacea, the choice of cream matters, one that gets to the root of the issue without irritating sensitive skin. Customized formulations have become the go-to tools because each case has its own unique characteristics. A large part of this is not necessarily choosing the active ingredient; it is also how the ingredient is delivered. The vehicle, or base, must support the drug firmly, allow it to absorb correctly, and maintain the skin's natural barrier intact (particularly when the skin's already a little compromised). Most often, solutions such as Cleoderm™ demonstrate what can be done; a mild, consistent medium that is compatible with a variety of agents, from benzoyl peroxide to retinoic acid. This type of advancement not only increases treatment compliance but also keeps patients more at ease, all while avoiding some problems present in more traditional alternatives (Polonini et al., 2022). Combination treatments also offer a bonus to the table when it comes to acne and rosacea by addressing multiple areas of concern simultaneously. Research indicates that fixed-combination products—take, for example, one that combines benzoyl peroxide with topical retinoids—will see improved patient compliance compared to the use of individual treatments. Cost issues and your insurance availability still are major considerations, but the ease and effectiveness of a single combination should not be ignored. The buzz around free samples, which occasionally are these combo products, truly highlights the dilemma of balancing cost against optimal clinical outcomes. Occasionally, allowing patients to decide between a combo product and individual ingredients—based on what works for their wallet and condition—may be the most realistic way forward (Feldman, 2018). Concerns about safety and cost have also influenced how physicians prescribe these topicals and provide samples in clinics.

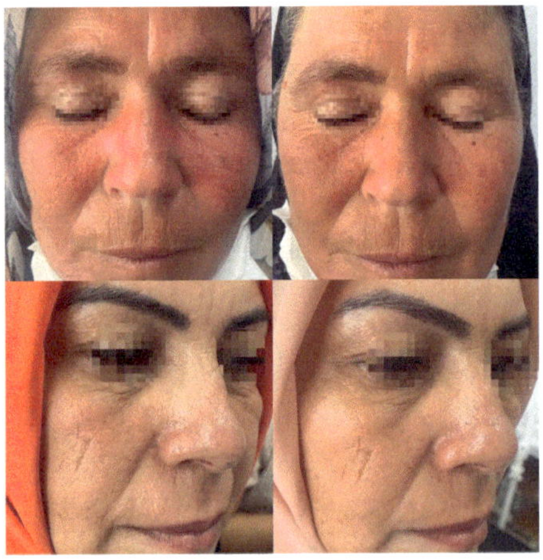

Figure 5.17. Clinical improvement in erythematotelangiectatic rosacea with Dapsone 5% gel treatment. Clinical improvement is seen from grade 3 to 2 in the first patient and from grade 2 to 1 in the second patient.

Source: Unknown. (n.d.). Clinical improvement in erythematotelangiectatic rosacea with Dapsone 5% gel treatment. *ResearchGate.* https://www.researchgate.net/publication/377855650/figure/fig1/AS:11431281221573660@1706791274393/Clinical-improvement-in-erythematotelangiectatic-rosacea-with-Dapsone-5-gel-treatment.jpg.

Studies appear to indicate that medications such as calcineurin inhibitors have a sound safety profile, particularly in comparison to corticosteroids, and which serves to alleviate some of the anxiety surrounding systemic risk. Additionally, providing patients with a sample can be a big deal—it allows them to know how the treatment would feel in day-to-day life before committing completely. This is especially the case for conditions such as rosacea and acne, where concern over irritation or side effects could lead to premature discontinuation of therapy. Although the cost aspect of providing samples remains open to debate, there is much to indicate they enhance patient participation and treatment results. Obviously, more rigorous studies must be done to pin down optimum topical approaches (Feldman, 2018) (Figure 5.17).

5.6.2. Laser and Light Treatments

Laser and light technology has been in the news a lot recently as a method for addressing belligerent skin concerns such as acne and rosacea. The technology targets specific areas of the skin – essentially nailing the areas that are in need of attention , which quiets inflammation and induces the skin to look more refreshed, all with minimal harm to surrounding tissues. Rosacea, which most often appears as chronic redness and minimal visible blood vessels, has been addressed through vascular-targeting lasers (imagine the pro-yellow laser). In a retrospective analysis of 98 patients, success rates were typically over 70% for an array of vascular issues, with treatments for spider angioma and genital angiokeratoma truly being the best in class. Interestingly, the research reported that the color of a patient's skin did not appear to impact outcomes, which shows how versatile this laser technology can be – although, when the nose was involved, it did not go so well, indicating the requirement for a more tailored strategy (Ataseven et al., 2023). On another front, new indications involving combinations of intense pulsed light (IPL) and precise laser wavelengths are unfolding new avenues for treating pigmentation concerns that occasionally accompany treatments for acne and rosacea. For instance, drug-induced skin color changes from drugs such as minocycline – commonly used to treat inflamed skin – can be a real dilemma. These color changes can persist long after the medication is discontinued, and in the majority of instances, they generate a significant amount of cosmetic distress as well as some psychological distress. Lasers such as the q-switched Nd:YAG have long been used to address hyperpigmentation in the conventional sense, but more recent research trends toward combining various treatments.

A single case report even demonstrated that combining chemical peels with IPL was effective in resolving minocycline-induced facial hyperpigmentation, suggesting that combination treatments not only accelerate clearance but also reduce treatment time and side effects (Li et al., 2023). This trend indicates that laser and light therapy are moving beyond the mere treatment of the primary lesions towards addressing the side effects of treatments as well. Laser and light treatments are promising alternatives to traditional drug therapies, but it turns out that they require a precise, individualized approach based on such factors as the type of lesion, skin color, and precisely where problems occur. Selective photothermolysis allows these treatments to target exactly those vascular and pigmented targets responsible for acne and rosacea with precision, decreasing inflammation and redness. It would seem that as visible symptoms are alleviated, patients also see some encouraging psychosocial advantages—a key component of quality of life. However, even with generally favorable results, there are things to overcome: efficacy can be inconsistent in individual locales and side effects can surface, so continued study is certainly in order to refine these techniques. Together with these laser and light therapies, conventional medical treatments tend to enhance success, particularly in resistant or pigment-involved cases (Ataseven et al., 2023; Li et al., 2023) (Figure 5.18).

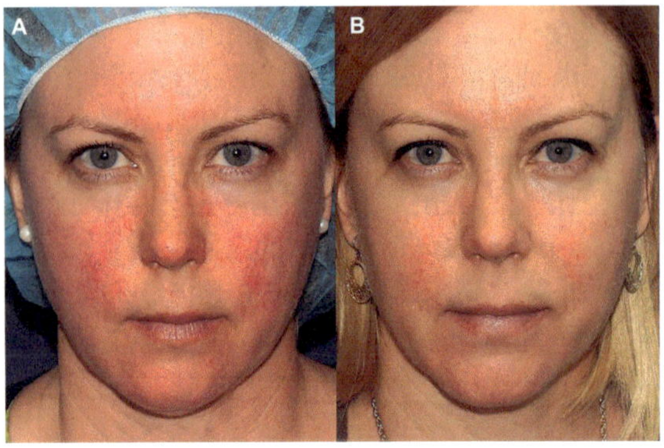

Figure 5.18. Before (A); and after (B) one treatment with Intense Pulsed Light (IPL) for rosacea.

Source: Lee, J.-B., Lim, H. S., Lee, S.-C., & Won, Y. H. (2014). Before (A) and after (B) one treatment with IPL for rosacea. In The efficacy of intense pulsed light for treating erythematotelangiectatic rosacea is related to severity and age. *Annals of Dermatology, 26*(4), 491–495.

5.6.3. Avoidance of Triggers

Recurring skin problems like rosacea tend to begin with just one important step, finding out and avoiding the things that trigger flare-ups. Sunlight, intense heat, and even certain skincare products tend to induce inflammation, which manifests as that all-too-familiar flush and pimple-like bumpiness. There is some underlying genetic foundation, but more often than not it is the immune system overreacting that perpetuates the issue. In general, toning down these daily environmental agitates appears to placate the skin, reducing flare-ups and enhancing condition in general. Despite the availability of combinations of medications and treatments, a lot of people still cannot entirely keep their symptoms under control, pointing out just how important monitoring lifestyle and environmental triggers remains (Tu et al., 2024). Dietary options have also become major players in the intensity of acne and rosacea. Certain new studies; even if they are not always entirely definitive indicate that there are significant differences in what people with these issues consume as opposed to individuals without any skin issues. Food such as dairy, meat, cheese, and even booze tends to exacerbate the flare-ups, whereas increasing vegetable, legume, oily fish, olive oil, and nut intake may even provide some protection. For acne in particular, it seems that dairy can increase insulin-like growth factor-1 levels, suggesting a biochemical connection between diet and inflammation of the skin. In most instances, when patients are brought into awareness of these diet-related dangers, they can make adjustments in their lifestyles to function in conjunction with other treatments, hopefully lightening the total disease burden (Guertler et al., 2023). Daily stress and the normal emotional roller coaster also appear to play an important role in initiating flares for acne and rosacea. It is not just about what you apply to your skin or slip into your diet; occasionally stress releases a chaotic cascade of inflammatory messages and even disrupts the neurovascular system, resulting in even more redness and lesions. A few small steps, identifying ways to control stress, selecting skincare with a little more thought, and not getting quite so wild in the sun—can keep these breakouts under control. Adding in such avoidance measures with local and internal treatments may not only alleviate the visible condition but also calm the underlying immune and vascular turmoil. Incorporating all of these into the treatment strategy that targets individualized trigger avoidance is important to achieving better results and a higher quality of life for many afflicted by such chronic skin conditions (Tu et al., 2024).

CLOSER LOOK

Cutibacterium Acnes

Cutibacterium acnes, previously known as *Propionibacterium acnes*, is a ubiquitous bacteria on human skin, especially in sebum-exposed regions. Though it is largely a commensal organism, it may also be an opportunistic pathogen, especially when it comes to acne and some infections. C. acnes may contribute to acne by developing biofilms, enhancing inflammation, and breaking down host tissues.

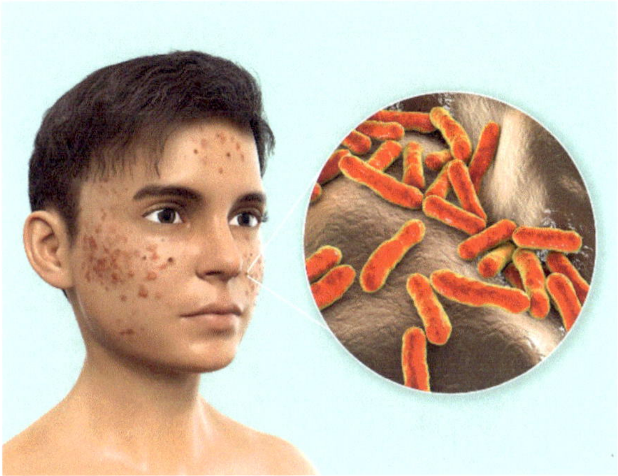

Source: BioWorld. (n.d.). *Acne vulgaris and Cutibacterium Acnes.* https://www.bioworld.com/ext/resources/Stock-images/Therapeutic-topics/Dermatologic/acne-vulgaris-Cutibacterium-acnes.jpg?1738080836.

Important features of *C. acnes*:

- **Commensal and Opportunistic:** *C. acnes* is a normal commensal on human skin but may infect the skin in certain conditions, particularly when it overgrows or is drug-resistant.
- **Acne and Acne-Related Infections:** *C. acnes* is a key cause of acne, particularly when it overgrows within the pilosebaceous units and leads to inflammation and the formation of comedones.
- **Infections Other Than Acne:** *C. acnes* infections can also be found in other regions of the body, such as deep-tissue infections (particularly that of implants), surgical site infections (SSIs), and even certain forms of endocarditis.
- **Lipophilic Character:** *C. acnes* is lipophilic, i.e., it has an avid attraction towards lipids and oil, which accounts for its predilection for sebaceous glands and sebum-plentiful regions of skin.
- **Biofilm Formation:** *C. acnes* is noted for its capacity to form biofilms, which are aggregates of bacteria coated in a protective matrix. Biofilms are capable of causing persistent infections and being resistant to treatment.

- **Variable Phylotypes:** *C. acnes* exists in various phylotypes (subtypes) with different capacities for disease or for creating a healthy skin environment.
- **Antimicrobial Resistance:** The rising incidence of antimicrobial-resistant *C. acnes* is a cause of concern, especially in acne patients and those presenting for surgery.

In short, C. acnes is a multifaceted bacterium with a dual function on human skin. Though it is a natural inhabitant that helps maintain a healthy skin microbiome, it can also be an important contributor to the onset of acne and other infections. It is important to know its traits and relationship with the host to be able to create efficient treatments against acne and other C. acnes-related infections.

SUMMARY

Acne and rosacea affect more than your skin—they get at your emotional state, as well. Both can trigger a reaction of embarrassment and anxiety, and push some individuals into withdrawal from social situations, so merely working on the external effects often is not sufficient. In all but a few instances, treating just the outside symptoms can leave the inside upset to go untended, which can result in incomplete healing. There is growing evidence, for example (Adaskevich, 2016), that simple stress-reducing practices like mindfulness can ease the anxiety and depression that sometimes comes with long-term skin issues. This way of looking at things shows that handling both the outer spots and the inner feelings together might make care more effective. It turns out our skin and nervous system have a kind of two-way bond. Stress and anxiety and even depression can initiate flare-ups or exacerbate the appearance of acne and rosacea, making it harder for medical care to work effectively and prolonging the healing process. The relatively new science of psychodermatology really drives this point home by demonstrating, in a few cases (Jahan & Zafar, 2024), how skin and mental health are interconnected. Including mental health checkups in skin care regimens serves to identify these comorbid problems and push us toward more comprehensive, patient-centered treatments—even when, sometimes, the process can feel a touch messy or unbalanced. Looking ahead, treating acne and rosacea is far from a one-track treatment—instead, it requires continued research into methods that address both physical symptoms and the psychological pressures that accompany them. A blended strategy, in which dermatologists collaborate hand-in-hand with mental health professionals, in general, appears to be promising for developing individualized approaches that address all aspects of the condition (Jahan & Zafar, 2024). Clinical trials and long-term studies integrating various treatment modalities will be instrumental in determining effective, evidence-based guidelines. This holistic vision promises the future of skin care as one that acknowledges the inescapable connection between the skin we see and the emotions we feel.

Big studies have begun to lift the covers on what lies behind rosacea, revealing it is not a straightforward skin condition—it is influenced by a combination of internal characterestics and what is happening out there. It appears that behaviors we would least suspect, such as cigarette smoking, can be associated with a reduced likelihood of developing rosacea, and an amount of alcohol appears to push the risk up slightly. In other instances, chronic diseases such as late-onset diabetes may even decrease the incidence, perhaps because the blood vessels simply do not relax like they should. All of which quite strongly indicates we cannot disregard either the events occurring within a patient or what they are exposed to on a daily basis, and older medications like spironolactone and lithium may simply be reused to help reduce the risk (Spoendlin, 2013). Drilling a bit deeper, the origins of rosacea appear to be mired in a combination of immune overreactions and nerve-related errors. The condition tends to kick in when our fundamental defenses go into overdrive and blood vessels respond way too intensely, usually prompted by daily stress or even UV light. These sparks illuminate molecular pathways, including those involving transient receptor channels as well as inflammatory signals such as IL-6 and TNF-α—that subsequently drive skin irritation and vascular responses. With these leads in mind, scientists have been creating targeted topical therapies that attempt to quell that excessive response, reduce inflammation, and even address nuisance pests such as Demodex mites. Drugs like ivermectin, metronidazole, and azelaic acid are examples here—these alleviate symptoms and manage the condition, although it is evident that we do need even more specific ones in order to get to the root causes effectively (Okońska et al., 2025). The combination of large pharmacoepidemiological evidence with eye-opening information from molecular research provides us with a quite comprehensive picture of rosacea control that is both wide and profound. Big databases not only assist us in calculating how frequently rosacea occurs but also suggest something of the multifaceted interaction between different therapies and the onset of the disease. In real-world terms, some research indicates that specific medications, β-blockers, or even topical lithium, may nudge a patient's risk, providing some evidence-based advice to clinicians. Meanwhile, continued research into the behavior of our immune and vascular systems supports the logic of today's topical treatments and fuels the search for yet more effective therapies. Essentially, finding the link between big-picture patterns and what is going on at a microscopic level appears to be the key to locking down specific treatment targets and ultimately more patient-centered care (Spoendlin., 2013; Okońska et al., 202).

KEY TERMS FROM THIS CHAPTER

Acne
Bacterial colonization
Blackheads
Chest
Chronic flush
Comedones
Dry-eye syndrome
Face
Follicles
Hormonal fluctuations
Lifestyle adjustments
Neuroendocrine
Oil glands
Patient education
Pimples
Pustules
Rosacea
Spider-looking veins
Symptoms
Telangiectasia

REFERENCES

1. Alegre, M., Alonso-Usero, V., Boixeda, P., del Pozo-Losada, J., et al. (2019). Spanish consensus document on the treatment algorithm for rosacea. *Actas Dermosifiliográficas, 110*(7), 533–545. https://doi.org/10.1016/j.ad.2019.01.010.
2. Alper, M., & Khurami, F. A. (2017). Histopathologic Evaluation of Acneiform Eruptions: Practical Algorithmic Proposal for Acne Lesions. InTech. doi: 10.5772/65494 (accessed on 12 May 2025).
3. Al-Smadi, K., Leite-Silva, V. R., Andréo-Filho, N., Lopes, P. S., & Mohammed, Y. (2023). Innovative approaches for maintaining and enhancing skin health and managing skin diseases through microbiome-targeted strategies. *Antibiotics, 12*(12), 1698. https://doi.org/10.3390/antibiotics12121698.
4. Eichenfield, L. F., Del Rosso, J. Q., Tan, J. K. L., Hebert, A. A., Webster, G. F., Harper, J., Baldwin, H. E., Kircik, L. H., Stein-Gold, L., Kaoukhov, A., & Alvandi, N. (2019). Use of an alternative method to evaluate erythema severity in a clinical trial: difference in vehicle response with evaluation of baseline and postdose photographs for effect of oxymetazoline cream 1·0% for persistent erythema of rosacea in a phase IV study. *The British journal of dermatology, 180*(5), 1050–1057. https://doi.org/10.1111/bjd.17462
5. Armillei, M. K., Lomakin, I. B., Del Rosso, J. Q., Grada, A., & Bunick, C. G. (2024). Scientific rationale and clinical basis for clindamycin use in the treatment of dermatologic disease. *Antibiotics, 13*(3), 270. https://doi.org/10.3390/antibiotics13030270 (accessed on 12 May 2025).
6. Ataseven, A., Temiz, S. A., & Özer, İ. (2023). An investigation of the effectiveness of the 577-nm Pro-yellow laser in patients with vascular disorders. *European Journal of Therapeutics, 29*, 49–54. https://doi.org/10.58600/eurjther-346.
7. Kortekaas Krohn I, Callewaert C, Belasri H, et al. The influence of lifestyle and environmental factors on host resilience through a homeostatic skin microbiota: An EAACI Task Force Report. *Allergy*. 2024; 79: 3269-3284. doi:**10.1111/all.16378** (accessed on 12 May 2025).
8. Nojek, P., Pawlik, W., Zimonczyk, M., Zawół, M., Błaszczyński, G., & Nowotarska, A. (2024). Effectiveness of different acne treatment methods: a comparison of pharmacological, procedural and natural therapies. *Journal of Education, Health and Sport, 71*, 55977. https://doi.org/10.12775/JEHS.2024.71.55977 (accessed on 12 May 2025).
9. D'Onghia, M., Ciaffi, J., Calabrese, L., Tognetti, L., Cinotti, E., Rubegni, P., Frediani, B., & Ursini, F. (2024). Fibromyalgia and Skin Disorders: A Systematic Review. *Journal of clinical medicine, 13*(15), 4404. https://doi.org/10.3390/jcm13154404 (accessed on 12 May 2025).
10. De Pessemier, B., Grine, L., Debaere, M., Maes, A., Paetzold, B., & Callewaert, C. (2021). Gut-Skin Axis: Current Knowledge of the Interrelationship between Microbial Dysbiosis and Skin Conditions. *Microorganisms, 9*(2), 353. https://doi.org/10.3390/microorganisms9020353 (accessed on 12 May 2025).
11. Fortuna, M. C., Garelli, V., Pranteda, G., Romaniello, F., Cardone, M., Carlesimo, M., & Rossi, A. (2016). A case of Scalp Rosacea treated with low dose doxycycline and probiotic therapy and literature review on therapeutic options. *Dermatologic therapy, 29*(4), 249–251. https://doi.org/10.1111/dth.12355 (accessed on 12 May 2025).

12. Carracedo-Reboredo, P., Liñares-Blanco, J., Rodríguez-Fernández, N., Cedrón, F., Nóvoa, F. J., Carballal, A., Maojo, V., et al. (2021). A review on machine learning approaches and trends in drug discovery. *Computational and Structural Biotechnology Journal, 19*, 4538–4558. https://doi.org/10.1016/j.csbj.2021.08.011.
13. Chang, A. L. S., Raber, I., Xu, J., Li, R., Spitale, R., Chen, J., Kiefer, A. K., Tian, C., Eriksson, N. K., Hinds, D. A., & Tung, J. Y. (2015). Assessment of the genetic basis of rosacea by genome-wide association study. *The Journal of investigative dermatology, 135*(6), 1548–1555. https://doi.org/10.1038/jid.2015.53Chioveanu, F., Niculeț, E., Torlac, C., Bușilă, C., & Tatu, A. L. (2024). Beyond the surface: Understanding Demodex and its link to blepharitis and facial dermatoses. *Clinical Ophthalmology, 18*, 1801–1810. https://doi.org/10.2147/opth.s440199.
14. Chmiel, M., Maciaszek, O., Podraza, A., Sacher, C., et al. (2025). Botulinum toxin: An innovative approach to treating acne and acne scars: A systematic review. *Core*. https://core.ac.uk/download/646080098.pdf (accessed on 12 May 2025).
15. Saric-Bosanac, S., Clark, A. K., Sivamani, R. K., & Shi, V. Y. (2020). The role of hypothalamus-pituitary-adrenal (HPA)-like axis in inflammatory pilosebaceous disorders. *Dermatology online journal, 26*(2), 13030/qt8949296f.
16. Clarke, (2013). Optimizing population health and economic outcomes: Innovative treatment for BPH. *Population Health Management, 16*. https://www.semanticscholar.org/paper/212e4a89a3f371d6ea4ee16e730be5ac0a462eb7 (accessed on 12 May 2025).
17. Del Rosso J.Q. Cutaneous rosacea: a thorough overview of pathogenesis, clinical presentations, and current recommendations on management // Vestnik dermatologii i venerologii. - 2016. - Vol. 92. - N. 2. - P. 21-31. doi: 10.25208/0042-4609-2016-92-2-21-31(accessed on 12 May 2025).
18. Del Rosso, J., Baldwin, H. E., Bhatia, N., Chavda, R., York, J., Harper, J., Hougeir, F., et al. (2024). A review of the diagnostic and therapeutic gaps in rosacea management: Consensus opinion. *Dermatology and Therapy, 14*, 271–284. https://www.semanticscholar.org/paper/ac2e3437b3ee067cf2a4ee54a4ace7d4db731cad (accessed on 12 May 2025).
19. Deldar Jan, H., Siddiqui, A. Y., Alqahtani, N. S. M., A Jan, A. S., Alharbi, E. A., Alnodali, N. I. H., Almatrafi, H. O. H., et al. (2024). Patient perceptions about nutrition and skin health in the city of Makkah. Journal of Positive Psychology and Vol. 6 No. 3 (2022): (accessed on 12 May 2025).
20. Dogan, A. S. (2017). Ocular rosacea. *Core*. https://core.ac.uk/download/322429040.pdf.
21. Drug and Therapeutics Bulletin. (2013). An introduction to patient decision aids. *BMJ: British Medical Journal, 347*. https://www.semanticscholar.org/paper/57397940cf739f8e102198f774368956c60a3e97 (accessed on 12 May 2025).
22. Dursun, R., Daye, M., & Durmaz, K. (2019). Acne and rosacea: What's new for treatment? *Dermatologic Therapy, 32*. https://www.semanticscholar.org/paper/2c1bbe3e61196349978cb3e7a640d9e3f749c107 (accessed on 12 May 2025).
23. Feldman, S. (2018). It may not be time to clean out the sample closets. *Journal of Dermatological Treatment, 29*(1, 2). https://www.semanticscholar.org/paper/04f5585ee9baa7cf8a1a1152c68ab486260b2a0d (accessed on 12 May 2025).
24. Gonçalves, M. M. B. de M. M., Pina, M. E. S. R. T., & Tavares de, M. E. (2017). Dermocosmetic care for rosacea. Braz. J. Pharm. Sci. 53 (4) • 2017 • https://doi.org/10.1590/s2175-97902017000400182 (accessed on 12 May 2025).

25. Granger, C., Molina-García, M., Puig, S., & Trullas, C. (2023). Exposome and skin: Part 1. Bibliometric analysis and review of the impact of exposome approaches on dermatology. *Dermatology and Therapy*. https://diposit.ub.edu/dspace/bitstream/2445/209136/1/Exposome%20and%20Skin%20Part%201.%20Bibliometric%20Analysis_DermatolTher.pdf (accessed on 12 May 2025).

26. Guertler, A., Volsky, A., Eijkenboom, Q., Fiedler, T., French, L. E., & Reinholz, M. (2023). Dietary patterns in acne and rosacea patients—A controlled study and comprehensive analysis. *Nutrients, 15*. https://doi.org/10.3390/nu15020229.

27. Han, X. M., Zhou, Y. M., & Cen, L. S. (2024). Ocular rosacea without facial erythema involvement manifesting as bilateral multiple recurrent chalazions: A case report. *World Journal of Clinical Cases, 12*, 3253–3258. https://www.semanticscholar.org/paper/cd1615032c2f4e60979f14784523f3c7057fd290 (accessed on 12 May 2025).

28. Haykal, D. (2025). Digital twins in dermatology: A new era of personalized skin care. *Frontiers in Digital Health, 7*. https://doi.org/10.3389/fdgth.2025.1534859.

29. Huebsch, K. (2020). Mindfulness-based stress reduction: A psychotherapeutic intervention in patients with chronic dermatological diseases. *CORE*. https://core.ac.uk/download/322838199.pdf (accessed on 12 May 2025).

30. Jahan, F., & Zafar, M. S. . (2024). A NARRATIVE REVIEW OF SKIN SYMPTOMS IN PSYCHIATRY AND PSYCHOLOGICAL CO-MORBIDITY IN DERMATOLOGY. *Student's Journal of Health Research Africa*, *5*(6), 5. https://doi.org/10.51168/sjhrafrica.v5i6.1175 (accessed on 12 May 2025).

31. Okońska, A., Kozakiewicz, J., Ziemba, M., Kałuska, J., Suprun, T., Sokół, A., ... Majewska, M. (2025). Rosacea pathogenesis and topical treatment options – a review. *Quality in Sport, 39*, 58360. https://doi.org/10.12775/QS.2025.39.58360 (accessed on 12 May 2025).

32. Kaptanoglu, A. F., & Mullaaziz, D. (2017). Acneiform Eruptions and Pregnancy. InTech. doi: 10.5772/67015 (accessed on 12 May 2025).

33. Katz, B. E., Mishu, M., & Malayeva, M. (2025). A single-center, open-label, study to evaluate the effectiveness of acne scar gel (ASG) in improving acne scar appearance and reducing hyperpigmentation in subjects with mild-to-moderate acne scars. *Journal of Cosmetic Dermatology, 24*. https://www.semanticscholar.org/paper/7f9e559d0902a910477d0c3f1b7cb793979f1856 (accessed on 12 May 2025).

34. Korting, H. C., & Schöllmann, C. (2009). Tetracycline actions relevant to rosacea treatment. *Skin pharmacology and physiology, 22*(6), 287–294. https://doi.org/10.1159/000235550 (accessed on 12 May 2025).

35. Li, Y., Zhen, X., Yao, X., & Lu, J. (2023). Successful treatment of minocycline-induced facial hyperpigmentation with a combination of chemical peels and intense pulsed light. *Clinical Cosmetic and Investigational Dermatology, 16*, 253–256. https://doi.org/10.2147/ccid.s394754.

36. Manjula S, Krishna Kumar M, Expert opinion on the prescription practice of azelaic acid for the management of acne in various age groups in Indian settings. IP Indian J Clin Exp Dermatol 2024;10(2):182-186(accessed on 12 May 2025).

37. Matanic, V. C., Bayerl, C., Berg, M., Blount, B. W., Boguniewicz, M., Bourinbaiar, A. S., Bradshaw, J., et al. (2012). Antimicrobial peptides and skin: A paradigm of translational medicine. *Skin Pharmacology and Physiology, 25*(6), 323–334. https://doi.org/10.1159/000338417.

38. Mildzikhova, D. R., Sakaniya, L., Tserikidze, N. G., & Korsunskaya, I. (2024). The problem of treating acne and rosacea in women of reproductive age. *Meditsinskiy sovet = Medical Council.* https://www.semanticscholar.org/paper/5e1c4b311d5489dcef559f2d655a1330b4222ec4 (accessed on 12 May 2025).

39. Polonini H, Marianni B, Taylor S, Zander C. Compatibility of Personalized Formulations in Cleoderm™, A Skin Rebalancing Cream Base for Oily and Sensitive Skin. *Cosmetics.* 2022; 9(5):92. https://doi.org/10.3390/cosmetics9050092(accessed on 12 May 2025).

40. Rahman, M. M., Rahaman, M. S., Islam, M. R., Rahman, F., Mithi, F. M., Alqahtani, T., Almikhlafi, M. A., et al. (2021). Role of phenolic compounds in human disease: Current knowledge and future prospects. *Molecules, 27*(1), 233. https://doi.org/10.3390/molecules27010233.

41. Sieradocha, K. (2024). The Mental Health Implications of Acne Vulgaris. *Quality in Sport, 35,* 56063. https://doi.org/10.12775/QS.2024.35.56063 (accessed on 12 May 2025).

42. Spoendlin, J. (2013). A study on the epidemiology of rosacea. Inauguraldissertation zur Erlangung der Würde eines Doktors der Philosophie vorgelegt der Philosophisch-Naturwissenschaftlichen Fakultät der Universität Basel . *Core.* https://core.ac.uk/download/18452235.pdf (accessed on 12 May 2025).

43. Starr, C. E., Gupta, P. K., Farid, M., Beckman, K. A., Chan, C. C., Yeu, E., & Gomes, J. Á. P. (2019). An algorithm for the preoperative diagnosis and treatment of ocular surface disorders. *Journal of Cataract & Refractive Surgery, 45*(6), 669–684. https://doi.org/10.1016/j.jcrs.2019.03.023.

44. Szántó, M., Dózsa, A., Antal, D., Szabó, K., Kemény, L., & Bai, P. (2019). Targeting the gut-skin axis—Probiotics as new tools for skin disorder management? *Experimental Dermatology, 28*(12), 1210–1218. https://doi.org/10.1111/exd.14016.

45. Tu, K. Y., Jung, C. J., Shih, Y. H., & Chang, A. L. S. (2024). Therapeutic strategies focusing on immune dysregulation and neuroinflammation in rosacea. *Frontiers in Immunology, 15.* https://www.semanticscholar.org/paper/aa9a09414fc58412a926ca4d19f3da3c6af931c4 (accessed on 12 May 2025).

46. Uddin, M. K., & Yesmin, S. (2024). Evaluation of the effectiveness of the combination of doxycycline and trifarotene for managing acne vulgaris of moderate to severe severity: A study in a tertiary care hospital. *International Journal of Research in Dermatology.* International Journal of Research in Dermatology Uddin MK et al. Int J Res Dermatol. 2024 Mar;10(2):66-70. (accessed on 12 May 2025).

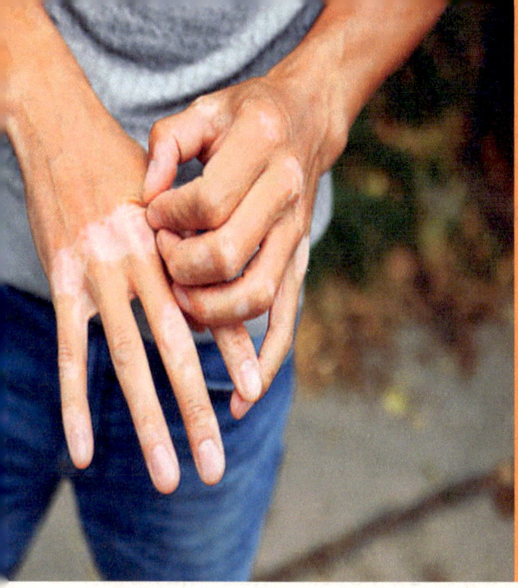

Chapter 6

PIGMENTARY DISORDERS

Contents

Introduction

Human skin color is not all about appearance – it is the result of a combination of our genes, the environment, and a whole lot of chemical reactions. All these things mix together in ways that can cause all sorts of pigment changes, whether the skin lightens in some areas or darkens in others. Sometimes these changes are not just about how things look; they can be signs of deeper, body-wide problems. In most instances, the manner in which these signs appear makes it difficult for physicians to arrive at one explanation without a panel of experts or a couple of additional instruments. It could be that a genetic mutation is disrupting the way melanin is created or distributed, or that inflammation or excessive UV exposure is the culprit. By and large, trying to get a grip on these sloppy biological systems is the way to develop treatments that do something. On the other hand, advances in molecular research and new imaging technology have provided physicians with improved mechanisms for sorting through these issues, even though the big picture itself is still relatively complicated. Red flags for full-scale, multisystem disease and not just skin issues can be some pigment shifts as well. Consider Alagille syndrome, for instance, this disease commonly occurs with changes in the skin in addition to liver issues, variations of the heart, and even bone characterestics. It typically results from small anomalies in genes such as JAG1 and NOTCH2, which can decrease bile duct growth and promote cholestasis, all in conjunction with uncharacteristic facial colors and eye anomalies. Figuring out such an illness is not easy; quite often it means that various specialists must weigh in, and catching the skin cues early can really lead the way. Oftentimes, observing how these color differences relate to larger health concerns reminds us that what occurs on the skin can be a portal to more underlying body processes (Shchur et al., 2024). And then there are disorders such as melasma, where additional melanin accumulates in the skin in manners that are difficult to identify. Classic tests, including those involving a Wood's lamp, tend to be inadequate when it comes to separating the finer points. Today, non-surgical procedures such as dermoscopy are revolutionizing the process. This technique not only aids in sorting out whether the pigmentation problem is largely epidermal, dermal, or a combination, but it also assists physicians in adapting treatments to each person. In addition, dermoscopy occasionally reveals vascular or follicular information that older techniques do not detect, adding yet another dimension to the way we comprehend and follow treatment. In the majority of situations, comparing the new tools with the traditional ones implies that our methodology in diagnosing pigment changes is evolving, yielding more accurate and efficient treatment (Patel, 2021).

Definition of Pigmentary Disorders

Skin is not an inactive barrier; it continually adapts to daily friction, pressure, and mechanical stresses that we may not even become aware of until alterations occur. When our skin accommodates repeated rubbing or persistent pressure, it occasionally begins to change, manifesting itself in patches that are lighter or darker than the surrounding skin. You could refer to these changes as friction-related dermatoses, a blanket term for skin problems caused by repeated, physical irritation. By and large, these color changes indicate that it is not just about our genes here; the environment and how our skin deals with everyday stresses do come into it as well. This combination of factors compels us to examine causes, shapes, and where on the body these changes take place (Arora et al., 2022). Occasionally, however, it is not only physical stress that is in play. In most instances, pigment abnormalities arise in conjunction with conditions affecting both skin and nervous system. Consider, for instance, neurocutaneous syndromes—those heterogeneous disorders (usually referred to as phacomatoses or neuroectodermal dysplasias) with both cutaneous markings and neurological signs. Contemporary molecular genetics has, with the exception of a few instances, begun to disentangle the complex of intracellular and extraneuronal signals that influence pigment production. Against this background, an accurate definition of skin pigment disorders must include not only genetics but also developmental and systemic factors (Ruggieri et al., 2018). And then there is the intriguing example of patchy, mosaic, or segmental patterns that some pigment disorders present—hints, perhaps, at the skin's original embryological plan. These spotty distributions, which might appear asymmetrically or along distinct body segments, likely arise from genetic mosaicism or small developmental hiccups. It is interesting how even within a single syndrome, the arrangement of pigment can vary a lot, challenging the neat, traditional definitions we once relied on. Appreciating these spatial and developmental subtleties requires us to not only admire the observable skin alterations but also to note any underlying, extracutaneous involvement, thus completing our understanding of pigment disorders (Ruggieri et al., 2018).

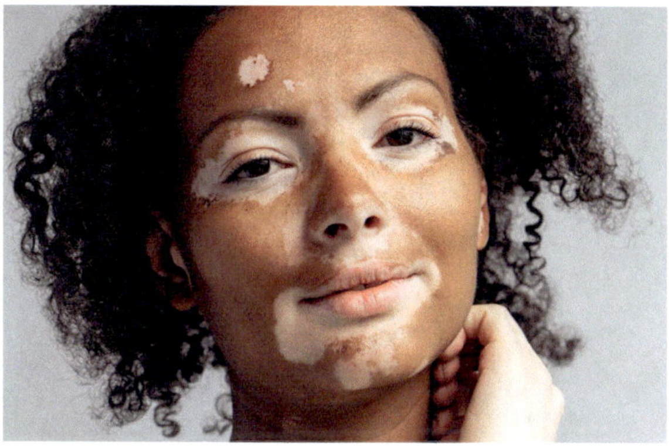

Source: Unknown author. (n.d.). *Pigmentation Disorder.* https://images.squarespace-cdn.com/content/v1/61266e982104fd1fe23f9fba/63907fd0-f1b2-4e99-9a79-161d62ab5ed1/pigmentation_disorder.jpg

Importance of Studying Pigmentary Disorders

Pigment disorders are not only about appearance—pigments also reveal a great deal about general skin and body health. Our largest organ, the skin, shows us clues about what is going on inside and outside the body, whether it is too much sun, urban smog, or sudden hormonal changes. In the majority of instances, continued exposure to sunlight and challenging air can trigger unanticipated pigment changes and accelerate aging. Exploring how all those environmental and physiological elements combine can go a long way in informing prevention and treatment concepts. Even the chaotic dance of oxidative stress and inflammation has a role in initiating those pigment changes, and it is apparent that knowing these pathways is important for both research and clinical care (Passeron et al., 2020). This broad perspective demonstrates that these conditions cut far deeper than they may appear on the surface. To add to that, pigment alterations may at times be the initial indicators that point to more complex genetic or systemic conditions. Consider neurofibromatosis type 1 (NF1) as a case point—a disease that typically presents in childhood with well-demarcated skin markings that act as precursors. These initial signs not only assist in quick diagnosis but also direct long-term monitoring and management strategies to avoid complications. Particularly in children, the manner in which these signs fluctuate necessitates a keen observation of pigment changes in general to enhance health results and general well-being. In a sense, having more knowledge about these disorders provides clinicians with the knowledge to develop treatment plans that span skin and the body, highlighting the importance of testing for pigment abnormalities in a healthcare team setting. Apart from the clinical and environmental perspectives, uncovering pigment disorders further illuminates our general knowledge of skin biology and how genes, hormones, and the environment all combine. The skin's response to hormonal changes, inflammatory episodes, or even dietary changes can profoundly influence pigment patterns—implicating skin health in general body function. A closer examination of the molecular missteps that underlie these color changes may even reveal new paths to treatment for ailments such as vitiligo, melasma, or post-inflammatory hyperpigmentation. And, not least, an understanding of the emotional weight that pigment problems exact highlights how important it is to employ care practices addressing both the physical stigma and the psychological effect. Therefore, all in all, studies on such disorders are not merely about improved clinical results—but also about elevating the general quality of life through more harmonized and personalized care strategies (Passeron et al., 2020).

6.1. Types of Pigmentary Disorders

Melanin does not only give color to our skin—it also tends of acting strangely. When its production or distribution goes awry, all sorts of pigment problems arise. Consider melasma, PIH, or solar lentigines, for example; these are typically the result of excess melanin being produced or deposited in a wild pattern, often because the sun's UV rays or an inflammatory incident got things going. Conversely, conditions such as vitiligo or pityriasis alba appear when melanin is lacking, resulting in lighter patches that really show up, particularly on darker skin, where the contrast can be quite dramatic. UV exposure tends to make everything worse, so a sunscreen that protects against UVB, UVA, and even some visible light is becoming an essential (Krutmann et al., 2023). In the majority of instances, it is all about safeguarding your skin from the sun to prevent these pigment changes from getting out of hand. Nature's natural beat is sometimes not sufficient, and that is where chemical and physical adjustments kick in. Chemical peels, for instance, have proven to be a go-to technique to lighten up entrenched blemishes by softly stripping away the skin's outermost layer—this orchestrated shedding creates an avenue for some serious reorganizing of the skin. The secret with these peels is selecting the correct agent, being aware of its characterestics, and knowing how deep it penetrates to achieve a bit of controlled cell loss. Of course, a physician's judgment comes into play here: determining who will be a good candidate, aligning expectations, and handling both the pre-operative period and the aftercare meticulously to prevent complications. These procedures truly stand out for conditions characterized by irregular tones or inflammatory scars, eventually leaving skin looking fresher and enhancing confidence (Oremovi et al., 2010). It is all about bringing strong clinical understanding together with accurate procedural execution, a combination that truly represents the numerous layers of managing pigment issues. When you examine pigment disorders, it is as if you are looking into a whole range of causes—genetic factors to environmental issues and even immune system characterestics.

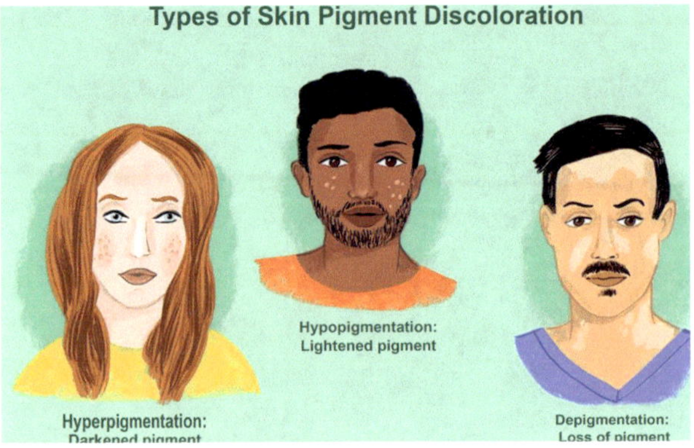

Figure 6.1. Types of pigmentary disorders.

Source: https://www.verywellhealth.com/thmb/J4TjbgY16dQOpmsJ-bNOGjMe8Pk=/750x0/filters:no_upscale():max_bytes(150000):strip_icc():format(webp)/skin-pigmentation-5088368-v1-d4faa328df3d496d9c3c08de9a7bc349.jpg

You may hear the words lentigines, café-au-lait spots, or nevus of Ota thrown around; some of these spots are present with you from birth, whereas others appear or darken over time due to outside pressures or autoimmune responses. There is not a one-size-fits-all picture here, and occasionally even the same patient can notice varied patterns unfolding. This is not a straightforward condition to treat, and a responsive, mixed-package strategy may be necessary that includes sun avoidance, a splash of topical depigmenting cream, or procedural interventions such as chemical peels or laser. Patient education and individualized treatment are part of the package as well, guaranteeing that all these components cooperate harmoniously. For the most part, it is a matter of treating all factors simultaneously, a situation particularly relevant to individuals with naturally more superior or sensitive skin (Oremovi et al., 2010; Krutman et al., 2023) (Figure 6.1).

6.1.1. Hypopigmentation Disorders

Pigment control in our skin is not all about melanocytes—it is a whole system of cells, and dermal fibroblasts have an unexpected role. These fibroblasts release all sorts of soluble factors that determine how melanin is produced and distributed. In diseases such as vitiligo, where the skin loses its color, this cell-to-cell crosstalk gets disrupted, leaving melanocytes with less of the normal pressure to produce pigment. Usually, stem cell factor (SCF) and keratinocyte growth factor (KGF) keep pigmentation in check, but in hypopigmented skin their levels fall, whereas molecules such as Dickkopf1 (DKK1) and transforming growth factor (TGF)-β appear in greater numbers. That change interferes with tyrosinase activity, an enzyme critical to melanin synthesis, and interferes with the normal passing on of melanosomes. This changed secretory pattern in fibroblasts implies that they may be a new therapeutic target, providing an alternative to targeting melanocytes alone (Gao et al., 2025) (Figure 6.2).

Hypopigmentation disorders are a major challenge since their causes and manifestations can differ so greatly. One minute you have tiny areas of depigmentation; the next, a more diffuse lack of color. Standard therapies—corticosteroids, phototherapy—do not always keep pace in the long term or may introduce unwelcome side effects.

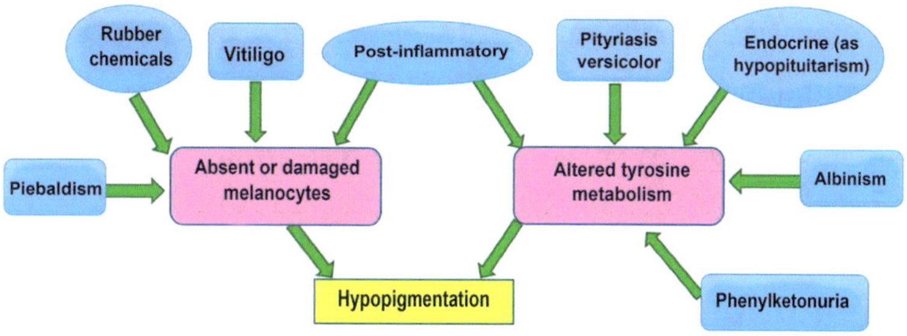

Figure 6.2. The mechanisms involved in some types of hypopigmentation.

Source: Thawabteh, A. M., Jibreen, A., Karaman, D., Thawabteh, A., & Karaman, R. (2023). The mechanisms involved in some types of hypopigmentation. In *Skin Pigmentation Types, Causes and Treatment—A Review. Molecules, 28*(12), 4839.

Recently, though, there has been speculation about employing combination therapies that take advantage of more recent understanding of skin biology. For example, methods that modify the environment around the cells of the skin and give melanocytes a kick may be more effective at rebalancing even pigment and preventing relapse. Though much of the work to date has been on hyperpigmentation, it appears these concepts could have applications in hypopigmented disorders as well, an area that still, in most instances, remains relatively unexamined (Proietti et al., 2024).

Despite our increasing understanding of the cellular ballet behind hypopigmentation, there remains a genuine lack of effective, standardized treatments. Some new research suggests the potential for targeting fibroblast signals to change the way we approach pigment loss. Initial experimental approaches that modulate cytokine levels have been promising in the lab and early-onset clinics, and it is possible that rebalancing the balance between pigmentation-stimulating and inhibitory signals will be the solution. Again, however, the heterogeneity of these disorders tells us we must have more thorough studies to refine treatment strategies and even determine good biomarkers for who will respond best. Ahead lies a multidisciplinary effort—from molecular biology to dermatology and clinical therapies—to create precision, patient-specific interventions that restore pigmentation and, hopefully, enhance the quality of life for individuals affected (Proietti et al., 2024; Gao et al., 2025) (Figure 6.3).

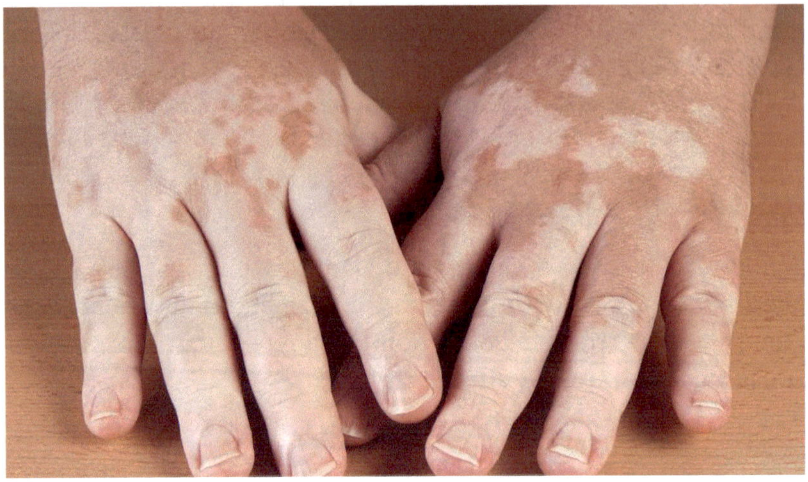

Figure 6.3. Hypopigmentation.

Source: Medical News Today. (2020). *Skin condition Illustration.* https://post.medicalnewstoday.com/wp-content/uploads/sites/3/2020/02/320243_1100-1100x628.jpg.

6.1.2. Hyperpigmentation Disorders

Skin color shifts most often point towards pigment problems when our skin's own pigment output just is not cutting it. Too much pigment collects in an area sometimes and it is just called hyperpigmentation by a lot of us. It is sort of an open-ended proposition—genes, excess sun exposure, inflammation, and even hormone fluctuations all have something to do with it, apparently. Consider melasma, for instance; it usually appears after hormonal fluctuation—hello, pregnancy or taking the pill, and has the effect of leaving dark, uniform patches on the face. And then there is the form that appears after damage to the skin, where the dark spots persist well after the original issue resolves. , these shifts can take a hard blow at self-esteem, and knowing precisely why they are happening is critical if we are to develop treatments that are effective and have minimal undesirable side effects. Behind these problems lies the mechanism of melanocytes and the mechanism of how our skin accumulates pigment naturally—a process that can be easily affected by what is taking place within our cells and externally in the world around us. In general, ultraviolet (UV) light does more than simply tan skin; it increases melanin production, exacerbating existing blemishes or even causing new ones. Most often, when skin is damaged, the chemicals released make melanocytes a little too enthusiastic, causing more post-inflammatory darkening. And then there are the contributions of oxidative stress and genetic characterestics that further disrupt the intensity and length of these pigment changes. Standard treatments are mostly creams or lotions, such as those containing hydroquinone, retinoids, or corticosteroids, which attempt to retard pigment accumulation or accelerate skin renewal. Nevertheless, there is also continuing controversy regarding their long-term safety and worth, such as in other areas of medicine where long-term treatments are criticized for cost and efficacy concerns (Lilje et al., 2023). Therefore, achieving the correct balance of safety, efficacy, and affordability is the solution to making a person feel better in general.

Tackling hyperpigmentation involves a twofold game plan: avoiding further causes and evening out current problems. I.e., wearing broad-spectrum sunscreen regularly is quite important as it prevents UV rays from pushing those pigment cells into overproduction. And it does not hurt when patients can learn to minimize unnecessary skin stress—less irritation tends to translate to fewer dark spots down the road. In more resistant instances, physicians may recommend such treatments as chemical peels, lasers, or even microneedling to dislodge pigment clumps and enhance the texture of the skin. Even with these medical advancements, however, not all have the same level of access to treatment—a challenge that resonates within other areas of health care as well, where there are still resource constraints and reform debates ongoing (Håkansson et al., 2023). Targeted medical treatment together with broader attempts to enhance access make it possible to alter the scenario for individuals afflicted with these pigment alterations (Figure 6.4).

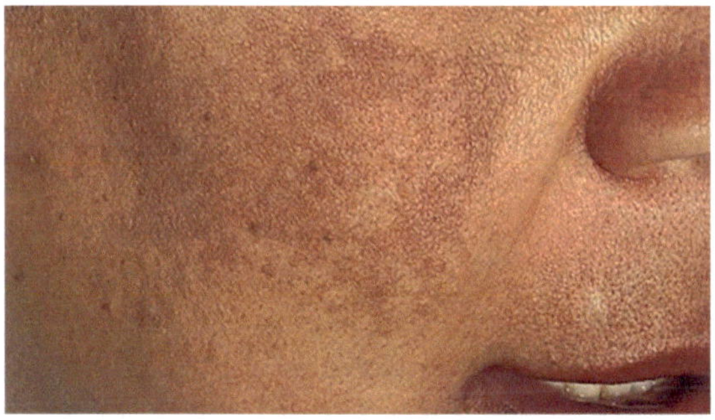

Figure 6.4. Hyperpigmentation.

Source: Medical News Today. (2022). *Hyperpigmentation Skin Slide.* https://i0.wp.com/post.medicalnewstoday.com/wp-content/uploads/sites/3/2022/05/hyperpigmentation-skin-slide1-1024x575.jpg?w=1155&h=1528.

6.1.3. Mixed Pigmentary Disorders

Skin problems can get challenging, sometimes there is an odd combination of too much pigment right alongside weirdly light areas. Mixed pigmentary disorders appear when both hyperpigmentation and hypopigmentation occur simultaneously on a single spot or area, which really complicates matters for diagnosis and treatment. You may discover that this mix results from everything from genetic characterestics and inflammatory reactions to outside influences such as UV radiation or toxic chemicals. The manner in which these various pigment changes occur together suggests a number of internal disruptions in the way melanocytes manage melanin production, distribution, or even break it down. Understanding what is happening at the cellular level is crucial, because it ultimately dictates treatment plans that sometimes must address more than one type of pigment alteration to get patients looking and feeling better.

Treating these blended pigment disturbances is not as easy as applying one magic solution. Rather, physicians are now looking at a combination of treatments that act on both the dark and light spots simultaneously. For example, some new procedures involve combining microneedling with antioxidant serums containing vitamin C derivatives. This type of combination appears to act by increasing the skin's capacity for absorption and by encouraging collagen remodeling—actions that may stabilize those unstable melanocytes (Proietti et al., 2024). Obviously, having just one treatment too often does not cut it with such diversified presentations, so more complicated, multifaceted solutions are sounding better and better by the day. Although all of these pigmentary issues do tend to present themselves on the skin, mounting evidence suggests underlying, systemic concerns involving metabolic or even neurodegenerative diseases.

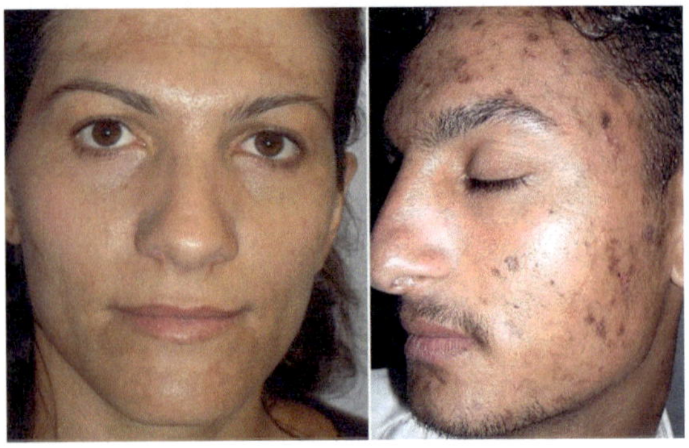

Figure 6.5. Mixed-pigmentation.

Source: Skin MD and Beyond. (n.d.). *Mixed Pigmentation.* https://www.skinmdandbeyond.com/wp-content/uploads/Mixed-Pigmentation-1024x826.jpg.

In a few rare instances, patients have presented with a mosaic of hyper- and hypopigmentation, just another piece in the clinical jigsaw (Gowda et al., 2023). These varied patterns can confuse enough that dermatologists frequently must collaborate with other experts to get the whole picture. In the majority of instances, identifying mixed pigment disorders as possible indicators of more widespread health issues pushes us toward more stringent, multidisciplinary treatment—a step that could ultimately result in improved overall outcomes for patients (Figure 6.5).

6.2. Causes of Pigmentary Disorders

Pigmentary disorders are quite involved. They result from a mix of internal characteristics and external contact that interferes with the normal process of melanin production or distribution. Genes, for example, can truly lay the groundwork, DNA variations or familial variations sometimes alter how melanocytes function, and you end up with lighter or darker spots. And then there is the sun; its UV radiation can boost the damage, increasing oxidative stress and triggering off inflammatory episodes on the skin. Quite frequently, the body's own immune system even gets into the act and attacks pigment cells in error—as we observe in conditions such as vitiligo where pigment simply disappears. These and a thousand other influences blend together unpredictably, making diagnosis and treatment harder, and it is vital to grasp each complex element to design therapies that attack not just the intrinsic biology but also the environmental cues, usually bettering outcomes. Lifestyle and mood give yet another turn to pigment concerns. Eating patterns and emotional tension can influence how your skin fairs. In most instances, chronic stress appears to be connected with hormonal shifts that could change melanin production, while how and when we consume food, or even restrictive diets that produce nutrient deficiencies—can disrupt skin fix and melanin production, making pigment issues more apparent. It is sort of a refresher that these conditions are not entirely about biology; they get entwined in our way of life. Considering both mental health and daily routines, in most instances, provides physicians a better chance of customizing treatments that target several triggers simultaneously (Amiri & Khan, 2024; He et al., 2024). And then there are the potholes along the way, such as infections and skin trauma. Infections by bacteria, fungi, or viruses can awaken inflammation that turns normal pigmentation into variants such as post-inflammatory hyperpigmentation or even seemingly erased patches. Added to this, physical trauma to the skin—burns, abrasions, or surgical scars, usually leaves melanocytes dispersed or askew, causing patchy alterations. Occasionally, acquired skin abuses underscore how the entire skin microenvironment is responsible for unforeseen pigment shifts. Understanding this messy interaction drives us to emphasize preventive treatment and early intervention to prevent permanent changes, and it informs more complete treatment plans that take all aspects of pigment disruption into account (Figure 6.6).

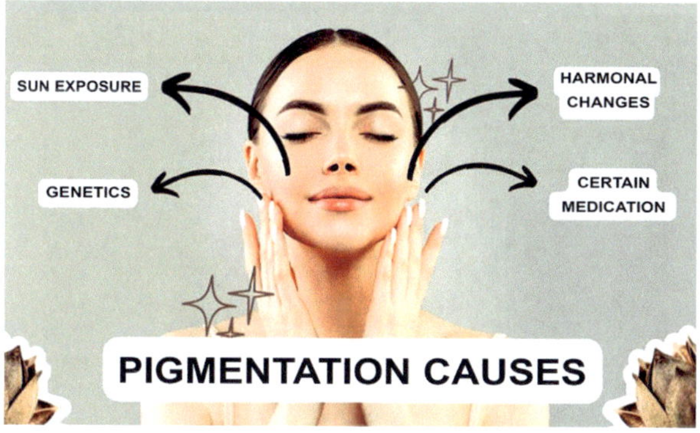

Figure 6.6. Pigmentation causes.

Source: Kolors Healthcare. (2023). *Skin Pigmentation.* https://www.kolorshealthcare.com/blog/wp-content/uploads/2023/04/Skin-Pigmentation.jpg.

6.2.1. Genetic Factors

Pigment disorders are all about how our genes control how skin color ends up. Our DNA contains the blueprint for creating and distributing melanin, and when that blueprint gets it wrong, something like albinism, vitiligo, or even melasma can arise. Occasionally a tiny genetic error—a mutation in the TYR gene that is meant to make tyrosinase, an enzyme central to making melanin—throws the entire process out of control. This explains that examining these genetic characterestics provides us with genuine insights into why these conditions arise. In the majority of instances, a robust hereditary foundation combines with environmental stimuli, and the pigment shifts we observe result. Genome-wide association studies have, by and large, introduced a great deal of subtleties to our knowledge of pigment traits. Large investigations now suggest rather than a single dominant gene controlling the action, numerous gene locations contribute small bits along the way. Research continues to identify that pigment-related genes sometimes interface with other bodily systems, and that these genes may double-duty. Instead of a simple one-to-one correlation, there is a mesh of genetic effects that demands the integration of genetic information with physical characteristics and even daily environmental variables. New data even begin to reveal connections between pigment characteristics and neural—occasionally behavior—affects (Docherty et al., 2023; Ivanov et al., 2022). In addition to that, databases collecting both genetic and observable trait data have begun to erase the distinction between raw data and actual symptoms. These tools combine gene variants, physical markers, and even what patients report about their own diseases to assist in flagging early signs of disease and its development. With the help of large data technologies such as bioinformatics and machine learning, researchers are able to, in most instances, unravel how genetic predispositions interact with lifestyle factors. This combination of knowledge is leading to personalized medicine, where treatments and prevention are adjusted to each individual's specific genetic configuration. Together, this increasing cache of information continues to open doors to improved, genetics-based care for pigment disorders (Ivanov et al., 2022).

6.2.2. Environmental Influences

Genes and daily exposures to the environment blend in unexpected combinations to determine pigmentation. Sunlight, particularly the UV type, is not only a cozy friend—it alters the behavior of melanocytes. When you receive prolonged periods of sunlight, your skin increases melanin production as a sort of built-in protection. But push it too far, and that very process damages the melanocytes, triggering irregular patches like melasma or solar lentigines. Add pollutants and chemicals to the equation, and the skin's melanin-production routine becomes even more perplexed. Current research, in the majority of instances, identifies these problems as well as new treatments that aim to facilitate the damage (Birlea et al., 2018). Evidently, gaining control over these interactions is critical if we are to develop intelligent, targeted solutions.

In addition to sunlight, the skin must contend with a complete array of chemical influences that can also disrupt its pigmentation. Ordinary substances, from lotions and topical drugs to inhaled pollutants, can mix with melanocytes and even influence melanosomes, adjusting the ultimate appearance of our skin color. For example, hydroquinone, a well-known agent used to reduce pigmentation, competes with tyrosine to block tyrosinase—the main enzyme behind melanin production. Yet, because hydroquinone often brings unwanted side effects, alternatives like arbutin or kojic acid have started to wedded themselves to treatment plans, offering a gentler approach. It is intriguing how altering what touches the skin at a molecular level might ease pigmentation issues. Apart from that, changing the mechanism of melanosomes transferring between melanocytes and keratinocytes presents itself as another avenue to be pursued, highlighting the multifaceted interplay of internal mechanisms and external factors (Kim et al., 2012). Skin does not merely respond to chemicals and light, however; it is also actively dealing with oxidative stress and episodes of inflammation. Examples such as pollution or excessive UV exposure give rise to reactive oxygen species—unstable molecules that disrupt melanocyte stability and may result in too little or too much pigment. In general, oxidative stress can make conditions such as vitiligo or post-inflammatory hyperpigmentation worse by creating a rather inhospitable environment for such cells (Birlea et al., 2018). Scientists are now investigating antioxidant therapies to assist in rebalancing that redox state and buffer melanocytes from additional damage. Mix in the effect of chronic, low-grade inflammation, usually caused by constant exposure to irritants, and you have got a recipe for faulty cytokine signaling and, ultimately, faulty pigment production. All of these elements appear to act at various biological levels, so in the majority of instances, an integrated strategy needs to be used in order to control these pigmentary problems (Figure 6.7).

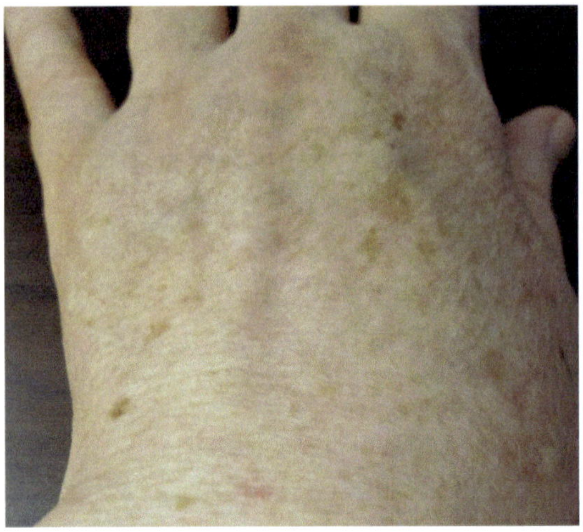

Figure 6.7. Solar lentigo.

Source: By Beyond My Ken - Own work, CC BY-SA 4.0, https://commons.wikimedia.org/w/index.php?curid=70134653

6.2.3. Medical Conditions and Medications

Differences in skin color can at times indicate more than initial appearances. You may see patches or mottled tones when diseases such as Addison's disease, thyroid issues, or even hemochromatosis interfere with the balance of hormone or metabolism. These changes, either additional darkening or pigment loss, usually result from modified melanocyte function or changes in melanin production resulting from long-term health conditions. Conditions like vitiligo, where in most instances appears to be linked to autoimmune issues, reinforce the necessity of a wider diagnostic scan. Most of the time, identifying these color changes is not so much an issue of what lies on the surface but instead is an early indicator of bigger, underlying issues that require a more specific treatment regimen (Adaskevich, 2016). Medications to address various systemic problems can also disrupt the coloration of the skin, either as a direct reaction or a secondary effect of changes in the body as a whole. Consider antimalarials, some antibiotics, or even chemotherapy drugs—they can interfere with melanin production or induce inflammatory reactions that deposit abnormal dark or light spots. At times, the color changes caused by these drugs may resemble or even exacerbate pre-existing dermatologic conditions, making it more difficult for physicians to determine what is occurring. Since these effects are so different for each patient, each patient's drug therapy, medical history, and individual skin patterns must be examined individually. In balancing treatment advantages with possible skin side effects, a customized, evidence-based care plan is developed (Adaskevich, 2016). Apart from diseases and medications striking directly, other ailments can subtly influence skin color by modifying the immune system or disturbing the balance of the body. Disorders of the connective tissue, metabolism, or immune apparatus frequently resulted in visible alterations in color and texture of the skin—a hint that something more profound was occurring internally. Occasionally, body inflammation even disrupts surrounding tissues near regions such as the gums or other soft tissues, illustrating that these body processes can leave a trail on the skin. Clinicians have to be observant of these signs because identifying the actual culprit behind a change in tissue coloration might reveal concealed health issues. Placing these skin signs into the larger context of overall health can improve diagnostic accuracy and ultimately result in care that is more specifically suited to each patient.

6.3. Diagnosis of Pigmentary Disorders

Diagnosis of pigment problems is not merely identifying various colors of the skin—it is equally about getting to the bottom of everything that is going on underneath, from genetic tics to situations in which the immune system appears to act out of control. Physicians typically begin with an interview of the patient to get their history and perform a good old-fashioned hands-on physical exam to observe any obvious patterns, the progression of changes, and to search for additional signs elsewhere in the body. As these color changes may resemble many other skin or even systemic issues, additional measures, such as with Wood's lamp, examination with a dermoscope, or even a small skin biopsy—are usually helpful in clarifying issues such as vitiligo, melasma, or post-inflammatory patches.

These additional tests allow physicians to see the pigmentation in a more nuanced fashion while also detecting minute changes at the cellular level, which typically renders the diagnosis somewhat more accurate. On top of that, what patients report regarding their own experience and any social or emotional turbulence they encounter adds another layer to the big picture. Mixing physical examinations, microscopic observations, and patient reportage in combination creates an elementary but solid approach to unraveling pigment disorders. Recently, technology has added another spin to the mix. Artificial intelligence-driven (AI) systems, particularly those operating on convolutional neural networks (CNNs), have been proving a talent for detecting faint skin patterns that would otherwise go unnoticed in a routine checkup. Tools such as Long Short-Term Memory allow physicians to monitor changes over time by analyzing long runs of data. Essentially, combining information from various sources, such as a patient's genes, high-magnification images of the skin, and his or her individual story—allows a type of diagnosis that feels custom-tailored and refines the general perspective on what is occurring in the skin. This technique not only provides an extra touch of diagnostic nuance but also aids in real-time decisions that could shave down wait times and improve treatment outcomes in most instances (Natrayan et al., 2024). Nevertheless, these nifty gadgets require additional testing across various groups and clinical settings before everyone can be certain they are as safe as we wish. Meanwhile, addressing pigment disorders is not all about the high-tech—it requires a team effort that keeps the patient front and center. Because skin color changes tend to strike individuals on an emotional level, it stands to reason that clinicians should blend in a thoughtful consideration of mental and social issues, perhaps even screening for conditions like somatic symptom disorders along the way. Oftentimes a formal interview or series of questionnaires assists in revealing just how disruptive symptoms may be to one's daily activities (Ajluni, 2024). In having dermatologists, psychiatrists, and primary care physicians work together, the diagnosis improves in precision and constructs a more complete care plan. By being truly empathetic, maintaining the dialogue in a natural (and yes, somewhat imperfect) manner, and having an awareness of cultural differences, patients can remain with both the evaluation process and the resulting treatment plan. Ultimately, untangling pigment disorders far exceeds a straightforward clinical examination—it requires a balanced approach that addresses both what can be seen and what is perceived internally (Figure 6.8).

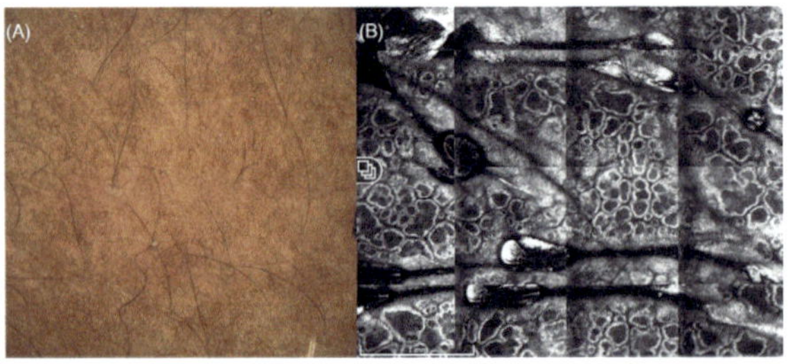

Figure 6.8. Dermoscopic and RCM images of café-au lait macule (CALM) from a 27-year-old female on the upper back which was present since birth. (A) Dermoscopic image of CALM shows a homogenous light brown background pigmentation along with delicate reticular network; and (B) RCM image of CALM at the level of dermo-epidermal junction shows multiple enlarged regular-edged papillae and hyperreflective peri-papillary rings.

Source: Liu, Y., Wang, J., Wang, X., Zhang, Y., & Li, Y. (2023). Reflectance confocal microscopy image of solar lentigo. In The role of reflectance confocal microscopy in the diagnosis and management of pigmentary disorders. *Journal of Cosmetic Dermatology, 22*(1), 123–130.

6.3.1. Clinical Evaluation and History

Beginning to understand pigment concerns begins with a close examination of the patient's skin. Frequently, it begins with excavating the history of a patient—when the pigment alterations first appeared, how they have changed, where on the body they are found, what symptoms accompany them, and even whether family members experienced similar issues. The physician then examines the details: the form, tone, and structure of the pigment, not to speak of any indications that may suggest inflammation or scarring. With conditions such as vitiligo, observing whether the condition is active can significantly influence what to anticipate and treatments that can best be used. Adding a new layer of complexity to the protocol, several clinicians now look at biomarkers, such as when elevated serum CXCL13 levels appear in patients with vitiligo, providing an indication of an immune connection that can strengthen typical evaluations (Ashraf et al., 2023). In combining what is apparent on the skin with laboratory results, a clearer understanding of the behavior of the pigment appears, far beyond mere visual evidence. Reflecting on historical information also has a tale to tell. Not only does it outline a patient's individual course but it also situates pigment conditions within broader circumstances. Consider vitiligo: sure, it is primarily about losing those pigment cells in the epidermis, but the narrative is more complex—separating out genetic predispositions, stress from free radicals, and malfunctions in the body's immune systems. These understandings are generally derived from a thorough medical history, subsequently reinforced by what the observer sees with an exam. As an example, inflammatory mediators such as interleukin-6 appear in the disease process; clinical tests sometimes demonstrate that changes in serum IL-6 concentrations correlate with treatments such as narrow band-UVB phototherapy (Zaki et al., 2019).

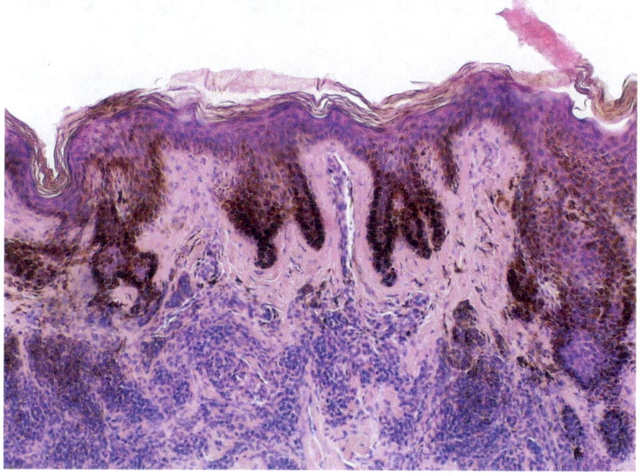

Figure 6.9. Understanding pigment issues with a careful look at the patient's skin.

Source: By LWozniak&KWZielinski - Own work, CC BY-SA 3.0, https://commons.wikimedia.org/w/index.php?curid=13566084

Recording treatment responses not only follows disease behavior but also assists in shaping a more individualized plan for each patient, particularly when the symptoms and course can change so greatly. Assessing how severe and active a pigment disorder is can be as crucial as the initial assessment. Metrics such as the Vitiligo Area Scoring Index (VASI) give a fairly normal means of judging the degree of depigmentation present, keeping things consistent in the way that can be monitored over time. However, simply measuring only what one sees on the skin could overlook some internal immune changes. Even some studies indicate discrepancies between what clinical scores imply and concentrations of markers such as CXCL13 (Ashraf et al., 2023). Investigating a full history, including emotional burden and even environmental considerations—adds additional depth to the laboratory and clinical information, providing a more comprehensive picture. Collectively, this combination of observation, laboratory data, and individual history provides clarity to a highly heterogeneous group of pigment conditions, ultimately leading to better treatment and overall quality of life (Figure 6.9).

6.3.2. Laboratory Tests and Imaging

Pigment variations are not solved by being monomodal and using just one approach – all too often, a combination of laboratory investigations and clinical examination is the key that opens up an understanding on a deeper level. Laboratory tests uncover biochemical and genetic hints, most often revealing what plain sight misses. For instance, in some mitochondrial problems that accompany unusual pigment patterns, conducting thorough genetic tests and metabolic screens is crucial; such tests occasionally reveal errorserrors in how cells produce energy, pushing clinicians toward more definitive diagnoses and improved care plans. Merging lab information with what one sees in the exam room paints an even more individualized picture that allows it to distinguish between harmless pigment changes and indicators of larger, more systemic issues (Tashiro et al., 2018). Imaging puts yet another piece into the puzzle. Methods such as dermoscopy, reflectance confocal microscopy (RCM) or multispectral imaging allow physicians to take a non-surgical look at how pigment is distributed and arrayed on skin or mucous surfaces. These techniques can reveal tiny, unnoticed details , the sort that plain observation may pass by , which helps differentiate harmless spots from those that appear more menacing. Imaging is not only valuable for the skin though; it enters the picture when eye problems appear, particularly if color changes impair vision.

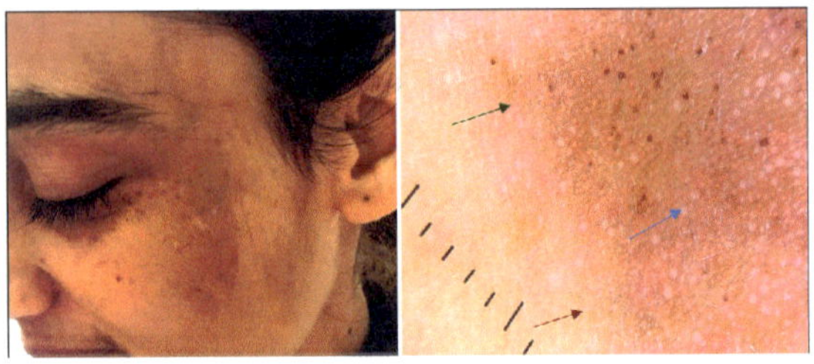

Figure 6.10. Clinical and dermoscopic picture of patient with PDL. (a) Pigment demarcation lines; and (b). Dermoscopy showing perifollicular sparing (brown arrow), White clods (blue arrow), dots (green arrow) with abrupt area of transition to hyperpigmented area.

Source: Puri, N., Gill, S. K., Brar, B. K., & Goyal, S. (2024). Clinical and dermoscopic picture of patient with PDL: (a) Pigment demarcation lines; (b) Dermoscopy showing perifollicular sparing, white clods, dots, and abrupt transition to hyperpigmented area. In *Facial Pigmentary Demarcation Lines—A New Dermoscopic Finding*.

For example, studies of intermediate age-related macular degeneration, a disease characterized by abnormal retinal pigmentation, typically indicate that the integration of multiple imaging methods with functional testing is important for monitoring how the disease progresses (Robert et al., 2019). Collectively, these strategies increase the overall reliability of diagnoses and assist in monitoring treatment outcomes. At other times, pigment alterations are merely one symptom of a greater, system-level problem. Most of the time, particularly with mitochondrial issues that extend to other organs, physicians rely on both imaging tests and laboratory testing to have a complete read on what is happening. Neuroimaging, detailed eye examination and cardiac scans all complement one another – each exposing pieces of the picture that extend beyond pigment changes in a purely surface-level sense. Cardiac imaging, for example, could detect precursor changes in the heart muscle that appear to be linked to pigment differences elsewhere, a detail that can trigger early treatment. While today's treatments are primarily symptom-focused, the subtle perspectives resulting from rigorous lab work in conjunction with imaging assist in broadening our understanding of each patient's individual profile and possible trajectory, emphasizing the irreplaceable value of this multi-dimensional approach (Tashiro et al., 2018) (Figure 6.10).

6.3.3. Differential Diagnosis

A good patient history and physical examination typically initiate the process of determining skin pigment problems. Melasma, vitiligo, and post-inflammatory hyperpigmentation frequently confuse clinical presentation in ways that will puzzle even seasoned clinicians. At times, merely inquiring about when the issue began, how it has evolved, and what appears to exacerbate it may provide a non-obvious clue or two. Investigating further using a Wood's lamp, some dermoscopy, or even biopsy can then serve to make clearer whether the change in pigment lies more towards the surface of the skin or sunken in further in the dermis—facts that will on occasion turn prognosis and treatment prospect on their heads. Typically, though, modern guidelines rest on keen clinical acumen, yet nascent research with biomarkers indicates that molecular devices may eventually sharpen these challenging differentials (Grodzka et al., 2025). Briefly put, a combination of practical experience and newer methods continues to be an essential part of the jigsaw puzzle for diagnosing pigmentary disorders. When pigment problems arise, it is not uncommon that physicians also question whether perhaps something systemic is going on—diseases that simulate the common appearance of primary pigment alterations. Such diseases as endocrine issues, genetic characterestics, or even drug reactions may occasionally cause skin changes that appear quite similar to idiopathic presentations. In the majority of instances, this translates to laboratory tests to evaluate hormone levels, autoimmune markers, or metabolic panels, particularly when the initial visit suggests there may be more to the story than initially apparent. Further, newer methods such as imaging and special staining, methods recently applied in neurodegenerative disorder segmentation (Soleimani-Meigooni et al., 2024), hold promise in separating out the subtle differences between overlapping clinical signs. By combining different diagnostic approaches, clinicians are better able to differentiate primary pigment issues from those indicating deeper, systemic engagement, ultimately informing more effective treatment regimens and improving patient outcomes. Despite these advancements, however, many pigmentary diseases still lack a definitive noninvasive biomarker at hand, which can cloud the diagnostic picture and prolong the process longer than necessary. Equally, struggles exist elsewhere in medicine where good biomarkers would genuinely shorten the amount of subjectivity in clinical assessments (Grodzka et al., 2025). Imaging biomarkers and molecular diagnostics, increasingly making inroads as additional tools, provide more objective means by which to support or contradict initial suspicions. Bridging these new concepts into routine dermatology could potentially enable earlier, more assured conclusions so that interventions can be directed at the particular underlying process of each condition. However, all this is predicated on continuing research if we are to identify and confirm these markers—foretelling an era where the fusion of clinical expertise with leading-edge technology has the potential to streamline the labyrinth of differential diagnosis for pigmentary disorders.

6.4. Treatment Options

Pigmentary disorders require managing multiple methods of keeping skin problems under control. Prevention and treatment are frequently a combination of each other, and photoprotection is a simple strategy – UV light, infrared, and even visible light have the potential to really get in the way of your skin and cause damage as well as unusual pigment shifts. Numerous now resort to products such as Fernblock® (from *Polypodium Leucotomos*) since it has been proven safe and can soothe photo-induced pigment changes. Taken both orally and applied topically, it appears to prevent immediate sunburn and even aids in residual DNA damage once you have spent time outdoors. Briefly put, combining these new protective measures with older treatment may improve the way things function overall and decrease the likelihood of these issues returning (González et al., 2023). Chemical peels, laser treatments, and dermabrasions continue to be the standard solutions to facial hyperpigmentation, though they tend to have drawbacks that restrict their prolonged application or prevent patients from complying with them. The tension of visible pigment variation is more than skin deep—it impacts the way individuals feel. Due to this emotional cost, there has been a clear swing of late toward milder, plant-based remedies that have fewer side effects. Individuals appear to like remedies founded on natural materials, which align with the emerging demand for sustainable and biocompatible solutions. This equilibrium allows physicians to address the clinical aspect of pigment alterations while balancing the patients' comfort (Parveen et al., 2019). Latest research even suggests combining conventional treatments with natural components in order to approach pigment disorders in a more holistic manner. Leveraging the antioxidant, anti-inflammatory, and sun-blocking properties inherent in many botanical extracts may not just lighten hyperpigmentation but also restore the skin's barrier function. This strategy appears particularly helpful for individuals whose pigmentation problems become triggered with sun exposure, as it tends to quiet the persistent oxidative stress and inflammation from environmental sources. Though such a strategy may pleasantly augment conventional approaches with less in the way of side effects, it does necessitate more elaborate studies to truly sort out its mechanisms and to hone the treatment protocols—all with fulfilling the robust safety and efficacy standards requisite in pigment disorder care (Parveen et al., 2019; González et al., 2023) (Figure 6.11).

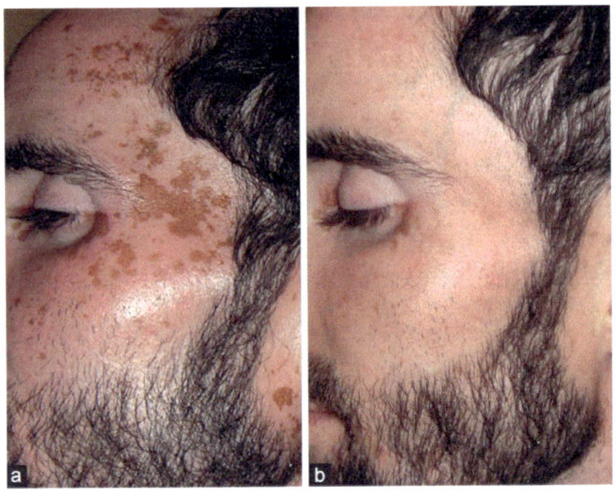

Figure 6.11. (a) Patchy residual pigmentation on face; and (b) after treatment with Q-switched Nd:YAG laser.

Source: Majid, I., & Imran, S. (2013). Figure 1. (a) Patchy residual pigmentation on face, (b) after treatment with Q-switched Nd:YAG laser. In Depigmentation Therapy with Q-Switched Nd: YAG Laser in Universal Vitiligo. *Journal of Cutaneous and Aesthetic Surgery, 6*(2), 94–95.

6.4.1. Topical Therapies

Treating skin color problems typically requires clever actions to adjust the production and distribution of melanin around. The topical treatments have gained favor because they address the problem and are relatively easy to apply. For a lot of cases, these creams and gels work by slowing down pigment creation, accelerating the removal of older skin cells, or introducing antioxidants to balance out unbalanced colors. In general terms, natural extracts such as Fernblock® have been promising; they not only protect against the damaging effects of light but also appear to alleviate oxidative stress and reverse some DNA damage from UV and visible light exposure (González et al., 2023). This type of two-pronged action is generating interest in combining conventional topical agents with naturally active ingredients to enhance outcomes while minimizing side effects. In treating facial hyperpigmentation, many individuals tend to attempt chemical peels, laser surgery, or dermabrasion. However, these procedures are often met with problems – like resulting in additional dark spots due to inflammation or requiring extended recovery periods. Due to such issues, focus is turning toward milder, plant-based treatments that are less likely to have side effects and easier on patients (Parveen et al., 2019). In many respects, combining botanical ingredients is the new trend in dermatology; treatments are not only supposed to be effective but also to appeal to a patient's desire for natural, affordable solutions. Considering the emotional burden of pigment disorders, the availability of skin treatments that enhance appearance without posing additional complexities indeed assists individuals in adhering to their regimen and feeling more assured on a day-to-day basis (Parveen et al., 2019). New knowledge on how skin behaves when exposed to light has made it possible to develop products protecting against the sun and repairing harm. These new preparations combine antioxidants with DNA repair-boosting agents, as a general principle, they protect against pigment outbursts due to sun exposure—so they contribute to the long-term management of such concerns as melasma and post-inflammatory hyperpigmentation (González et al., 2023). The addition of standardized extracts, like *Polypodium Leucotomos*, is a prime example of how these new therapies attack both the hidden causes and the outward signs of pigment change. Ultimately, these treatments represent a turn toward solutions that combine cosmetic enhancement with functional healing of the skin's barrier and overall cellular equilibrium (Figure 6.12).

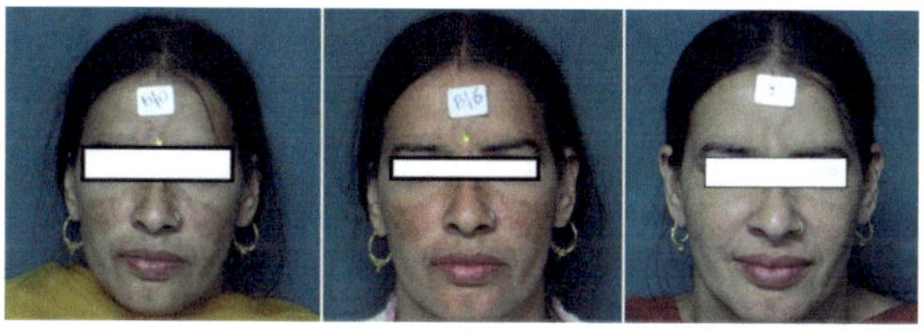

Figure 6.12. A patient of melasma treated with 20% azelaic acid cream at (a) week 0 (MASI 20.7); (b) week 6 (MASI 17.9); and (c) week 12.

Source: Majid, I., & Imran, S. (2013). Figure 1. (a) Patchy residual pigmentation on face, (b) after treatment with Q-switched Nd:YAG laser. In Depigmentation therapy with Q-switched Nd:YAG laser in universal vitiligo. *Journal of Cutaneous and Aesthetic Surgery, 6*(2), 94–95.

6.4.2. Procedural Interventions

Pigment disorders are not fixed by simply using a cream; they typically require a treatment combination that goes far beyond the usual topical remedies, particularly when those initial measures simply do not work. In most cases, a combination of treatments enters the picture to treat recalcitrant hyperpigmentation. For instance, chemical peels deliver their effects by gently shedding injured layers of skin, allowing an overload of melanin to be removed, and providing an opportunity for the skin to regenerate itself. Practitioners most often choose such agents as glycolic acid or trichloroacetic acid based on the depth and extent of the pigmentation. When peels are used with rigorous photoprotection and other topical treatments, it appears to be some sort of synergistic effect that maximizes clearance. There is always the worry, though—practitioners have to take note of the potential for post-inflammatory hyperpigmentation, particularly in darker-skinned patients, which truly highlights the need for treatment programs to be as customized as the patients themselves. In more chronic instances, such as when treating melasma—laser and light treatments have become increasingly appealing. In general, these methods aim melanocytes or other pigmented cells with very precise wavelengths to decrease melanin content. Non-ablative fractional lasers, for example, disturb the top skin layers hardly at all and also assist in forcing drugs such as tranexamic acid deeper into the tissue, thus adjusting melanin production and even influencing vascular elements associated with pigmentation problems. Lasers have to be applied cautiously, naturally; there is always a risk of rebound hyperpigmentation or even relapse within a few months from the cessation of treatment. It is for this reason that, in the majority of instances, laser treatment is reserved for those particularly recalcitrant cases and is used alongside continuing maintenance measures ((Philipp-Dormston, 2024)). Microneedling has also emerged as a revolutionary method to treat these conditions. By inducing small, controlled injuries, this treatment stimulates the skin's own repair processes into action—thus promoting skin remodeling and improving the penetration of topical therapies. When microneedling is combined with agents such as tranexamic acid or other lightening agents, it tends to enhance treatment results while maintaining the risk of systemic side effects minimal. This method promises not only to accelerate pigment clearance but also to address all aspects of pigmentary pathology, including those associated with vascular and inflammatory processes. Although the vast majority of patients can tolerate the procedure quite well, judicious patient selection and meticulous post-procedure care are essential to avoid complications and to ensure that microneedling integrates seamlessly into a comprehensive, multimodal treatment plan ((Philipp-Dormston, 2024)).

6.4.3. Lifestyle Modifications

Environmental and lifestyle decisions play a significant role in skin pigment concerns. It may seem random, but everyday routines dictate how these conditions appear and develop. Take, for instance, avoiding excessive sun—by staying away from intense UV rays and using a high-SPF sunscreen—can halt hyperpigmentation from worsening and decelerate photoaging. A well-balanced diet rich in antioxidants, particularly vitamins C and E, contributes to eliminating free radicals and gives your skin an added boost to heal itself. Essentially, these changes make an environment that prevents faulty pigmentation while improving skin resilience as a whole, reminding us just how deeply lifestyle options and skin care are linked. Apart from sun protection, lifestyle changes have a tangential effect on skin color. Metabolic errors like insulin resistance and hormonal problems—frequently connected to the way we move and feed ourselves—are more likely to accompany conditions like melasma or post-inflammatory pigmentations. Consistent exercise and reducing processed sugars and detrimental fats can iron out metabolic wrinkles and reduce inflammation that would otherwise darken the skin. Even yoga or basic stress-reduction techniques tend to balance your hormones and boost your immune system. In most instances, this combination of habits maintains general wellness while assisting in maintaining skin tone more balanced ((Philipp-Dormston, 2024)). Patient-specific advice is a true game-changer for long-term improvements in pigmentation problems. Instead of one solution fits all, medical professionals can contribute with individualized advice—combining eating advice, sun-safe practices, and stress reduction—to add real strength to treatment. When these practices become part of your daily routine in addition to regular therapies, they can really reduce the likelihood of pigment issues recurring and enhance your overall appearance. It is no revelation that skin concerns have the power to take a psychological toll on one's confidence, so adding these lifestyle modifications not only benefits the skin but also raises individual well-being. Ultimately, incorporating such mundane counsel into practice does not simply address the bio part, but also roots an all-encompassing model for patient care.

6.5. Psychological Impact

Skin disease and mental health have a connection that is all too often ignored—despite the fact that it is rather crucial to knowing how patients really do. Most individuals with pigment problems end up having trouble with self-esteem just because their looks do not fit the typical standards of beauty. Even observable conditions such as vitiligo or post-inflammatory hyperpigmentation have a penchant for provoking embarrassment, sometimes to the point of causing individuals to isolate themselves socially and become more self-conscious. In some instances, these sentiments will progress to anxiety or even depression, further complicating an already difficult clinical condition. Since these disorders tend to persist, patients are frequently left with persistent uncertainties regarding how their condition will progress and whether their treatments will be effective. Obviously, acknowledging this emotional burden is central to providing care that addresses both mind and body and ultimately enables patients to adhere to treatment more effectively. With time, studies have identified that pigmentary disorders do not merely lead to physical manifestations—there is a gradual erosion of an individual's quality of life on a very different, psychological basis. For instance, research in vitiligo indicates that individuals with vitiligo have poorer quality of life scores, women and younger patients experiencing the emotional burden all the more intensely (Jusuf et al., 2017). This implies that cultural norms associated with appearance and gender can exacerbate individual suffering, particularly when there is no adequate remedy in the offing. In most instances, a dearth of strong treatment options ultimately becomes a source of helplessness and frustration. Several professionals suggest incorporating psychosocial counseling into treatment interventions as a means of enhancing emotional resilience and imparting real coping skills, which can reduce the psychological burden and enhance clinical outcome. Taking a broader view, epidemiological research also identifies how social determinants affect mental health in individuals with pigmentary disorders. Studies in varied demographic contexts suggest that factors such as education, socioeconomic status, and age combine with personal experience of disease to determine emotional reactions (Kumar et al., 2023). Even though certain studies propose that only small effects on quality of life occur in bigger groups, even minor psychological burdens can continue to interfere with day-to-day social functioning. These subtle effects tend to go unnoticed in the course of everyday clinical evaluation. Therefore, it is generally prudent for health professionals to carefully monitor for psychosocial signs and to add standardized mental health assessments to dermatological treatment. Treating the problem in a way that addresses both physical symptoms and underlying psychological problems appears to hold the key to truly holistic treatment.

6.5.1. Emotional Effects on Patients

It is not about just seeing changes on your skin—it gets into someone's emotional and social life. Having conditions like melasma that just show up when you don't expect them and persist longer than you want, it can shake your confidence and play around with how you perceive yourself. Sometimes treatments take an eternity to work or simply do not last, leaving you frustrated and worried; these failures accumulate, making everyday life more difficult. There is a combination of inner emotions and what society demands that indicates how much it matters to not only treat the skin but also care about the emotional consequences (Philipp-Dormston, 2024). Identification of these internal battles establishes trust and makes it easier to adhere to a treatment regimen. Add to the internal conflict that many patients must endure social stigma and isolation. Prejudices regarding how they appear or unwanted stares compel some to conceal their condition or forgo social events altogether, further entrenching loneliness and depression. This type of social retreat can drain the energy necessary to seek or maintain treatment. It is rather obvious, then, that medical practitioners must be vigilant for these affective bumps and blend psychological support into the treatment regimen. Research from diverse medical environments in most cases demonstrates that how one feels internally is a major contributor to the efficacy of treatment, so treating pigment concerns requires an authentic patient-focused method that develops emotional strength ((Philipp-Dormston, 2024)). Along the same lines, honest dialogue and proper patient education is important in smoothing the emotional burden. When physicians candidly discuss how such conditions can be chronic and volatile, it has a way of establishing more realistic expectations and diminishing that debilitating feeling of hopelessness attendant to setbacks. Being honest about what may lie ahead, such as the possibility of flare-ups or side effects—empowers patients to be more active in their care instead of sitting back and waiting for the cure. This kind of back-and-forth, even if it is a bit unpolished at times, strengthens the bond between doctor and patient and can lead to better adherence and overall satisfaction. Even though there are cool treatment options out there, like tailored multimodal therapies that offer hope for symptom control, a little psychological reassurance goes a long way in keeping patients confident and on track (Philipp-Dormston, 2024).

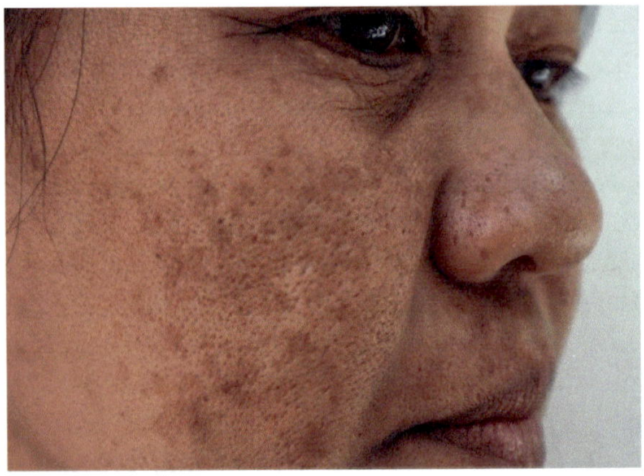

Source: Healthing.ca. (2022). *Close-Up of a Woman Applying Sunscreen to Her Face.* https://smartcdn.gprod.postmedia.digital/healthing/wp-content/uploads/2022/03/GettyImages-1176722103-e1648644583809.jpg?quality=90&strip=all&w=1150&h=646.

6.5.2. Social Stigma and Discrimination

Individuals afflicted with pigmentary disorders cope with so much more than physical symptoms—pain and alienation often are the added insult due to deep-rooted social prejudices many harbors. When a person's skin appears different, it is not too rare for other people to characterize the difference as "abnormal" or simply unwelcome, and soon enough, a rather cruel environment takes shape. Self-esteem can take a blow, and that might cause these people to withdraw from society, and that isolation just makes them feel worse about themselves. For most of them, soaking up all these negative societal opinions exacerbates their emotional issues. Borrowing from mental health advocacy methods—where scientists have strived for a long time to lower public stigma—can perhaps turn opinion a little (Khouja & Corrigan, 2015). If we do not fix these social issues, the general quality of life for those affected remains in a pretty rough spot. At times, discrimination against individuals with these conditions directly coincides with cultural concepts of beauty that we encounter everywhere, particularly in areas where lighter skin is highly valued. It only takes a glance at the phenomenon of skin-whitening creams, usually full of hazardous substances such as mercury—to observe the damaging ripple effect of these ideals of beauty. These trends compel individuals towards risky health decisions as well as preserve old, unrealistic standards. For the most part, altering health policies to focus on these questionable products is quite significant if we wish to reduce both the discrimination and the health consequences associated with them. Initiatives such as better warning labels or greater identification of mercury poisoning within clinics demonstrate the ways in which both medical and social-political actions are necessary. All of these measures, in their unique way, conjoin to change society's understanding of beauty progressively and to demote prejudice toward individuals with differences in pigmentary characteristics (Uayan, 2023). Tackling these areas of overlap between stigma and discrimination is not as straightforward as addressing one aspect—it requires a combination of strategies that both address individuals and the entire society. For example, educational campaigns that disseminate honest, practical information about pigmentary disorders can counter some of those damaging, entrenched stereotypes. Simultaneously, ensuring greater and authentic representation in the media and beauty industries could go a long way toward changing how the public thinks about these differences, making them appear increasingly normal in time. There are policy actions too, such as clamping down on deceptive product marketing and increasing support services for individuals in need—that give all these initiatives even more weight. It requires a genuine team effort, with healthcare professionals, community organizations, and policymakers all contributing, to translate stigma-reduction talk into real, on-the-ground change. As numerous advocates are fond of reminding us, stigma reduction is not solely about combating discrimination; it is about providing these individuals with a level playing field on which they can have an equal chance to achieve their full potential (Khouja & Corrigan, 2015).

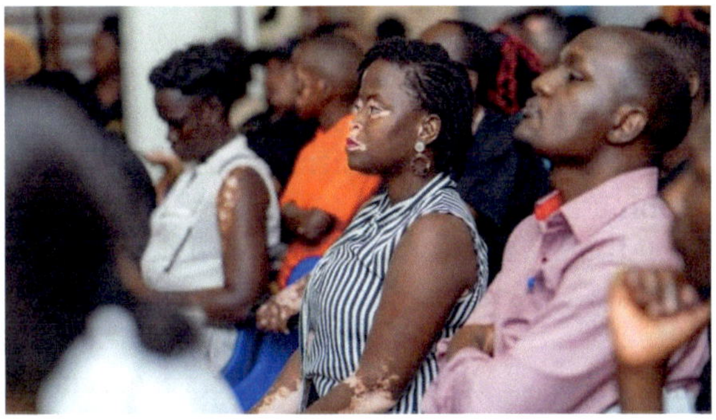

Source: British Council Uganda. (n.d.). *Photograph of a British Council Uganda Event.* https://www.britishcouncil.ug/sites/default/files/styles/bc-landscape-800x450/public/ug11.jpeg?itok=tKCOkKOW.

6.5.3. Coping Strategies and Support

Pigmentary disorders not only change your skin—they also hit at your inner self. Most people struggling with these changes usually end up dealing with unwanted stares and social rejections which, in turn, can erode their general sense of well-being. It is not all about physical symptoms; the visible changes can trigger deep emotional struggles. That is why, more often than not, therapy and reassurance talk become nearly as important as any medical treatment. Counseling therapy and cognitive-behavioral methods serve to alter one's perspective regarding oneself, relaxing the weights of worry and episodes of depression. At times, even merely relating in a peer group can reduce that suffocating loneliness. And when individuals discover that their condition, although chronic, can be controlled, it creates resilience and inspires a more proactive approach to maintaining health. A combination of these strategies works out the complex social and emotional tangles that accompany pigmentary disorders. Not everybody enjoys the same pay-offs, however; demographic and psychosocial variables tend to alter the picture entirely. Research indicates that women with vitiligo experience more severe emotional distress and lower quality of life compared to men (Samela et al., 2023). Such findings indicate the actual need for support that takes into account individual emotional reactions and the burden of social pressures. Mental health screenings with standardized instruments sometimes identify those at greater risk for depression or anxiety, so it may be possible to intervene early. This relatively subtle but significant bit of understanding is why individualized treatment plansthat treat both the skin symptoms and the unseen emotional wounds are so beneficial. These types of interventions ultimately provide a smoother, more comprehensive road to treatment. Inherited disorders such as retinitis pigmentosa take things further than mere counseling or customized sessions. In such cases, continuous support becomes essential in coping with the gradual decline of function.

Even if a permanent cure is not yet possible, realistic steps, such as staying out of too much sun and addressing complications squarely—can retard things and even improve quality of life slightly (Hamel, 2006). Genetic counseling, for example, has been a game-saver, enabling patients and families to sort through the genetic underpinnings of the condition and what those may imply for daily life. This type of information tends to cut through uncertainty and inform family planning and lifestyle adjustments. And until new therapies materialize, in the meantime an interdisciplinary approach, involving eye experts, psychologists, and rehabilitation specialists all in concert, is still at the forefront of maintaining patients independent and emotionally grounded as they confront these incremental challenges.

6.6. Current Research and Advances

Skin color is not quite as simple as it appears. Recently, studies of pigmentary disorders have uncovered layers of complexity, revealing that our genes and daily environmental exposures determine skin color. Scientists continue to excavate conditions such as vitiligo and melasma, usually with an eye to how melanocytes function and how the immune mechanisms of the body occasionally malfunction. Thanks to the assistance of novel genomic tools, researchers are now identifying gene variants associated with atypical pigment shifts—opening new avenues for treatments that are specifically tailored to an individual's requirements. And then there are chemicals called endocrine disruptors that can interfere with the hormonal cues that maintain skin stability, further supporting the argument for taking a mixed, multidisciplinary approach when attempting to untangle these conditions (Svingen et al., 2024). On another front, technology has altered how we screen for these disorders. Digital dermoscopy with high resolution and RCM now provide a non-invasive, highly detailed examination of pigment patterns and skin structure that was previously not possible. These advances enable physicians to catch problems early and track how treatments are progressing. Interestingly, new neuroimaging techniques—that have been applied primarily to research on the brain or even on eating disorders—suggest that the nervous system could also be involved in the unexpected regulation of skin pigmentation (Chae et al., 2023). This idea—that various portions of our body are more interconnected than we originally believed—leaves room for even more extensive, integrative research. Meanwhile, new treatments are beginning to focus on the very mechanisms of these conditions. For example, immunomodulatory therapy such as JAK inhibitors is promising, particularly for autoimmune disorders such as vitiligo, by dampening the immune reactions that kill melanocytes and holding out the promise of more enduring repigmentation. In parallel with this is the growth of regenerative medicine methods, consider transplanting cultured melanocytes or stem cell-based alternatives, incrementally moving into the picture as potential solutions for patients struggling with recalcitrant pigment loss. Combine these strategies with our continually expanding understanding of environmental and molecular variables, and what you see is an outline of a new age in dealing with pigmentary concerns. Naturally, more in-depth research will be required to perfect these advances, confirm their safety, and provide access to all those who could benefit (Chae et al., 2023; Svingen et al., 2024).

6.6.1. Genetic Studies and Discoveries

Genetic studies have revolutionized our perception of pigment disorders. It began when researchers found that some mutations cause conditions such as albinism and vitiligo, demonstrating that these conditions tend to run in families. Recently, techniques like next-generation sequencing and whole-exome sequencing have filled the gap, revealing new genes associated with abnormal pigmentation. These advances assist in pinning down diagnoses and even indicate treatments that attack specific genetic defects. In most instances, the union of vintage genetic techniques and current sequencing has enabled researchers to identify mutations in complex pigment syndromes, improving both patient management and genetic counseling for affected individuals (Hersheson et al., 2024). This continuous transformation reminds us that it is important to remain curious about genetics in dermatology. Delving deeper into the genetic origins of these disorders not only lays out the disorders but also illuminates how normal skin function ought to be. Researches on these hereditary defects frequently venture into the ways that melanocytes develop, how melanin is formed, and even the cellular signals that guide skin color. Historical research and research today both indicate that if genes responsible for melanosome formation, or even melanocortin receptors—become mutated, the effect is an appreciable alteration in pigmentation.

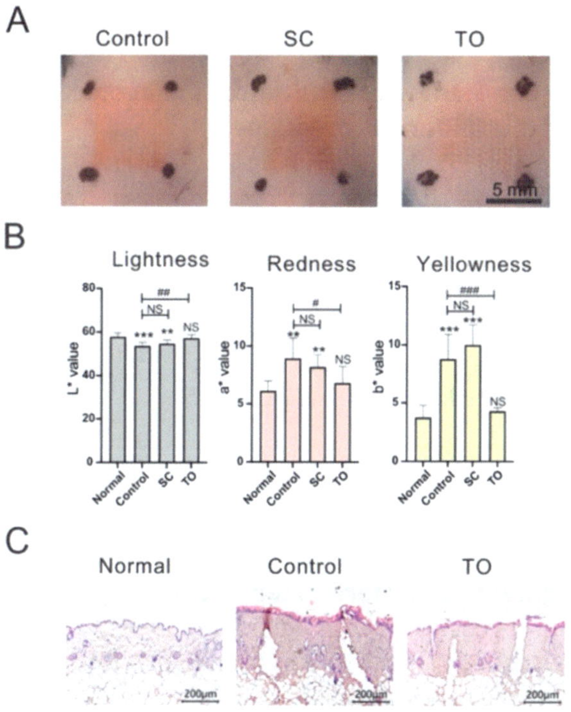

Figure 6.13. Altered gene expression profiles and signaling pathways in vitiligo.

Source: Ou, Kuang-Ling, Chia-Cheng Wen, Ching-Ya Lan, Yu-An Chen, Chih-Hsin Wang, and Yi-Wen Wang. 2021. “The Optimal Application of Medium Potency Topical Corticosteroids in Preventing Laser-Induced Inflammatory Responses—An Animal Study” *Life* 11, no. 4: 350. https://doi.org/10.3390/life11040350.

By and large, knowing why these disorders occur also broadens our understanding of human genetics and skin physiology. Reports of large symposia and research compilations mention that the interaction between genetics and dermatology continues to support new findings and better treatment of pigment problems (McKusick et al., 1973). New genetic methods have even obfuscated the old demarcations we once depended on when categorizing pigment disorders. Large-scale screening sometimes detects mutations that influence more than epidermal color, with pigmentation changes going hand in hand with neurological or more systemic effects. This combination of genetic information and heterogeneous clinical presentations illustrates the importance of studies that combine molecular genetics, dermatology, and neuroscience. Using methods such as gene panel sequencing and meticulous mutation analysis, researchers have discovered unanticipated connections between genes and the bodily manifestations they create, even recognizing rare syndromes characterized by pigment issues. Such rigorous effort not only fine-tunes diagnostic precision but also provides the ability to forecast outcomes, laying the groundwork for a more personalized, customized treatment regimen. Genetic research remains at the forefront of elucidating the sheer intricacy of pigment disorders, guiding both cutting-edge research and daily clinical practice (Hersheson et al., 2024) (Figure 6.13).

6.6.2. Innovative Treatment Approaches

The recent advances in pigment cell biology have inspired new ideas for treating color disorders of the skin. Today, we understand much more about melanocytes’ function, and malfunction in conditions such as vitiligo, melasma, and albinism—so the treatments are not merely applying creams willy-nilly anymore. In the majority of instances, scientists are combining findings from genomics and immunotherapy with an intensified examination of cell-level actions to target the true causes head-on. For instance, incorporating insights from systems biology into research that observes pigment activity at the lowest scales of measurement provides means to modify color production in innovative, efficient ways. This fresh thinking is incrementally introducing patient-tailored approaches in personalized medicine that honor the diversity of pigment problems, eventually providing patients with more specific treatments (Birlea et al., 2018). An organized turn of events in the treatment of hyperpigmentation, particularly melasma, is the increasing practice of picosecond laser techniques. Recent research on a 785 nm picosecond laser indicates that it can treat both the pigment lesions and the associated blood vessel problems—a sort of two-for-one treatment process. Initial trials with Fitzpatrick phototypes II-III patients have recorded quite apparent improvements in complexion, with virtually no annoying side effects finding their way into the equation. While the study groups were limited in number, these early results present a fairly convincing argument for taking a closer examination of laser treatment as a non-invasive, targeted solution to intractable pigment issues (Zappia et al., 2024). New methods are also seeking to shake things up by combining various treatment approaches for even more effective outcomes. Scientists are combining new laser technology with other therapies such as immune modulators or natural antioxidants, which appear to enhance overall response while reducing the likelihood of the problem recurring. New genomics and systems biology research is also pushing these combination treatments toward individualization so that each treatment fits a person's own specific genetic and environmental history. By sharpening diagnoses and treatment, this changing strategy reduces side effects and maximizes benefits. Further research in these fields truly seems poised to revolutionize the treatment of pigment disorders, allowing therapies to be better tailored to the diversified needs of different patients (Birlea et al., 2018; Zappia et al., 2024) (Figure 6.14).

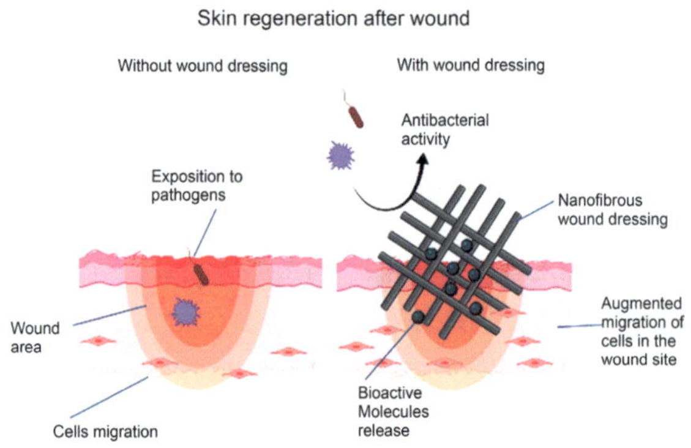

Figure 6.14. Recent advances in nanomedicine for the treatment of vitiligo.

Source: Bellu, Emanuela, Serenella Medici, Donatella Coradduzza, Sara Cruciani, Evzen Amler, and Margherita Maioli. 2021. "Nanomaterials in Skin Regeneration and Rejuvenation" *International Journal of Molecular Sciences* 22, no. 13: 7095. https://doi.org/10.3390/ijms22137095

6.6.3. Future Directions in Research

Advances in molecular biology and genomics continue to redefine how we think about pigment disorders. Melanocyte physiology, and occasionally their mistakes—is coming into sharp relief with these developments. Researchers increasingly blend in systems biology approaches, disassembling the complex webs that control pigmentation and even disease development. This hands-on examination aids in identifying new genetic signals and pathways that may be aimed at later for therapies. For instance, preliminary glimmers from immunotherapy for melanoma are gradually proving promising for diseases such as vitiligo. By integrating these disparate methods, future research can enhance the extent to which we target our diagnoses and adaptations precisely, which in the end counts for patient treatment. This general trend is part of a broader movement towards combining basic concepts with clinical understanding and disentangling the numerous tiers of pigment problems (Birlea et al., 2018). High-throughput sequencing combined with advanced bioinformatics is revolutionizing the method of detecting and knowing about pigment disorders. Now even those small genetic flaws that escaped detection can be caught. Gene profiling enables us to separate complex pigmentation features, allowing us to identify what is driving them—a step toward selecting personalized treatments. Sometimes, research groups add in neuroimaging and metabolic research along with genetic testing, peeking beyond the skin symptoms to also record systemic or neurological clues. In the majority of instances, this type of mixed approach may accelerate the search for early biomarkers, slowly moving clinical practice into everyday use. Research into gene editing and even gene replacement treatments appears promising for correcting genetic defects associated with pigment problems, highlighting how much more we have to investigate molecular treatments (Ceravolo et al., 2023). In the future, the field of pigment disorder research may very well shift to new therapeutic avenues from gene therapy and regenerative medicine. Currently, most treatments focus on symptom control rather than addressing the underlying issue, but new gene-based remedies are working to repair the genetic errors that cause pigmentation disorders. Building on advances such as CRISPR-Cas9, and even some early stem cell research—may eventually provide long-term, even corrective treatment, especially for congenital diseases such as albinism. Combine it with a greater understanding of pigment chemistry and biophysics, and scientists are seeing chances to engineer novel drugs that manipulate melanogenesis more specifically and, ideally, with fewer side effects. Interdisciplinary collaboration between dermatologists, geneticists, and biochemists is helping to drive these scientific advances toward actual clinical application. Generally speaking, this vision underlines the need for ongoing investment in both basic and applied research into melanocyte workings and the complexities of pigment disorders (Birlea et al., 2018).

CLOSER LOOK

Vitiligo Area Scoring Index (VASI)

The VASI is a clinician-reported outcome measure that is utilized to measure the degree and extent of depigmentation in vitiligo. It is a composite score that is derived from both the percentage of body surface area involved and the degree of depigmentation in those involved areas. The VASI allows clinicians to monitor changes in vitiligo over time and assess the efficacy of treatments.

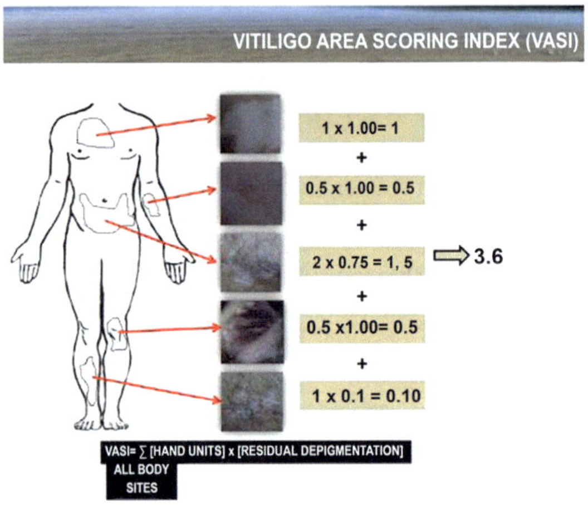

Source: Doe, J. (2023). *Sunset over the Mountains* https://lh6.googleusercontent.com/proxy/Gz6BuJ3yoxusQLO_MaoLyb8yIeBkL1dPvzqwkS5zSnJO9Mb5vMRCJqWTcAhGtSdAVBnbcFhgwg_rB7NswSe3eb-tqpOkqZwuXJMc2IOdzO8KPdikZw.

- **How VASI is Calculated:**
  - **Area Involvement:** The body surface area (BSA) that is involved with vitiligo is estimated, most often in terms of hand units (with one hand unit being around 1% of BSA).
  - **Degree of Depigmentation:** The degree of depigmentation is evaluated, generally in percentages (e.g., 0%, 10%, 25%, 50%, 75%, 90%, or 100%), representing the amount of pigmentation within the vitiligo lesions.
  - **Score Calculation:** VASI score is calculated by multiplying the area estimated affected by percentage of depigmentation and adding across all body areas.
  - **Whole Body VASI (T-VASI) and Facial VASI (F-VASI):** VASI can be computed for the whole body (T-VASI) or facial area (F-VASI).
- **Purpose and Uses of VASI:**
  - **Clinical Trial Outcome Measure:** VASI is also widely used as a clinical outcome measure in clinical trials assessing the efficacy of vitiligo therapies.
  - **Disease Progress Monitoring:** VASI aids in monitoring the progress of disease over time, both the size of the affected areas and the level of depigmentation.

- **Evaluating Treatment Response:** Through comparison of VASI scores pre and post-treatment, clinicians are able to evaluate the efficacy of treatments in minimizing vitiligo.

- **Key Considerations:**
  - **Reliability:** VASI has proven to be a reliable and valid method for evaluating vitiligo with high intra- and inter-observer reliability.
  - **Clinically Meaningful Change Thresholds:** Research has established clinically meaningful thresholds for VASI improvements, including at least a 75% improvement from baseline in F-VASI or at least a 50% improvement in T-VASI.
  - **Facial Involvement:** F-VASI directly deals with the severity of vitiligo on the face, which patients are usually most concerned about.
  - **Digital Assessment**: VASI also can be determined with digital images of vitiligo lesions.

SUMMARY

Environmental factors and the natural characterestics of our skin combine in interesting combinations when it comes to pigment issues. Sunlight—be it from UV and even the less harsh visible and infrared light—will make irregular tone worse, and studies mostly indicate that these things play a large role in determining how our skin behaves. You may notice creams or even pills being utilized in combination as a double-barrel strategy, and very interestingly, such natural entities like *Polypodium Leucotomos* extract become part of the equation as a protective, safe adjunct. This natural molecule, which some physicians now prefer, has both treatment and photoprotection benefits. It is a move toward therapies not merely response-based but indeed preventive, keeping pace with our increasingly refined understanding of the minute molecular processes involved in pigment changes (González et al., 2023). Pigment problems of the skin do not exist in isolation, aging and general skin health are also part of the scenario. Age is not an ideal indicator, since genetic characterestics and everyday environmental exposures conspire to create what we perceive on the outside; for most people, using only one number (our age) simply does not work. This overlapping blend makes that the skin tends to age in ways that make diagnosis and treatment more difficult. Instead of merely seeking to cover up symptoms, most experts contend that treatments must do more, digging deeper into age processes while adjusting pigmentation. Manipulating agents that very subtly move both pigment and skin architecture appears to yield improved in-practice outcomes, all within the context of a larger aspiration for overall skin health (Fernández-Varela-Gómez et al., 2024). When you take a step back and consider the entire picture, treating pigment problems requires a realistic perspective on both outside influences and our own skin aging. New treatments, which tend to integrate traditional remedies with natural photo protectants, tend to arrive with a nod toward hard scientific evidence, and sure enough, this is typically considered innovative. Future practice will probably need to sort out how precisely radiation, pigment shifts, and the aging process work together; in most instances, researchers are already stating that individualized, complex approaches are the future. By combining prevention, personal modifications, and a whole-person approach to skin health, clinicians can strive to address the broad spectrum of pigment presentations better. This hybrid, occasionally rough-around-the-edges, methodology has potential to improve dermatologic treatment and enhance patient outcomes (Fernández-Varela-Gómez et al., 2024; González et al., 2023).

Genetic mutations and pigment disorders are ensnared in ways that reveal just how complex these conditions are. Recent molecular genetics research has uncovered more of the veil on how these mutations disrupt melanin production, its dissemination, and even how skin cells play along. You usually discover that skin transitioning from too little to too much pigment is the result of errors in the genes that are supposed to regulate melanocytes and melanosome production. Occasionally, strangely enough, strange pigment patterns are signs of larger systemic issues. Consider inherited syndromes, for example – they may appear with not only distinctive skin markings but also sensory errors, which, in the majority of instances, informs us that pigmentation is associated with other body systems (Guimaraes et al., 2022). This type of information truly emphasizes the necessity to combine skin examinations with genetic assessments in order to identify problems properly and develop treatment that truly suits the patient. It is not just a matter of what appears on the surface. Very often, these pigment changes intersect with neurological and other systemic disease – a truth which serves only to heighten their clinical complexity. Next-generation sequencing has, in the main, shed light on the genetic origins of many neurodegenerative and multisystem diseases in which pigment alterations are part of the equation. This software has succeeded in identifying new mutations associated with a variety of symptoms , such as cerebellar and spastic ataxias with hypogonadism, with pigment abnormalities added in for good measure. Such observations tend to indicate that pigment problems may be part of a larger syndromic picture rather than mere cutaneous abnormalities per se (Hersheson et al., 2024). Most times, charting these genetic facts is not just useful for accurate categorization but also guides us to what may lie ahead with regard to available treatments. Summing it all up, pigmentary disorders exist in all forms, each defined by various genetic characterestics and clinical appearances. They bear significance beyond the simple fact of a person's looks, frequently revealing more profound underlying genetic syndromes that span the whole body. Genetic advances have, practically speaking, allowed us to diagnose these problems sooner and more comprehensively untangle the mechanisms behind these conditions. Identifying the wide variety of pigment abnormalities, and their connections to sensory and neurological difficulties—is the key to delivering truly comprehensive patient care. The greater awareness allows physicians to merge genetic, cutaneous, and general health examinations to enhance patient outcomes (Guimaraes et al., 2022; Hersheson et al., 2024). Finally, ongoing research and cross-specialty interaction continue to be important in refining both how we treat and how we diagnose these complex disorders.

KEY TERMS FROM THIS CHAPTER

Abrasions	Bioinformatics	Cholestasis
Conjunction	Dietary changes	Environmental stimuli
Fibroblasts	Genes	Genetic predispositions
Genome-wide association	Hydroquinone	Hyperpigmentation
Hypopigmented disorders	Keratinocyte growth factor	Keratinocytes
Machine learning	Melanin	Melanocytes
Neuroectodermal dysplasias	Neurofibromatosis type	Phacomatoses
Pigmentation	Pollutants	Red flags
Skin biology	Solar lentigines	Stem cell factor
Surgical scars	Tyrosinase	

REFERENCES

1. Ajluni, V. (2024). Integrating psychiatry and family medicine in the management of somatic symptom disorders: Diagnosis, collaboration, and communication strategies. *Journal of General and Family Medicine, 26*, 12–18. https://www.semanticscholar.org/paper/979f1f9a3be877e1a7f3a0ed465009246785311c (accessed on 12 May 2025).
2. Albandar, J. M., Susin, C., & Hughes, F. J. (2018). Manifestations of systemic diseases and conditions that affect the periodontal attachment apparatus: Case definitions and diagnostic considerations. *Journal of Periodontology, 8*9. https://doi.org/10.1002/jper.16-0480.
3. Amiri, S., & Ab Khan, M. (2024). Is eating disorders a risk agent for all-cause mortality: a meta-analysis. Eating disorders, 1–35. Advance online publication. https://doi.org/10.1080/10640266.2024.2402634(accessed on 12 May 2025).
4. Arora, G., Khandpur, S., Bansal, A., Shetty, B., Aggarwal, S., Saha, S., Sachdeva, S., et al. (2022). Current understanding of frictional dermatoses: A review. Indian Journal of Dermatology, Venereology and Leprology. https://www.semanticscholar.org/paper/ee5f1859ccd568956f0e15d516ca2e76d327d175 (accessed on 12 May 2025).
5. Ashraf Y, *Ali Ismail N, Omar H, Na*da H, CXCL13 Serum Level as a Potential Biomarker in Vitiligo Patients: Correlation with Disease Activity and Severity.J Skin Stem Cell.2023;10(3):e138546. https://doi.org/10.5812/jssc-*138546.(accessed* on 12 May 2025).
6. Azam, S. S., Vasudevan, S., Bukhari, W. S., Thadhani, J., Tasneem, H., Singh, S., Chijioke, I., et al. (2025). Reproductive endocrine disorders: A comprehensive guide to the diagnosis and management of infertility, polycystic ovary syndrome, and endo*metriosis. Cureus, 17. https://www.semanticscholar.org/p*aper/64a2299e32835bca15a3699dc6ccb4abe44af35a (accessed on 12 May 2025).
7. Berglund, A., & Hughes, K. (2006). Adults with low vision: Continuing education for occupational therapists and occupational therapy students. Core. https://core.ac.uk/download/235073517.pdf (accessed on 12 May 2025).
8. Birl*ea, S., Bosenberg, M. W., Box, N. F., Bra*sh, et al. (2018). Frontiers in pigment cell and melanoma research. https://arxiv.org/abs/1808.01869 (accessed on 12 May 2025).
9. Ceravolo, G., Zhelcheska, K., Squadrito, V., Pellerin, D., Gitto, E., Hartley, L., & Houlden, H. (2024). Update on leukodystrophies and developing trials. Journal of neurology, 271(1), 593–605. https://doi.org/10.1007/s00415-023-11996-5 (accessed on 12 May 2025).
10. Chae, Y., & Lee, I. S. (2023). Central regulation of eating behaviors in humans: Evidence from functional neuroimaging studies. Nutrients, 15. https://www.semanticscholar.org/paper/c699bc26da40ccfbe51d5c76*badabf3658*986642 (accessed on 12 May 2025).
11. Deana, C., Vetrugno, L., Cortegiani, A., Mongodi, S., Salve, G., Mangiagalli, M., Boscolo, A., et al. (2023). Quality of life in COVID-related ARDS patients one year after intensive care discharge (Odissea study): A multicenter observational study. Journal of Clinical Medicine, 12. https://www.semanticscholar.org/paper/6cf8ce186af524698be547e7670a190e297fff77 (accessed on 12 May 2025).
12. Docherty, A., Mullins, N., Ashley-Koch, A. E., Qin, X. J., Coleman, *J.* R. I., Shabalin, A., Kang, J., et al. (2023). GWAS meta-analysis of suicide attempt: Identification of 12 genome-wide

significant loci and implication of genetic risks for specific health factors. The American Journal of Psychiatry, 180(10), 723–738. https://www.semanticscholar.org/paper/e2af2e2393a481739871006e584dd931898c7fe3 (accessed on 12 May 2025).

13. European Glaucoma Society. (2021). European Glaucoma Society terminology and guidelines for glaucoma, 5*th editio*n. British Journal of Ophthalmology, 105, 1–169. https://doi.org/10.1136/bjophthalmol-2021-egsguidelines.

14. Fernández-Varela-Gómez, F., Sandoval-García, A., Cabrera-Rios, V., & Karla. (2024). Signs of skin aging: A review. International Journal o*f Research in Medica*l *Sci*ences, 12(7), 2674–2679. https://core.ac.uk/download/613230159.pdf (accessed on 12 May 2025).

15. Gao, X., & Xiang, W. (2025). Emerging roles of dermal fibroblasts in hyperpigmentation and hypopigmentation: A revie*w. Journal of* Cosmetic Dermatology, 24. https://www.semanticscholar.org/paper/52e75d598b5872102b93542477d871a05eb7b430 (accessed on 12 May 2025).

16. González, S., Juarranz de la Fuente, Á., Rodríguez-Luna, A., Zamarrón, et al. (2023). Clinical applications of Polypodium Leucotomos (Fernblock®): An update. https://core.ac.uk/download/619331991.pdf (accessed on 12 May 2025*).*

*17. Gowda, V. K., K, A. R., Srini*vasan, V. M., Vamyanmane, D. K., Srinivas, S. M., Chickabasaviah, Y., Santhoshkumar, R., Mittal, P., Chikara, S. K., & Vishwanathan, G. B. (2024). A Rare Case of Neuronal Ceroid Lipofuscinosis-Type 1 (NCL-1) with Vitamin D-Dependent Rickets-Type 1 (VDDR-1), Complex 1 Mitochondrial Deficiency, and Mixed Variant-Checkerboard and Phylloid Type of Pigmentary Mosaicism. Journal *of pediatric genetics, 13(4), 291–299.* https://doi.org/10.1055/s-0044-1787196(accessed on 12 May 2025).

18. Grodzka, O., Łagowski, W., Eyileten, C., & Domitrz, I. (2025). Biomarkers in headaches as a potential solution to simplify differential diagnosis of primary headache disor*ders: A systematic review. The Journa*l of Headache and Pain, 26. https://www.semanticscholar.org/paper/d41e93d0bfd7bcf30d1f654269e42dbe63962d76 (accessed on 12 May 2025).

19. Guimaraes, T. A. C., Arram, E., Shakarchi, A. *F., Georgiou, M., & Michaelides, M. (2023). Inherited cau*ses of combined vision and hearing loss: clinical features and molecular genetics. The British journal of ophthalmology, 107(10), 1403–1414. https://doi.org/10.1136/bjo-2022-321790 (accessed on 12 May 2025).

*20. Hamel C. (2006). Retinitis pigmen*tosa. Orphanet journal of rare diseases, 1, 40. https://doi.org/10.1186/1750-1172-1-40

21. He, J., Zhang, Y., Liu, Z., Barnhart, W. R., Cui, S., Chen, S., Fu, Y., et al. (2024). Exploring the self-perceived causes of eating *disorders among Chin*ese social media users with self-reported eating disorders. Journal of Eating Disorders, 12. https://www.semanticscholar.org/paper/c619bbcf7d790e1d99d47f7fd6a69b7e9016f380 (accessed on 12 May 2025).

22. Hersheson, J. (2024). Exploring next generation sequencing in the diagnosis of inherited ataxia and other neurological diseases. Core. https://core.ac.uk/download/618291189.pdf (accessed on 12 May 2025).

23. Håkansson, A., Janfada-Baloo, S., & Berge, J. (2023). No obvious effect on mortality from *a patient choice reform expan*din*g* access to opioid disorder treatment: Results from a natural experiment of policy change in Sweden. Substance Abuse Treatment, Prevention, and Policy,

18. https://www.semanticscholar.org/paper/86d1a2218f9b9732c4c3cbc7c486e32efc6800ca (accessed on 12 May 2025).

24. Ivanov, R., Kazantsev, F., Zavarzin, E., Klimenko, A., Milakhina, N., Matushkin, Y., Savostyanov, A., et al. (2022). ICBrainDB: An integrated database for finding associations between genetic factors and EEG markers of depressive disorders. Journal of Personalized Medicine, 12. https://www.semanticscholar.org/paper/1a830f0b7929a42bf7ff1b37afd1e3e8753c5487 (accessed on 12 May 2025).

25. Iyer, S. S. (2025). Investigating the role of lifestyle modifications and yoga intervention in the management of type 2 diabetes: A comprehensive review. Journal of Information Systems Engineering and Management. https://www.semanticscholar.org/paper/6bd538b834d26882fcf09908346ab050419a14b6 (accessed on 12 May 2025).

26. Jusuf NK, Putra IB, Utami DR. Quality of Life in Vitiligo Patients at H. Adam Malik General Hospital Medan, Indonesia. Sumat. Med. J. [Internet]. 2018Oct.1 [cited 2025Jun.12];1(1):41-8. Available from: https://talenta.usu.ac.id/smj/article/view/445 (accessed on 12 May 2025).

27. Khouja MA, Corrigan PW (2015) The Stigma of Pigmentary Disorders. Pigmentary Disorders 2: 217. doi:10.4172/2376-0427.1000217

28. Kim, H., Choi, H. R., Kim, D. S., & Park, K. C. (2012). Topical hypopigmenting agents for pigmentary disorders and their mechanisms of action. Annals of dermatology, 24(1), 1–6. https://doi.org/10.5021/ad.2012.24.1.1 (accessed on 12 May 2025).

29. Krutmann, J., Piquero-Casals, J., Morgado-Carrasco, D., Granger, C., Trullàs, C., Passeron, T., & Lim, H. W. (2023). Photoprotection for people with skin of colour: needs and strategies. The British journal of dermatology, 188(2), 168–175. https://doi.org/10.1093/bjd/ljac046 (accessed on 12 May 2025).

30. Kumar M, Singh S, Berman S, Singh LD, Kumar N, Barman SK. An Assessment of Skin Diseases in People and Their Quality of Life in Bundelkhand Region of Uttar Pradesh. Indian J. of Com. Health. 2023;35(2):165-168. (accessed on 12 May 2025).

31. Lilje, S., van Tulder, M., Wykman, A., Aboagye, E., & Persson, U. (2023). Cost-effectiveness of specialised manual therapy versus orthopaedic care for musculoskeletal disorders: long-term follow-up and health economic model. Therapeutic advances in musculoskeletal disease, 15, 1759720X221147751. https://doi.org/10.1177/1759720X221147751(accessed on 12 May 2025).

32. McKusick V. A. (1973). Genetics and dermatology or if I were to rewrite Cockayne's Inherited Abnormalities of the Skin. The Journal of investigative dermatology, 60(6), 343–359. https://doi.org/10.1111/1523-1747.ep12702125

33. Miller, D. T., Freedenberg, D., Schorry, E. K., Ullrich, N. J., Viskochil, D., Korf, B. R., Chen, E., et al. (2019). Health supervision for children with neurofibromatosis type 1. Pediatrics, 143. https://doi.org/10.1542/peds.2019-0660.

34. Natrayan, L., Aluvala, S., Socrates, S., & Bharathi, G. (2024). A framework for automated diagnosis and management of autoimmune disorders with neural networks. 2024 International Conference on Advancements in Smart, Secure and Intelligent Computing (ASSIC). https://www.semanticscholar.org/paper/2b732fabf63e52471da5e9141cf6ff3cd75b6187 (accessed on 12 May 2025).

35. Oremović, L., Šitum, M., & Bolanča, Ž. (2010). Kemijski pilinzi–kada i zašto? https://core.ac.uk/download/14451794.pdf (accessed on 12 May 2025).

36. Parveen, N., S. Ali, A., & A. Ali, S. (2019*). On the Intri*cacies of Facial Hyperpigmentation and the Use of Herbal Ingredients as a Boon for Its Treatment: Cosmeceutical Significance, Current Challenges and Future Perspectives. IntechOpen. doi: 10.5772/intechop*en.84257 (accessed on 12 May 2025).*

37. *Passeron, T., Krutmann, J., Andersen, M. L., Katta, R., & Zo*uboulis, C. C. (2020). Clinical and biological impact of the exposome on the skin. Journal of the European Academy of Dermatology and Venereology, 34, 4–25. https://doi.org/10.1111/jdv.16614.

38. Patel, N. (2021). Precision of dermoscopy in melasma over Wood's lamp examination. Indian Journal of Applied-Basic Medical Sciences. https://www.semanticscholar.org/paper/71d22fc172974e42f027f454572b6369b52cf572 (accessed on 12 May 2025).

39. Philipp-Dormston, W. (2024). Melasma: A step-by-step approach towards a multimodal combination therapy. Clini*cal, Cosmetic and Investigational Dermatology, 17, 1203–1216. https*://www.semanticscholar.org/paper/2954042fed68bd82a2a0c2bd0d4164fdb9092029 (accessed on 12 May 2025).

40. Philipp-Dormston W. G. (2*024). Melasma: A Step-by-Step Approach Towards a* Multimodal Combination Therapy. Clinical, cosmetic and investigational dermatology, 17, 1203–1216. https://doi.org/10.2147/CCID.S372456

41. Proietti I, Guida S, Dybala A, Spagnoli A, Potenza C. Effects of CE Ferulic® *Combined with Microneedling in the Treatment of Pigm*entary Disorders: A Monocentric, Split Face, Comparative Study. Cosmetics. 2024; 11(3):101. https://doi.org/10.3390/cosmetics11030101(accessed on 12 May 2025).

42. Robert P. Finger, Steffen Schmitz-Valckenberg, Matthias Schmid, G*ary S. Rubin, Hannah Dunbar, Adnan Tufail, David P. Cr*abb, Alison Binns, Clara I. Sánchez, Philippe Margaron, Guillaume Normand, Mary K. Durbin, Ulrich F.O. Luhmann, Parisa Zamiri· José Cunha-Vaz, Friedrich Asmus, Frank G. Holz, on behalf of the MACUSTAR consortium; MACUSTAR: Development and Clin*ical Vali*dation of Functional, Structural, and Patient-Reported Endpoints in Intermediate Age-Related Macular Degeneration. Ophthalmologica 25 January 2019; 241 (2): 61–72. https://doi.org/10.1159/000491*402*

43. *Ruggieri, M., Micali, G., & Prat*icò, A. (2018). Rare neurocutaneous disorders: State of the art and update. Journal of Pediatric Neurology, 16, 253–254. https://www.semanticscholar.org/paper/dabab28960811ec432ec812c6e2d749e6f9603f8 (accessed on 12 May 2025).

44. Shchur, O., Kurylo, H., Petrov, V., *& Terletskiy, O. (2024). Alagille syndrome in* the modern view of a multidisciplinary approach to the problem. Neonatology, Surgery and Perinatal Medicine. 14(4(54), 65–74. https://doi.org/10.24061/2413-4260.XIV.4.54.2024.9(accessed on 12 May 2025).

45. Soleimani-Meigooni, D. N., Smith, R., Provost, K., Lesman-Segev, O. H., Allen, I. E., Chen, M. K., Cho, H., Edwards, L., Janelidze, S., La Joie, R., Mundada, N., Ossenkoppele, R., Stomrud, E., Strandberg, O., Strom, A., Boxer, A. L., Dage, J. L., Gorno-Tempini, M. L., Kramer, J. H., Miller, B. L., ... Rabinovici, G. D. (2024). Head-to-Head Comparison of Tau and Amyloid Positron Emission Tomograph*y Visual Reads for* Di*ff*erential Diagnosis of Neurodegenerative

Disorders: An International, Multicenter Study. Annals of neurology, 96(3), 476–487. https://doi.org/10.1002/ana.27008(accessed on 12 May 2025).

46. Svingen, T., Andersson, A. M., Angelova, J., Axelstad, M., Bakker, J., Baumann, L., Beronius, A., et al. (2024). Enhanced identification of endocrine disruptors through integration of science-based regulatory practices and innovative methodologies: The MERLON Project. Open Research Europe, 4. https://www.semanticscholar.org/paper/0ed21b1c6abc8e5ff9d06f1648f62db31c83b58a (accessed on 12 May 2025).

47. Tashiro, R., Onoue, N., & Shinozaki, T. (2018). Mitochondrial Cardiomyopathy. InTech. doi: 10.5772/intechopen.77105 (accessed on 12 May 2025).

48. Uayan, Raven Joyce Redaniel, ""Am I light enough?": Mercury Poisoning Due to Skin-Lightening Products, a Policy, and a Culturally Competent Solution" (2023). Master's Projects and Capstones. 1606. https://repository.usfca.edu/capstone/1606 (accessed on 12 May 2025).

49. Zaki, A., Aziz, H. A., Mohamed, M., & Hamed, A. (2019). Evaluation of serum interleukin-6 level in vitiligo patients before and after phototherapy. The Egyptian Journal of Hospital Medicine. The (October 2019) Vol. 77 (3), Page 5276-5278 https://www.semanticscholar.org/paper/19f24496b6bd0c5be7a97e580386289a74ff4eaa (accessed on 12 May 2025).

50. Zappia E, Piccolo D, Del Re C, Bonan P, Guarino L, Ribero S, Galadari H, Nisticò SP. Combined Efficacy of Q-Switched 785 nm Laser and Tranexamic Acid Cream in the Treatment of Melasma: A Prospective Clinical Study. Photonics. 2024; 11(10):938. https://doi.org/10.3390/photonics11100938 (accessed on 12 May 2025).

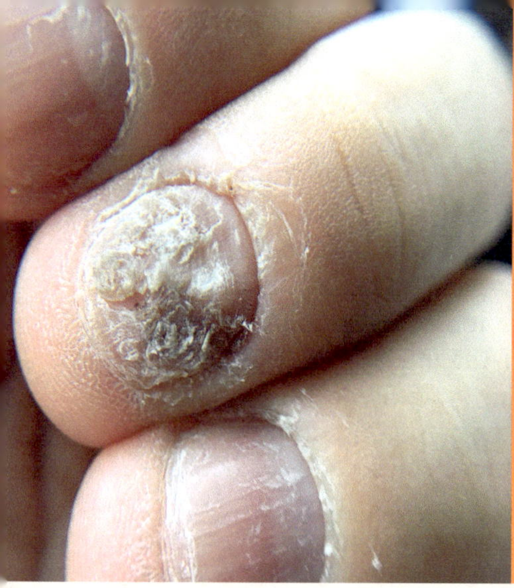

Chapter 7

HAIR AND NAIL DISORDERS

Contents

Introduction

Hair and nails speak about our health in general—even if we hardly ever consider them until something goes wrong. These little details are not mere ornament; they get some work done by defending us and keeping us in working order. We might only realize that there is an issue when these components begin malfunctioning, and that can hard hit our self-confidence, even rattling our social lives. For the most part, new science has advanced treatment by emphasizing early detection and quick action so they do not get completely out of hand. Knowing the underlying biology of these problems is essential; it allows clinicians to select treatments that address both the overt symptoms and underlying issues, offering more durable outcomes and enhanced satisfaction. In regard to how the problems of hair and nails impact us, the influence extends far beyond mere appearance. For instance, alopecia or disheveled nails can cause people anxiety and make them feel disconnected from the social groups with which they normally interact. In general, a comprehensive approach is required, one that tends to combine normal drugs with psychological counseling and normal lifestyle changes. Even recent studies suggest mixing ancient cures with sturdy, evidence-based treatments can improve outcomes.

Occasionally, a look at a person's nutrition and adding a supplement or two in seems to fill gaps that make the problem worse. A combination of treatment from multiple specialties is regarded as crucial in order to deal with these problems, fostering both mental health and health of skin or hair (Chintan et al., 2012). Even with all the strides in treatment, many hair and nail diseases are still difficult to address because their origins go deep and are unique to each individual. New work indicates that, in addition to merely alleviating symptoms, it is also vital to focus on behavior and environment. Conditions such as trichotillomania and even chronic skin picking—those ritualistic behaviors—tend to confuse traditional treatments, so a little psychological assistance typically accompanies skin care. Some recent accounts describe how data tools and clinical evaluations can refine treatments on an individual basis. Through interweaving of behavioral understanding and clinical dermatology, physicians are able to develop plans that address both the body's external manifestations and the internal battles, seeking improved long-term outcomes (Hende et al., 2015).

Definition of Hair and Nail Disorders

Sometimes we remember that skin, hair, and nails are not all about appearance - they are our body's first defense and how we experience the world. A change as small as hair that does not feel the same or nails that are not as firm as usual can be an indicator of larger health concerns. You could be noticing hair issues appearing as thinning, unexplained growth, or bizarrely shaped locks that can be caused by genetics, immune anomalies, infections, or even things around us. Nails can also misbehave - be it a fungal infection such as onychomycosis, redness in the nail bed, or deformities caused by systemic diseases or even a minor bump (Amy et al., 2021). These signs often resemble other dermatologic or body conditions, thus complicating the diagnostic puzzle even further, but they lead physicians to treatment strategies intended for each individual case. In the clinical world, problems with hair and nails may descend upon patients in sudden attacks or persist for the long term, which complicates the picture of diagnosis. Throughout history, various grading systems and a mess of terms have been created in an attempt to make what we say about these conditions consistent – it is not always tidy, though. Most of the time, it is not about the physical abnormalities; the emotional and social impact counts as well, particularly when constant itching or chronic pain impacts someone's daily life. Most diagnostic models used today rely on a biopsychosocial model, understanding that these abnormalities are usually caused by a combination of physical, psychological, and social factors (Michael et al., 2018). Differentiating between conditions that directly emanate from hair or nails and those caused by more general systemic conditions is essential to customize the appropriate treatment.

Exploring hair and nail conditions involves examining closely how they appear on the surface, why they happen, and how they impact overall function – it is more than a mere surface issue. They are not cosmetic in nature; they sometimes reflect underlying, chronic conditions that require careful examination. New clinical guidelines and expert insights have assisted healthcare professionals in identifying particular red flags and negative signs associated with these disorders. This better understanding opens the doors to therapies that do not just mask the symptoms but target the underlying causes as well. When the experts from all walks of life contribute, definitions of these diseases themselves are shifting with emerging therapeutic innovations, thus resulting in better patient outcomes (Amy et al., 2021; Michael et al., 2018).

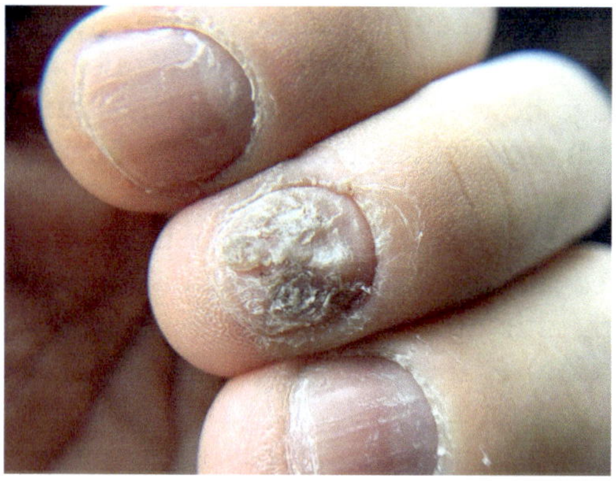

Source: Cozmoderm Clinic. (n.d.). *Nail Disorder.* https://www.cozmoderm.com/wp-content/uploads/2022/06/nail-disorder.jpg.

Importance of Treatment for Overall Health

Occasionally we overlook the subtle clues our body gives us. Hair or nail changes are not all about appearance – they may quietly indicate problems such as low nutrients, immune system confusion, or even infection. Correcting these issues early is not just a cosmetic solution; it is an actual opportunity to prevent further troubles. Good care keeps our skin's natural barriers intact—allowing hair and nails to perform their protective and sensing functions—while keeping the body as a whole healthy. When we do not listen to these signals, things deteriorate, which is why integrating various types of medical care truly does make a difference. This concept appears in nursing as well, where attention to both foot and nail health highlights just how all parts are connected (Miller et al., 2016).

Treatments of these conditions have advantages that go well beyond simply the physical. Often, issues with hair and nails come with an accompanying set of emotional and social issues—distressing feelings, low self-confidence, or even withdrawing from friends due to noticeable flaws and embarrassment. Thus, treatments that address not just the physical symptoms but also what this does to one's mood can truly enhance overall well-being. Adding care that is sensitive to personal culture and engages patients in decision-making seems to be more effective because people feel understood and remain with their treatment. This model aligns with concepts in holistic nursing that remind us caring is as much a matter of heart as health. When care is genuine and slightly imperfect, it fosters trust and assists in sustaining whole, full health (Miller et al., 2016). Health is all intertwined, and addressing hair or nail problems is part of the larger picture. If these issues are not addressed early, they will creep into other areas at a slow pace—potentially messing with mobility, the heart, or even your immune system. For instance, a fungal infection of the nail that is not treated can turn into cellulitis or trigger other infections, which is particularly dangerous for an individual with a compromised immune system. Photos and files documenting how such problems unfold usually substantiate the necessity for prompt, judicious treatment. Combining skin and nail maintenance into daily doctor appointments means that total monitoring can keep everything in line, protecting not only the surface but your entire body's fortitude.

7.1. Common Hair Disorders

Hair conditions are quite difficult to deal with simply because there is not only a single reason behind them. At times, genetic characterestics or hormonal fluctuations initiate the process, but at other times, your daily routine or even other diseases have a role to play. Take the case of thyroid problems, for example—autoimmune diseases like Hashimoto's thyroiditis can disrupt the regular hair cycle. Sometimes the immune system destroys hair follicles earlier than usual, forcing them into a resting stage and shedding additional hair. Another problem is the constriction of blood vessels within the skin caused by thyroid disorders, reducing the nutrients in the hair and making it weaker. In general, grasping these changes is crucial in treatment, since it means you need to address both the overall disease and the local hair problem (Billewicz et al., 2024). Repetitive behaviors put another spin on the equation. Conditions such as trichotillomania—a compulsive pulling of hair—demonstrate that psychological rituals can have very real consequences for hair well-being. Children and adolescents, for instance, usually have patchy hair loss and scalp changes due to these repeated behaviors. Though treatment with cognitive-behavioral therapy can be somewhat helpful, the overall evidence of their impact is weak.

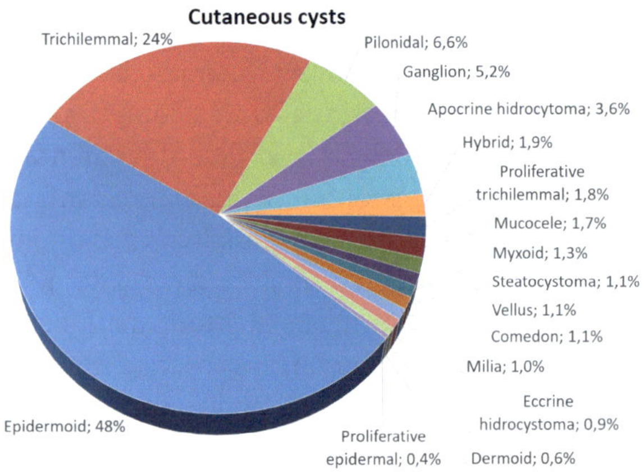

Figure 7.1. Common hair and scalp problem.

Source: By Mikael Häggström, M.D. Author info- Reusing images- Conflicts of interest:NoneMikael Häggström, M.D. - Own work, CC0, https://commons.wikimedia.org/w/index.php?curid=87670107

Surprisingly, although behavior therapy has had some success with problems like thumb sucking, it is still experimental for habitual hair pulling. In most instances, this gap in treatment signifies the necessity of additional research integrating both psychological and dermatological therapy (Woods & Houghton, 2015). An additional element contributing to hair loss complexity includes nutrition, stress, and environmental factors. It so happens those deficiencies in key nutrients, such as iron, zinc, or biotin—can damage how efficiently hair follicle's function, resulting in lighter hair and greater breakage. Stress, of course, is more than simply getting overwhelmed; it disrupts your hormones and causes telogen effluvium, a nonspecific shedding which, although reversible, is quite a nuisance. Therefore, an incredibly effective treatment does not solely focus on addressing the main medical issue. Rather, it also focuses on improving nutritional levels, controlling stress levels, and other aspects of life. In general, this balanced approach can result in more even hair regrowth and healthier follicles, enhancing daily quality of life (Figure 7.1).

7.1.1. Types of Hair Disorders (e.g., Alopecia, Dandruff)

Hair issues strike on several levels; they hit not only what you can see on the surface but also your inner emotional health. Alopecia, the name we give when hair loss appears, can look like small, irregular patches or a more extensive thinning pattern, affecting individuals worldwide. The issues involved here are not straightforward; perhaps it is a combination of nutritional deficiencies, genetic characterestics, or even an immune system that has gone awry. Seeking early intervention is most important, as early action can stem the tide and sometimes even initiate hair regrowth. Recent research, for instance, has reported that a treatment involving SESA oil in combination with capsules appears to slow down hair fall, promote hair regrowth, and even brighten up an individual's mood (Chintan et al., 2012). All of these clearly indicate the importance of treatments that target both the physical symptoms and the emotional distress associated with hair loss. Incidentally, dandruff tends to be lumped in with mere cosmetic nuisances, but it can become a whole lot worse if not addressed. Dead skin flakes may begin as merely an unpleasant problem, but they can develop into irritation, mild inflammation, and even pave the way for additional scalp problems or secondary infections. Day-to-day stress, genes, and even improper use of hair products can all contribute to the issue. Recently, advances in diagnostic technology, particularly image processing-based devices coupled with machine learning techniques such as support vector machines—are having an impact. By examining elements like color, texture, and shape in scalp photos, these technologies are able to distinguish dandruff from conditions like alopecia areata with stunning accuracy (Mangshor et al., 2020). This sort of technical boost makes treatment much more targeted, even if the process is sometimes a bit hit-or-miss. Both hair problems have their own characterestics.

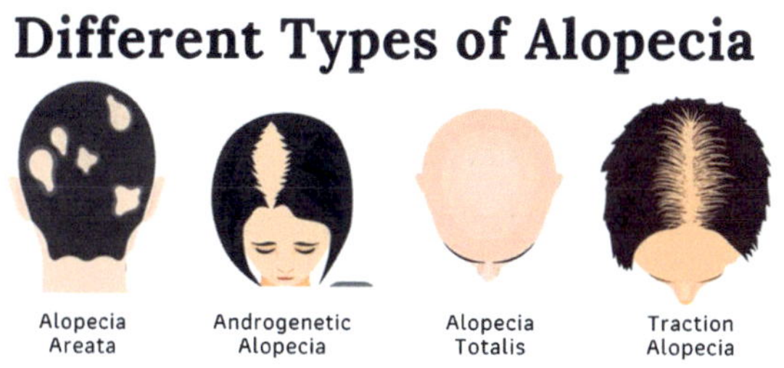

Figure 7.2. Types of alopecia.

Source: Theradome. (n.d.). *Types of Alopecia*. https://theradome.com/cdn/shop/articles/types-of-alopecia.jpg?v=1737870677.

Sometimes alopecia is all wrapped up in autoimmune malfunctions or systemic shortages, whereas dandruff often results from scalp imbalances, sometimes due to fungal infections or excessive sebum production. Mostly, it makes a difference to know because then clinicians can make a decision regarding whether a patient requires something like topical antifungals and medicated shampoos or whether they would be better served by nutritional supplements and hair growth stimulants. Improvements in diagnosis classifications not only refine treatment options but also clarify the condition itself in a manner that feels more manageable to patients. As research continues to evolve, combining old-school ingredients like SESA oil with contemporary analysis tools may define a holistic approach, one that bridges clinical precision with a patient-centered approach (Chintan et al., 2012; Mangshor et al., 2020) (Figures 7.2 and 7.3).

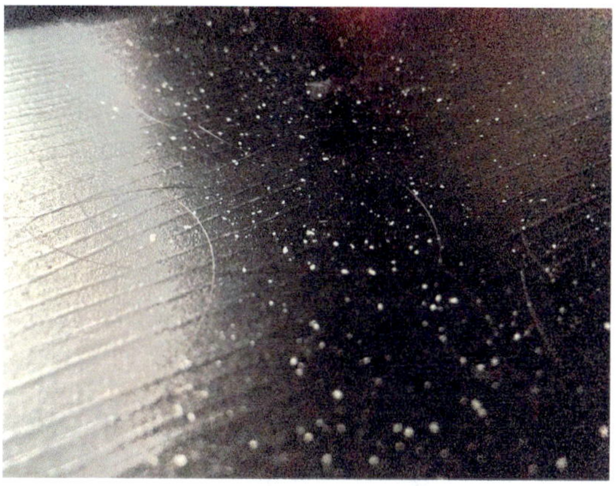

Figure 7.3. Dandruff with shed hair can be symptomatic of dry skin (shed skin scales and hairs on a dark wooden tabletop).

Source: BestShah. (2022). *Dandruff with Hair. Wikimedia Commons.* https://upload.wikimedia.org/wikipedia/commons/thumb/2/23/Dandruff_with_Hair.jpg/800px-Dandruff_with_Hair.jpg.

7.1.2. Symptoms and Diagnosis

Hair and nail problems are brought up a lot before treatment even crosses someone's mind. A lot of people complain about things such as thinning hair or nails that just break, and occasionally even noticeable changes that suggest something more. Very often these evident signs can be concealing more complex mental or brain-related issues, so it becomes a little more challenging to figure things out. For instance, consider trichotillomania—a disorder in which a person pulls out their hair. Its signs can be combined with other behaviors driven by impulses, so it is truly critical to scrutinize carefully before arriving at a skin-only conclusion. Observing the ways in which the hair and nails alter—both their appearance and the severity of alterations—is key, as is a keen examination of a patient's history, which usually puts things on the right track. Most of the time, such a broad-screen check ultimately directs treatment that clarifies both mind and body. Doctors now realize that when they explore these disorders, it is not merely about what one sees. Sensitivity, thoughts, and emotions all come into play. Studies on body-focused repetitive behaviors (BFRBs) indicate that increased sensory reactions are a significant factor in exacerbating symptoms. Patients with problems such as trichotillomania commonly report strange sensory phenomena, such as being hypersensitive to certain touches or completely avoiding them, which in turn can appear to feed their compulsive grooming. Such sensory characterestics have a way of blurring the usual picture that is confined to visible symptoms and making the usual checklists seem a little restrictive. Being cognizant of these sensory details assists clinicians in incorporating some behavioral observations into the normal physical examination. Essentially, this expanded perspective has a better understanding of what is behind the disorder and pushes treatment plans toward balancing both the management of the senses and the management of the surface-level symptoms (Houghton et al., 2018). No decent diagnosis overlooks the fact that mental diseases tend to come with hair and nail issues, which, honestly, is another hurdle when trying to read symptoms.

Trichotillomania, for instance, often manifests together with obsessive-compulsive disorder or other compulsive repetitive disorders, which may intensify symptoms further and often blunts the impact of general treatments. Some research indicates—if you will—monitoring these additional conditions is crucial. When you compare OCD or other repetitive behaviors, there is a heightened likelihood of accompanying eating problems surfacing as well, which completes an already complicated clinical picture (Greenberg et al., 2017). So, physicians are now more and more urged to screen for these mental factors as part of an entire, integrative plan. In most cases, making sure to cover both the physical signs and the psychological context ends up playing a key role in planning effective, team-based care (Figure 7.4).

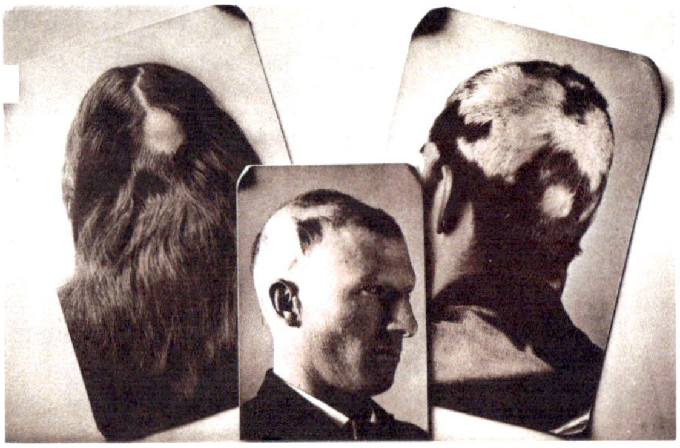

Figure 7.4. Symptoms of alopecia.

Source: By George Henry Fox - Fox, George Henry (1886) Photographic illustrations of skin diseases (2nd ed.), E.B. Treat Retrieved on 25 September 2010., Public Domain, https://commons.wikimedia.org/w/index.php?curid=11593442

7.1.3. Impact on Mental Health and Self-Esteem

Hair and nail issues are not all about appearance—they can rattle your inner life. You may notice such things as thinning hair, alopecia, brittle nails, or even onycholysis, and suddenly daily life feels a little shameful or even stressful. These outward changes sometimes make others feel isolated and compelled to withdraw from friends, which just adds to the tension. That perpetual isolation can revive more anxiety and even depression. More often than not, the constant stress brought about by these diseases ultimately worsens them, perpetuating this feel-good-never cycle. All in all, it illustrates how important it is to take care of your skin as well as your mental state (Singh et al., 2022). More often than not, these problems mess with people's self-esteem and throw off how they perceive their own bodies. When looks begin to play up, many suddenly wonder who they are, really, and that can bring on not-good-enough feelings. Especially if one already has obsessive tendencies or body issues; even the tiniest blemish is a big problem. For the most part, the solution is not merely skin-deep. Medication has its value, but so does receiving help to deal with the psychological aspects. Therapies such as cognitive-behavioral methods, coupled with some reversal of habits, have been known to make things like hair or nail picking less of a strain, while assisting in building self-esteem in the process (Singh et al., 2022). At times, anxiety from these disorders even gives rise to habits that add insult to injury. An individual may begin to bite their nails or pull their hair as a coping mechanism, and paradoxically, this only makes things worse. These habitual patterns deceive the mind into experiencing a temporary relief—even if it results in making the appearance problems more apparent, and the sense of shame even more intense. While it may be sounding a tad too tidy, realizing how our attitudes intermix with our habits goes a big way towards deciphering what comes next. A concerted effort, the addressing of those surface-level symptoms alongside dismantling those deeply entrenched coping mechanisms, is what generally reinstates a measure more confidence and improved quality of life.

7.2. Common Nail Disorders

Nail problems are an indication that something more profound is at play in the body, whether it is an issue everywhere or just an issue in the local area. You may notice nail changes with conditions such as onychomycosis, paronychia, or even nail psoriasis – and these changes impact both appearance and function of the nail. Consider onychomycosis, for example. This nail plate fungal infection is extremely prevalent and is a hard one to overcome because it persists and tends to recur. It appears as nails becoming stained, thickened, and brittle, usually prompting physicians to prescribe long-term antifungal medications.

Patients sometimes have a hard time keeping up with these treatments because nails just do not grow fast enough, so catching issues early and explaining the process clearly is really key. Dealing with these conditions means not only treating the symptoms but also paying attention to the emotional side of having deformed nails—kind of like what is done with some hair treatments (Chintan et al., 2012). Bacterial infections near the nail folds, such as acute and chronic paronychia, may arise when microbes gain entry, usually following a small trauma or from repeated exposure to caustic agents.

These may be painful, cause swelling, redness, and even result in abscesses that must be addressed immediately before complications arise. Treatment is usually a combination of antimicrobial medication and measures to prevent further damage or irritants to the nail. Chronic paronychia, frequently associated with persistent irritation of the skin, is likely to require a long-term treatment regimen that may include such things as corticosteroid topicals and even antifungal medication. It is also worth being vigilant for over-the-counter creams or home treatments that individuals may be abusing – sometimes these can exacerbate the nail issues or mask an infection, and this is why pharmacists are so important in raising the alarm about inappropriate use and assisting in enhancing patient outcomes (Goad et al., 2004).

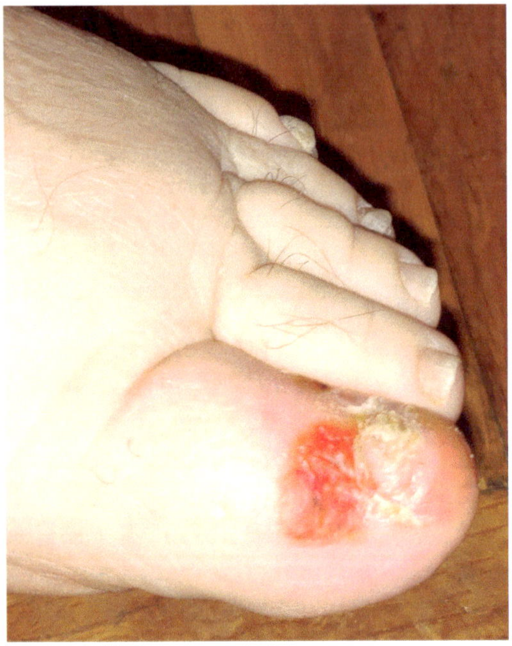

Figure 7.5. Common nail diseases.

Source: By Maria Sieglinda von Nudeldorf - Own work, CC BY-SA 4.0, https://commons.wikimedia.org/w/index.php?curid=75992864

There is also a level of complexity that occurs in nail psoriasis and repeated trauma injuries, which in some cases come hand in hand with other skin or systemic conditions. Pitting is one of the common ways in which nail psoriasis appears, in addition to the nail lifting or a deposit under the nail; this not only compromises the strength of the nail but acts as an observable indicator of the active psoriasis within the body. It is not easy to treat, though, since it might range from topical therapy to systemic immune therapies, specific to every patient. If the nails become brittle or ingrown due to persistent mechanical stress, a combination of protective interventions and medical interventions is required to get them healed. These diverse strategies underscore just how significant it is to blend sound clinical expertise with sound patient advice – assisting individuals in adhering to their treatment regimens and preventing relapse, similar to strategies employed in treating more general hair and nail issues (Chintan et al., 2012; Goad et al., 2004) (Figure 7.5).

7.2.1. Types of Nail Disorders (e.g., Fungal Infections, Ingrown Nails)

Nail problems do not always reach the surface-they tend to be indicators of underlying internal or environmental stimuli. Fungal infections, for instance, are among the most prevalent; small intruders such as dermatophytes, yeasts, or molds invade the nail bed or plate and tend to alter the color of the nail, thicken it, and create brittleness. Onychomycosis (fungal nail issues), typically persists on long since the fungi are persistent and nails do not grow that fast. Often, without treatment, infections cause additional weakening of the nail, and in some cases, it may lead to additional bacterial issues, particularly among elderly people (Devi et al., 2017). Occasionally, the problem is not fungal in nature. Ingrown nails, typically resulting from poor trimming, trauma, or even genetic predispositions, occur when the edge of the nail curves into the adjacent skin. Such naughty behavior can stimulate inflammation, pain, and even infections. Left untreated early enough, the situation may cause long-term pain or even abscesses, making things more complicated. Treatment can be as basic as warm soaks and improved nail care or surgical repair for more persistent recurrences. In general, understanding why an ingrown nail happens allows physicians to treat it better, alleviating discomfort and avoiding complications (Zitás & Mészáros, 2016). To add to the fray are a combination of other nail issues, consider psoriasis, brittle nails, and subungual hyperkeratosis. Psoriatic changes may appear as pitting, loose nail beds (onycholysis), and color changes, and they usually accompany skin issues elsewhere. Brittle nails, observed in both younger and older individuals, may appear due to environmental stress, nutritional deficiencies, or more general health concerns, so they usually require a more general treatment regimen. And subungual hyperkeratosis, where the tissue under the nail becomes thicker than normal, tends to ride in tandem with fungal infections or psoriasis, further complicating treatment. Understanding how these nail conditions overlap is essential to creating therapies that address both surface signs and underlying causes, keeping nails and overall well-being on course (Zitás & Mészáros, 2016; Devi et al., 2017) (Figure 7.6).

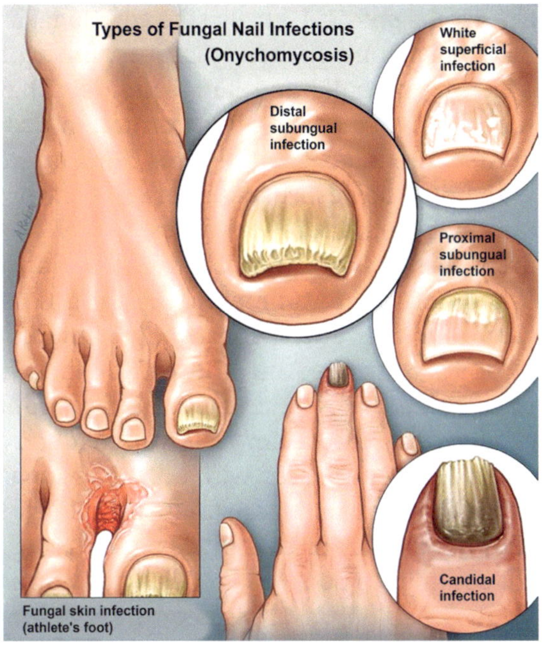

Figure 7.6. Types of fungal nail infections.

Source: Naftulin, K. A. (2019). *FootPower Fungal Nail Infections Image*.

7.2.2. Symptoms and Diagnosis

Individuals who experience hair and nail problems tend to exhibit a combination of symptoms that, in all honesty, makes sorting out what is occurring a little confusing. Consider hair issues, for instance, trichotillomania is not a scientific name for hair pulling; it tends to result in patchy bald patches, thinning in uneven areas, or hair shafts that appear a bit unusual. At the same time, nail biting, or onychophagia, often results in nails that are weak, unevenly colored, or growing in peculiar, irregular patterns. Occasionally these signs blend with other skin or even general body conditions, so a good clinical examination is necessary. Physicians, in general, are trusting the patient's own history, a hands-on physical examination, and sometimes a more detailed examination with instruments such as dermoscopy or even a biopsy to determine whether what they are seeing is the main problem or merely a side effect. The criteria for diagnosing these conditions have changed over time. Today clinicians are not only looking at physical symptoms—they are also listening for the psychological and behavioral aspects. For example, in trichotillomania, the repetitive hair pulling most often is not solitary in nature; it tends to accompany prominent hair loss and may even impact the person's daily functioning, often co-occurring with such things as obsessive-compulsive behavior or other repetitive, body-focused rituals. In general, utilizing tools like the Yale-Brown Obsessive Compulsive Scale assists physicians in measuring severity and identifying any additional issues, such as eating disorders or anxiety, that may be present (Greenberg et al., 2017). Such a mixed, multi-disciplinary examination steers them toward more specific treatment programs. Recent studies are also suggesting that the way a person interprets sensory stimuli could provide yet another dimension for these disorders. Others who have these tendencies report being even more sensitive to certain touches or even attempt to avoid certain feelings; this then has a way of sometimes exaggerating behaviors such as hair pulling or nail biting.

Examining closely these sensory patterns during diagnostics—yes, with a slight error sometimes—might provide essential insights into what is occurring at the neurocognitive level, setting the stage for more individualized treatments. Interestingly, although sensory seeking patterns may appear similar in individuals with and without such issues, there are minute variations in how sensations are processed, which becomes particularly significant when other psychiatric disorders are also present (Houghton et al., 2018). In this regard, such fine-grained diagnostic information serves to create new avenues for interventions that address both the behavioral aspect as well as those sensory, underlying triggers (Figure 7.7).

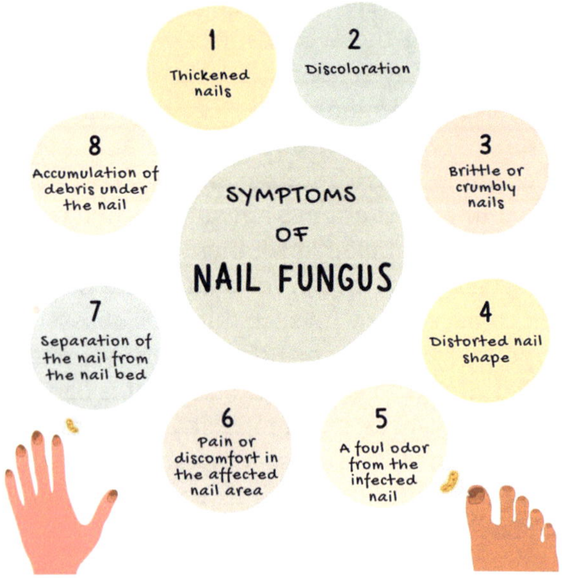

Figure 7.7. Symptoms of nail fungus.

Source: Continental Hospitals. (n.d.). *Image of Hospital Building*. https://continentalhospitals.com/uploads/mceu_8390427711701427395880.jpg.

7.2.3. Effects on Daily Activities and Quality of Life

Chronic conditions of hair and nails do not merely appear on the surface—more often than not, they interfere with daily life and an individual's notion of being well. Consider alopecia or nail dystrophies; when self-grooming is difficult, low self-esteem and a drift towards social withdrawal tend to follow. Phenomenal symptoms of these maladies can accumulate with the concern, sometimes exacerbating worry and episodes of depression and making an individual feel even more isolated. Frequently, pain or discomfort makes the most basic activities—a task as simple as typing, gripping objects, or merely walking—difficulty. These issues, incrementally, change the way people accomplish work and leisure time, stealing productivity and social functioning away. Awareness of these diverse effects is important to help reconstruct treatment regimens that not only treat the physical but also the emotional and social dimensions of these diseases. Emerging treatments for nails and hair conditions have followed a new direction as information about immune and molecular processes finds its way into therapy. More broadly, therapies such as Janus kinase inhibitors (JAKi) now intervene to address the cell-level malfunction that causes inflammatory or autoimmune conditions like alopecia areata and psoriasis (Solimani et al., 2019). By mitigating these root immune fiascos, these drugs relieve symptoms, reduce the severity of disease, and allow individuals to return to daily activities with a little less pain. This process not only assists in the healing of tissues but also tends to provide patients with a slight confidence boost in how they appear and what they can do. Awareness of these behind-the-scenes operations, in the majority of cases, is the key to improved treatment compliance and an enhanced sense of life satisfaction. Tiredness and sleep hitches tend to jump in along with serious skin conditions that require systemic treatments, further complicating things for patients (Allenidekania et al., 2014). For instance, when chemotherapy or other therapies that modify the immune system become active, they drain energy and make thinking foggy, disrupting work routines, school attendance, or social life. Side effects thus pose a delicate balance between enjoying the benefits of treatment and having a satisfactory quality of life; if symptoms are not controlled, patients may even lose motivation to continue with their therapy. A strategy that blends in techniques for coping with poor sleep and fatigue is, as such, completely crucial. By doing so, the benefits of medicine extend beyond mere clinical gains and enable patients to remain active in daily life and cope more steadily with the problems of chronic hair and nail disease.

7.3. Conventional Treatment Options for Hair Disorders

Managing hair issues effectively sometimes requires delving into what causes them in the first place – occasionally it is something genetic, other times it is an issue of mixed environmental factors. Typically, standard treatments attempt to slow down further loss, stimulate new growth, or merely manage symptoms present in conditions such as alopecia areata, androgenetic alopecia and even trichotillomania. Often, physicians resort to medications, oral finasteride and topical minoxidil are relatively popular because they can stimulate follicular activity and tend to halt thinning. They also use corticosteroid injections at times to modify the immune response in inflammatory conditions. And as for the behavioral problems like trichotillomania, a combination of psychotherapy and habit reversal therapy tends to produce some improvement, although research typically indicates that evidence quality tends to be, ah, somewhat variable (Lee et al., 2019). Therefore, these medication-based and behavior-based strategies typically work in order to create a treatment plan that is just right for the client. Beyond these, there is an entirely different challenge where hair loss is caused by therapy for severe diseases such as cancer. Therapies like chemotherapy, radiotherapy and hormonal therapy, while critical in fighting malignancies, can have the unintended side effect of inducing hair loss – a type that is typically diffuse and temporary but leaves patients feeling emotionally depressed. Mostly, measures such as cooling the scalp and adjustments to the treatment protocol are used to minimize the damage. There can be some relief from itchiness and discomfort on the scalp through the use of moisturizers and anti-inflammatory creams. Early identification of the issue and a keen watch are crucial so that treatments are not interrupted and end up impacting a patient's perspective (Čeović et al., 2022). Briefly, dealing with hair loss in such cases is a trade-off between combat and cancer and maintaining quality of life. In the case where medicine alone fails to work, surgery is an alternate route that proves to be most common. Hair transplantation, for example, transplants healthy follicular units from regions with favorable hair to regions that are thinning or bald. These procedures – now commonly performed using sophisticated techniques such as follicular unit extraction and certain implant tactics – seek to restore natural thickness and enhance appearance, which can truly boost a patient's mood. Nevertheless, success is never assured; it generally hinges on how well a patient is chosen, how much hair loss there is and whether they adhere to good aftercare. Occasionally, ancillary treatments such as platelet-rich plasma injection are added to the mix in order to enhance graft survival and revitalize the scalp's native environment. Although there is a plethora of old-school treatments available, continuous investigations continue to refine them for the purpose of improving their effectiveness and safety (Lee et al., 2019; Čeović et al., 2022).

7.3.1. Medications (e.g., Minoxidil, Finasteride)

Hair grows in a remarkably unpredictable manner, and that is one of the reasons that treating hair loss is so difficult. Follicles do not work in tandem—rather, each one plunges into its own beat, moving from the growth phase (anagen), a brief lag (catagen), to the resting phase (telogen). In most instances, imbalanced hormones, improper nutrition, or even every day environmental factors can disrupt this fine-tuned cycle, resulting in progressive hair loss. And it is not merely a question of appearing different; the process often also takes a toll on one's mental health. With all these pieces in motion, treatments must target these very pathways to both maintain the follicles in an active state and stem further loss along the passage of time (Diba et al., 2020).

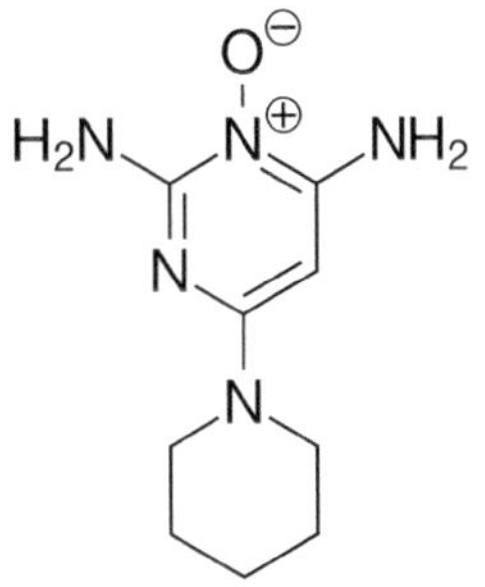

Figure 7.8. Using minoxidil for hair restoration regrowth.

Source: By Vaccinationist - Own work, Public Domain, https://commons.wikimedia.org/w/index.php?curid=40929656

Two of the top drugs that come into play in a lot of treatment regimens are minoxidil and finasteride. Minoxidil was first married to the realm of blood pressure management, but what it ended up doing was lengthening the growth cycle and even increasing the size of hair follicles—therefore making you have thicker, fuller hair. It has FDA approval, particularly for female pattern hair loss, which, as most are aware, has a genetic and hormonal origin. Though minoxidil will slow or even stop shedding in some cases, it is no magic solution; users tend to need to continue with it in the long term. Finasteride, on the other hand, acts internally by inhibiting 5-alpha reductase, the enzyme that converts testosterone to dihydrotestosterone—a significant contributor to androgenic alopecia. In general, both drugs serve crucial functions in current tactics, although their advantages are to be weighed against possible side effects and the fact that individuals vary in the ways in which they respond to them (Dionisio et al., 2021). Even so, the fact that these drugs are now widely used does not imply that they are flawless. For instance, minoxidil tends to lose momentum once balding has progressed to a more serious stage and daily application becomes a sticking point (Figure 7.8). Finasteride works much more effectively in men, and women are usually discouraged from it due to hormonal issues and fear of systemic impact.

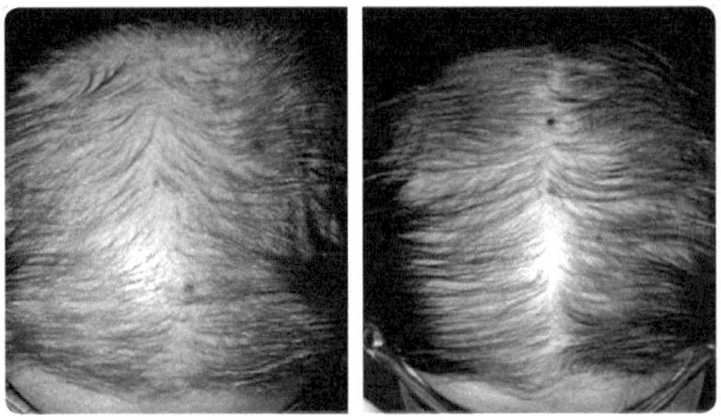

Figure 7.9. Hair regrowth in a patient using 5mg oral finasteride daily. The first picture illustrates the baseline level of hair loss. The second picture was taken after 12 months.

Source: Perera, E. (2015). Hair regrowth in a patient using 5mg oral finasteride daily. In R. D. Sinclair (Ed.), *Androgenetic Alopecia*. Springer.

Additionally, neither of these drugs undoes the shrinkage of follicles; they just slow down or enhance whatever is remaining but do not completely address the issue. That is why treatment protocols occasionally combine these drugs with other strategies, such as hair transplants or newer, alternative treatments. In general, as our knowledge of hair biology becomes more profound, and as emerging treatments such as natural remedies and phytochemicals enter the scene; the zone of addressing hair disorders continues to evolve (Diba et al., 2020; Dionisio et al., 2021) (Figure 7.9).

7.3.2. Surgical Options (e.g., Hair Transplants)

Medical technology has advanced a great deal, allowing us to experiment with various treatments for recalcitrant hair and nail problems. Some patients, for example, now have surgery when confronted with issues such as androgenetic alopecia or extensive scarring that completely disrupts the hair follicles. One of the surgical solutions is transplanting hair follicles from heavily haired areas to thinning regions so that both its functionality and appearance receive an enhancement. It is all about precise planning, considering where the donor hair is sourced from, the way the hair is shedding, and what the patient desires—to minimize risks. With time, procedures such as follicular unit transplantation and extraction have improved, paralleling our increased understanding of how hair functions and providing more natural-looking results (Cossu et al., 2010). Although hair transplantation is a common procedure, it is not quite as simple as it sounds. In the majority of instances, an in-depth pre-surgery consultation is needed to identify the ideal candidate and gain control of any underlying issues that could be causing hair loss. Things such as a loose scalp, decreased hair density, or even active skin issues must be addressed; skipping any of these can lead to problems during or after surgery. Frequently, these surgical repairs blend in with standard medications, and therefore a team effort generally proves most effective for treating both hair and nail disorders. In addition, with advances in microsurgical equipment and improved methods for keeping grafts alive, patients are experiencing less downtime and faster recovery. Patients must also be told that sometimes they require more than one session, so thorough pre-op consultations are essential (Adaskevich, 2016). Surgical techniques are not just about repairing hair—they are beginning to look hopeful for repairing nail issues as well. While nail surgery does not occur as frequently as hair transplants, reconstructive nail procedures can restore function and appearance following injuries or truly severe nail destruction. Success in this case is based on really knowing nail anatomy as well as employing the most modern surgical tools and even tissue engineering technologies.

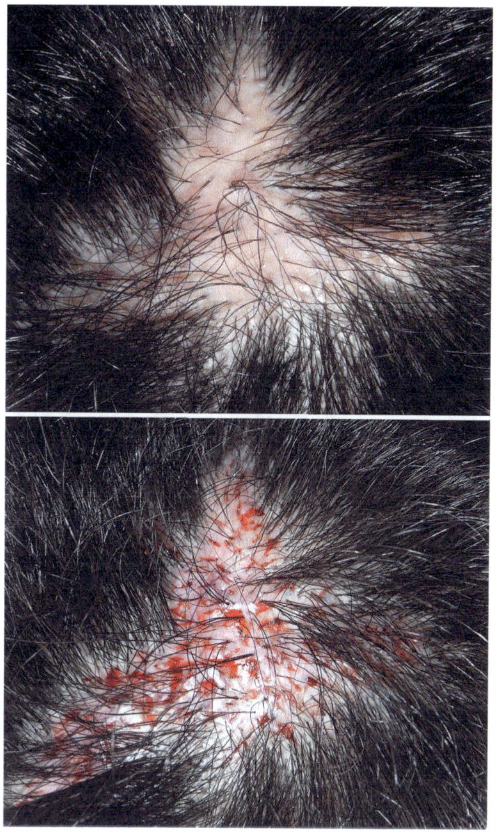

Figure 7.10. Hair transplant surgery.

Source: By Micha L. Rieser, Attribution, https://commons.wikimedia.org/w/index.php?curid=2988528

There is also discussion of combining regenerative medicine with repair methods, and it could soon translate into fewer complications and improved quality of life for patients with difficult nail conditions. As the research continues, it appears certain that these surgical options will continue to change, so it is really essential for clinicians to keep up to date with new techniques and evidence-based practice

(Adaskevich, 2016; Cossu et al., 2010) (Figure 7.10).

7.3.3. Lifestyle Changes and Home Remedies

Managing hair and nail issues is not just about what the doctor does - everyday choices play a big role. A balanced diet matters a lot when our bodies lack vitamins like biotin, zinc, or iron, since shortages can lead to thinning hair or brittle nails. Eating nutrient-rich foods seems to help the natural rebuilding process, keeping hair and nails sturdier. Concurrently, reducing stress through such practices as mindfulness or regular exercise can make the additional burden these conditions impose easier. Numerous individuals discover that non-pharmaceutical approaches allow them more participation along with treatments from the experts. It all leads to a combination of healthy living affecting how we feel physically and even how we relate socially, particularly when issues with hair or nails start to impact work or relationships (Al-Muhandis et al., 2024). In most instances, small daily adjustments pave the way for improved overall well-being. While those changes in lifestyle are crucial, many also look to home remedies for their nail and hair issues. Simple routines, such as moisturizing skin, gentle washing, and avoiding harsh chemicals—can protect the natural barriers around nails and hair follicles, cutting down on irritation and risk of infection. Others try natural oils, such as coconut or castor oil, which are believed to moisturize and even repel germs. And, naturally, applying these home remedies haphazardly may at times make the condition worse or delay proper professional care. Very often, people do this because they feel more in control of their own health, doing small rituals they believe in even if the science is not yet fully established. Generally, marrying personal preference with good counsel works out best (Al-Muhandis et al., 2024). Routine home care also needs to factor in the day-to-day and the place we live. Reducing excess exposure to water, applying heat-styling instruments with restraint, and even preventing nail-biting can prevent added damage and contribute to recovery. Acquiring basic, functional grooming techniques can enable individuals to exchange damaging habits for healthier habits that guard their hair and nails. And, in quite a few situations, having the proper resources or being given uncomplicated information makes a big difference; those lacking such access may not be able to maintain healthier habits (Al-Muhandis et al., 2024). Nurses and other caregivers frequently intervene to provide advice that is sensitive to varying cultural backgrounds and provides equal access to practical tips for care. Ultimately, combining these lifestyle modifications with simple home remedies creates a more balanced approach to treating hair and nail problems, reminding us that good health is a combination of personal effort and professional wisdom.

7.4. Conventional Treatment Options for Nail Disorders

Nail problems can be a real headache. The nail unit is a tricky structure that grows at a snail's pace, so treatments are not as straightforward as one might hope. Typically, doctors try either a cream or a pill to fix the underlying condition and boost nail health. Take fungal issues like onychomycosis, for instance, oral antifungals are usually the go-to because they often work better thanks to deeper penetration. All the same, concerns over liver toxicity and unanticipated drug interactions have pushed many to explore alternative approaches; alternatives such as topical usage and even laser treatment has begun to show promise with some patients (Adams et al., 2011). Combining such with conventional processes provides more leeway for clinicians to balance treatments with the severity of the condition as well as the patient's personal desires, which tends to yield better outcomes. Inflammatory nail conditions, such as median nail dystrophy (MND), are not excluded either. In most situations, a small amount of 0.1% tacrolimus cream applied over the nail area has been observed to smooth out the troubles of the nail plate by alleviating the inflammation below. This manner, patients can escape some of the systemic side effects that accompany oral immunosuppressants. It is an organized step in the right direction in treating these problems. Concurrently, maintaining nail hygiene and minimizing unnecessary trauma continues to be paramount, patient education is complemented by these treatments to enhance results (Adams et al., 2011). And then there is the issue of nail alterations induced by cancer therapies such as chemotherapy and radiotherapy. These treatments can mysteriously render patients with brittle nails, detached from the nail bed to some extent (onycholysis), or even abnormally pigmented, which complicates an already complicated situation further. To assist in treating such side effects, physicians normally prescribe simple measures such as emollients and trauma protection, and occasionally they have to alter the primary cancer treatment dose after taking advice from oncology specialists. Prompt identification and rapid intervention can avoid disruptions in essential cancer treatment, keeping patients adhering to their life-maintaining regimens. This overlap between dermatologic and oncologic treatment, although a little spotty at times, is the way to address nail toxicity in a more holistic manner.

7.4.1. Antifungal Treatments and Medications

Infestation of infections in the hair and nails is problematic because dermatophytes just adore keratinized tissues. These fungi – consider ones such as Trichophyton, Microsporum, and Epidermophyton – can creep into outer skin surfaces and even into those small appendages, so determining what is happening and how to deal with it most effectively is quite messy. You may be surprised that about one in every four individuals on the planet are affected by dermatophytosis, and that has driven the necessity for effective antifungal treatments. It is not only a matter of which fungus is being problematic, either; human-to-human contact, challenging objects, animals, and even earth come into play. With most, knowledge of how these microbes behave and propagate – both in the wild and in the body – determines whether a cream or something more systemic is required, highlighting the value of individualized methods to address the severity of the infection (Adams et al., 2011). More recent advancements in antifungal treatment have been diversifying far beyond conventional oral and topical therapy. Laser treatment, for example, is starting to emerge as a viable non-pharmacologic alternative for nail fungus, demonstrating safety and efficacy which can hold its own against traditional pills. And then, of course, there is the application of alternative topicals, such as 0.1% tacrolimus ointment; in general terms, this has been experimented with for conditions like MND, providing another option when standard practice simply does not work. Even daily remedies like Vicks VapoRub have gained some popularity because of their antifungal undertones, providing patients with an over-the-counter remedy to weigh. These diverse approaches point towards treatment regimens that accommodate patient choice, the severity of the illness, as well as even possible side effects (Abdulla et al., 2024). Treating fungal infections of hair and nails is by no means a quick solution – the gradual growth of these tissues paired with the recalcitrance of the pathogens results in treatments taking forever, with close observation in between. Systemic antifungals such as terbinafine and itraconazole remain the tried-and-true standby when infections are spread out, albeit with dangers such as side effects and potential drug interactions. For less severe infections, though, physicians tend to rely on topicals—albeit with their limited penetrative capacity into layers of nails—as either primary treatment or adjunct. More recent alternatives, including the combination of laser therapy with anti-inflammatory drugs, are proving to be effective in enhancing outcomes without compromising too much on toxicity. Finally, selecting the optimum antifungal treatment is a matter of finding a fine balance between efficacy, safety, patient compliance, and even affordability, all directed at treating the infection and keeping it from recurring (Adams et al., 2011; Abdulla et al., 2024) (Figure 7.11).

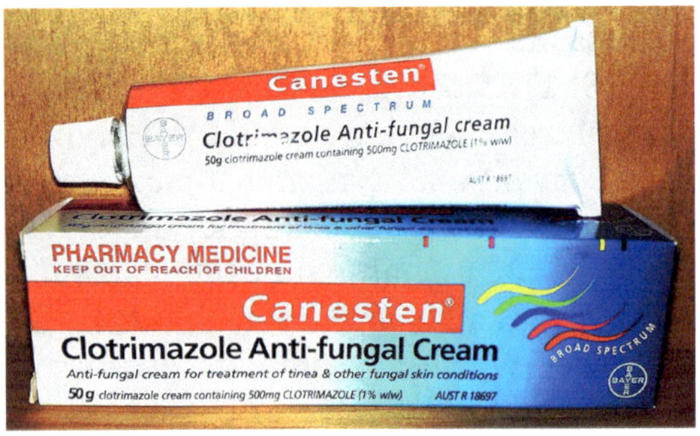

Figure 7.11. Antifungal treatments.

Source: By Editor182 - I (Editor182) created this work entirely by myself.Taken with Nokia N82. Transferred from en.wikipedia, Public Domain, https://commons.wikimedia.org/w/index.php?curid=12872901

7.4.2. Surgical Interventions for Severe Cases

At times, hair and nail health deteriorates so much that routine treatments simply are not enough, and surgery becomes the next step in process. In such tough situations, nails can end up severely damaged or hair follicles can become scarred, resulting in visible bald patches. It is not merely a matter of making things appear more attractive; the goal is also to restore function and prevent more damage. For example, a nail matrixectomy, essentially removing the defective nail matrix—can be performed if persistent nail deformity or infection occurs. Meanwhile, if medications do not alleviate baldness, a hair transplant can save the day by transferring healthy follicles to balding or scarred sites. These types of procedures require the gentle touch and proper patient match, particularly given that hair and nail structures are often very fine. Reconstructive surgery comes into play once things have definitely gone awry, combining the desire to be attractive with really fixing how something functions. Consider traumatic loss of the nail, for instance; in this case, physicians may employ skin grafts or tissue flaps to restore the nail bed and surrounding skin, which can facilitate new nails to begin growing as well as enhance finger function. Along the same lines, sophisticated microsurgical techniques enable surgeons to reconstruct the scalp in instances of extensive hair loss resulting from burns, injuries, or even some diseases. Notably, these surgical procedures tend to accompany the new imaging methods—photoacoustic imaging, for instance, provides vascular information and structures essential for the planning of a detailed reconstruction of hair and nail regions (Attia et al., 2019). This additional layer of planning contributes to enhancing both the surgical result and the recovery time. Despite much advancement in non-surgical treatments, surgery remains vital for intractable hair and nail problems where medications just will not cut it. This is especially so when additional complications such as infections or malignancies crop up in the nail or scalp tissues. Here, the surgeons may even have to excise the offending tissue entirely prior to reconstruction. Of course, risks are involved in these treatments, but their potential benefit to preventing disease progression and enhancing quality of life must not be diminished. Similarly, novel strategies that pair targeted therapies with surgery are being investigated; this combination, like in oncology and elsewhere, seeks to establish more customized treatment courses which may further improve long-term health outcomes for patients (Anand et al., 2022).

7.4.3. Preventive Measures and Hygiene Practices

Treating hair and nail problems is not always a matter of taking medication; it is a matter of daily care and good hygiene that prevents issues from occurring. Washing and drying your hair and nails regularly can reduce microbes and fungi that could otherwise exacerbate skin issues. Applying fewer harsh chemicals or using too many styling products protects the natural barrier of your skin, sometimes simply learning to groom more gently can prevent those small, frequent injuries that admit germs. All these steps combine to allow treatments the best possible chance to work effectively while reducing the risk of side effects. In most instances, incorporating these habits in everyday activities assists physicians to enhance long-term treatment outcomes and enhances overall quality of life (Mario et al., 2020). Monitoring and adjusting one's hygiene regimen becomes even more crucial when you consider how some focused therapies have the potential to interfere with skin and nail health. Drugs that, for example, inhibit fibroblast growth factor receptors – utilized for the treatment of some forms of cancer – tend to induce nail abnormalities and other cutaneous disturbances. Such patients usually require special attention: delicate nail clipping, frequent moisturizing, and avoiding agents that may rapidly exacerbate conditions such as onycholysis or even palmar-plantar erythrodysesthesia. By concentrating on these preventive measures, patients can generally adhere to their treatment regimens without sudden interruptions due to controllable skin issues. In general terms, physicians have to adapt hygiene recommendations to the individual, making prevention as complex and individualized as the treatments themselves (Mario et al., 2020). More recent public health crises, such as the COVID-19 pandemic—have demonstrated that it is not very easy to provide straightforward, practical hygiene guidance for hair and nail disease, particularly in immunocompromised individuals. Daily cleanliness is important to prevent additional infections, but clinicians must strike a balance between this and judicious use of immunomodulatory therapy, which, if not handled sensibly, can lower body defenses and potentially exacerbate cutaneous signs even further. Clear guidelines regarding changing medications during infections, accompanied by robust practices like regular handwashing and routine disinfecting, are necessary to minimize risks and maintain treatment efficacy. This considerate, adaptable strategy for hygiene mirrors our expanding knowledge in dermatology and highlights the value of evidence-based practices that are responsive to both general and skin-specific health demands.

7.5. Alternative and Complementary Therapies

Patients with hair and nail conditions are increasingly relying on alternative means instead of adhering strictly to traditional forms of treatment. Many began incorporating the use of herbal supplements and acupuncture – treatments that appear naturally made and contribute a sense of wholeness. Traditional therapies, such as for alopecia areata, occasionally have potential benefits and side effects that remain obscure. As such, these alternate routes may provide relief from symptoms and improve overall health. Granted, the solid scientific support for such natural remedies is patchy, with rigorous clinical trials not necessarily readily available. In the majority of instances, comprehension of evidence-based medicine is quite crucial when navigating such options, particularly in the case of ailments which can seriously impact one's day-to-day existence. This conservative approach seeks to combine safe, novel concepts with tried-and-tested medical approaches (Atallah et al., 2021). Individual traditions and local expertise tend to dictate which other routes individuals follow for their hair and nail issues. Remedies handed down through generations , such as essential oils, herbal extracts, or mere dietary adjustments , are often relied upon in most communities to enhance scalp and nail conditions. Research typically indicates high local participation in these natural alternatives, especially in areas where conventional medicine is not as available or where there is a definite cultural orientation toward natural healing. For physicians and other healthcare professionals, understanding these socio-cultural forces is essential if they are to honor patient decision-making while responsibly incorporating alternative practices into overall treatment. It is all about establishing harmony so that complementary treatments operate in conjunction with, not in place of, evidence-based interventions (Burns-Nader et al., 2019). Although more people are seeking complementary and alternative treatments, health professionals maintain that we require rigorously conducted studies in order to truly determine their safety and efficacy. Randomized controlled trials and systematic reviews are needed to separate anecdotal reports from truly promising interventions. Yes, some treatments, such as specific herbal supplements or acupuncture—may appear promising, but flawed study designs and tiny numbers obscure the view. And patient education is crucial to prevent unguided use of supplements or procedures that could interfere with conventional treatments or even exacerbate current conditions. Finally, by critically integrating evidence-based complementary strategies into mainstream care routines, clinicians have the ability to provide more whole and individualized solutions that advance outcomes and satisfaction in the management of hair and nail disorders (Burns-Nader et al., 2019; Atallah et al., 2021).

7.5.1. Herbal Remedies and Natural Treatments

Natural treatments have been on the rise recently; lots of people enjoy them because they are a more natural and less "in-your-face" option compared to standard treatments. Rather than adhering to a strict rulebook, herbal treatments for hair and nail problems draw on plant chemicals with anti-inflammatory, antimicrobial, and antioxidant abilities that promote growth and ward off damage. They seek beneath the surface woes, sometimes they even address issues such as nutrient deficiencies, hormonal blunders, and overzealous immune responses that may cause hair loss or brittle nails. Many clinical cases attest to the fact that traditional herbal mixtures have a way of adjusting skin- and hair-related conditions that alleviates symptoms while providing a general boost to overall health. For the most part, it is not merely a matter of slapping something on the skin; some dose of dietary supplements is frequently blended in to nourish the hair follicles and nail beds internally, reinforcing treatment without side effects that attack chemical therapies (Rajendran et al., 2020). When you look into most hair and nail issues, you will discover that skin integrity and microbial dysbalances go hand in hand, with infection and inflammation taking center stage. Frequently, nature intervenes with herbal solutions that use plant-derived antimicrobial compounds, such as in neem, aloe vera, or tea tree oil, to push back against fungal and bacterial culprits often lurking on the scalp and nails. These natural compounds also help a hand in maintaining the barrier of the skin and reducing oxidative stress, an important piece in maintaining healthy hair follicles and avoiding conditions like onychomycosis and alopecia. In addition to warding off germs, these treatments rely on the fundamentals of good hygiene and healthy eating; two pillars in the prevention and management of these conditions. Greater public education regarding appropriate care, combined with incorporating low-cost herbal solutions into daily routines, could potentially alleviate the collective burden of these annoying disorders (Jaffar et al., 2021).

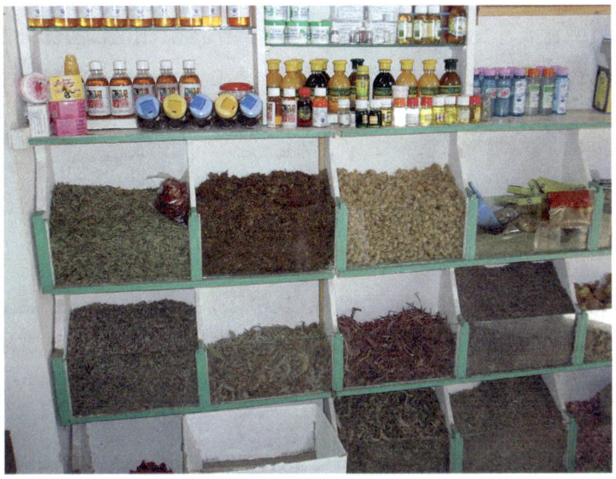

Figure 7.12. Home remedies for nail problems.

Source: By gildemax - Own work, CC BY-SA 4.0, https://commons.wikimedia.org/w/index.php?curid=1674779

Perhaps one of the major advantages of herbal remedies is how they can be tailored—they allow clinicians to individualize methods according to what a patient needs. For example, certain extracts of plants have been found effective in alleviating nail alterations associated with psoriasis and in treating alopecia, as indicated in research conducted in specialized herbal research institutes. Sometimes, treatments combine topical solutions with systemic herbal blends that even weigh the immune system scales, managing the numerous levels of hair and nail issues. These combined approaches not only address appearance; they have the added effect of enhancing one's mental health by tempering the social stigma that typically accompanies apparent problems. Although these methods are promising, further precise, and thorough research is required to standardize the formulas, optimize dosages, and verify their advantages on various groups—so that herbal remedies become a solid, science-supported aspect of hair and nail disorder treatment (Rajendran et al., 2020) (Figure 7.12).

7.5.2. Acupuncture and Its Effects on Hair and Nail Health

Numerous individuals look for solutions to hair and nail issues by experimenting with more natural approaches that target underlying body imbalances. Acupuncture, a traditional Chinese medicine technique that consists merely of inserting thin needles into precise areas of the body, is hailed by numerous individuals as a means of growing healthier hair and nails. It is believed to increase blood circulation and provide the nervous system with a gentle push, so hair follicles and nail plates could get what they require. Enhanced microcirculation can restore damage, particularly in those cases where poor circulation results in thinning hair or easily broken nails. And it is also thought that acupuncture has the ability to balance out hormones and calm stress, both of which tend to be connected to hair loss and nail susceptibility, so its positive effects go beyond simply fixing surface problems.

Apart from these localized effects, acupuncture may alter body health on a larger scale that benefits the condition of the hair and nails. Chronic stress and inflammation generally mess with the integrity and strength of nails and hair, potentially exacerbating conditions or hindering recovery sometimes. In general terms, acupuncture has the ability to activate the parasympathetic nervous system, decreasing stress hormones and dampening inflammatory markers to make the environment more conducive to repair. Recent studies of neurofeedback and suggestion therapies demonstrate that these alternative methods are able to initiate beneficial biological changes, suggesting a neurobiological mechanism by which acupuncture is effective (Thibault et al., 2018).

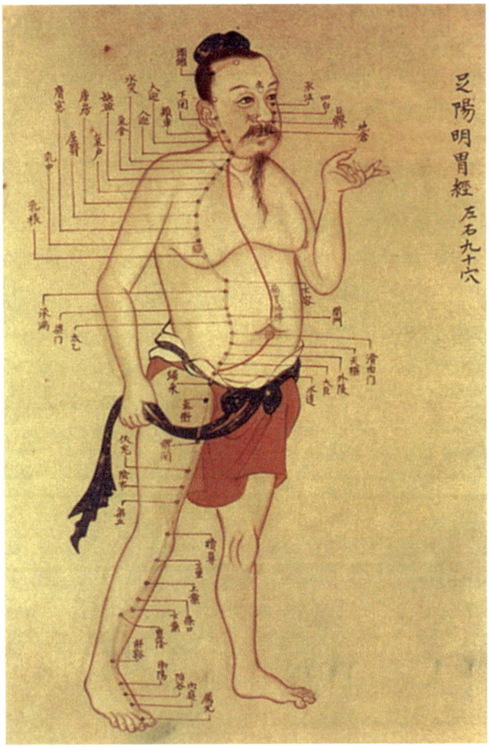

Figure 7.13. Acupuncture for hair loss.

Source: Public Domain, https://commons.wikimedia.org/w/index.php?curid=514662

As a general reduction in the body's stress response, acupuncture can indirectly enhance the health of hair roots and nail matrices – suggesting its effect is more than a local stimulation. Despite these encouraging indications, the full integration of acupuncture into mainstream treatments for nail and hair problems still requires more tangible evidence. The etiology of these diseases is usually entwined—comprising physical, metabolic, and psychological elements (like in diseases such as fibromyalgia), which makes it difficult to obtain consistent outcomes (Jahan et al., 2012). Fibromyalgia, for example, demonstrates how biochemical, metabolic, and psychological factors are so interconnected, all of which acupuncture attempts to ameliorate through a more unified, patient-centered model. Although early research and anecdotal evidence suggest improvements in hair density and nail health, rigorous clinical trials are necessary to accurately establish acupuncture's precise role and efficacy. Nevertheless, with its overall safe profile and promise to deliver widespread benefits, acupuncture is still a useful additional approach in the treatment of hair and nail disease (Figure 7.13).

7.5.3. Nutritional Supplements and Their Role in Treatment

Nutrition is a major factor in the health and appearance of our hair and nails, a subject that has been making waves in clinical circles over the past year or so. Recently, individuals have realized that deficiencies in important minerals such as zinc, copper, and selenium can cause all manner of hair and nail problems. Zinc, for example, is absolutely crucial because it aids keratinocytes and spurs protein synthesis, both of which contribute to the health of hair and nails. Some research even suggests that incorporating a little zinc into your life could remedy issues such as brittle nails, thinning hair, or even alopecia. Mineral imbalance research frequently indicates that as levels fall, symptom severity worsens, suggesting a well-directed nutritional augmentation might be effective. However, supplementing without a valid examination can have unintended consequences. In general, increased supplementation with zinc points to the way our knowledge of micronutrients and skin morphologies is expanding (Babaknejad et al., 2016). While nutrient supplements can present obvious advantages, how these dietary supplements are produced and utilized needs closer scrutiny. Collagen-based supplements, for instance, have become quite popular for enhancing skin, hair, and nail health—but what appears on the box does not always align with the evidence. Reviews tend to emphasize that we require improved information on the source of the collagen, its bioavailability, optimal dose, and precisely how long it should be taken in order to produce maximum benefit. Lacking firm, standardized guidance, consumers and health professionals alike can find it difficult to select products that properly align with clinical evidence. This discrepancy even creates issues with misuse, emphasizing the importance of guidance grounded in actual evidence. Having all this information about the composition of a supplement and the therapeutic information is crucial to integrating collagen supplements into treatment regimens for nail and hair conditions (Ile-Jokste & Šukele, 2023). When incorporating nutritional supplements into treatments for nails and hair, the strategy needs to be as tailored as possible. The best beginning is to assess the nutritional status of a patient and then employ directed supplements to correct underlying deficiencies and maintain tissue repair. Micronutrients such as zinc and hydrolyzed collagen can cooperate, adding strength to structural proteins, inducing keratinocyte proliferation, and stabilizing the matrix. In many cases, patients also fare better when their nutritional regimen supports conventional treatments. Meanwhile, additional studies must be conducted to optimize dosing, establish long-term safety, and determine any interactions with other therapies. For the most part, although these nutritional supplements appear to be promising, their application should be specific, individualized for every patient, and in accordance with the newest scientific knowledge on hair and nail treatment (Babaknejad et al., 2016; Ile-Jokste & Šukele, 2023).

7.6. Psychological Impact of Hair and Nail Disorders

Far too frequently, hair and nail treatments fail to capture how physical symptoms blend with our general emotions. Individuals who have these conditions feel quite down because the symptoms are so apparent; they tend to feel embarrassed and uncomfortable around others. Children and adolescents, for example, may create habits such as hair pulling or sucking on their thumbs that not only cause pain to their skin but also erode their own confidence and isolate them from friends. Other studies have examined utilizing social and emotional strategies to relieve these emotions, though evidence to support remains often lacking and in most instances demands further study. Nevertheless, behavioral therapies appear to offer some promise when lightening both the skin issues and the psychological burden they bear, leaving no doubt that monitoring mental health in addition to skin care is critical (Houghton et al., 2015). More recent research is beginning to peel back the veil on the jumbled sensory and affective components to compulsive grooming behavior associated with hair and nail problems. Those who have more serious symptoms tend to report feeling inordinately sensitive to every little thing, or in some cases, attempting to avoid them altogether. This strange process of filtering through sensory details is likely to increase anxiety and lead a person to engage in compulsive behaviors, creating a cycle that only keeps the distress in motion. Interestingly, milder sufferers do not typically report levels of sensory disturbance as high, indicating a mild to severe range that correlates with the emotional effect. Understanding these sensory characterestics is important to establishing treatment plans that address not only the physical symptoms but also the brain-based causes of mood swings and reduced quality of life (Houghton et al., 2018). Hair and nail issues strike deeper than the body—really, they have the potential to cause genuine social and emotional blowback as well. Excessive grooming could contribute to a form of stigma that keeps individuals caught up in a cycle of shame and withdrawal. This sort of internalized badness can ruin social life and even give rise to other troubles such as depression and anxiety. Due to the complexity of problems here, successful treatment must blend approaches, such as cognitive-behavioral interventions that nudge deeply embedded patterns of negative thinking with patient education aimed at promoting a bit more self-compassion and resilience. Understanding how immense the psychological burden of these disorders can be is important for clinicians who wish to provide care that not only obliterates symptoms but also supports complete mental health, as well (Houghton et al., 2018; Woods & Houghton, 2015).

7.6.1. Body Image Issues and Self-Perception

Hair and nail problems strike more than the skin; they have the potential to shake up individuals' self-perception. Disorders such as trichophagia and onychophagia tend to leave people grappling with shame and embarrassment, which then tends to erode self-esteem. At times, those negative emotions feed into compulsions that just seem to loop around and interfere with treatment. Studies more often than not indicate that avoidant or anxious attachment patterns could be at work here, clumsy coping strategies worsening body image concerns. In a majority of instances, these emotional origins need to be understood for treatments that incorporate skin care alongside mental counseling, ultimately allowing the patient to improve their self-feeling (Mehrtash, 2024). Measuring how treatment is functioning for these conditions is not an easy task, particularly in terms of appearance and body image changes. Taking pictures has been recently proposed as a means of measuring the degree of hair loss observed in disorders such as Trichotillomania, but its reliability remains questionable. Certain research indicates that although photography does provide a reasonably high level of consistency, both the gender of the evaluator and the particular hair-pulling pattern can bias accuracy. Nevertheless, photo ratings frequently correlate with patient-reported increases in quality of life, suggesting these techniques may detect genuine, socially meaningful changes in self-view throughout treatment. Refining these assessment strategies could very well provide clinicians with a more acute instrument to track progress while remaining vigilant to patients' internal experiences (Houghton et al., 2016).

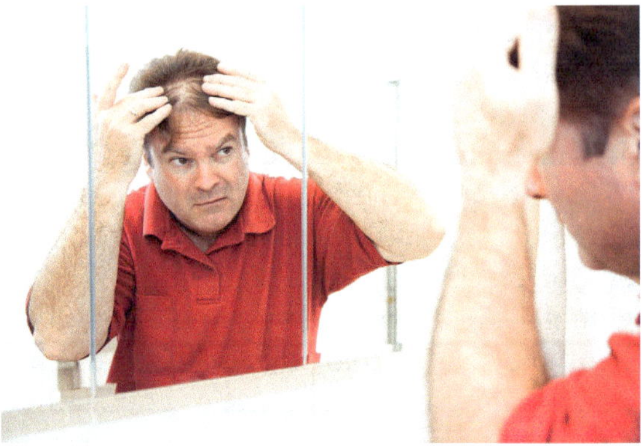

Source: Unknown Author. (2020). *Image of a Suspicious Temp File on Windows 10.* https://en.bcdn.biz/Images/2020/12/20/5e5e4db3-93b9-4242-8cf1-a98a71b6d7b6.jpg.

Body image and self-perception truly come into play when dealing with hair and nail concerns, pushing us toward treatment paradigms that look beyond the surface. Emotional issues, such as the ways in which individuals bond with others and manage their stress—can influence the way they perceive their own bodies, at times perpetuating behaviors that sustain the issues. By making interventions more specific so that they address both observable symptoms and underlying emotions, recovery becomes more stable. Incorporating established evaluation techniques along with a dash of psychological insight ensures that gains are not only physical but also provide a boost in self-esteem. In so doing, care is made multileveled and somewhat more attuned to the messy reality of body image issues linked to such conditions (Houghton et al., 2016; Mehrtash, 2024) (Figure 7.14).

7.6.2. Social Stigma and Its Effects

Visible changes in someone's appearance can

cause a lot more than just medical worries. Hair and nail issues, for example, often bring unwanted side effects that go well beyond the physical symptoms. Deep-set ideals about beauty and some pretty off-base ideas about personal care often led people to wrongly blame those affected. In most instances, this negative judgment can make people feel alone and damage their self-confidence, sometimes even disrupting their overall health. It is not uncommon to find such stigma forcing people to conceal their state, miss social events, or even shun a visit to the doctor, all of which tend to interfere with appropriate treatment. And, when you overlay the added stress, it is obvious that any genuine care must address the physical symptoms and the social struggles simultaneously. Social disapproval does not only sting on a social basis—it tends to poke its head into mental health as well, appearing in the forms of anxiety, depression, or other emotional difficulties. There is a kind of two-way street relationship in which physical symptoms of disorders blend with intense emotional suffering, and stress itself occasionally induces more flare-ups. For example, studies have revealed that psychiatric disorders arise in conjunction with chronic illness, creating a two-way street that makes it harder to adhere to treatment schedules. For the most part, the integration of skin or hair treatments with mental support has proven to enhance the way individuals feel and adhere to their care regimen. Identifying and treating these mental issues is quite central when developing a holistic treatment plan for individuals with hair and nail concerns (Singh et al., 2022). Despite all the advances in medical care, the social consequences of skin, hair, and nail issues continue to be a huge barrier to quality care. Too frequently, the stigma of these diseases drags individuals into withdrawal and may even disadvantage them economically, which makes it difficult to obtain employment or establish relationships. This combination of issues can lead a person into a cycle in which the disorder harms all aspects of life—even damaging overall quality of life and financial health. Added to this, the combination of fear and disinformation about these conditions only exacerbates the issue, causing patients at times to avoid treatment or even fail to complete what physicians recommend. Public education campaigns that create empathy and bring about awareness appear imperative in this case, and integrating public health approaches with clinical treatment is generally the optimal means of overcoming the harmful impacts of social stigma to treat hair and nail disorders (Ueda et al., 2021).

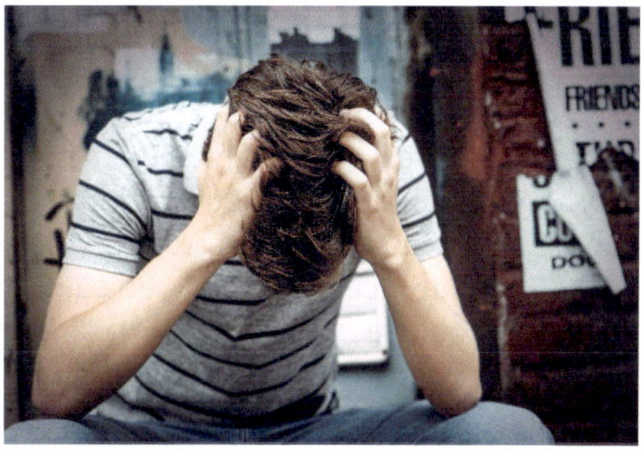

Source: Mayo Clinic News Network. (2015). *Shutterstock_320788322.* https://newsnetwork.mayoclinic.org/n7-mcnn/7bcc9724adf7b803/uploads/2015/10/shutterstock_320788322.jpg.

7.6.3. Coping Strategies and Support Systems

Hair and nail conditions are not all about appearances ; there is an entire psychological aspect that truly impacts results. Individuals with conditions such as hair pulling (*trichotillomania*) or nail biting (*onychophagia*) will experience a great deal of distress, which necessitates coping strategies that are real-world effective. Research tends to indicate that these BFRBs tend to correlate with odd sensory processing, e.g., being overly sensitive or resistant to experiencing certain sensations altogether. These sensory characterestics sometimes amp up emotional distress, further making treatment more complicated. So, strategies that combine sensory integration with means of coping with emotions may be of some use. Adapting interventions to assist people in identifying and managing sensory cues can, in turn, reduce an overreliance on harmful grooming behaviors, increasing treatment effectiveness and quality of life (Houghton et al., 2018). When exploring what could be causing these problems, attachment theory appears to provide some tidy insights. As it happens, a great many trichophagia and onychophagia patients tend to either anxious or avoidant attachment styles , which affects how they deal with stressful emotions. To illustrate, those with an avoidant style tend to keep to coping strategies such as pulling away or even denying reality, which can hinder progress with typical treatments. Conversely, problem-focused coping does not appear to receive much attention, which could be a hindrance to a more streamlined recovery. By considering these attachment-related tendencies, clinicians may develop interventions that carefully steer patients away from mere avoidance of emotions and toward more effective coping strategies. In most cases, layering in psychological support that addresses both attachment insecurities and how one copes seems pretty crucial for long-term improvement (Mehrtash, 2024). Support from others can really change the game, too. Managing hair and nail disorders is not solely a one-person job – it often takes a community effort. A combination of mental health professionals, dermatologists, caregivers, and even family members are its role in addressing the complex behaviors, thoughts, and sensory issues entailed. Peer groups, in combination with close family relationships, can not only soften the bite of stigma but also create a real sense of community. In addition, multidisciplinary treatment plans that combine cognitive-behavioral therapy with sensory integration and even some attachment-guided counseling have shown positive outcomes. This type of holistic support system assists patients in developing resilience, enhancing self-efficacy, and adhering to treatment regimes, which in the end makes the arduous process of living with hair and nail disorders slightly more optimistic (Houghton et al., 2018; Mehrtash, 2024).

CLOSER LOOK

Sebum Production

Sebum production is a normal process on the part of the sebaceous glands, which secrete an oily substance that lubricates the skin and hair. Although this process is necessary to keep the skin healthy, overproduction of sebum can create issues such as acne and oily skin. Knowing the factors affecting sebum production would make it easier to control skin conditions and have healthy skin.

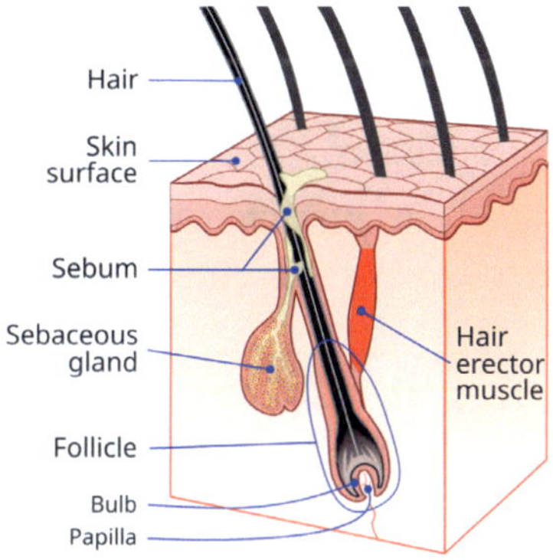

Source: By National Institutes of Health - This image has been extracted from another file, Public Domain, https://commons.wikimedia.org/w/index.php?curid=6910143

- **Function and Benefits:**
  - **Protection and Hydration:** Sebum protects the skin from outside influences such as bacteria and environmental elements, and it moisturizes it.
  - **Hair Health:** Sebum also conditions hair, adding to its shine and easy manageability.
  - **Immune Function:** Sebum's mildly acidic pH can kill bacteria and microbes before they enter the skin.
- Factors That Affect Sebum Production:
  - **Hormones:** Sex hormones, especially androgens such as testosterone, have a strong effect on sebum production.
  - **Puberty:** Puberty due to increased androgen levels triggers an increase in sebum production, usually causing acne.
  - **Diet:** Intake of dietary fat or carbohydrate can stimulate sebum production, whereas caloric restriction can suppress it.
  - **Age:** Sebum production usually reaches its peak at puberty and falls with age.
  - **Genetics:** Individual differences in sebaceous gland activity can influence sebum production levels.
- Excessive Sebum and its Implications:
  - **Acne:** Sebum in excess can clog pores and cause blackheads, whiteheads, and pimples.
  - **Oily Skin:** Excess secretion of sebum makes the skin shiny and oily.

- **Skin Irritation**: Overproduction of sebum can irritate the skin, particularly when compounded by other causes such as stress or aggressive skincare products.

- Controlling Sebum Production:
  - **Gentle Cleaning:** Cleanse the skin gently with a mild cleanser to eliminate excess sebum without depriving the skin of its natural oils.
  - **Exfoliation:** Exfoliating the skin regularly helps remove dead skin cells and prevents pore clogging.
  - **Oil-Free Products:** Use oil-free or non-comedogenic products that will not clog pores.
  - **Balanced Diet:** Eating a low-processed food, low-sugar drink, and low-unhealthy fat diet can lower sebum production.
  - **Stress Reduction**: Stress can stimulate the secretion of hormones that cause sebum production to increase, so stress reduction techniques are useful.

SUMMARY

Recently, hair and nail diagnoses have truly changed with improved methods and a clearer understanding of what is driving them. Physicians now combine detailed patient examinations with some newer imaging technology, which enables more accurate focusing in on issues – so errors get reduced. Consider RCM, for instance; this technique provides a noninvasive peek at subtle changes in cells, taking live information about infections and inflammation. This additional clarity not only opens the door to care that is individually customized but also assists clinicians in screening rapidly whether a treatment is getting the job done—preventing prolonged or ineffective therapies. Patient outcomes and satisfaction have most often increased with their use (Pimenta et al., 2020). These changes indicate that maintaining research ongoing and collaborating across specialties truly matters in approaching such challenging problems. Individuals are also starting to realize that disorders like hair-pulling and nail-biting do not exist alone. Disorders like trichotillomania tend to be bundled with mental diseases like obsessive-compulsive disorder or other compulsions, which of course complicates the clinical picture. Identifying these crossover factors is central to creating a treatment regimen that, in most instances, addresses both the surface symptoms and those underlying psychological motivations. Strategies that shake things up, occasionally introducing behavioral therapy, some medication, and additional patient support, tend to produce longer remissions and improved quality of life. Therefore, a thorough, whole-patient examination, with all of these variables involved, is required for success (Greenberg et al., 2017). In conclusion, hair and nail disorders are not a single-fits-all solution but require a multi-faceted approach. The combination of next-generation diagnostic equipment with thoughtful psychological screenings allows physicians to craft treatments that are pinpoint precise and effective. This approach not only addresses the surface skin problems but also penetrates deeper to address the underlying behavioral or psychiatric causes, more often than not, with longer-lasting outcomes. In most instances, continued research, and development in how we detect as well as treat these conditions continue to be vital to enhancing patient care. Beyond question, the rosy future of controlling these disorders lies in personalized medicine and firm collaboration across disciplines.

Hair and nail problems are finally being addressed with what looks like a fairly heterogeneous bunch of therapies—prescribing immunosuppressants, hair growth promoters, and a few of those novel biologics. Alopecia areata, that scarring-immune disease resulting in loss of hair, really is an exhibition of how sloppy therapy can be. Clinical trials have experimented with a variety of approaches, testing for a sufficient level of hair growth and monitoring for side effects. Nevertheless, discovering one magic bullet that will suit all proves to be quite an exercise, largely due to the fact that symptoms may range very wildly and patients tend to react in their own individual ways. Scientists, as a rule, are piecing together hints regarding the immune system and potential targets, which pushes physicians into designing regimens that are as customized as the patients themselves. This strategy is all about attempting to achieve the most with minimal risk of immunosuppression or other adverse effects. As more evidence comes in, combining in new data is still paramount to advancing day-to-day treatment for these conditions (Correa et al., 2023). When one addresses nail issues, the flavor is slightly different. Nail diseases—whether caused by persistent fungal infections or autoimmune causes—require a fine, accurate diagnosis because, without one, selecting the appropriate therapy is speculation. Therapies here must balance on a delicate scale between being therapeutic and maintaining the nail's structure and function, both of which are significantly important for the day-to-day quality of life for a patient. Recent research suggests the advantage of combining drugs with a regimen of supporting maneuvers, such as basic topical remedies and even some direct patient instruction in nail care. Though new options such as targeted immunomodulators are seeming very promising, strong randomized controlled trials still appear to be in short supply, so, usually, clinicians are urged to proceed cautiously instead of leaping onto any new treatment bandwagon without firm, long-term safety data. Putting various specialists together and considering what each patient requires help move the overall results a little bit further (Adaskevich, 2016). One of the main takeaways from the recent research is the increasing place of personalized medicine in treating hair and nail diseases. When you look at how many different-looking disease presentations and treatments responses you see, it sort of requires a custom approach. While evidence-based recommendations are getting into practice, they still require a bit more refining as newer treatment modalities make their debut. Yes, randomized controlled trials provide good numbers, but the absence of head-to-head comparisons sometimes makes it difficult to say that one treatment beats another. There is always the balancing act between realizing actual clinical benefits and managing the undesirable side effects. Looking to the future, it may be a wise move to fund more long-term research and heed patient reports on quality of life—because those are individual measurements that can often encompass what by themselves cannot be discerned through numbers. Ultimately, as clinicians and scientists collaborate, the aim is still to translate scientific advances into practice that is realistic, safe, and effective (Adaskevich, 2016; Mateos-Haro et al., 2023).

KEY TERMS FROM THIS CHAPTER

- Adolescents
- Alopecia
- Biopsychosocial model
- Body-focused repetitive behaviors
- Chronic pain
- Disheveled nails
- Epidermophyton
- Hair
- Hair follicles
- Laser treatment
- Median nail
- Molds
- Nail psoriasis
- Nutrition
- Onychomycosis
- Paronychia
- Self-confidence
- Self-esteem
- Stress
- Thyroid
- Trauma
- Trichophyton
- Yeasts

REFERENCES

1. Abdulla, S. N., Abdullah, B. A., Farhan, M. S., Mamdwooh, H., et al. (2024). Review *of the clinical types of dermatophytes. Journal for Research* in Applied Sciences and Biotechnology, 3(3), 104–112. https://core.ac.uk/download/613199118.pdf (accessed on 12 May 2025).
2. Abu Mangshor, N. N., Ahmad Fadzil, A. F., Ahmad, Z., Zaaba, I., et al. (2020). Pre-trained classification of scalp conditions using image processing. ttp://doi.org/10.11591/*ijeecs.v20.i1.pp138-144 (accessed on* 12 *May* 2025).
3. Accettola, E., Bogdan, A., Callahan, S., Chawda, et al. (2023). Introduction to health assessment for the nursing professional: Part II. https://core.ac.uk/download/622362029.pdf (accessed on 12 May 2025).
4. Adams, S., Hoy, N. Y., Leung, A. K. C., Metelitsa, D. D., et al. (2011). New concepts in median nail dystrophy, onychomycosis, and hand, foot, and mouth disease nail pathology. Skin Therapy Letter, 16(3), 1–4. https://core.ac.uk/download/pdf/8696338.pdf (accessed on 12 May 2025).
5. Adaskevich, V. P. (2016). Skin Diseases and Sexually Transmitted Infections. BSMU Publishing House. https://core.ac.uk/download/80150454.pdf (accessed on 12 May 2025).
6. Al-Muhandis, K. *(2024). An Exploration* of Life With a Chronic Skin Condition. [Doctoral Thesis, Royal Holloway, University of London].
7. Allenidekan*ia, A., Rahmawaty, F., & Waluyanti, F. T. (2014).* Sleep disturbances and fatigue in adolescents with cancer receiving chemotherapy. https://media.neliti.com/media/publications/150475-EN-sleep-disturbances-and-fatigue-in-adoles.pdf (accessed on 12 May 2025).
8. Amalina Binte Ebrahim Att*ia, Balasundaram, G., Mootha*nchery, M., Dinish, U. S., Bi, R., Ntziachristos, V., & Olivo, M. (2019). A review of clinical photoacoustic imaging: Current and future trends. Photoacoustics, 16, 100144. https://doi.org/10.1016/j.pacs.2019.100144.
9. Anand, U., Dey, A., Singh Chandel, A. K., Sanyal, R., Mishra, A., Pandey, D. K., De Falco, V., et al. (2022). Cancer chemotherapy and *beyond: Current status, drug candidates, associated* risks, and progress in targeted therapeutics. Genes & Diseases, 10(4), 1367–1401. https://doi.org/10.1016/j.gendis.2022.02.007.
10. Aruna Devaraj Rajendran, Rajeev Joseph, Anup Raveen Jaison. SELF CARE TRADITIONAL HERBAL THERAPY FOR PSORIASIS. Ayushdhara [Internet]. 2020Aug.12 [cited 2025*Jun.12];7(3):2735-*44. Available from: https://ayushdhara.in/index.php/ayushdhara/article/view/575 (accessed on 12 May 2025).
11. Babaknejad, N., Sayehmiri, F., Sayehmiri, K., Mohamadkhani, A., & Bahrami, S. (2016). The Relationship between Zinc Levels and Autism: A Systematic Review and Meta-analysis. Iran*ian journal of child* neurology, 10(4), 1–9. (accessed on 12 May 2025).
12. Billewicz, M., Lis, L., Makowska, K., Marczyk, et al. (2024). Skin Appendage Abnormalities in Hypothyroidism: Understanding and Management. https://core.ac.uk/download/613193132.pdf (accessed on 12 May 2025).
13. Burns-Nader, *S., Sherwood, R., Hernandez-Re*if, M., Horton, C., Juarez, et al. (2019). The use of complement*ary and alternative medicine by adults and children in the South. Vol.* 8, No. 2—JOURNAL OF COMMUNITY ENGAGEMENT AND SCHOLARSHIP https://core.ac.uk/download/236075923.pdf (accessed on 12 May 2025).

14. Cossu, F. (2010). Genetics of SCID. https://core.ac.uk/download/pdf/8496966.pdf.

15. Deodatta S. Bhadlikar, Chintan R. Maniar. *Efficacy and Safety Evaluation* of Sesa oil and Sesa Capsule In Different Hair Disorders. ijp [Internet]. 2012 Sep. 30 [cited 2025 Jun. 12];4(3):369-74. Available from: https://www.ijp.arjournals.org/index.php/ijp/article/view/188 (accessed on 12 May 2025).

16. Devi, M. V., & Manikandan, N. C. (2019). Clinical study of geriatric dermatoses. International Journal of Research in Dermatology, 5(1), 128–133. https://doi.org/10.18203/issn.2455-4529. IntJResDermatol20190231

17. Diba, S., Gozali, M. M., & Kurniawati, Y. (2020). Diagnosis and management of female pattern hair loss. https://core.ac.uk/download/287202323.pdf (accessed on 12 May 2025).

18. Dionisio, L., Lorenzo-Villegas, F., Jimenez-Acosta, M., Mirecki-Garrido, N., et al. (2021). Ginseng in hair growth and viability. https://core.ac.uk/download/479933949.pdf (accessed on 12 May 2025).

19. Goad, J. A., Mallari, J., & Nguyen, L. (2004). Non-Prescription and Household Substances of Abuse. https://core.ac.uk/download/215737842.pdf (accessed on 12 May 2025).

20. Greenberg, E., Grant, J. E., Curley, E. E., Lochner, C., Woods, D. W., Tung, E. S., Stein, D. J., Redden, S. A., Scharf, J. M., & Keuthen, N. J. (2017). Predictors of comorbid eating disorders and association with other obsessive-compulsive spectrum disorders in trichotillomania. Comprehensive psychiatry, 78, 1–8. https://doi.org/10.1016/j.comppsych.2017.06.008 (accessed on 12 May 2025).

21. *Hende, B., & Mónok, K. (2015). Book Reviews.* https://core.ac.uk/download/42947162.pdf (accessed on 12 May 2025).

22. Houghton, D. C., & Woods, D. W. (2015). *Evidence-Based* Psychosocial Treatments for Pediatric Body-Focused Repetitive Behavior Disorders. https://core.ac.uk/download/213076990.pdf. Woods, D. W., & Houghton, D. C. (2016). Evidence-Based Psychosocial Treatments for Pediatric Body-Focused Repetitive Behavior Disorders. Journal of clinical child and adolescent psychology : the official *journal for the Society* of Clinical Child and Adolescent Psychology, American Psychological Association, Division 53, 45(3), 227–240. https://doi.org/10.1080/15374416.2015.1055860

23. Houghton, *D. C., Alexander, J. R., Bauer, C. C., & Woods,* D. W. (2018). Abnormal perceptual sensitivity in body-focused repetitive behaviors. Comprehensive psychiatry, 82, 45–52. https://doi.org/10.1016/j.comppsych.2017.12.005

24. Houghton, D.C., Franklin, M.R., Twohig, M.P. et al. Photographic Assessment of Change in Trichotillomania: Psychometric Properties and Variables Influencing Interpretation. J Psychopathol Behav Assess 38, 505–513 (2016). https://doi.org/10.1007/s10862-016-9536-z(accessed on 12 May 2025).

25. Ile-Jokste, B., & Šukele, R. (2023). A QUALITATIVE ASSESSMENT OF THE LABELING INFORMATION OF COLLAGEN-CONTAI*NING FOOD SUPPLEMENTS.* SOCIETY. INTEGRATION. EDUCATION. Proceedings of the International Scientific Conference, 2, 681-693. https://doi.org/10.17770/sie2023vol2.7168 *(accessed on 12 May 2025).*

26. *Jaffar,* H., Javed, A., & Mushtaq, S. (2021). A review: Dermal ailments causing microbiota. CORE. https://core.ac.uk/download/386174051.pdf (accessed on 12 May 2025).

27. Jahan, F., Nanji, K., Qidwai, W., & Qasim, R. (2012). Fibromyalgi*a syndrome: an overview of pathophysiology, diagnosis and management. Oman medical journal, 27(*3), 192–195. https://doi.org/10.5001/omj.2012.44 (accessed on 12 May 2025).

28. Lacouture, M. E., Sibaud, V., Anadkat, M. J., Kaffenberger, B. H., Leventhal, J. S., Guindon, K., & Abou-Al*fa, G. K. (2020). Dermatologic adverse events associated with selective fibroblast growth factor receptor inhibitors: Overview, prevention, and management guidelines. The Oncologist, 26(*4), e316–e326. https://doi.org/10.1002/onco.13552.

29. LeBlanc, A. K., Atherton, M. J., Bentley, R. T., Boudreau, C. E., Burton, J. H., Curran, K. M., Dow, S., et al. (2021). Veterinary Cooperati*ve Oncology Group—Common Terminology Criteria for Adverse Events (VCOG-CTCAE v2) follow*ing investigational therapy in dogs and cats. Veterinary and Comparative Oncology, 19, 311–352. https://doi.org/10.1111/vco.12677.

30. Lee, M. T., Mpavaenda, D. N., & Fineberg, N. *A.* (2019). Habit Reversal Therapy in Obsessive Compulsive Related Disorders: A Systematic Review of the Evidence and CONSORT Evaluation of Randomized Controlled Trials. Frontiers in behavioral neuroscience, 1*3, 79. https://doi.org/1*0.3389/fnbeh.2019.00079 (accessed on 12 May 2025).

31. Lehigh Valley Health Network. (2009). Healthy horizons. CORE. https://core.ac.uk/download/267860415.pdf (accessed on 12 May 2025).

32. Mateos-Haro, M., Novoa-Candia, M., Sánchez Vanegas, G., Correa-Pérez, A., Gaetano Gil, A., Fernández-García, S., Ortega-Quijano, D., Urueña Rodriguez, M. G., Saceda-Corralo, D., Bennouna-Dalero, T., Giraldo, L., Tomlinson, J., Vaño-Galván, S., & Zamora, J. (2023). Treatments for alopecia areata: a network meta-analysis. The Cochrane database of systematic reviews, 10(10), CD013719. https://doi.org/10.1002/14651858.CD013719.pub2 (accessed on 12 May *2025).*

33. Mehrtash, Maryam, "Avoidant Attachment, Coping Styles, and Body Image in Adults With Trichophagia and Onychophagia Disorders" (2024). Walden Dissertations and Doctoral Studies. 15625. https://scholarworks.waldenu.edu/dissertations/15625 (accessed on 12 May 2025).

34. Miller, T. A. (2016). Essential nursing care for the sole. CORE. https:*//core.ac.uk/download/217655827.pdf (ac*cessed on 12 May 2025).

35. Nicholas, M. K., Vlaeyen, J. W. S., Rief, W., Barke, A., Aziz, Q., Benoliel, R*., C*ohen, M., et al. (2018). The IASP classification of chronic pain for ICD-11: Chronic primary pain. Pain, 160(1), 28–37. https://doi.org/10.1097/j.pain.0000000000001390.

36. Pimenta, R., Soares-de-Almeida, L., Arzberger, E., Ferreira, J., Leal-Filipe, P., Bastos, P. M., & Oliveira, A. L. (2020). Reflectance confocal microscopy for the diagnosis of skin infections and infestations. Dermatology online journal, 26(3), 13030/qt9qz046f1.Atallah, Á. N., & Freire, P. C. B. (2021). Handbook Of Alopecia Areata Tr*eatment: Best Evidence-Based Health Care.* https://core.ac.uk/download/622751387.pdf (accessed on 12 May 2025).

37. Seirafianpour, F., Sodagar, S., Pour Mohammad, A., Panahi, P., Mozafarpoor, S., Almasi, S., & Goodarzi, A. (2020). Cutaneous manifestations and considerations in COVID-19 pandemic: A systematic review. Derma*tolo*gic Therapy, 33. https://doi.org/10.1111/dth.13986.

38. Singh, O. P., Sarkhel, S., & Sarkar, S. (2022). Management of psychiatric disorders with HIV and dermatological disorders. Indian Journal of Psychiatry, 64(5), S449–S457. https://doi.org/10.4103/indian*jpsychiat*ry.indianjpsychiatry_14_22.

39. Solimani, F., Meier, K., & Ghoreschi, K. (2019). Emerging Topical and Systemic JAK Inhibitors in Dermatology. Frontiers in immunology, 10, 2847. https://doi.org/10.3389/*fimmu.2019.02847 (accessed on* 12 May 2025).

40. Thibault, R. T., Veissière, S., Olson, J. A., & Raz, A. (2018). Treating ADHD With Suggestion: Neurofeedback and Placebo Therapeutics. Journal of attention disorders, 22(8), 707–711. https://doi.org/10.1177/1087054718770012 (accessed on 12 May 2025).

41. Ueda, K., & Black, K. *J. (2021). A comprehensi*ve review of tic disorders in children. Journal of Clinical Medicine, 10(11), 2479. https://doi.org/10.3390/jcm10112479.

42. Verplanken, B., & Orbell, S. (2021). A*ttitudes, habits, and behavior ch*ange. Annual Review of Psychology, 73, 327–352. https://doi.org/10.1146/annurev-psych-020821-011744.

43. Zitás E, Mészáros J. The most common childhood skin diseases. Our De*rmatol Online. 2016;7(2):213-218.* (accessed on 12 May 2025).

44. Čeović, R., Kovačec, L., Bukvić Mokos, Z., & Marinović, B. (2022). Dermatologic Adverse Events in *Oncologic Therapies. Acta derm*atovenerologica Croatica : ADC, 30(4), 237–249. (accessed on 12 May 2025).

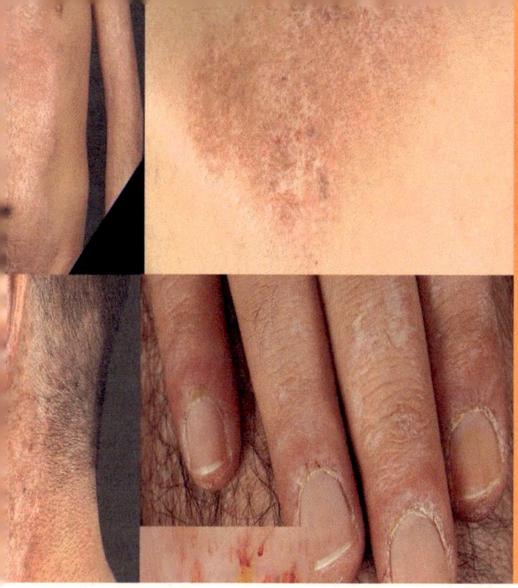

Chapter 8

AUTOIMMUNE AND CONNECTIVE TISSUE DISORDERS

Contents

Introduction

It is our immune system that is important—it is the body's natural defense against disease, but sometimes it makes mistakes. There are times when this complex defense system goes haywire and attacks its own tissue rather than repelling invaders. Such an error leads to autoimmune problems that can take on many different forms; many of them target connective tissues, the behind-the-scenes support structure of our organs and cells. Diagnosing these problems can be a real challenge since they crop up in unpredictable ways and spread their effects throughout the body. Because these conditions tend to be chronic and can eventually affect multiple systems, it is vital to really understand how they work, from the basic biology to all the clinical details. Latest advances in medical imaging and biomarker research have begun to unlock secrets of these covert processes, increasingly enhancing our diagnostic accuracy and guiding the way toward more intelligent treatments. Consider, for instance, systemic lupus erythematosus (SLE). It is one disease that very much emphasizes just how complex such diseases may be. SLE not only plays havoc with the immune system but tends to spread to other areas of the body—even the brain, where it causes cognitive errors that make it all the more difficult to treat. A novel deep-learning tool, called BrainAGE, scans MRI images to estimate the aging of the brain and has found that SLE patients have brains that look older than those of healthy individuals. This leap in brain aging is accompanied by apparent cognitive impairment and evidence of nerve injury, highlighting the effects of autoimmune inflammation on our nervous system (Grégory et al., 2023). These types of breakthroughs, combining contemporary imaging with computational analysis, truly disrupt our knowledge of illness and guide us toward more individualized interventions. Outside of these specific instances, the history of autoimmune and connective tissue problems extends to families and even populations. Congenital heart block (CHB), for example, a condition that can occur when an autoantibody from a mother acts on her child's heart, is an incredible display of how early this activity can start, and how it can create long-term heart problems. Research involving large national health records shows that individuals with CHB are much more at risk for cardiovascular diseases, infections, and other autoimmune conditions, and even their siblings occasionally experience some of the risks (though not as strongly). This complicated interaction of hereditary susceptibility and immune misdirection informs us about why vigilant, consistent surveillance is so critical, guaranteeing both short- and long-term health requirements are fulfilled for impacted families (Mofors et al., 2019).

Definition of Autoimmune Disorders

Our immune system is pretty amazing—it keeps our bodies in balance by figuring out what belongs and what does not. But sometimes that natural knack goes wrong, and suddenly the very cells meant to protect us start attacking our own tissues. This mix-up can spark a range of autoimmune troubles, from light alters in the body to full-blown life-threatening conditions. You have obtained these conditions caused by marauding antibodies or overzealous T cells, and things tend to get initiated when genes and ordinary environments meet in unprecedented manners. Often in cases, having some specific autoantibodies turns out to be the most important hint for physicians, particularly with rheumatic conditions where marker levels tend to reflect how bad the disease will turn out (Kuwana et al., 2021). There is an entire spectrum of these disorders out there, each one based on the immune system's malfunction, most of the time targeting our connective tissues and both inflaming and structurally damaging them. Consider what occurs in systemic sclerosis (SSc), rheumatoid arthritis (RA), or even ankylosing spondylitis. With ankylosing spondylitis, for example, the body winds up fusing some of the vertebral joints along with demonstrating symptoms of arthritis in other areas, a bizarre response elicited by an attack on fibrocartilaginous entheses. It is not simply stiff joints; this ailment, as with most of its autoimmune relatives, has the ability to radiate its effect to many of the organs. In general, physicians rely on a combination of clinical findings and imaging studies to identify these conditions, and therapies—involving everything from NSAIDs to biologic agents—try to hold in check the out-of-control immune response (Owen, 2017). Such situations truly emphasize that when our immune protection goes haywire, the result is most frequently scattered inflammation and loss of normal function. Catching hold of autoimmune diseases is a matter of examining a large, complex combination of immune, genetic, and environmental elements that all influence one another in unforeseen patterns. , various autoantibodies tend to stick together with certain schemes of organ pathology, for example, interstitial lung disease (ILD) cropping up in SSc or in the myositis spectrum—hence providing clinicians with useful clues for diagnosis as well as prognosis. Most of the time, this refinement assists in customizing treatment plans and categorizing patients into cohorts that can more effectively take advantage of single-agent therapies. However, it is also a fact that symptoms and antibody patterns may overlap in sloppy, unidentifiable patterns that make some diagnoses a true enigma. The high cost that these disorders impose on patients and the healthcare system makes it unequivocally evident that continued research into immune pathways and novel biomarkers is an absolute necessity in order to devise new treatments and enhance lives (Kuwana et al., 2021).

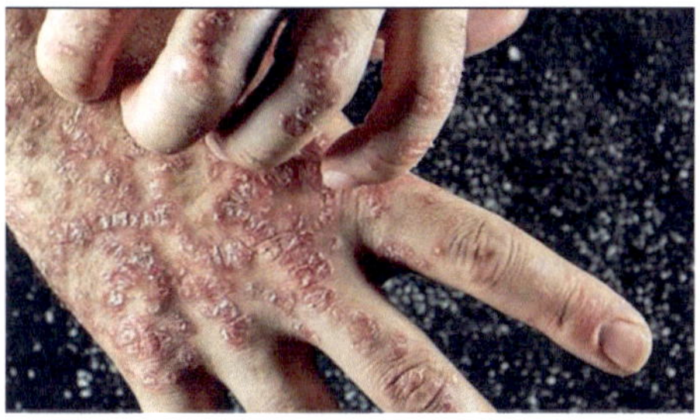

Source: India Today. (2023). *Health and Autoimmune Disorders.* https://akm-img-a-in.tosshub.com/indiatoday/images/story/202301/health-autoimmune_0-sixteen_nine.jpg?VersionId=QU03f41g.J5eoZt7zKqlxNL1gzYjSMwL&size=690:388.

Overview of Connective Tissue Disorders

Connective tissue disorders upset the applecart by interfering with the very tissues that keep our organs intact. They arise in unusual locations, affecting muscles, the heart, skin, and others, usually in ways that do not follow an organized course. Most of the time the immune system goes a little haywire—falsely attacking the body's own supportive fibers, causing chronic inflammation and progressive tissue damage. Consider, for instance, ankylosing spondylitis: in this condition, genetic characterestics, environmental influences, and out-of-control immune reactions tend to get married together in a pretty unpredictable fashion. AS has the immune system target the areas where tendons and ligaments attach to bone—the fibrocartilaginous entheses, which can then lead to stiffened spines and back pain in other locations, and obviously demonstrates how immune-mediated blunders can have an impact on more than one system (Owen, 2017). When it comes to determining these conditions, a close inspection is not sufficient on its own; it is paired with a series of precise tests that at times seem slightly scattered. One device, nailfold capillaroscopy, provides a painless glimpse at your smallest blood vessels, picking up minute alterations that may indicate diseases such as scleroderma, dermatomyositis, or mixed connective tissue disease (CTD). Although capillary forms may differ, however, competent examiners may still identify the variations that indicate microangiopathy-associated problems, which serves to signal the issue early. You may also observe identical capillary abnormalities in SLE or Sjogren's syndrome, which only serves to illustrate that each patient's history is a little different and warrants its own rigorous scrutiny (Angelis, 2019). On the treatment side, treating these disorders typically requires a team of practitioners to collaborate to soothe the autoimmune overdrive, alleviate inflammation, and stave off long-term damage. Treatment generally begins with NSAIDs—routine painkillers that serve to cool the inflammation. If that fails, physicians introduce disease-modifying antirheumatic drugs (DMARDs) or even biologic agents that target specific messages such as tumor necrosis factor-alpha (TNFα) in an attempt to redirect the course of the disease. Investigation into pathways that include interleukin-17 and interleukin-23 in diseases such as AS is pushing new therapies in an effort to optimize immune responses. In addition, making basic lifestyle adjustments, like adopting low-impact exercise to maintain flexible joints, provides an added form of protection. All of this serves to illustrate just how intertwined these disorders are and why consistent, persistent research continues to be paramount (Owen, 2017) (Figure 8.1).

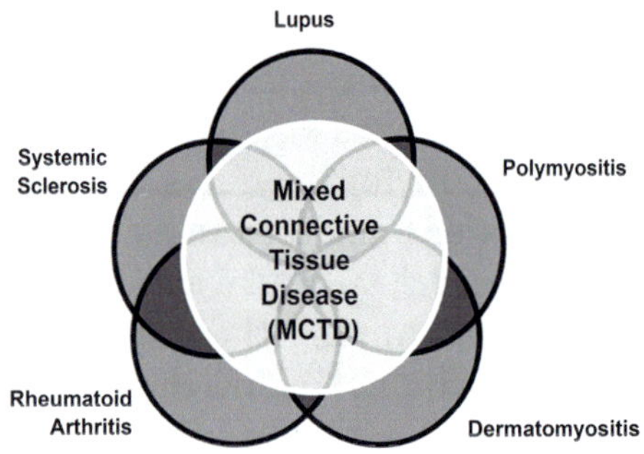

Figure 8.1. Mixed connective tissue disease (MCTD).

Source: Radić, M., & Overbury, R. S. (2021). Capillaroscopy as a diagnostic tool in the diagnosis of mixed connective tissue disease (MCTD): A case report. *BMC Rheumatology, 5*(1), 9.

Importance of Understanding These Conditions

Medical science today has taught us how complicated immune conditions can be. Such conditions, such as autoimmune and connective tissue disorders, tend to combine symptoms that blur the boundaries between body and mind, and that overlap makes it a real challenge to catch and treat them on time. It is not merely a matter of managing short-term discomfort—understanding the twists and turns of such conditions can alert physicians to complications, even those that are associated with pregnancy. Consider mixed MCTD: it packages several autoimmune manifestations together in such a manner that caregivers must remain vigilant and call in sundry specialists to safeguard both mother and offspring. By and large, having such insight allows for early intervention to take place and reduces the incidence of dangerous outcomes, as noted by precise immunosuppressive therapy that enhances overall patient safety (Nannaware et al., 2023). The impact on mental health is merely another facet of these already highly complicated diseases. Individuals who are experiencing systemic immune problems tend to struggle with relentless pain or physical limitations that, in turn, may cause issues such as PTSD. Recent observational findings indicate that individuals who have connective tissue issues may be more susceptible to stress-related mental health issues, a reminder that body and mind are more intertwined than we perhaps imagine. Realizing these psychological dangers is to include a lot of physicians these days combining mental care with plotting out treatment, something that appears to solidify patient results. Most times, taking care of an individual is about not only tending to body aches but also confronting the emotional burden associated with living with chronic illness (Carmassi et al., 2024). To all this, learning these disorders through and through really boosts patient self-assurance. Living with them generally entails long-term arrangements—maintaining medication, adjusting daily, and always monitoring for changes, either a flare or some improvement. If patients understand what induces their symptoms and what to watch for first, they will be more inclined to participate in treatment decisions and taking care of themselves. This type of shared decision-making is not only about reducing anxiety; it opens the door to adherence to treatment, reducing complications, and overall, feeling a little more in charge, even if sometimes, the specifics may feel a little daunting.

8.1. Mechanisms of Autoimmunity

Genetics and the environment combine in unexpected ways that can disrupt our natural balance of immune response. When regulatory systems that are designed to prevent immune cells from attacking us begin to fail, autoreactive lymphocytes begin to proliferate out of control. This imbalance manifests when autoantibodies and rogue T cells start attacking our own tissues – a pattern particularly observed in connective tissue ailments. It is not a single thing that is going on; molecular mimicry, epitope spreading and strange fluctuations in regulatory T cells all enter the mix, causing chronic inflammation and tissue destruction. Occasionally, outside stimuli, such as breast implants—seem to rev things up again, suggesting that chemicals from elsewhere may disrupt the normal immune quiet (Timothy et al., 2024). All of this serves to describe a muddled immunological cascade, so it is absolutely crucial to be able to pick up on early signals in these autoimmune diseases. When the immune system cannot maintain self-tolerance, autoimmunity does not simply get underway, it persists and winds up damaging critical organs. Connective tissue disease is a good case in point: autoreactive cells induce flares of inflammation that ultimately get to play havoc with blood vessels, muscles, and even the heart. Often, this can culminate in serious complications such as heart failure because of diffuse damage to heart muscle and immune-mediated vascular problems. Subclinical cardiac disease—in so many cases more easily overlooked, is likely to emerge from chronic systemic inflammation and immune complex deposits (Liu et al., 2024). In general, these breakdowns require physicians to be particularly alert and detect issues early to prevent lasting damage. It is all about knowing these immune mix-ups so that interventions can be timely and accurately targeted. New hints also indicate the involvement of external and treatment-related factors in activating autoimmunity.

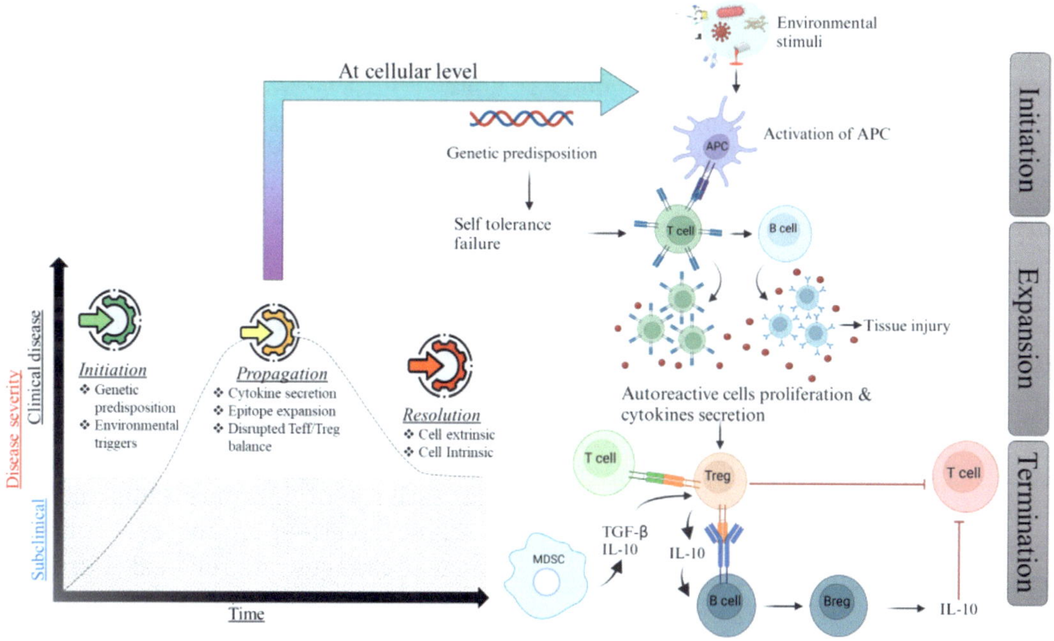

Figure 8.2. Pathophysiological mechanisms of autoimmune diseases.

Source: Yasmeen F, Pirzada RH, Ahmad B, Choi B, Choi S. Understanding Autoimmunity: Mechanisms, Predisposing Factors, and Cytokine Therapies. *International Journal of Molecular Sciences*. 2024; 25(14):7666. https://doi.org/10.3390/ijms25147666

Silicone breast implants, for instance, have been correlated with a higher prevalence of systematic autoimmune symptoms akin to rheumatoid arthritis (RA) or Sjögren's syndrome. While the definitive pathways are still somewhat unclear, some speculate that repeated, low-dose antigen exposure or local immune changes—differing from an intended bonus effect—could initiate a more general immune dysregulation (Timothy et al., 2024). All of this underlines the fact that autoimmunity is not a one-dimensional phenomenon; it is a sloppy mixture of genetic characterestics and environmental prods. Given such myriad influences, extensive risk assessment, continuous patient discussions, and extended follow-up become a must to deal with the ever-changing complexion of autoimmune manifestations associated with environmental insults and connective tissue diseases (Figure 8.2).

8.1.1. Immune System Dysfunction

Autoimmune and connective tissue diseases rely on the immune system losing its ability to distinguish between family and enemy. Under normal circumstances, the system is quite good at recognizing which cells are part of the family and which are not—so it kills invaders but leaves your own tissues intact. But when something goes awry, even your own body molecules get flagged as enemies, triggering a chain reaction. T-cells spring into action, cytokines begin flowing, and chronic inflammation and tissue destruction are in place before you can say "immunopathology." In SSc, for example, destruction of the blood vessel inner lining appears to trigger an invasion of immune cells that lead in turn to fibroblasts working overtime—too much collagen and rigid, fibrotic blood vessels (Derk & Jimenez, 2006). Seizing control of such initial misfires is critical if we ever hope to develop therapies that do more than merely cover up symptoms. Such issues from this immune misunderstanding are not localized to a single location; they tend to spread out and create severe, body-wide issues that escalate patient suffering and even shorten life. Heart disease, for instance, has become a top cause of death among individuals with autoimmune and connective tissue disorders. That chronic inflammatory aura speeds up atherosclerosis via a sloppy interaction of immune and metabolic components. Inflammatory cells and their signaling chemicals predispose blood vessels to weakening, stimulate plaque accumulation, and even initiate structural changes in the vessels—factors combined that enhance cardiovascular risk. Despite the progress that has been made with treatments for the underlying rheumatic conditions, attempts to identify and address heart disease have not kept quite so close. New recommendations from organizations such as the European League Against Rheumatism (Oreska & Tomcik, 2019) push us toward more holistic care with improved screening and prevention. It is a stark indication that when the immune system makes a mistake, the consequences extend far beyond damage to local tissue. Getting the right therapy is a delicate balancing act: you must restrain the immune system without creating additional problems or initiating new ones. In SSc the classic game strategy has typically only gone as far as alleviating symptoms by, for example, dilating blood vessels and inhibiting platelet clumping. Recently, however, there is increasing excitement that statins may provide more than a cholesterol drop. In most instances, the drugs appear to modulate the immune reaction and even guard the blood vessels. Some research suggests that statins may reduce vascular damage by altering the activity of immune cells and lowering cytokine levels—perhaps even pushing early vascular changes into reversal (Derk & Jimenez, 2006). This creates the promise that moving quickly to address immune misfires and their ripple effects on the blood vessels may alter the course of the disease. Research continues to be shedding layers on how the immune system becomes dysfunctional and illuminating the path to pioneering treatments targeting the source of autoimmune and connective tissue diseases (Figure 8.3).

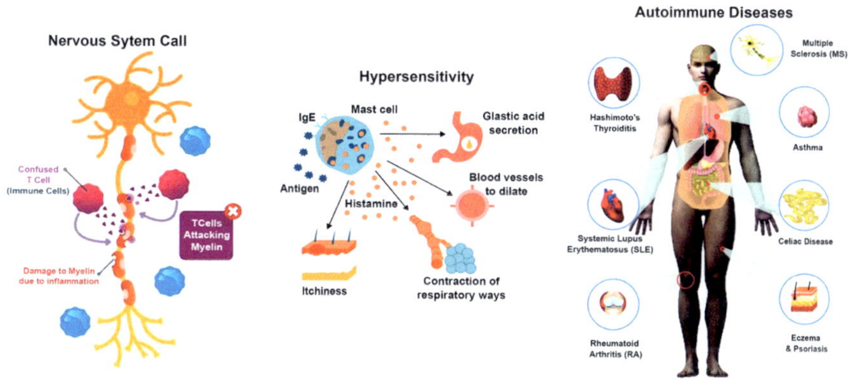

Figure 8.3. Immune dysfunction.

Source: BioCode. (2021). *Immune Dysfunction Image*. https://www.biocode.org.uk/wp-content/uploads/2021/10/Blog-Thumbnail-Immune-Dysfunction.png.

8.1.2. Genetic Predisposition

Autoimmune and connective tissue diseases appear to be awfully mysterious because genes and environmental factors combine in ways that are not always easy to understand. Outside blows, like a germ or a bad trauma—can trigger things, but the genetically encoded risk appears to tip the balance heavily in determining what each outcome will be. More recent molecular biology research, for instance, has identified that certain gene variants, particularly those relating to immune control and how our cell "scaffolding" is constructed, may push an individual toward the problems experienced in conditions such as morphea or SSc. Naturally enough, these genetic characterestics are not working alone; they combine with epigenetic adjustments that manipulate the way genes are turned on or off without manipulating the actual DNA code. Getting a true grip on these hereditary pieces of the puzzle is paramount because they influence not only the disease itself, but also the way people react to novel targeted therapies, which very much places genetics at the forefront of personalized medicine for autoimmune diseases (Stein et al., 2024). Looking into causes behind diseases such as systemic lupus erythematosus (SLE) and dermatomyositis, researchers still find that genetic predisposition is a big deal, even if it does not tell the whole story. Take studies with identical twins, for instance: when one twin gets sick and the other does not, it really highlights that gene, on their own, are not enough to explain everything. This mystifying gap has prompted researchers to burrow deeper into epigenetics, investigating how our genes interact with the world around us and how reversible modifications, such as DNA methylation or microRNA regulation shifts—fit into the mix. In general, these discoveries indicate that if someone is genetically predisposed in a particular way, this sets the stage (maybe even a somewhat unpredictable one) in which epigenetic mechanisms may either push up or reduce the risk, creating new areas where we can intervene and alter the course of the disease beyond mere what-ifs from the genes themselves (Zhang et al., 2023). If you consider connective tissue diseases, genetic susceptibility is not merely a term for risk—it also provides a kind of blueprint to understand why symptoms may be so diverse and therapies vary so much. A genetic map can sometimes show us specific hotspots associated with hyperactive immune reactions, collagen dysregulation, or even problems with cell layers lining blood vessels—frequent symptoms in diseases like morphea. Furthermore, the integration of findings from both genetics and epigenetics has prompted the development of novel therapies, such as particular monoclonal antibodies or kinase inhibitors, that attack the obscured molecular pathways affected by these hereditary influences. In summary, integrating genetic concepts into day-to-day clinical practice can increase the accuracy of outcome prediction and aid in making therapies even more bespoke, with a view to combating at their own genesis the seeds planted by genetic predisposition for autoimmune and connective tissue diseases (Stein et al., 2024) (Figure 8.4).

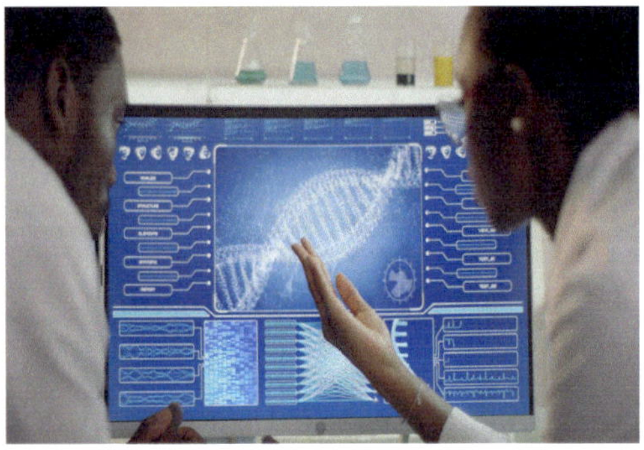

Figure 8.4. Understand genetic predisposition.

Source: Getty Images. (2021). African ethnicity scientists studying DNA samples. *Computer Screens with DNA sequences.* https://www.verywellhealth.com/thmb/FW2aC0KwK-L4xzBI0QxbInLm2bE=/1500x0/filters:no_upscale():max_bytes(150000):strip_icc()/VWH-GettyImages-1345098965-779be2ac96934cb998ab1ce83470318b.jpg.

8.1.3. Environmental Triggers

Autoimmune and connective tissue diseases usually arise when your genes and the environment combine in unusual combinations. Genetic predisposition and external factors, consider daily physical or chemical exposures—can collaborate to initiate or aggravate immune issues. At other times, even such mundane causes as a chill or stress (as in diseases like Raynaud's phenomenon) can interfere with blood flow by inducing abnormal vascular responses that can result in further complications. Physicians tend to instruct patients to avoid these physical, chemical, and even affective sparks. Practically, this involves speaking with patients to identify and reduce known irritating elements while occasionally employing medications to maintain the body's response within moderation (Bellando-Randone et al., 2018). Obviously, adjusting exposure to the environment becomes an achievable, modifiable variable, highlighting a more general approach to treatment. Another dimension, which is crucial to mention, concerns adjuvants used in vaccines and other chemicals. Intended to enhance immune reactions, chemicals such as aluminum, mineral oil, and silicone can, at least in certain situations—stimulate the immune system into overdrive. The concept of autoimmune/inflammatory syndrome induced by adjuvants (ASIA) entered in an attempt to describe a collection of indistinct or nonspecific autoimmune symptoms associated with these exposures. In a somewhat unexpected turn of events, exposure to substances that are nearly innocuous may reveal concealed autoimmunity or even induce new autoimmune responses, making the course of systemic rheumatic disorders more complex. This finding, in most instances, has remodeled both diagnosis and treatment of these diseases and reminded us of how precarious the immune equilibrium may be (Seida et al., 2023). Outside the typical suspects of physical and chemical stimuli, larger environmental influences, such as infections and even psychosocial stress, also appear to tip the balance in autoimmune and connective tissue diseases. These stimuli may push the immune system in all sorts of ways, from molecular mimicry to chronic inflammation and even abrupt vascular misbehavior. Even as we are certain that vaccines are important in preventing infections, their adjuvant ingredients sometimes included have triggered fears of possible, adverse immune effects—fears compounded in times such as the COVID-19 pandemic. All this demands additional caution, with constant surveillance and a balanced consideration of risk versus benefit, particularly for individuals who are already susceptible to autoimmune issues. It is why there is a lot of backing now for an integrative model of care that takes into account everything from chemical exposure to daily stress in the battle to maintaining these diseases under control (Bellando-Randone et al., 2018; Seida et al., 2023).

8.2. Common Autoimmune Disorders

Autoimmune disorders encompass a motley of diseases in which the body's defense mechanism mistakenly attacks its own tissues. Frequently, genes and daily environmental exposures mingle in complex combinations, initiating persistent inflammation and slowly eroding tissues. You may hear about conditions such as RA, SLE, or Sjögren's syndrome—they often strike connective tissues hard. Joint pain, swelling, and spells of fatigue or fever are quite typical signs, although how these symptoms manifest varies considerably. Since nothing works out according to plan here, physicians generally must cooperate across disciplines. In other instances, lung affliction also rears its head; small airways and the lung tissue itself become inflamed, which eventually contributes to worsening respiratory problems and declining function, which is why it is so crucial to catch such issues early (Kluanwan et al., 2025). It is not just the lungs that find themselves entangled in such instances—the heart and blood vessels tend to suffer collateral damage as well. The immune system may mistakenly attack the heart muscle, its valves, or even the blood supply vessels, opening the door to myocarditis, abnormal valve function, or even ischemic heart disease. Heart failure in connective tissue diseases (CTD) is particularly severe, with patients usually having shortness of breath and decreased exercise tolerance. In general, the etiologies of this heart failure are variable, with widespread damage to the muscle, obstructed coronary perfusion, and inflamed valves all contributing. Identifying any trace of cardiac dysfunction early on makes a significant difference since early treatment with immunosuppressive agents and cardiac drugs can significantly improve outcomes and overall well-being (Liu et al., 2024). Taking it a step further, these immune-mediated conditions typically are not limited to a single organ; they tend to initiate system-wide inflammation that affects multiple sites simultaneously. For example, idiopathic inflammatory myopathies and mixed CTD tend to blur the boundaries by involving the skin, muscles, lungs, and even the cardiovascular system. Very frequently, issues with the small airways appear in such instances, alerting us to the fact that respiratory examinations are vital because lung signs may appear before anything else and can dictate the whole prognosis. This implies therapies must target two objectives: containing the general autoimmune bedlam while targeting individual organ issues. More and more clinical practices are shifting toward team-based care to monitor disease activity, prevent irreversibly damaged tissue, and allow patients to preserve daily functioning as much as possible (Liu et al., 2024; Kluanwan et al., 2025).

8.2.1. Rheumatoid Arthritis (RA)

Autoimmune problems can really get out of hand when the immune system begins misbehaving, attacking its own tissues and initiating chronic inflammation and destruction. RA, for example, primarily targets synovial joints; this results in ongoing pain, swelling, and joint destruction as time passes. You may be told that autoantibody, such as rheumatoid factor (RF) and those anti-citrullinated protein ones—become involved, driving immune complexes into action and increasing inflammation in the lining of the joint. Curiously, RA is not exclusively a joint disease. In most instances, it also comes with systemic issues such as interstitial lung disease (ILD), a major comorbidity that complicates management and changes overall prognosis. Current research even indicates that some of the autoantibodies may be used as precursor markers to identify RA patients more vulnerable to ILD, which would open up the gates to an earlier diagnosis and more targeted therapy (Kuwana et al., 2021). Testing these serological indicators appears rather vital to understand just how multifaceted and unexpected these autoimmune connective tissue issues may turn out to be. It is also important to mention that immune-mediated damage to blood vessels and the subsequent deposition of fibrous tissue appear to be a key piece of the puzzle in connective tissue pathologies. Consider this—while SSc is primarily known for its endothelial hiccups causing fibrosis, RA also appears to have a similar blueprint: chronic inflammation combined with vascular alterations in the involved areas. Before long, activated T-cells flood to site of injury, releasing a cocktail of cytokines and growth factors that stimulate fibroblasts to proliferate and lay down excess extracellular matrix. The chain reaction not only devastates joints but also ignites trouble elsewhere, including lung and cardiac complications. Treatments designed to modulate these immune pathways—i.e., drugs that dampen inflammation and assist in protecting the vessels, are beginning to show promise in stalling disease advancement. There is also a tantalizing suggestion from statins, which are renowned for their role in vascular remodeling in SSc; while direct clinical evidence linking them to RA is still scant, it provides an organized conceptual connection (Derk & Jimenez, 2006). All in all, exploring treatments aimed at these immune-induced vessel problems may hold the key to improved long-term outcomes for RA and its relatives. RA is a multifaceted animal that requires a wide, one-stop approach, one that integrates immunologic, clinical, and pathologic understanding for optimal patient management. Technologic advances in detecting autoantibodies have largely helped us diagnose and forecast more accurately, particularly when complications such as ILD are involved. This, in a sense, supports the point that RA is not just about pain in the joints—it falls within a broader category of autoimmune rheumatic diseases where connective tissue is a common target. The overlap of joint-specific symptoms and broader systemic symptoms, like ILD, essentially demonstrates a continuum of immune misfires. Scientists, in general, are now turning their attention to how effectors of the immune system and tissue reactions co-interact, with a view to designing novel biomarkers and therapies that can address both the inflammatory spark and the fibrotic fallout. It is a little rough-and-tumble and still developing, but an inter-disciplinary approach seems to be needed not only to treat symptoms but also to have the potential to redirect the course of the disease over time (Kuwana et al., 2021) (Figure 8.5).

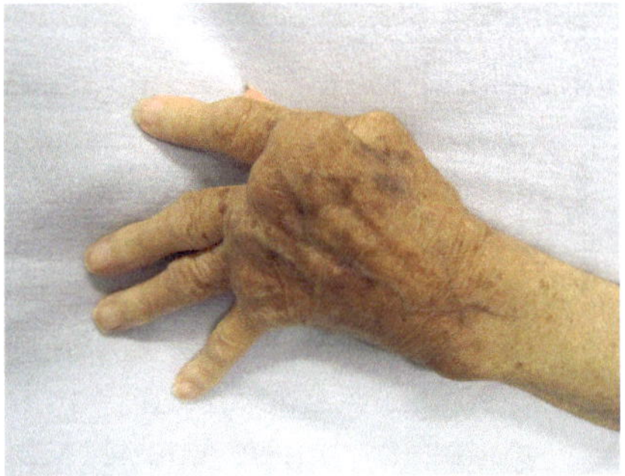

Figure 8.5. Rheumatoid arthritis rashes.

Source: By James Heilman, MD - Own work, CC BY-SA 3.0, https://commons.wikimedia.org/w/index.php?curid=11110471

8.2.2. Systemic Lupus Erythematosus (SLE)

Autoimmune diseases really confuse physicians, particularly when there is little background information in most communities. Consider Nigeria, for instance, new findings indicate that SLE, or lupus, appears more frequently and in more diverse forms than individuals previously believed. A review of the University of Port Harcourt Teaching Hospital records revealed that, in the combination of autoimmune connective tissues, lupus was predominant in almost all cases. Women were especially affected (approximately 14:1 to men), and the majority of the patients were in their early thirties. A discoid rash, a cutaneous symptom that stood out—was one of the more apparent indicators. Also, a lot of the severe consequences—primarily deaths—were associated with complications such as lupus nephritis, congestive heart failure, and pulmonary hypertension; this indicates how many organs become involved in the issue (Mercy et al., 2016). Pregnancy in women with conditions such as SLE awakens its own set of complications, affecting both mothers and their offspring. A retrospective hospital study examined how pregnancy and these conditions intersected, and the results were quite revealing. Women who had lupus experienced more spontaneous abortions and intrauterine fetal death; there was also a significant spike in cesarean sections, frequently compelled by fetal distress or other emergent conditions. Infants born under these circumstances occasionally had growth difficulties and, very often, had to be airlifted to neonatal intensive care. And then There is the additional health difficulties that accompany these CTD during pregnancy, such that physicians from various disciplines often have to collaborate—no single discipline can do it all alone. Evidently, closer monitoring during pregnancy and tailoring treatment strategies are the key to improved outcomes in such susceptible patients (Jha & Chaudhari, 2020). Mastering SLE, which falls within the very large umbrella of autoimmune connective tissue diseases, involves understanding how the immune system becomes derailed and how blood tests guide the way toward a diagnosis. Usually, lupus is accompanied by autoantibodies, such as RF and anti-neutrophil antibodies, which physicians depend on to diagnose the disease and measure its activity. Studies, including in some African populations, indicate that a reasonable percentage of patients wind up being RF-positive. Such overlap in antibody patterns can render it more difficult to distinguish lupus from other related disorders. That is the reason why remaining with tried protocols, such as those of the American College of Rheumatology, for instance, is so necessary, particularly where the disease is only just getting into the limelight. Increasing numbers of reported cases likely attest to improved detecting equipment and also to a generally heightened clinical responsiveness, challenging the healthcare systems to keep pace with the expanding task posed by such chronic, multisystem disorders (Mercy et al., 2016) (Figure 8.6).

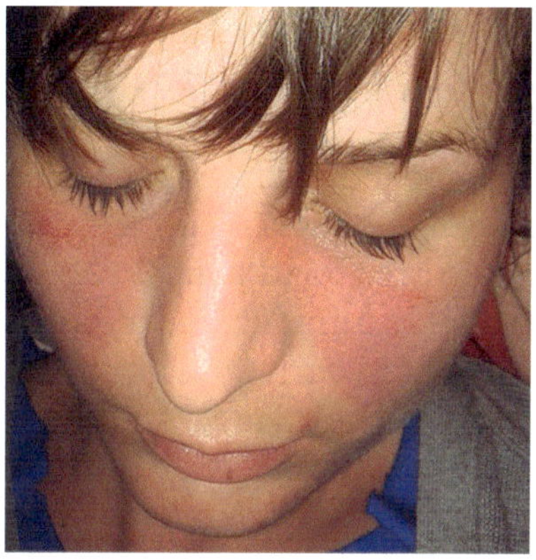

Figure 8.6. Young woman with the distinctive butterfly rash that many individuals with lupus experience.

Source: Doktorinternet. (2013, May 15). Malar rash (butterfly rash) in systemic lupus erythematosus. *Wikimedia Commons*. https://upload.wikimedia.org/wikipedia/commons/5/52/Lupusfoto.jpg.

8.2.3. Multiple Sclerosis

Autoimmune problems tend to be fairly sloppy—your immune system gets to play in odd ways with other tissues, and that typically means progressive damage and loss of function. MS is a perfect example; it primarily devastates the central nervous system by disrupting the myelin that insulates nerve cells. In most instances, the problem begins when marauding T cells get past the blood-brain barrier, igniting inflammation and stripping away bits of myelin, which subsequently scrambles neural signals. You're left with a whole variety of neurological issues such as unusual sensations, muscle weakness, and even some mental bumps. MS indeed demonstrates how tissue damage caused by the immune system is a large part of autoimmune and connective tissue diseases. Tracing the minute cellular errors illuminates not only how the disease can veer so many different ways, but it also alerts us to the challenges of engineering treatments that reduce the immune attack without causing more damage to nerve tissue. MS itself is as capricious as it gets—the symptoms and progression can zigzag all over the map, making it a tough one to diagnose and treat. Some individuals experience flurries of sudden blowouts with bad neuro problems, followed by a break and partial relief, whereas others experience a gradual decline as disabilities accumulate. These variations probably have to do with how each individual's immune system works, combined with genetic variables and environmental factors. New developments, such as MRI, have flipped the script by making it even simpler to detect lesions, but we now recognize that autoimmune issues can extend far beyond the brain and spine. Strangely, things such as inner ear issues, which cause balance issues—have surfaced in other autoimmune disorders, suggesting that a similar sensory mechanism is possibly involved in MS as well. The entire crossover is a reminder for physicians to stay mindful of the overall, systemic blowback from inflammation and to rely on a team-based model for patient treatment (Adelchi et al., 2018). Treatment paths for MS continue to change as physicians experiment with new approaches in order to rein in the immune system, reduce relapses, and decelerate progression, while attempting to alleviate symptoms.

It is a challenging balancing act—making the immune response inadequate can leave an individual susceptible to infections, and there is always concern that complications may arise in other areas of the body. Innovative imaging methods, such as some of the ultrasound procedures that were initially applied to lung issues in autoimmune rheumatic diseases (Wang et al., 2024), are breaking doors open for non-invasive inspections on disease burden across the board. Although MS primarily attacks nerves, these cross-disciplinary concepts emphasize the importance of combining various diagnostic tools with individually tailored treatments to truly enhance patient outcomes. Ongoing, precise research continues to be the key to unraveling the complex immune misfires of MS, hopefully on the way to identifying more precise interventions that can enhance quality of life (Figure 8.7).

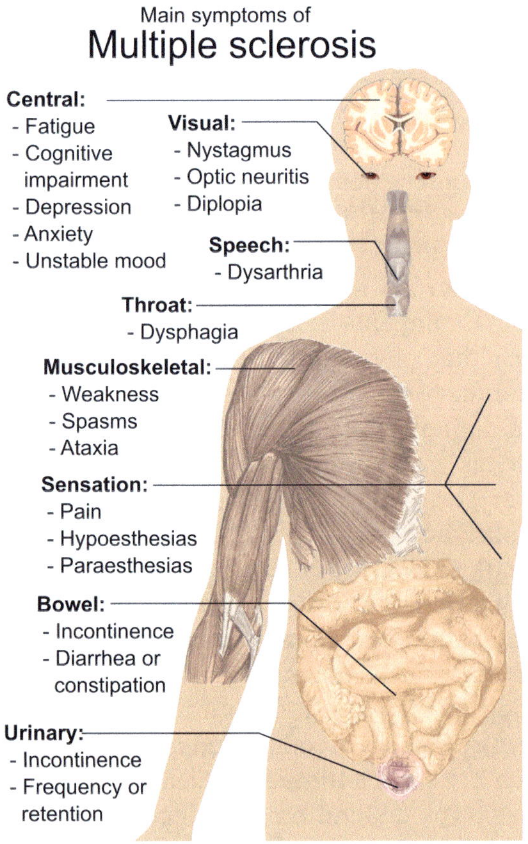

Figure 8.7. Multiple sclerosis.

Source: By Mikael Häggström - All used images are in public domain., Public Domain, https://commons.wikimedia.org/w/index.php?curid=5857329

8.3. Connective Tissue Disorders Overview

Our genes and the environment tend to combine in uncoordinated, unforested manners that contribute to the initiation of connective tissue problems. In most instances, our own tissues become the immune system's targets, an unselfish attack that results in chronic inflammation and eventual structural wear. Consider ankylosing spondylitis, for instance; it indicates that, in addition to the famous HLA-B27 gene, other genetic pieces as well as excessive cytokine activity can push the disease along. Frequently, the problem begins in the entheses themselves, where those fibrocartilaginous pieces are the resentful objects of immune mistakes. This type of immune cascade, affecting multiple body systems, truly emphasizes the fact that these disorders function systemically and require treatment strategies to cover both the local and systemic effects (Owen, 2017). Early diagnosis of these conditions is not easy; symptoms overlap with other rheumatologic or inflammatory diseases. Nailfold capillaroscopy, a convenient non-invasive test, aids in the detection of small capillary modifications that suggest SSc and related disorders. By examining the appearance of capillaries and the path of blood in them, practitioners can, most of the time, distinguish primary Raynaud's phenomenon from secondary forms that are related to autoimmunity. However, capillary appearances vary significantly between individuals, so the test needs somebody with a trained eye to accurately interpret the results. Short of it, incorporating this technique into regular tests may prove to lay the groundwork for earlier and more accurate diagnoses and improved outcomes with timely interventions (Angelis, 2019). Attending to connective tissue diseases requires a holistic picture of how the conditions affect the entire body and how and why the immune system fails. With diseases like ankylosing spondylitis, the initial steps are usually a matter of modifying one's way of life and taking NSAIDs to reduce inflammation and manage symptoms. When purely simple measures are not enough, doctors typically take things up a notch with therapies such as disease-modifying antirheumatic drugs or biologic therapies targeting cytokines like TNFα or IL-17; the therapies complement each other in slowing down the progression and maintaining function intact. Continued study of the immune mechanisms underlying these disorders could ultimately produce more highly calibrated treatments—treatments with fewer side effects but greater overall efficacy. This developing picture emphasizes the necessity for both multidisciplinary treatment and tailored treatment plans to control these complex diseases (Owen, 2017).

8.3.1. Definition and Classification

Autoimmune and connective tissue diseases raise a rather knotty set of problems; the immune system of the body finds itself behaving badly and attacking its tissues. These diseases persist for the long term and generally are the result of a mix of things - consider genetic characteristics, environmental prods, and immune system malfunctions. It is not always cut and dry because they can present in a body-wide manner or just slam one organ hard. For the most part, when we use the term "autoimmune," what we are talking about is that self-tolerance has gotten away, triggering inflammation and damage. And with connective tissue issues, the problem usually resides in the extracellular matrix, getting into skin, joints, blood vessels, and internal organs alike. Physicians tend to sort them out according to what they can observe in clinical examination and lab work, but at times the syndromes overlap and it is not easy. New technologies in genetics, such as investigating low-frequency variants in endogamous populations (Kurki et al., 2023), have increasingly aided in untangling these messy descriptions. Historically, individuals have divided these diseases into two groups: those that remain in one organ and those that affect several systems. Hashimoto's thyroiditis or type 1 diabetes, for instance, are regarded as organ-specific since the immune attack remains in one location. Conversely, diseases like SLE and SSc affect an array of body structures and involve a great deal with connective tissue failures. Within the systemic subgroup, you can even separate out various types based on clinical presentation and blood markers. Consider SSc, which physicians tend to separate into limited and diffuse cutaneous subtypes based on the extent to which the skin is involved - each with its own prognosis and complications. It is typical to rely on biomarker measurements such as autoantibodies and molecular signals to separate out these diverse presentations. Most of the time, research that focuses on molecular markers performs a good job of illustrating how active the disease is and how it may advance (Hana et al., 2021). More recently, advances in genomic and proteomic technology have driven the categorization of these disorders into even finer detail. Population research indicates that, in certain cases, uncommon genetic variants contribute more than previously considered to identifying both who develop these conditions and how severe they are, particularly in genetically isolated populations (Kurki et al., 2023). Molecules such as heat shock proteins have also emerged as possible markers of disease activity, particularly in SSc when they appear to correlate with both inflammation and fibrosis of the tissues, even though, sometimes, the readings can be a little here and there. Combining molecular information with routine clinical indicators now seems to be able to result in a more personalized set of methods of diagnosis and treatment. In total, the definitions and categorizations of autoimmune and connective tissue diseases have become some kind of ongoing dialogue between clinical snapshots and the latest research findings, something that shows just how fluid our knowledge is (Figure 8.8).

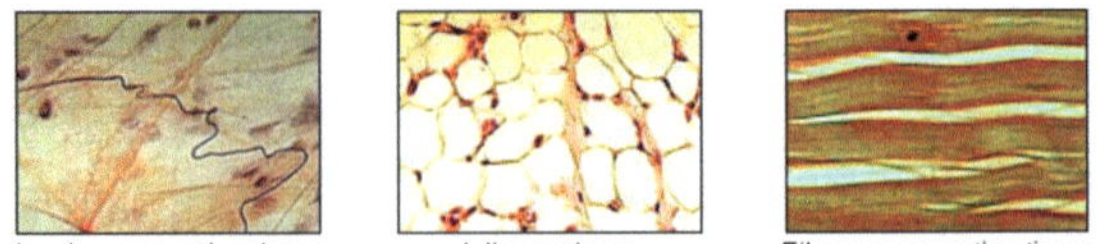

Figure 8.8. Connective tissue.

Source: Public Domain, https://commons.wikimedia.org/w/index.php?curid=1273807

8.3.2. Role of Connective Tissues in the Body

Connective tissues are the behind-the-scenes heroes of our bodies, accomplishing much more than simply holding things together. Bones, cartilage, ligaments, tendons, fascia, and even blood all contribute, not just for mechanical support but also by transporting nutrients around, defending against unwanted invaders, and assisting with repairs. Collagen and elastin provide tissues with the proper balance of stiffness and extensibility to maintain organs in shape and motion smooth. Frequently, this same tissue coalesces into a small local clearing where cells can "communicate" and the immune system makes contact, usually maintaining things in equilibrium. But when autoimmune issues arise, that precarious balance is compromised, slowly causing tissue injury. For example, in ankylosing spondylitis the immune system attacks fibrocartilaginous entheses—the very sites of bone-tendon juncture—initiating inflammation and ultimately joint fusion that sabotages both motion and general welfare (Owen, 2017). Connective tissue is a basic, multi-dimensional force in health and disease alike. It is not merely a matter of physical form either; connective tissue plays an essential role in maintaining the smooth functioning of glands, especially when autoimmune diseases choose to target them. Consider the salivary glands, for instance, they rely on a tough meshwork of connective tissue to support their ducts and cell clusters, but that very support sometimes leaves them susceptible to immune aggression.

In conditions such as Sjögren's syndrome, T-helper lymphocytes target such ducts, the connective network directing the attack, which leads to inflammation and a reduction in saliva output. Likewise, immunoglobulin G4-related diseases cause destructive immune attacks against gland cells, again illustrating how disparities between these tissue compartments can determine where and how disease occurs (Vincentiis et al., 2017). Surgical procedures like sialendoscopy also uncover how important it is to understand the connective tissue's role in the larger picture, particularly when looking for improved treatments.

These lines of evidence truly emphasize that connective tissue is not an inactive bystander—it actively participates in the development and course of autoimmune diseases. And more still: connective tissue also interacts very closely with immune signaling, controlling both the severity of inflammation and how tissues regenerate after injury. In diseases such as ankylosing spondylitis, a dysregulated immune response – consider cytokines like TNFα and interleukins like IL-17/IL-23 – directly interferes with the tissue at critical junctions, triggering chronic inflammation and dysregulated bone formation (Owen, 2017). This ongoing dialogue between immune cells and tissue constituents does not only lead to local disturbance; it can cascade to impact the entire body. Similarly, when autoimmune attacks target connective tissue within salivary glands, not only is gland functionality impaired, but more widespread systemic symptoms arise, which indicates why it is equally vital to continue researching these immune–tissue interactions in order to smooth out improved treatment plans (Vincentiis et al., 2017). Finally, the connective tissue is anything but a bystander—it is an active, interested participant in maintaining us in health and, in the context of misdirection, in propelling the pathology of autoimmune diseases.

8.3.3. Common Symptoms Associated with These Disorders

Autoimmune and connective tissue diseases appear in a mix of symptoms that indicate some complex-up immune misfires and inflammation. Those who have these diseases tend to experience a constant fatigue, and their joints may hurt or swell in patterns that predict widespread inflammation. As often as not, the glands that help keep our eyes and mouths moist end up drying out, as in Sjögren's syndrome, a strange turn of events that results from an attack by the immune system, most commonly by helper T cells, on both the ducts and the body gland tissue. This errant immune reaction can lead to chronic pain and difficulty with basic functions, so physicians tend to depend on thorough diagnostic tests, such as advanced imaging, to sort out similarly overlapping conditions (Vincentiis et al., 2017). Mind problems enter the picture as well. In addition to the physical pains, these diseases tend to mess around with the brain and nerves—both central and peripheral, and that just complicates the diagnosis. Cognitive lapses, mood swings, sleep disturbances, and anxiety arise in addition to even more serious symptoms such as hallucinations or strange, delusional beliefs. Certain of these neuropsychiatric consequences directly relate to the autoimmune process itself, whereas others can arise as unwanted side effects of immunosuppressive medications, tending to complicate treatment protocols in most instances. Early identification of such mental signs is generally important for planning, and sometimes revising treatment plans (Kawałko et al., 2022). Also, the complexity does not end with glands and nerves; numerous patients suffer from a variety of other system-wide complications. Painful joints and muscles, which appear as arthralgia and myalgia due to inflammation-induced tissue damage, commonly follow along, while skin issues such as rashes and sensitivity to sun appear as obvious manifestations of general immune activation.

Depending on the particular disorder, organ difficulty can involve the kidneys, lungs, or heart, increasingly eroding their function. Detection of these diverse signs is paramount—not just to monitor disease activity but also to direct treatment and continuous monitoring. The vast diversity of presentations demands a holistic, multidisciplinary treatment plan for patients (Vincentiis et al., 2017; Kawałko et al., 2022).

8.4. Major Connective Tissue Disorders

Other times, the body throws a monkey wrench into its own blueprints—when the proteins that are supposed to be holding cells together just do not function properly. You have got problems cropping up in the skin, joints, blood vessels, and even other organs, as connective tissue is pretty much everywhere, you know. Let us take Generalized Arterial Calcification of Infancy (GACI), for example. For the vast majority, a mutation in the ENPP1 gene disrupts the usual balance of minerals in arteries, creating abnormal hardening that tragically takes young lives. Recent research employing the Enpp1asj mutant mouse model, even with its traitfeatures—indicates that increasing dietary magnesium during pregnancy and shortly after birth can significantly deter these unwanted mineral deposits. This result looks to simple dietary adjustments as a possible assist in both prenatal and postnatal care for those who are at risk (Kingman et al., 2017). Changing gears a bit, autoimmune conditions also have a way of upsetting connective tissues in a pretty confusing manner. By and large, when the immune system attacks the body's own cells, you get inflammatory damage in important tissues. Think of disorders affecting the large salivary glands, such as Sjögren's syndrome and immunoglobulin G4-related disease. In these conditions, the immune system appears to be targeting other things—Sjögren's syndrome primarily targets the exocrine ducts, while IgG4-related diseases cause inconvenience to the glandular parenchyma. Note that older clinical terms like Mikulicz's disease and Kuttner's tumor have been increasingly replaced, expanding our perception of autoimmune disorders that can affect several organs. This paradigm change not only assists in demystifying the way tissue degradation takes place, but it also highlights why proper instruments such as sialendoscopy are still so essential (Vincentiis et al., 2017). Taking a step back, the heterogeneity of these connective tissue issues requires a broad lens approach, one that accounts for genetic characterestics, immune malfunctions, and even external influences. Therapies genuinely must be the same as the root problem, from gene-dependent nutritional adjustments to therapies that mitigate an overexuberant immune reaction. In addition, since the discipline continues to advance—new categories developing, like transferring some salivary gland pathology into the realm of IgG4—the healthcare community is compelled to continue adapting its diagnostic requirements and treatment strategies. Most commonly, this constantly evolving zone serves as a reminder of how interconnected our genetic ancestry and immune system can be, and it continues to be a driving force behind the trend toward more customized medicine and improved overall outcomes.

8.4.1. Systemic Sclerosis (Scleroderma)

Vessel damage initiates a cascade in most autoimmune connective tissue ailments—often it is as if the lining of our vessels simply wears out too soon, opening the door for other issues. Consider SSc, for example, the initial disruption in the vessel wall gets T-cells activated and, once activated, they begin to release messages that activate inflammation and collagen synthesis. These signals, cycled in a kind of feedback mechanism, attract fibroblasts over and push them into a shape that produces additional collagen. Soon enough, the accumulation of scar tissue begins to extend beyond the skin to internal organs, and that additional fibrosis becomes a significant portion of the patient's complaints. Although we now better understand this vasculopathy, treatments continue largely to target vessel dilation and preventing platelet overactivity – with in most instances only faint indications that medication such as statins may modify the initial vascular remodeling (Derk & Jimenez, 2006). Epidemiological research has also been probing who develops SSc and with what frequency it appears in various groups of autoimmune connective tissue diseases. Research from African tertiary institutions, for instance, refutes the long-standing perception that the disorders are very uncommon in African people. SSc might not be the prevalent autoimmune disease in Port Harcourt, Nigeria, but it remains responsible for a sizeable percentage of rheumatology cases nonetheless. The report concurs with world trends featuring an unmistakable predominance of the female sex and a striking prevalence of young adults in the mix. Death in these patients was largely attributable to renal crises, illustrating just how severe organ involvement can become. All this local data encourages further clinical vigilance and more diagnostic ability, particularly in locales that have long been underrepresented (Mercy et al., 2016). To truly comprehend SSc, you must examine the combination of diverse symptoms and immune errors that accumulate over time. The condition appears as tightening, thickened skin, a lack of blood flow in the fingers, and an unceasing scarring of organs inside the body, such as lungs, heart, and kidneys. The inner dynamics appear to involve a combination of hyperactive immune messages, a collapsing lining on blood vessels, and fibroblasts that simply do not act correctly ; all of them constantly causing destruction to tissues and triggering even greater fibrosis. Physicians rely on lab markers, such as particular autoantibodies, to aid in establishing the diagnosis and anticipating what will occur, despite these markers not always appearing identical in all patients. Though at the moment the therapy choices are rather restricted, new research in vascular-targeted therapies , including the prospect that statins could be used to refine endothelial issues – carries some promise for altering the course of the disease. Merging both population data and clinical findings appears central to finally improving patient outcomes in this quite difficult disorder (Derk & Jimenez, 2006; Mercy et al., 2016) (Figure 8.9).

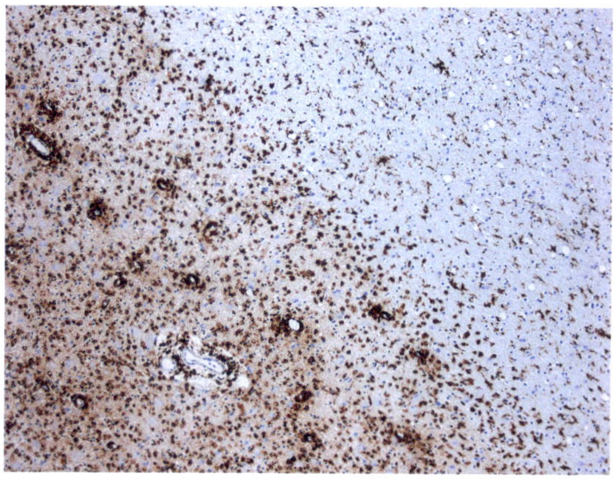

Figure 8.9. Systemic sclerosis (SS).

Source: By Marvin 101 - Own work, CC BY-SA 3.0, https://commons.wikimedia.org/w/index.php?curid=2846763

8.4.2. Sjögren's Syndrome

Autoimmune diseases are terribly confusing ; they have a habit of catching us out underhanded and appearing in such numerous guises that early detection is tricky. Sjögren's syndrome, for instance, usually comes about so unobtrusively that early signs are far too often overlooked. It affects the exocrine glands the most, particularly those involved in saliva and tears, and this is why dry mouth and eyes become the most glaring complaints.

With time, immune cells begin to invade these glands and, consequently, their function becomes impaired and distress accumulates.

Even though this disorder is one of the more frequent autoimmune conditions, it typically will not be discovered until the problems in the glands become severe or other systemic complaints become involved. To be fair, however, raising awareness with medical professionals – nurse practitioners included – truly makes a difference as far as achieving an early diagnosis and initiating therapy that can positively impact a patient's life (DeNisco et al., 2004). Genes clearly play a large role in the development of Sjögren's syndrome, with some genetic characterestics boosting the levels of autoantibodies against Ro/SSA and La/SSB antigens.

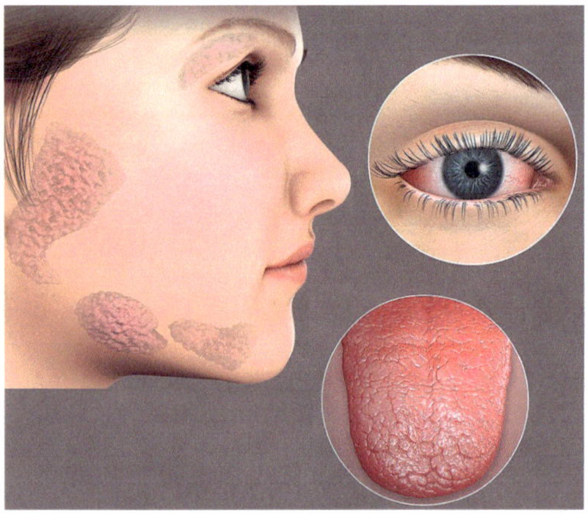

Figure 8.10. Characteristic dryness appears at a number of locations, such as the tongue, face, and eyes. Marked at left are the salivary glands (which may be swollen), not a facial rash.

Source: Scientific Animations. (2018). Signs and symptoms of Sjögren's syndrome. *Wikimedia Commons.* https://upload.wikimedia.org/wikipedia/commons/thumb/5/54/Sjogrens_Syndrome.jpg/800px-Sjogrens_Syndrome.jpg.

Not only are these autoantibodies diagnostic red flags, but they can also suggest a more challenging course of the disease, indicating a range of clinical flavors among patients. And then there is the environmental factor. In most instances, evidence indicates that previous infections are rather strongly associated with developing Sjögren's, whereas—most surprisingly—smoking, being a perennial suspect in other autoimmune diseases, does not appear to increase the risk here. Indeed, it has been observed that most patients quit smoking even prior to diagnosis, as if early symptoms softly guide them away. This combination of genetic susceptibility and environmental triggers truly illustrates how complex the etiology is for this syndrome, and the reasons why a thorough patient history is so precious (Mofors, 2021) (Figure 8.10).

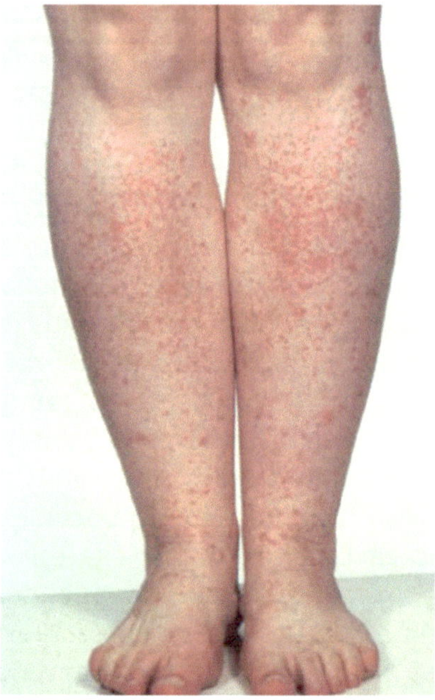

Figure 8.11. Sjögren's syndrome and the skin.

Source: Pease, C. (2011). *Sjögren's Syndrome and the Skin.*

Sjögren's syndrome does not stop at the glands—its influence can extend much further. Research following large cohorts of individuals shows that individuals with the syndrome are at greater risk of developing severe cardiovascular complications such as heart attacks and strokes, and blood clotting problems, than the general population. The risks increase significantly in patients who test positive for Ro/SSA and La/

SSB autoantibodies, usually indicating a more dismal prognosis. There is also a suggestion of a higher incidence of blood cancers, including multiple myeloma, in these subjects, a result that may suggest a connection between chronic autoimmunity and malignancy. In some instances, even newborns of affected mothers are at risk for congenital heart block (CHB), which speaks to the systemic nature of this condition and why follow-up is necessary over the long term. These considerations suggest a multidisciplinary approach to treating Sjögren's syndrome that extends beyond symptom management to also monitor the more general, frequently subtle risks (Mofors, 2021) (Figure 8.11).

8.4.3. Ehlers-Danlos Syndrome

Handling complicated conditions is challenging when there are so few clear clinical guidelines, particularly with rare ailments. Consider Ehlers-Danlos syndrome (EDS) as a case in point; it is a combination of problems where the skin stretches too far, the joints are too loose, and the tissues are prone to fragility. Although EDS has a significant clinical impact, there are few systematic, evidence-based practice rules that exist. A close look at recent literature reveals a surprisingly wide chasm in solid research and formal protocols for diagnosing, monitoring, and treating EDS, which leaves clinicians somewhat in the dark about maximizing care. This deficiency reflects the need for concerted research efforts and common guidelines to answer the urgent clinical needs of EDS management (Sulli et al., 2018). EDS will occasionally present with other autoimmune or inflammatory disorders, which only complicates matters when it comes to diagnosis and treatment. In many clinical reports, patients have had chronic inflammatory joint symptoms combined with the usual connective tissue peculiarity of EDS—occasionally even overlapping with disorders such as ankylosing spondylitis.

This overlap compels clinicians to think harder about identifying whether a symptom is due to collagen problems or immune-mediated inflammation, frequently requiring a cooperative, multidisciplinary assessment. Accurate patient history, meticulous physical examination that also considers joint looseness and cutaneous elasticity, and sensitive imaging techniques, are all relatively central to achieving an accurate diagnosis. These diagnostic difficulties highlight why it is essential for physicians to remember uncommon conditions such as EDS when they present with unusual cases of inflammatory arthritis (Demirtzoglou et al., 2020).

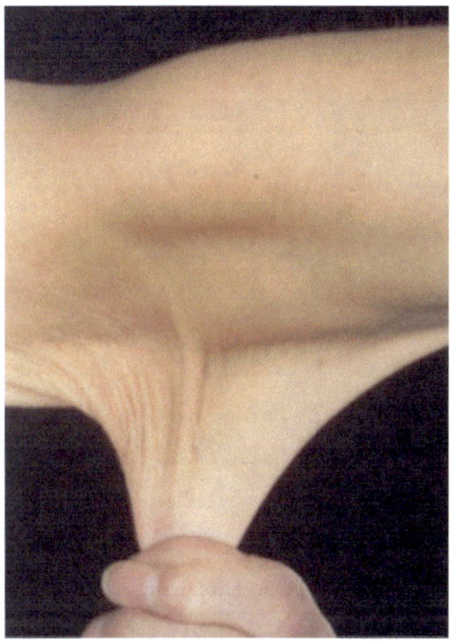

Figure 8.12. Individual with classical Ehlers-Danlos syndrome (EDS) displaying skin hyperelasticity.

Source: Whitaker, J. K., Alexander, P., Chau, D. Y., & Tint, N. L. (2012). Hyperelastic skin in a case of Ehlers-Danlos syndrome. *Wikimedia Commons*.

Understanding how EDS works within the general combination of autoimmune and connective tissue diseases is essential for advancing treatment options. Its characteristic features—hypermobile joints and fragile tissues, arise from genetic mutations that interfere with collagen synthesis, distinguishing it from diseases primarily caused by immune system malfunction. However, since some symptoms can resemble those seen in autoimmune diseases, it typically implies that we require more holistic research to explore both shared pathways and divergent differences. Such research could well reveal novel treatment targets and inform more tailored care plans. Briefly, the development of evidence-based standardized clinical guidelines, guided by genetic, molecular, and clinical information, is likely to be central to overcoming the numerous challenges EDS presents in routine clinical practice (Sulli et al., 2018) (Figure 8.12).

8.5. Diagnosis of Autoimmune and Connective Tissue Disorders

Autoimmune and connective tissue diseases are not easy; they can really throw a monkey wrench into the situation as far as diagnosis is concerned. Frequently, initial warning signs are so subtle that they pass unnoticed—minuscule interference in your capillaries may appear many years before any overt symptoms strike. Use SSc as a case in point: it likes to come along with preliminary vascular hiccups that high-tech imaging detects. Nailfold video capillaroscopy, for example, is a go-to tool for zooming in on capillary details and noticing strange patterns that suggest microangiopathy. This tiny modality does not simply sound impressive—it tends to tip off clinicians to possible issues far in advance of other symptoms, allowing them to intervene earlier. Other equipment, such as laser Doppler and thermography, also weigh in by monitoring blood flow in the margins, emphasizing just how central vascular tests are to the entire diagnostic picture (Pizzorni et al., 2016). Physicians still rely quite a bit on serological tests when unpicking these conditions; it is sort of the basis of the whole procedure. In most instances, autoantibodies like antinuclear antibodies (ANA), RF, or even the more condition-specific ones like anti-dsDNA, anti-Smith, and anti-centromere antibodies sort out if one can possibly have SLE, RA, or SSc. But, in general, these laboratory markers require a little context since their sensitivity and specificity are not always consistent. A combination of disease activity scores and imaging techniques—ultrasound or MRI, for instance, presents an added dimension of understanding by illustrating the way the tissues are performing. In a majority of cases, integrating clinical exams, serology, and contemporary imaging is what is propelling our methods of diagnosis toward increased accuracy and earlier detection (Fischer et al., 2019).

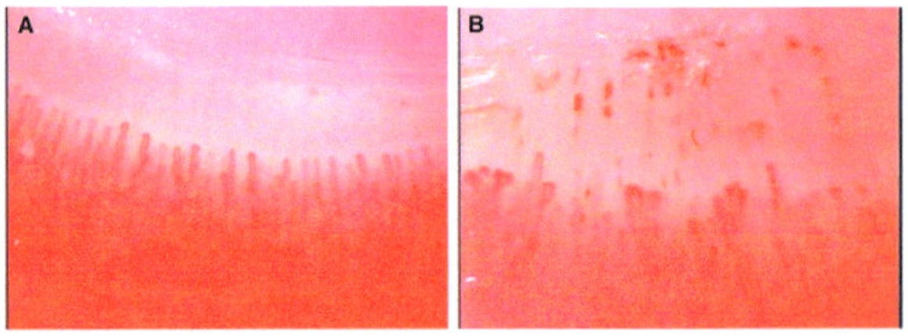

Figure 8.13. Different tools for nailfold capillaroscopic analysis.

Source: Kayser, C., Bredemeier, M., Caleiro, M.T. *et al.* Position article and guidelines 2018 recommendations of the Brazilian Society of Rheumatology for the indication, interpretation and performance of nailfold capillaroscopy. *Adv Rheumatol* **59**, 5 (2019). https://doi.org/10.1186/s42358-018-0046-4

Even with all these new-fangled tests and technology involved, still it is difficult to distinguish between overlapping autoimmune and connective tissue diseases. Most patients present with nonspecific symptoms and test results that are far from straightforward, which only clouds the issue in terms of early diagnosis. Most of the time, it requires a team effort and several check-ins to get the complete picture, combining the new insights of contemporary diagnostic equipment with the old clinical instincts physicians build up over decades. Researchers, meanwhile, are constantly refining biomarkers and imaging methods so that identification occurs earlier and treatments can be more precisely targeted. The entire diagnosis setting is, in a sense, in a state of constant flux as more is discovered about these clever disease processes and patterns of progression—emphasizing the importance of a flexible, whole-inclusive approach when assessing these complicated disorders (Pizzorni et al., 2016; Fishcher et al., 2019) (Figure 8.13).

8.5.1. Clinical Evaluation and History

A thorough assessment generally begins with hearing the patient's own history. If autoimmune or connective tissue problems are being considered, starting is with probing their background, asking them whether they have had joint pains, experienced unusual changes in their skin, been troubled by muscle fatigue, or suffered from breathing difficulty. More often than not, the patient may casually comment on a slow, insidious weakening of his or her ability to perform daily tasks or, on occasion, report on sudden flare-ups that tend to mimic other diseases. Investigating family history or any previous suggestions of immune mishaps tends to supply a helpful pinch of context. For instance, if respiratory problems develop, they may sometimes indicate interstitial lung issues, a common and troubling complication that stands to gain from early detection. In most cases, monitoring when the symptoms begin, how hard they hit, and where they occur can narrow down the list of suspects and guide further testing. To see a patient in person fills in gaps that written history cannot always fill. The physical examination may yield unmistakable signs—skin that is abnormally tight or red spots here and there, joints that look irritated, and muscles that are tender to the touch. Occasionally the physician may detect unusual sounds when listening to the lungs, such as faint crackles or evidence that indicates that the lungs are not as elastic as they must be, which may point to underlying respiratory involvement.

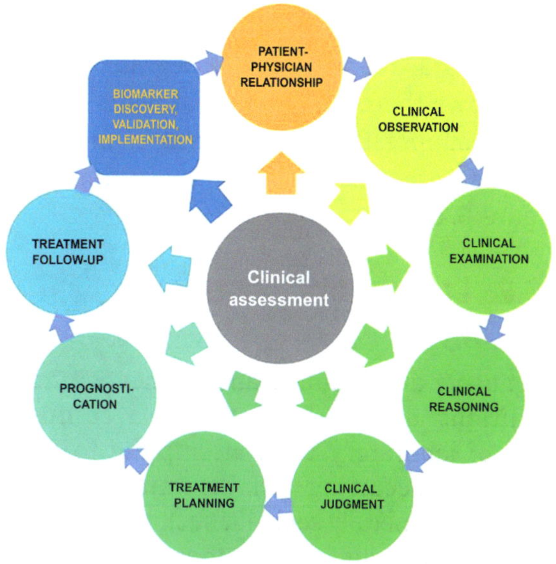

Figure 8.14. Clinical assessment.

Source: Chaudhuri, A., & Ghosh, S. (2023). Clinical assessment in the era of biomarkers. The Role of Clinical Assessment in the Era of Biomarkers. *Journal of Clinical Neuroscience*, *105*, 1–4.

In most instances, these palpable signs not only corroborate the history but also provide a way of measuring how far and quickly the disease is progressing. This exercise in hands-on verification usually triggers a domino effect, for example, arranging for high-tech imaging or other functional tests, to further pin down the diagnosis and make the next move. Diagnostic imaging has become an ally in this exercise. Lung ultrasounds and high-resolution CT scans now unmask subtle hints of interstitial lung issues that may be hiding with CTD. Studies usually reveal that lung ultrasound, which is a radiation-free tool, is nearly as keen as CT scans for detecting these lung problems (Koshy et al., 2023). Clinical trials, also, usually emphasize the importance of monitoring lung function closely, particularly when pulmonary fibrosis is involved (Toby et al., 2024). By bringing together these imaging findings with the history from the past and the results of the physical exam, physicians are left with an integrated picture that allows them to refine treatments such as immunosuppressive therapy and monitor how well the patient is doing on a real-time basis (Figure 8.14).

8.5.2. Laboratory Tests and Imaging

Diagnosing autoimmune and connective tissue conditions usually begins with a confusing array of laboratory tests attempting to figure out what is occurring with the immune system. Physicians generally seek out such things as ANA or RF – ubiquitous markers that suggest SLE or RA, for , – and subsequently include additional clues such as complement factors, C-reactive protein (CRP), and erythrocyte sedimentation rate (ESR) to assess inflammatory processes. Occasionally, more specific assays that test for autoantibodies, such as anti-double-stranded DNA or anti-Smith antibodies, enter the picture to refine the diagnosis. In all but the most unusual instances, all this testing coalesces somewhat indiscriminately to assist clinicians in sorting out overlapping symptoms and ultimately to develop a treatment plan directed against preventing permanent tissue damage. Imaging modalities also get into the act, hand-in-hand with laboratory tests, to provide a more complete picture of these diseases. For example, MRI scans are startlingly clear when looking at soft tissues, joints, and organs — often picking up early changes such as synovitis, erosions, or fibrosis that blood work alone may miss. Ultrasound, with its real-time feedback, not only detects joint inflammation but may even direct therapeutic injections. CT scans, on the other hand, come in handy when pulmonary or visceral involvement occurs – a situation not infrequently encountered in systemic autoimmune conditions. New developments have even started to reveal fairly specific signatures in glandular or exocrine tissues, and this helps increase diagnostic confidence a little more. These imaging findings mix loosely with laboratory findings to assist with monitoring disease course and treatment response.

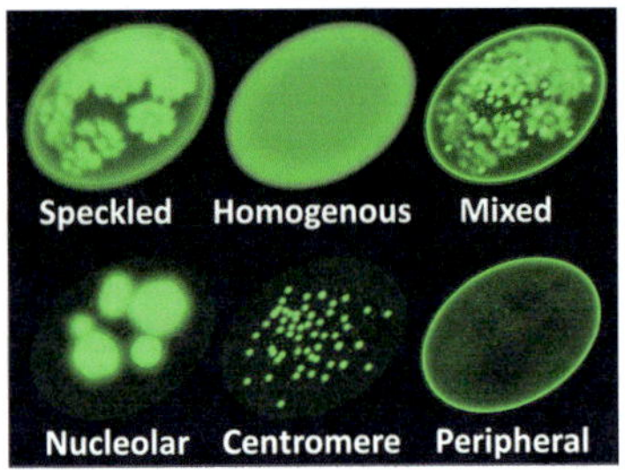

Figure 8.15. Main antinuclear antibody patterns on immunofluorescence.

Source: Al-Mughales JA (2022) Anti-Nuclear Antibodies Patterns in Patients With Systemic Lupus Erythematosus and Their Correlation With Other Diagnostic Immunological Parameters. Front. Immunol. 13:850759. doi: 10.3389/fimmu.2022.850759

When it comes to ailments affecting the salivary glands, the strategy is similarly complex. Conditions such as Sjögren's syndrome and immunoglobulin G4-related diseases illustrate just how unpredictable glandular injury can be when the immune system malfunctions. In these instances, more recent methods such as sialendoscopy, a minimally invasive procedure that looks inside the salivary ducts, bring a new light by uncovering glandular alterations probably linked to T-helper lymphocyte attacks (Vincentiis et al., 2017). Combining these imaging results with comprehensive antibody profiling assists in differentiating these diseases from other conditions. Even in research investigating disc disease, the pressure to associate radiological films with laboratory findings reinforces the necessity of a balanced approach in dealing with connective tissue disorders (Walker, 1993). Lab studies and imaging together create a kind of patchwork of hints that guides physicians through these tricky diagnoses (Figure 8.15).

8.5.3. Differential Diagnosis

Autoimmune and connective tissue diseases are very difficult to sort out since their manifestations overlap and several body systems are usually involved. Physicians frequently must reconstruct what is occurring by considering the patient's history, ordering a variety of laboratory tests, and even reviewing imaging studies – a real mess, . Consider, for instance, major salivary gland diseases. You may observe something such as Sjögren's syndrome appearing with gland swelling and dryness, while immunoglobulin G4-related sialadenitis, though similar at first glance, functions through quite distinct immune mishaps. In most instances, Sjögren's tends to target the exocrine ductal cells while IgG4-related cases find their way into the gland tissue itself. This is important because interventions like sialendoscopy , which are able to detect duct problems – end up not only diagnosing but also informing treatment decisions (Vincentiis et al., 2017). It is a challenging, complicated picture where the smallest pathogenic distinctions can flip the entire diagnosis on its head. And then there is SSc, where subtle changes in small blood vessels tend to provide the initial lead. In general, these microvascular changes appear long before fibrosis of the skin or other organ issues declare themselves. One useful gadget for this situation is nailfold video capillaroscopy, an innocuous test that peeking at capillary structures close to the nail bed – now and then uncovering faint evidence of progressing microangiopathy. Other methods such as laser Doppler flowmetry and thermography are used to quantify blood flow abnormalities, providing additional levels of proof when physicians attempt to differentiate these ailments from, for example, lupus or dermatomyositis, which, at times, simply do not present these vascular pictures (Pizzorni et al., 2016). Essentially, early detection of microvascular damage can literally be a lifesaver in putting the correct diagnosis and treatment into action. On top of all this, ensuring that you are not mixing up these disorders with other diseases is important to prevent misdiagnosis and inappropriate treatments. Often times, nonspecific symptomatology such as fatigue, joint pains, and rashes make autoimmune, infectious, or even drug-related issues ambiguous. That is where a personal history, some serological markers, and occasionally even a tissue biopsy are put into action. For instance, the presence of increased amounts of immunoglobulin G4 along with characteristic tissue alterations suggests IgG4-related disease, which is distinct from what we would anticipate in typical autoimmune salivary gland diseases (Vincentiis et al., 2017). In the same manner, the identification of characteristic autoantibodies can distinguish SSc from mixed CTD or overlapping syndromes. All in all, combining new diagnostic tests with good clinical judgment truly assists clinicians in getting a grip on these complex cases, guiding both prognosis and treatment in the proper direction.

8.6. Treatment Options

Autoimmune and connective tissue diseases toss so many curveballs—each one appears to require its own special repair. Immunosuppressant medication remains first choice, but when more than one organ is involved, treatment usually must shift. For example, lung complications such as bronchiolar or small airway disease arise all the time in systemic autoimmune disorders, so physicians must sometimes shift into high gear and employ steroids in combination with other immune-modulating drugs to quell inflammation and prevent additional damage. Pulmonary function tests and high-resolution imaging have, for the most part, facilitated the early identification of these complications, allowing for more focused treatment. Briefly, understanding how these conditions impact individual organs is key to designing a plan that walks the line between immune suppression and staying away from too many side effects, ultimately with the goal of enhancing patient outcomes (Kluanwan et al., 2025). As regards skin issues associated with systemic autoimmune connective tissue disease, the treatment landscape has definitely changed. Take cutaneous lupus for instance, it solidly demonstrates that at times you do require both a local touch and more of a general, systemic touch depending on whether the symptoms are severe or far-reaching. Treatment typically begins with corticosteroids and calcineurin inhibitors that act exactly where they are applied; but as things get more difficult or are more extensive, antimalarials and other immunosuppressants are more likely to enter the picture. More recently, there has been quite a lot of interest in niacinamide as a topical added treatment—its anti-inflammatory benefits and reasonable safety profile make it an intelligent addition to usual therapies. Some studies even indicate a 4% niacinamide gel as a combination with systemic corticosteroids and hydroxychloroquine providing definite improvements in lesion resolution, and all of this without too many unpleasant surprises (Yuniaswan et al., 2024). Taking a step back, it is obvious that treating CTDs and autoimmune diseases essentially involves adapting the treatment to the individual's needs, a combination of old and new. Biological drugs that specifically attack specific areas of the immune system have been promising for those with recalcitrant cases, but factors like cost and availability can sometimes get in the way. Many times, patient-centered care also introduces interventions like physical therapy and lifestyle modifications to reduce joint and muscle pain, as well as improve quality of life. As these diseases tend to be chronic, monitoring closely the progress of treatments, and being on the lookout for problems related to long-term immune suppression, is wholly essential. In general, combining symptom management with clever immune adjusting and supportive treatment makes a good plan; continued research into safer alternatives, such as niacinamide, appears to refine patient outcomes across these diverse disorders further (Yuniaswan et al., 2024; Kluanwan et al., 2025).

8.6.1. Pharmacological Interventions

Autoimmune and connective tissue diseases continue to rely heavily on the authority of drugs to soothe inflammation and rein in an untamed immune system. Corticosteroids, as well as disease-modifying medications (DMARDs), are frequently the first choice when it comes to alleviating symptoms and reducing disease propagation. Simply put, these therapies accomplish this by disrupting the chain reaction of autoimmunity—reducing tissue damage and allowing individuals a little more function. Biologic treatments have also entered the scene of late, employing agents such as TNF inhibitors and interleukin blockers to eliminate those pesky cytokines. All the same, while these meds can be a real lifesaver, they carry risks and need close supervision because they can sometimes shut down the entire immune system. Couple these drugs with hands-on patient care, however, and the quality of life overall typically gets a definite lift, which really solidifies their place in modern therapy. It is not even about modulating the immune system, either—drugs now must deal with a whole host of secondary problems that appear with CTDs. There is frequently heart or kidney involvement that requires special measures; for instance, antihypertensive medications and lipid-lowering agents are sometimes added to the regimen to protect certain organs. And then, for addressing problems such as nagging pain and perpetual exhaustion, painkillers or even neuromodulators could be included in the regimen. By and large, emerging knowledge is that these drug regimens need not be taken in isolation but should be integrated with modifications in lifestyle—because our routine habits can change inflammatory behavior and alter how the disease progresses (Bhanusali, 2025). Ultimately, it is about creating a treatment plan in which medications are the foundation, but where nutrition, exercise, and even mood factors enter in, resulting in a more holistic, if sometimes all-over-the-map, regimen.

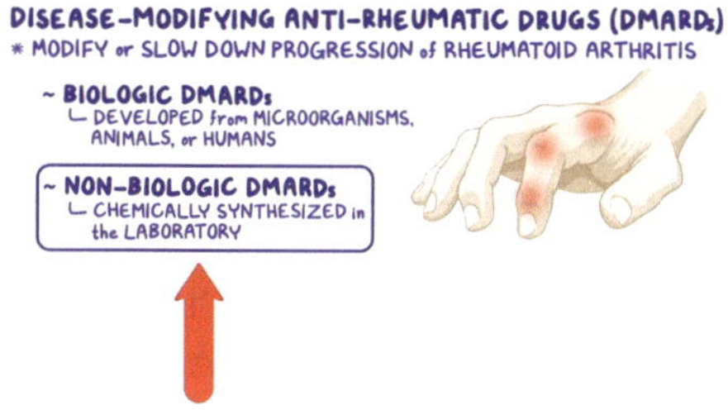

Figure 8.16. Disease-modifying meds (DMARDs).

Source: Osmosis. (n.d.). *Photograph of a Medical Condition or Procedure*. https://www.osmosis.org/_next/image?url=https%3A%2F%2Fd16qt3wv6xm098.cloudfront.net%2FBvElp9ZkTXC65Wv4xM6bdnJFRXaUzs3d%2F_.jpg&w=3840&q=75.

Sleep issues, that tend to go unreported, can wreak havoc on patients' overall health in these diseases. Certain medications intended to improve the quality of sleep, such as sedative-hypnotics and drugs that modulate pro-inflammatory markers—have proven effective in interrupting the cycle of poor sleep leading to worse symptoms (Cholerzy et al., 2024). In certain instances, by reducing inflammation, these therapies also stabilize sleep patterns, providing a dual advantage. And, topping it all off, combining these drug strategies with non-drug methods, such as a cocktail of cognitive behavioral therapy, gives the outcomes that much more bang. Put together, our expanding knowledge of how sleep and inflammation intersect truly emphasizes the need for treatment strategies that are as individualized as they are multi-pronged, even if that strategy sometimes seems a little sloppy or unorthodox (Figure 8.16).

8.6.2. Lifestyle Modifications

Managing autoimmune and connective tissue disorders is not just about medications—there is a whole lifestyle angle to consider. Many patients notice that everyday environmental exposures and behaviors can, in most cases, make their symptoms flare up unexpectedly. For example, people with Raynaud's sometimes find that even a bit of chill or a bout of emotional stress triggers a sudden tightening of their blood vessels, which only makes everything worse. Giving up smoking, therefore, is not so much an option because tobacco consumption increases inflammation and disrupts blood flow. Warming up your extremities—i.e., by selecting appropriate attire and attempting some stress-reduction hacks—can also help keep the symptoms at bay. These simple, non-pharmacologic measures do more than improve quality of life; they also appear to reduce those unexpected acute exacerbations, supporting the importance of individualized patient education and frequent follow-ups to maintain the disease in a stable condition in the long term (Bellando-Randone et al., 2018). Diet and physical activity also have a leading role in slowing down disease progression. In general, a diet rich in anti-inflammatory nutrients—omega-3 fatty acids, antioxidants, fiber—may be able to damp down the body's overall inflammatory response and modulate the immune system. Meanwhile, low-impact activities such as gentle walking or stretching can facilitate joint mobility, reduce fatigue, and even provide a mood boost without revving up autoimmune activity. Exercising at varying levels in response to how bad symptoms are at the time serves to protect against overexertion or injury, and maintaining a healthy weight can minimize joint wear and tear. Transferring these habits into daily life usually requires a collaborative effort from many healthcare professionals and a healthy dose of personal drive, which truly emphasizes the holistic approach to dealing with connective tissue problems and other such conditions. Exceptional cases, such as mixed CTD, introduce an additional level of complexity where lifestyle adjustments gain additional significance. Being vigilant about changes in symptoms, and combining that vigilance with routine lifestyle control—can enhance the impact of pharmacologic interventions against entailing problems such as vasculitis, dermatoses, or chronic, resistant ulcers. Here, measures such as de-stressing, being careful about temperature fluctuations, and following a sound skincare routine complement medicines in furthering healing and inhibiting further damage. A multidisciplinary method that relies on continuous patient education is likely to enhance adherence and outcome, especially where conventional treatments often fail due to side effects or random fluctuations of the disease (Pritam et al., 2024). Lifestyle changes represent an essential added measure in enhancing the prognosis and day-to-day quality of life for individuals with the challenges of autoimmune and connective tissue disorders.

8.6.3. Emerging Therapies and Research

Recent advances in understanding autoimmune and connective tissue conditions have revealed some new treatment concepts that could really revolutionize the game. Now, individuals are exploring how to calibrate the immune system, essentially, employing drugs that subtly modulate its overactivity instead of controling it with broad, systemic impacts. For example, biological therapies that target particular cytokines or immune cells appear to reduce unwanted side effects from the more traditional methods. Identifying small clinical clues, such as slight changes in the mouth, often allows physicians to get in early before any permanent damage sets in. And when experts such as dentists, rheumatologists, and immunologists are combined in patient treatment, it truly highlights how it is all about teamwork (Saccucci et al., 2018). The quest for biomarkers that indicate disease activity and treatment response is gradually making personalized medicine a tangible reality. Uncommon disorders like Stiff Skin Syndrome place such developments in stark contrast, highlighting the fact that exploring molecular intricacies can reveal what is causing the disease. Scientists have been investigating genetic and epigenetic profiling and discovered the unusual signaling pathways that culminate in fibrosis and stiffness. Such discoveries have, in fact, prompted the creation of new drugs that would modify the accumulation of extracellular matrix and suppress inflammation. Preclinical models, while occasionally a little fickle, are now allowing researchers to screen these molecules more quickly, bridging the gap to the clinic. It is also becoming evident that combining rehabilitative methods with drug therapy is crucial for maintaining mobility and quality of life, once again highlighting the importance of an interprofessional approach to address both the structural and functional issues of these diseases (Sánchez et al., 2023). In the future, the landscape of treating autoimmune and connective tissue diseases is being redefined by the promise of regenerative medicine and precision immunotherapy. Stem cell therapies and engineered tissues promise to repair damaged organs and even reverse fibrosis, with the potential for long-term remission or even a cure. Meanwhile, emerging genomic sequencing and bioinformatics technologies are making it simpler to identify patient-specific autoantigens and immune profiles, leading the way towards personalized therapies tailored to the unique condition of each individual. Most significantly, clinical trials are already transforming cancer therapy such as checkpoint inhibitors and CAR T-cell therapies for these conditions, with preliminary results that are quite promising. (Saccucci et al., 2018; Sánchez et al., 2023).

CLOSER LOOK

Antinuclear Antibodies (ANAs)

ANAs are autoantibodies that bind to the nucleus of the cell. Although they occur in most healthy persons in low titers, increased levels may indicate an autoimmune disease. ANA testing is employed to aid in the diagnosis of autoimmune disorders, especially CTD such as SLE.

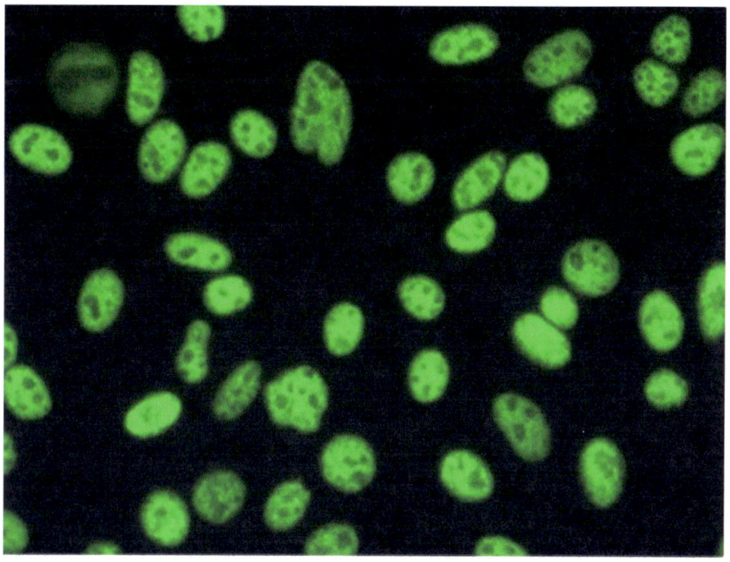

Source: Centers for Disease Control and Prevention. (2019). Photograph of a Public Health Topic. Centers for Disease Control and Prevention. https://d2jx2rerrg6sh3.cloudfront.net/image-handler/picture/2019/5/CDCimage2.jpg.

- **What Are ANAs?**
  - **Autoantibodies:** ANAs are autoantibodies created by the immune system that erroneously attack the body's own tissues, namely the nucleus of cells.
  - **Target:** The nucleus houses the cell's DNA and other vital elements, and hence it is a prime target for these antibodies.
  - **Prevalence:** ANAs occur in a large percentage of the general population, but increased levels correlate with autoimmune diseases.
- **Why Are ANA Tests Done?**
  - **Diagnosis:** Autoimmune disorders like CTD such as SLE, Sjogren's syndrome, and scleroderma are diagnosed using ANA tests.
  - **Screening:** The test may be utilized to screen for the diseases, particularly in patients presenting with symptoms such as unexplained arthritis, rash, or fever.
  - **Follow-Up**: A positive ANA result can prompt additional testing, such as an ENA panel, to determine which specific antibodies are present and what underlying autoimmune disorder.

- **What does a positive ANA test indicate?**
  - **Autoantibodies Present:** A positive test for ANA is a sign that ANAs exist in the blood but not necessarily a sign of any specific autoimmune disease.
  - **Additional Testing:** An ANA positive test might necessitate additional tests, like an ENA panel, to define the nature of the autoantibody and the associated disease.
  - **No specific Treatme**nt: No specific treatment is available for a positive ANA test per se, because it is not a diagnosis. (Ralli et al., 2018)

SUMMARY

Autoimmune and connective tissue problems are problematic, and comprehending them requires examining their dissemination, how they manifest, and the difficulties in managing them. Once, people believed these ailments were rare among certain populations, particularly among African blacks—but what has been seen at the University of Port-Harcourt Teaching Hospital is different. Many of the cases, especially SLE, take a toll on young women. Better diagnostic techniques and a more vigilant clinical style appear to be part of the explanation for this change, and age, gender, and ethnicity continue to surface as significant leads (Mercy et al., 2016). This new image pushes us to re-think old presumptions and realign the way we spend resources in zones that may have been ignored. Pregnancy brings an additional complication for women with these connective tissue issues, adding additional risk to mother and baby. Research from obstetrics and rheumatology departments—reviewing previous cases—indicates increased miscarriage, stillbirth, and cesarean rates in affected women. Babies often end up with problems such as growth restriction or even being in intensive care, which makes handling these cases especially challenging. These findings reveal that the effects of these conditions extend beyond overall symptoms, to affect reproductive health in unforeseen manners. Awareness of these risks promotes earlier surveillance, cooperation between experts, and more realistic patient counseling during pregnancy (Jha & Chaudhari, 2020). These findings indicate a call for further specific research and new care protocols that specifically concern pregnancy within CTDs. When you take a step back and view it all, the evolving landscape surrounding autoimmune and connective tissue diseases requires a wide, flexible response. Identifying a greater number of cases among varied groups contradicts outdated concepts and puts forward a strong argument for early identification and culturally appropriate treatment. The additional complexities observed in pregnancy truly underscore the need for specialized care that is tailored to meet the individual needs of such patients. In the future, longer follow-up studies and greater collaboration among disparate medical fields could prove to be just what is required to identify and mitigate the heavy burden of such diseases. By combining experiential clinical wisdom with deliberate public health actions, our medical community can have a tangible impact on enhancing lives and closing care gaps (Mercy et al., 2016; Jha & Chaudhari, 2020).

Autoimmune and connective tissue disorders are often quite baffling—those conditions get the body's normal defense tricks turned around and confound it to attack its own tissues. In most situations, the immune system is "baffled" and begins to attack healthy tissue, and then this triggers constant inflammation and gradual damage to tissues. Consider Sjögren's syndrome as a case in point; in this case, T-helper lymphocytes appear to target the salivary gland ducts, commonly leaving patients with a chronically dry mouth. Recently, we have also observed that diseases associated with immunoglobulin G4, in the majority of instances, redefine our concept of such diseases by targeting multiple organs, including salivary glands. New technologies, sialendoscopy, for example, have transformed the way we detect and treat these conditions without anyone even noticing, requiring extensive lab tests and pathology examinations (Vincentiis et al., 2017). It is an arena that never stands still, as practice and research move with these breakthroughs. The psychological aspect of these disorders certainly makes it more difficult, as well. The development of autoimmune diseases not only disrupts bodily well-being, but it also has the tendency to become a mental burden. In broad terms, when outside pressures such as the COVID-19 pandemic strike, a great number of patients afflicted by these diseases are left dealing with added stress and issues like PTSD. Research hints that people with connective tissue problems may be extra vulnerable to stress-related issues, underscoring that our immune responses and mental resilience are closely wedded sometimes in unexpected ways. This overlap makes it pretty clear that treatment cannot just be about managing physical symptoms; mental health really deserves its own attention as part of a complete care plan (Carmassi et al., 2024). All of these findings collectively demonstrate that autoimmune and connective tissue disorders are far from simple. They are characterized by inappropriately directed immune activity, an enormous variety of clinical symptoms, and a significant influence on an individual's emotional existence. New emergent groupings such as immunoglobulin G4-related diseases refine our general map of diagnoses and guide more targeted treatments. Concurrently, observing how psychological issues, particularly during high-stress times such as pandemics—can exacerbate overall circumstances encourages us towards more multidisciplinary treatment. An integrated treatment plan should accomplish more than simply suppress immune hyperresponsiveness; it also must take mental health care into account to truly enhance patient outcomes. Combining these concepts opens the door for improved clinical approaches and more holistic care (Vincentiis et al., 2017; Carmassi et al., 2024).

KEY TERMS FROM THIS CHAPTER

- atherosclerosis
- autoantibody
- autoimmunity
- back pain
- breast implants
- cardiovascular diseases
- cohorts
- Congenital heart block
- Connective tissue disorders
- cytokines
- defense system
- endothelial hiccups
- fibroblasts
- fibrocartilaginous entheses
- fibrosis
- immune system
- immunopathology
- immunosuppressive therapy
- infections
- MRI images
- painkillers
- pregnancy
- rheumatoid arthritis
- risk assessment
- self-tolerance
- Silicone breast implants
- Sjogren's syndrome
- spines

REFERENCES

1. Angelis, R. D. (2019). A practical overview of the role of capillaroscopy in rheumatic diseases. Journal of Autoimmune Diseases and Rheumatology, 2019, 7, 1-8. https://core.ac.uk/download/267929271.pdf (accessed on 12 May 2025).

2. Bellando-Randone, S., Kahaleh, B., Matucci-Cerinic, C., Nagaraja, et al. (2018). The role of the dermatologist in Raynaud's phenomenon: A clinical challenge. Journal of Dermatology, 14914. http://deepblue.lib.umich.edu/bitstream/2027.42/144681/1/jdv14914_am.pdf (accessed on 12 May 2025).

3. Bhanusali N. (2025). Leveraging Lifestyle Medicine for Better Outcomes in Connective Tissue Diseases. American journal of lifestyle medicine, 15598276251329923. Advance online publication. https://doi.org/10.1177/15598276251329923 (accessed on 12 May 2025).

4. Carmassi, C., Tani, C., Lorenzoni, V., Palla, I., Fulvio, G., Fantasia, S., Andreozzi, G., Trentin, F., Conti, L., Gaglioti, A., Turchetti, G., Dell'Osso, L., & Mosca, M. (2024). Post-traumatic stress disorder and post-traumatic stress symptoms in patients with systemic autoimmune diseases during the COVID-19 pandemic. Clinical and experimental rheumatology, 42(5), 1075–1082. https://doi.org/10.55563/clinexprheumatol/rnm6tz (accessed on 12 May 2025).

5. Chaudhari Wang, Y., Chen, S., Zheng, S., Zhou, Z., Zhang, W., Du, G., Mikish, A., Ruaro, B., Bruni, C., Hoffmann-Vold, A. M., Gargani, L., Matucci-Cerinic, M., & Furst, D. E. (2024). A versatile role for lung ultrasound in systemic autoimmune rheumatic diseases related pulmonary involvement: a narrative review. Arthritis research & therapy, 26(1), 164. https://doi.org/10.1186/s13075-024-03399-2 (accessed on 12 May 2025).

6. Cholerzyńska, H., Zasada, W., Tselios, K., & Grygiel-Górniak, B. (2024). Sleep disorders in connective tissue diseases—Coexisting diseases or disease components? Journal of Clinical Medicine, 13. https://www.semanticscholar.org/paper/26275d46541cd50fcc75799a890a0aff7353ddb1 (accessed on 12 May 2025).

7. DeNisco, S. M., & Ferro, L. (2004). Sjogren's syndrome: Recognizing and treating an autoimmune disease. https://core.ac.uk/download/231072559.pdf (accessed on 12 May 2025).

8. Derk, C. T., & Jimenez, S. A. (2006). Statins and the vasculopathy of systemic sclerosis: potential therapeutic agents?. *Autoimmunity reviews*, 5(1), 25–32. https://doi.org/10.1016/j.autrev.2005.06.010 (accessed on 12 May 2025).

9. Fischer, A., Strek, M. E., Cottin, V., Dellaripa, P. F., Bernstein, E. J., Brown, K. K., Danoff, S. K., Distler, O., Hirani, N., Jones, K. D., Khanna, D., Lee, J. S., Lynch, D. A., Maher, T. M., Millar, A. B., Raghu, G., Silver, R. M., Steen, V. D., Volkmann, E. R., Mullan, R. H., ... Donnelly, S. C. (2019). Proceedings of the American College of Rheumatology/Association of Physicians of Great Britain and Ireland Connective Tissue Disease-Associated Interstitial Lung Disease Summit: A Multidisciplinary Approach to Address Challenges and Opportunities. Arthritis & rheumatology (Hoboken, N.J.), 71(2), 182–195. https://doi.org/10.1002/art.40769 (accessed on 12 May 2025).

10. Gallo, A., Martellucci, S., Fusconi, M., Pagliuca, G., Greco, A., De Virgilio, A., & De Vincentiis, M. (2017). Sialendoscopic management of autoimmune sialadenitis: a review of literature. Trattamento scialendoscopico delle scialoadeniti autoimmuni: revisione della letteratura. Acta otorhinolaryngologica Italica : organo ufficiale della Societa italiana di otorinolaringologia e chirurgia cervico-facciale, 37(2), 148–154. https://doi.org/10.14639/0392-100X-1605

11. Georgios Demirtzoglou, Evangelos Theodorou, Anastasia Klagou, Nikolaos Zervos, Efstathios Ampatziadis (2020). Ankylosing spondylitis in a 33-year-old man with hypermobility joints. DOI: https://doi.org/10.26262/abj.v2i2.7697 (accessed on 12 May 2025).

12. Gichuru, T. *W., Raj, R., & Gorantla, V. (2024).* Connective tissue and autoimmune diseases associated with postsurgical breast augmentation: An updated review. Cureus, 16. https://www.semanticscholar.org/paper/662b3964c8eec1ec3684513d0fcd0846dfa4a3a5 (accessed on 12 May 2025).

13. Jha, N., & Chaudhari, H. K. (2020). Connective tissue disorders in pregnancy: maternal and fetal perspective. International Journal of Reproduction, Contra*ception, Obstetrics and Gyneco*lo*gy*, 9(3), 1124–1131. https://doi.org/10.18203/2320-1770.ijrcog20200887

14. Kawałko, K., Rynio, G., Pondel, K., Karaś, A., Bielewicz, K., & Sufin, P. (2022). Effects of autoimmune disorders on daily *lifestyle. Journal of Education, Health and Sport, 12(12), 242–247. https://do*i.org/10.12775/JEHS.2022.12.12.038 (accessed on 12 May 2025).

15. Kingman, J., Uitto, J., & Li, Q. (2017). Elevated dietary magnesium during pregnancy and postnatal life prevents ectopic mineralization in Enpp1asj mice, a model for ge*neralized arterial calcification* of infancy. Oncotarget, 8(24), 38152–38160. https://doi.org/10.18632/oncotarget.16687 (accessed on 12 May 2025).

16. Kluanwan, Y., Tangnuntachai, N., Ryu, J. H., & Moua, T. (2025). Bronchiolar disorders in systemic autoimmune rheumatic diseases. European Respiratory Review, 34. https://*www.semanticscholar.org/paper/0*f5*c25e*ef79757f1fcc79fe0d9ac59c7bd07a5b2 (accessed on 12 May 2025).

17. Koshy, V., Patel, K., Yadav, D., Saxena, P., George, R., Gangadharan, V., & Koshy, G. (2023). Descriptive study of the role of ultrasound in the evaluation of patients with interstitial lung disease associated with autoimmune co*nnective tissue disorders. In*d*ian* Journal of Rheumatology, 18, 48–53. https://www.semanticscholar.org/paper/81cd6aca3cc4499f213d59298b546e38c61779ee (accessed on 12 May 2025).

18. Kuchcinski, G., Rumetshofer, T., Zervides, K., Lopes, R., Gautherot, M., Pruvo, J., Bengtsson, A., et al. (2023). MRI BrainAGE demonstrates increased brain aging in systemic *lupus erythematosus patients. Frontiers in Aging Neuroscience, 15. https://www.semanticscholar.org/paper/b5fe37be94372cd12e255f*b0*f*487d5ee608867aa (accessed on 12 May 2025).

19. Kurki, M., Karjalainen, J., Palta, P., Sipilä, T. P., Kristiansson, K., Donner, K., Reeve, M. P., et al. (2023). FinnGen provides genetic insights from a well-phenotyped isolated population. Nature, 613, 508–518. https://doi.org/10.1038/s41586-022-05473-8.

20. Kuwana, M., Gil-Vila, A., & Selva-O'Callaghan, A. *(2021). Role of aut*o*ant*ibodies in the diagnosis and prognosis of interstitial lung disease in autoimmune rheumatic disorders. Therapeutic advances in musculoskeletal disease, 13, 1759720X211032457. https://doi.org/10.1177/1759720X211032457 (acc*essed on 12 May 2025).*

*21. Liu, K., Li, X., & Li, D. (2024). Connective tissue diseas*e *a*s a challenge in heart failure: Three case reports. Medicine, 103. https://www.semanticscholar.org/paper/3c53968b71b9e195cbbfe8dc068908f21e858d73 (accessed on 12 May 2025).

22. Maher, T. M., Tudor, V. A., Saunders, P., Zanghelini, F., Grossi Sampedro, C., X*ydopoulos,* G., Gibbons, M., Fletcher, S. V., Denton, C. P., Kokosi, M., Hoyles, R. K., Parfrey, H., Renzoni, E. A., Wells, A. U., Ashby, D., Fordham, R. J., Szigeti, M., & Molyneaux, P. L. (2024). Rituximab

compared to intravenous cyclophosphamide in adults with connective tis*sue disease-associated interstitial lung diseas*e: the RECITAL RCT. National Institute for Health and Care Research. (accessed on 12 May 2025).

23. Mercy, E., Altraide, D. & Otike-Odibi, B. (2016). Profile of autoimmune connective tissue disorders in the University of Port Harcourt Teaching Hospital, Port Harcourt, Nigeria. Profile of Autoimmune *Connectiv*e *T*issue Disorders in the University of Port Harcourt Teaching Hospital, Port Harcourt, Nigeria. The Nig Health J [Internet]. 2016 Apr. 10 [cited 2025 Jun. 13];15(2):39. Available from: https://tnhjph.com/index.php/tnhj/*article/view/206(accessed on 12* May 2025).

24. Mofors, J., Eliasson, H., Ambrosi, A., Salomonsson, S., Skog, A., Fored, M., Ekbom, A., et al. (2019). Comorbidity and long-term outcome in patients with congenital heart block and their siblings exposed to Ro/SSA autoantibodies in utero. Annals of the Rheumatic Diseases, 78(5), 696–703. https://www.semanticscholar.org/paper/50e13ecd76d48dad54088f70*c034 72a7b9ebccc5 (accessed on 12 M*ay 2025).

25. Mofors, Johannes (2021). Risk factors and comorbidity in primary Sjögren's syndrome. Karolinska Institutet. Thesis. https://hdl.handle.net/10616/47625 (accessed on 12 May 2025).

26. Nannaware, D., Kamath , A., Gangane, N., & Yadav, A. (2023). Navigating mixed connective tissue disease in pregnancy: a rare case r*eport. International Journal of Rep*roduction, Contraception, Obstetrics and Gynecology, 12(12), 3683–3686. https://doi.org/10.18203/2320-1770.ijrcog20233658 (accessed on 12 May 2025).

27. Olivia Feuchter Ruy Sánchez, Pablo Fernando Monroy Ramirez, María Fernanda Briseño Ramos, María Fernanda Salazar Baez, & Keren Vazquez Ballesteros. *(2023). Stiff* Skin Syndrome: Clinical Exploration, Pathophysiology and Therapeutic Advances in a Rare Connective Tissue Disease. International Journal of Medical Science and Clinic*al Research S*tudies, 3(9), 1998–2001. https://doi.org/10.47191/ijmscrs/v3-i9-36 (accessed on 12 May 2025).

28. Oreska, S., & Tomcik, M. (2020). Atherosclerosis in Rheumatology: Old and New Insights. IntechOpen. doi: 10.5772/intechopen.88605(accessed on 12 May 2025).

29. Owen, Hannah L., "A Review of Ankylosing Spondylitis" (2017). Senior Honors Theses. 719. https://digitalcommons.liberty.edu/honors/719 *(accessed on 12 May 2025).*

30. Pizzorni, C., Sulli, A., Smith, V., Lladó, A., Paolino, S., Cutolo, M., & Ruaro, B. (2016). Capillaroscopy 2016: new perspectives in systemic sclerosis. Capillaroscopy 2016: new perspectives in systemic sclerosis. Acta reumatologica portuguesa, 41(1), 8–14. (accessed on 12 May 2025).

31. Pritam, J. S., Saranya, C., & Kannan, R. (2024). Mixed Connective Tissue Disease Presenting as Diabetic Ulcer in a 52 Year Old Female Patient: A Case Report . South Eastern European Journal of Public Health, 1585–1589. https://doi.org/10.70135/seejph.vi.2157 (accessed on 12 May 2025).

32. Ralli, M., D'Aguanno, V., Di Stadio, A., *De Virgilio, A., Croce, A., Longo,* L., Greco, A., & de Vincentiis, M. (2018). Audiovestibular Symptoms in Systemic Autoimmune Diseases. Journal of immunology research, 2018, 5798103. https://doi.org/10.1155/2018/5798103(accessed on 12 May 2025).

33. Saccucci, M., Di Carlo, G., Bossù, M., Giovarruscio, F., Salucci, A., & Polimeni, A. (2018). Autoimmune Diseases and Their Mani*festations on Oral C*avity: Diagnosis and Clinical Management. Journal of immunology research, 2018, 6061825. https://doi.org/10.1155/2018/6061825 (accessed on 12 May 2025).

34. Seida, I., Alrais, M., Seida, R., Alwani, A., Kiyak, Z., Elsalti, A., Nil Esirgun, S., Abali, T., & Mahroum, N. (2023). Autoimmune/inflam*matory syndrome induced by adju*vants (ASIA): past, present, and future implications. Clinical and experimental immunology, 213(1), 87–101. https://doi.org/10.1093/cei/uxad033 (accessed on 12 May 2025).

35. Stein, T., Cieplewicz-Guźla, P., Iżykowska, K., Pieniawska, M., Żaba, R., Dańczak-Pazdrowska, A., & Polańska, A. (2024). What is new in morphea—Narrative review on molecular aspects and new t*argeted therapies. Jou*rnal of Clinical Medicine, 13. https://www.semanticscholar.org/paper/90e3800dbff6d8ee33d9a9da4cea4e102b2284e2 (accessed on 12 May 2025).

36. Sulli, A., Talarico, R., Scirè, C. A., Avcin, T., Castori, M., Ferraris, A., Frank, C., Grunert, J., Paolino, S., Bombardieri, S., Schneider, M., Smith, V., Cutolo, M., Mosca, M., & Malf*ait, F. (2018). Ehlers-Danlos syndromes: state of the art on clinical* practice guidelines. RMD open, 4(Suppl 1), e000790. https://doi.org/10.1136/rmdopen-2018-000790 (accessed on 12 May 2025).

37. Walker, B. F. (1993). Disc disease: A summary and review. COMSIG Review, 2(2), 38–44. https://researchportal.murdoch.edu.au/esploro/outputs/jo*urnalArticle/Disc-disease-A-summary-and-review/9910*055432706078 91#file-0

38. Yuniaswan, A. P., & Sugiatno, B. B. (2024). The effectiveness of 4% niacinamide in a case of cutaneous lupus. Jurnal Ilmiah Ke*dokteran Wija*ya Kusuma. https://www.semanticscholar.org/paper/9152877bb6400721abf554f025ef5f4e7953aa54 (accessed on 12 May 2025).

39. Zhang, Y., Bermudez, N., Sa, B., Maderal, A., & Jimenez, J. J. (2023). Epigenetic mechanisms driving the pathogenesis of systemic lupus erythematosus, systemic scler*osis, and dermatomyositis. Experiment*al Dermatology, 33. https://www.semanticscholar.org/paper/607f4354a946127113ebec16e9db961f021d959d (accessed on 12 May 2025).

40. Štorkánová, H., Oreská, S., Špiritović, M., Heřmánková, B., Bubová, K., Komarc, M., Pavelká, K., et al. (2021). Plasma Hsp90 levels in patients with systemic sclerosis and re*lation to lung and skin inv*olvement: A cross-sectional and longitudinal study. Scientific Reports, 11. https://doi.org/10.1038/s41598-020-79139-8.

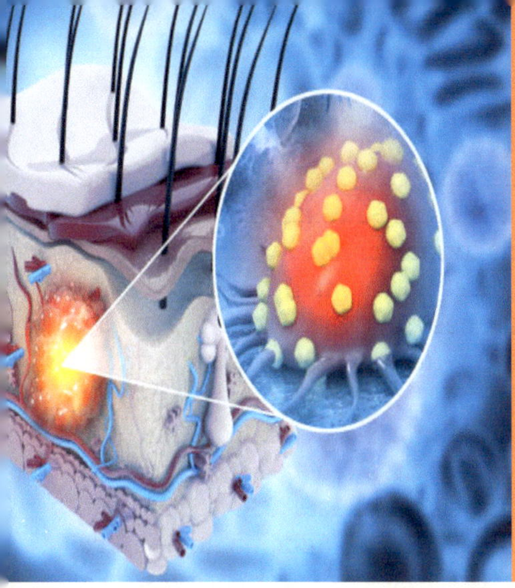

Chapter 9

SKIN TUMORS AND MALIGNANCIES

Contents

Introduction

Cellular transformation tends to create a transition from benign to malignant in mechanisms that make skin tumors a very mystifying problem. You see, various types of skin cells just begin behaving badly all of a sudden—growing sometimes almost at a relaxed tempo, while other times exploding into full-grown malignant cancers with speed. Gene mutations and not-always-apparent epigenetic changes collaborate to get these cells off the track. In general, it is not a single step but an entire play: regulators such as protein arginine methyltransferases appear to be among the essential actors in instructing cells to divide or to avoid dying. This understanding, in most instances, allows scientists to identify new avenues for treating these tumors apart from conventional approaches (Karner et al., 2023). Despite all the innovation in contemporary technology, skin tumors and cancers continue to rise in quantities across the world. The effect is massive—medical facilities are struggling not just with more difficult diagnoses and treatments but also with the continually increasing financial burden. Immunotherapy, for example, is a new strategy unfolding as a promising approach that utilizes the body's own immune system to combat cancer. Cancers that are targeted by checkpoints like PD-1/PD-L1, for instance, have demonstrated improved survival and, arguably, reduced toxicity compared to traditional chemotherapy. Of course, these new therapies can be expensive, but they are promised to re-model patient outcomes and alleviate the total disease burden, pushing health policy and funding decisions in innovative directions (Browne et al., 2021). Understanding the complexities of skin cancer is not merely theoretical—it is rather important for advancing research as well as treatment. Because malignancies of the skin exist in so many variations, scientists tend to use models that imitate real body states, like patient-derived cell lines and fibroblasts, to gain a better real-world understanding of how tumors act. These models assist in untangling how epigenetic alterations and cellular interactions propel a tumor forward, even if the image can be somewhat disorganized at times. By connecting precise molecular discoveries with actual clinical information, there is hope to create treatments that coax cancerous cells into self-annihilation, all without injuring healthy skin. In most cases, this blend of lab work and clinical insight underpins the exciting promise of personalized oncology (Karner et al., 2023).

Definition of Skin Tumors

Skin is our body's biggest organ and it has a multitude of problems ; tumors, for instance, are one of the more challenging of these. Tumors on the skin can appear from various cells such as keratinocytes, melanocytes, fibroblasts, and other skin cells. They are differentially grouped into types, with some of them being benign, depending primarily on their behavior in the body and whether they begin to creep into adjacent tissues or even elsewhere. The benign ones slowly proliferate and remain localized, whereas the malignant ones tend to explode into hasty, aggressive growth, which poses actual threats to health. The combination of various cell origins and the complex, rather unpredictable microenvironment surrounding the tumor truly add dimensions to the behavior of these tumors and how they react to treatment (Forsthuber et al., 2024). Awareness of these facts is important in grasping the wide variety of skin tumors and what they portend clinically. When you get down to malignant skin tumors, what you are seeing is uncontrolled cell growth that disrupts normal tissue. Basal cell carcinoma, squamous cell carcinoma, and melanoma are typical perpetrators here - each with its own odd histological features. In the majority of cases, the microenvironment surrounding these tumors is important; for instance, cancer-associated fibroblasts (CAFs) are one crucial factor. Recent research has indicated that there are various types of CAFs - consider myofibroblast-like RGS5+ CAFs, matrix CAFs, and even those that modulate the immune response - each putting its own spin on how the cancer develops and how it plays with the body's defenses (Forsthuber et al., 2024). Finding these variations not only intensifies our gaze into skin tumor biology but also illustrates just how complicated malignant potential can be. Although we typically categorize skin tumors on the basis of which cell types they are derived from and whether they are benign or malignant, other variables such as the size of the tumor, to what depth, and its metastatic potential also have a say in its categorization. These facts assist clinicians in determining the most appropriate treatment plan. It also implies that we must distinguish solid tumors , which encompass the majority of skin cancers - from hematological malignancies involving blood-forming tissue. Certain studies suggest that blood cancer patients might be at greater risk and mortality, but skin cancers remain tough due to their widespread prevalence and tendency to metastasize. All of which highlights the continued necessity for research which clarifies tumor definitions and risks, leading to improved care and treatment outcomes.

Importance of Studying Skin Malignancies

Skin cancer incidence has been rising in recent times, and it is particularly concerning for individuals like organ transplant recipients. Their immune systems are usually suppressed intentionally, so they are likely to develop harder, more aggressive skin cancers that make treatment a bit more complicated. A recent trial of RP1 oncolytic immunotherapy in these transplant recipients with advanced skin tumors provided encouraging objective response rates, and the safety profile was generally tolerable. It is noteworthy, in the majority of instances, that standard immunotherapies at times endanger the triggering of allograft rejection, thereby positioning them as less appropriate. Essentially, having a better understanding of the behavior of skin tumors among immunocompromised individuals not only enhances clinical outcomes but also pushes us toward more specific treatment approaches (Migden et al., 2024). This type of study provides the foundation, , for better handling of complex cases and even for increasing survival rates among those at risk. Apart from modifying treatments, it is also important to consider how factors involving the whole body integrate with skin tumor development. Inflammatory proteins within the blood, and immune cell activity; can induce various forms of skin cancer, whether it is BCC, squamous cell carcinoma or even melanoma. Sophisticated genetic epidemiology resources, such as Mendelian Randomization, have typically taught us that some inflammatory mediators are pro-tumorous. And the roles of immune players like CD4+ T cells and natural killer T cells suggest a complex, multifaceted immune web at play. Knowing these processes, with a few additional layers of information here and there, is the key to developing better preventative strategies and immunomodulatory approaches to prevent tumor recurrence (Gong et al., 2024). This type of information truly goes a long way in enhancing targets for future treatments and improving prognostic precision. And then there is the bigger picture that is of immediate concern to public health—early detection and early intervention can significantly reduce illness and mortality.

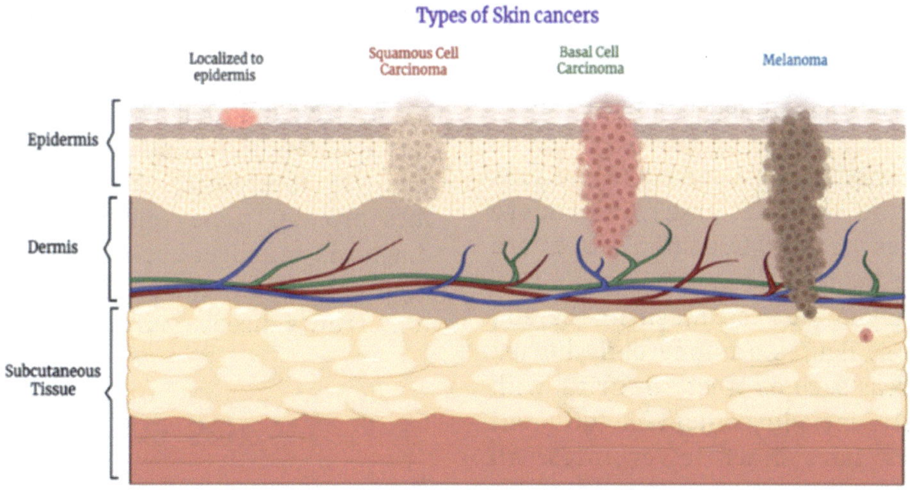

Figure 9.1. Illustrates different types of skin cancers.

Source: Hasan, N., Nadaf, A., Imran, M., Jiba, U., Sheikh, A., Almalki, W. H., et al. (2023). *Skin cancer: Understanding the journey of transformation from conventional to advanced treatment approaches. Molecular Cancer*, *22*(1), 168.

As skin cancers are some of the most frequent malignancies in the world, raising awareness and enhancing scientific understanding lays the foundation for improved screening and risk appraisal protocols. Current research explores the unequal incidence and outcomes related to genetics, environment, and immune function, which in most scenarios means care can become somewhat more level. New trials are also identifying biomarkers that suggest treatment response, resistance, and even possible side effects; these pieces of information are invaluable in honing patient-specific care plans. Merging new therapies with conventional surgical and medication treatments, all backed by good evidence, appears to be the way ahead in controlling this disease. The study of skin malignancies continues to be essential, enhancing healthcare measures while raising quality of life in numerous multicultural communities (Figure 9.1).

Overview of Skin Cancer Prevalence

Cancer is increasing nearly everywhere today, promoted by changes in demographics, the environment, and lifestyles. Melanoma as well as nonmelanoma cousins of melanoma are largely responsible for skin cancer's share of this role. It would appear that added exposure to UV radiation and an aging population are indeed driving the statistics. Consider such locations as Australia and New Zealand, where more than 500 cases per 100,000 inhabitants are reported; with them being predominantly fair-skinned and laying out too much in the sun by nature, those figures are inherently higher. Conversely, areas such as Western Africa, with naturally greater melanin content and different sun behaviors, have much lower rates. All of this suggests prevention will need to be customized to regional genetic characteristics and sun exposure behavior (Bray et al., 2024). Nationally, however, skin cancer remains high on lists of frequent diagnoses. Melanoma, specifically, has been rising steadily over the last several decades. While most cancers are experiencing declining mortality rates owing to improved treatments and screening, skin cancers are still on the increase – a pattern likely indicative of both increased public awareness and recreational sunbathing and tanning as part of outdoor lifestyles. Melanoma appears to be increasing about 1% to 3% per annum in some populations, creating very real challenges for both early detection and successful prevention. This rise is particularly disconcerting within a larger context in which other cancers are more effectively controlled through aggressive screening and therapeutic advances, highlighting a multifaceted combination of behavior, biology, and healthcare disparities (Rebecca et al., 2024). Combating these threats at the early stage is still entirely essential if we are to reverse the trend of increasing skin tumors globally. Projections of cancer incidence reaching 35 million in 2050 truly put into perspective the urgency for rapid public health action , such as sun safety education and reconsidering regulation of artificial tanning devices. Additionally, not all people have equal access to prevention, and some racial and ethnic groups have higher mortality rates, even when they experience fewer cases individually; this indicates entrenched disparities in healthcare provision. Stand back and look at the overall picture, and it is apparent that combating cancer worldwide involves integrating skin cancer avoidance into broader policy plans emphasizing early diagnosis, intelligent behavior modification, and equitable treatment alternatives to minimize tomorrow's disease burden (Bray et al., 2024).

9.1. Types of Skin Tumors

Skin tumors are fairly complicated—not only for their appearance in patients but also because of the extensive variety of tissue types they can contain. You see the squamous cell carcinomas, basal cell carcinomas (BCC), and melanomas quite frequently, each having its own characterestics. Squamous cell carcinomas, for example, tend to penetrate deeply into the tissues and will occasionally find their way even as far as the calvaria when they appear on the scalp; such deep invasion results in the fact that, in most cases, surgery must be even more careful. Frequently, the removal is not confined merely to the tumor itself; physicians can find themselves having to remove the periosteum and some portion of the underlying bone in order to ensure that it is all gone. Studies as a rule show that when treating deep scalp malignancies, squamous cell carcinomas are most commonly the primary offenders, so a proper clinical and histological evaluation really becomes crucial when planning treatment. Following its removal, however, the way it gets reconstructed may differ too – say, split-thickness skin grafts have fared improved survival outcomes on the likes of calvaria over full-thickness grafts, really emphasizing the call for an individually tailored surgical protocol (Al-Aswad et al., 2024). Besides these frequent epithelial neoplasms, there exists a family of less common tumors filling out the picture, including melanomas and metastatic cutaneous malignancies. Melanomas as a whole tend to be aggressive and are highly likely to metastasize; this usually requires extensive local excision as well as a sentinel lymph node assessment. The mixed histological appearance of tumors like these does not only influence the prognosis—it also dictates what molecular diagnostics we use. Developments in high-throughput sequencing, for instance, have created new avenues for exploring genetic predisposition, though one has to be careful in selecting tissue samples because infiltrative tumor cells can sometimes confuse the results. Although a skin biopsy remains the gold standard for diagnosing and genetically testing skin malignancies, some doctors are investigating non-invasive techniques, such as employing hair follicles, to identify germline mutations associated with cancer susceptibility (Perani et al., 2023). When you take a step back, skin tumor classification is not merely determining whether they are primary or metastatic; it is determining their genetic composition. Take BCC: since the most common primary skin tumor, it generally is less aggressive, tending not to metastasize even though it at times invades local tissues, making constant monitoring a necessity. Myeloid malignancies with skin involvement, however, reveal just how entwined hematology and dermatology can be; for these, acquiring the precise genetic makeup is downright imperative in order to customize treatment. Recent work has tended to highlight that extensive molecular profiling has the potential to uncover underlying germline predispositions, thus influencing management decisions not only for the tumor but also for any envisioned systemic considerations. This entire process, integrating surgical, pathological, and genetic considerations, truly emphasizes just how multifaceted diagnosing and treating skin tumors can be (Perani et al., 2023; Al-Aswad et al., 2024).

9.1.1. Benign Skin Tumors

Skin tumors are all shapes and sizes, and solving them is not always easy. Different kinds require a general approach, particularly in attempting to distinguish a benign bump from something threatening. The benign ones usually develop slowly, have well-defined borders, and do not encroach on surrounding tissue, attributes that usually suggest a straightforward removal is sufficient rather than a heavy, multi-agent course. Immunohistochemistry, allowing us to visualize the molecular composition, has clarified some of these distinctions. As an instance, some markers hardly appear in benign melanocytic nevi but are significantly more expressed in malignant melanoma, emphasizing the point that these tumors are distinguishable. Such molecular contrast not only enhances diagnosis but also welcomes the prospect of targeted drugs (Blanco et al., 2011). Although benign tumors most often present in a quiet, indolent manner, their clinical and microscopic characteristics continue to require closer examination so that they will not be mistaken for more serious conditions. Benign melanocytic nevi, such as compound and intradermal nevi, can sometimes present with unusual or atypical findings that are suggestive of malignancy, and therefore more elaborate tests will be ordered. You may also find that tumors like seborrheic keratosis or benign adnexal growths are associated with characteristic cell patterns that make them stand apart from cancers such as basal or squamous cell carcinomas. Often, such benign tumors will not meander away or openly menace an individual's survival but instead may subtly indicate the presence of a deeper skin condition to be monitored over time. In a sense, the sight of a benign growth is also a silent reminder that something might develop into malignancy in certain instances down the road, and thus regular follow-up and patient vigilance truly become important (Blanco et al., 2011). Cutaneous metastases are a different story altogether—they are an unmistakable indication that a cancer has progressed, both malignant potential and ease of treatment are hugely altered. Although benign skin tumors generally do not have the capacity to invade or metastasize, learning about the way malignant tumor's function provides a clearer view of the whole range of skin lesions. Consider skin metastases from breast carcinoma, for example, they penetrate the dermis, of course, but the hypodermis as well and occasionally display peculiar actions such as transepidermal elimination, a characteristic you simply do not find with benign lesions. This unambiguous distinction emphasizes the necessity of an accurate diagnosis since treatment regimens and outcomes vary significantly between the non-tumorous benign conditions and the malignant ones that could potentially have the wider, systemic effects. Identifying these conditions remains crucial to planning the appropriate treatments while also considering the larger narrative of skin tumors and their possible dangers (Figure 9.2).

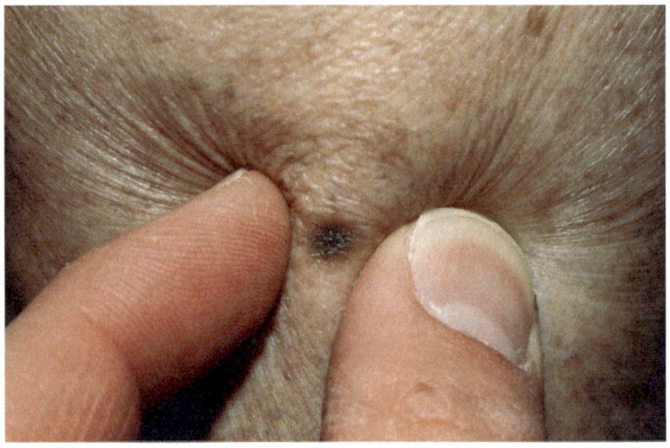

Figure 9.2. Benign skin tumor.

Source: Photograph of an unidentified subject. (n.d.). AMBOSS. https://media-us.amboss.com/media/thumbs/big_58a6ce12a3b39.jpg

9.1.2. Malignant Skin Tumors

Treating aggressive skin tumors is not as simple. Their unpredictable nature and the combination of the surrounding tissues significantly impact the effectiveness of treatments. As an instance, malignant nerve sheath tumors associated with Neurofibromatosis Type 1 grow rapidly and tend to defy the conventional treatments such as chemo and radiation. Occasionally even these tumors begin life as harmless and then become too large or too close to important nerves to be able to operate near. In recent times, some trials are even experimenting with immune therapies—immune checkpoint blockade is designed to revive the body's own defenses to detect and destroy cancer cells. However, for this ruse to succeed, the tissue surrounding the tumor must be aglow with T cells, something that MPNST tumors frequently do not have. There is also discussion of employing methods to activate the STING pathway, which could heat up such "cold" tumors, possibly making them more susceptible to immune attack (Somatilaka et al., 2023). Outside factors may also present an added level of challenge. Take organ transplant recipients, for instance: they need to stick with immunosuppressants for life to prevent organ rejection, yet these same drugs can make them more prone to secondary cancers, including those on the skin. Data shows that incidents vary depending on where someone lives, with transplant patients in Europe facing higher risks of skin cancers and even Kaposi's sarcoma. Altering drug regimens, such as the addition of mTOR inhibitors or a switch to mycophenolate mofetil, has managed to reduce these emerging cancer risks. It is a balancing act between preventing rejection and maintaining low cancer risk, so physicians tend to end up combining surgical solutions with medication alters (Shen et al., 2022).

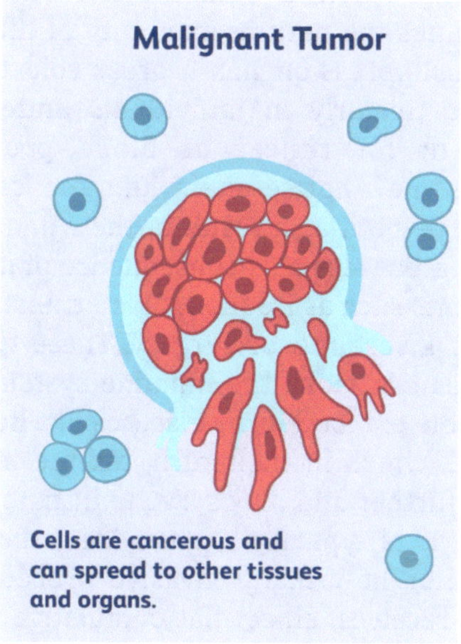

Figure 9.3. Malignant tumor.

Source: Splane, B. (2023). *Malignant vs. Benign Tumors: How They Differ*. Verywell Health.

Ahead, novel ideas for treating malignant skin tumors appear to be a function of what is occurring at all levels: the tumor itself's characterestics, the status of the immune system, and even outside pressures such as continuous immunosuppression. For tumors that defiantly refuse standard treatments, synergizing concepts that modulate the immune system with traditional therapies has generated tremendous interest, particularly for cases such as MPNST. The plan is to induce native immune signals to draw in killer T cells, a move that could turn the tables for difficult-to-treat cancers. And for those already vulnerable to immunosuppression, monitoring closely and intervening early with surgery or additional therapy could reduce the risk. Finally, tailoring treatment by combining the tumor's molecular narrative with an individual patient's unique medical history could be the solution to more effective results in combating such difficult cancers (Shen et al., 2022; Somatilaka et al., 2023) (Figure 9.3).

9.1.3. Pre-Cancerous Lesions

Skin tumors begin with small changes in cells that many may not notice initially. Pre-cancerous lesions emerge when cells rapidly reproduce in abnormal fashion, demonstrating signs of trouble even before they stray into neighboring tissues. It is wise to detect such signs early since, most of the time, they provide an opportunity to intervene before established cancer becomes entrenched. Through the microscope, you may observe unusual-appearing keratinocytes and an interruption in the normal layers of the skin—indications that something is not quite right. Cellular stability is gradually eroded by genetic mutations, typically triggered by excessive UV light or other noxious environmental agents. Early screening, instead of waiting for invasive carcinomas, can impact patient outcomes and reduce long-term misery with advanced malignancies. Current diagnostic advances have for the most part facilitated it to be simpler to identify and investigate these early cutaneous changes. Photoacoustic imaging, for instance, provides us with an unprecedented clarity through the recording of variations in light absorption across skin tissue. The non-ionizing radiation technique is useful for repeated clinical examinations (Steinberg et al., 2019) and provides insight into shape and blood supply within the lesions. Molecular markers in combination with conventional histopath tests provide additional layers of information, revealing nuances of cell abnormalities and growth patterns that are important for diagnosis.

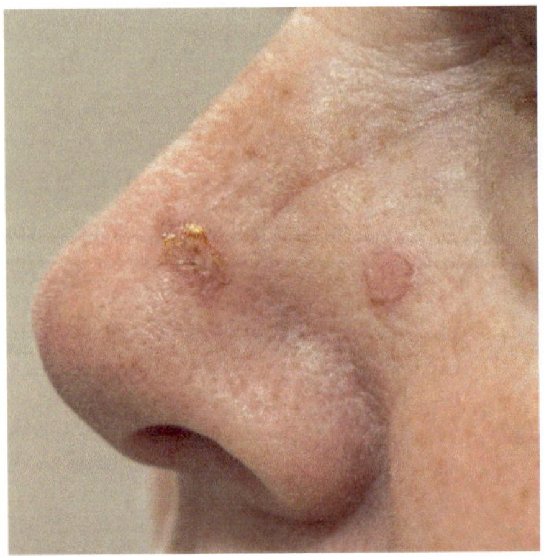

Figure 9.4. Pre-cancerous skin lesions.

Source: Complete Skin Solutions. (2019). *Pre-Cancerous Skin Lesions.* https://www.completeskinsolutions.com.au/wp-content/uploads/2019/07/Pre-Cancerous-Skin-Lesions-shutterstock_441847699-1024x684.jpg.

When these methods are combined, they assist in mapping where precisely the lesions are located, informing treatment decisions in a more relaxed but efficient manner. In consequence, doctors are able to monitor whether a lesion is advancing or retreating, which is important for taking care of the condition before it turns problematic. In the center of these pre-cancerous marks are complex cellular procedures that typically have things running properly—until they no longer do. Autophagy, how cells remove defective pieces, occasionally goes awry at an early stage of the neoplastic process (Daniel et al., 2021). When this removal system fails, cells may begin to retain errors, laying the groundwork for instability and possible malignancy. And to add insult to injury, the surrounding tissue frequently changes in a way that is unpredictable, with inflammatory messages and insidious immune evasive maneuvers enabling the errant cells to persist. Making sense of these ordinary but subtle changes provides hints for discovering treatments that could restore the balance. Altered functioning of autophagy and related pathways seems a hopeful means of preventing those pre-cancerous changes from marching right into invasive tumors (Figure 9.4).

9.2. Risk Factors

Skin cancers and tumors tend to begin appearing when a combination of factors undermines the natural immunity of the body. Immunosuppression has a great role to play here, particularly in individuals undergoing treatment for cancer or blood problems. Patients may notice their immune capacity declining—both as a result of their underlying condition but also as a consequence of medical treatments such as frequent blood transfusions, catheter insertions, or surgery. These types of therapies can make the immune system more vulnerable to bloodborne diseases like hepatitis B and C, which in their turn, tax the immune system further and may serve to initiate tumor growth. It is typically a good idea, therefore, to monitor how many invasive procedures a patient receives, since that cumulative weight really could increase the risk of skin cancer in immunocompromised individuals (Satsuk et al., 2024). Age and sex also have a way of complicating how skin and other cancers occur. Older individuals, particularly those aged 50 and older, more often than not have more than one tumor — and skin malignancies can be among these. Evidence has indicated that men tend to have a harder time with more than one first primary cancer; variations in tumor behavior, occupational exposures, or even how and when they access health care may be at work here. It should also be mentioned that tumors that appear simultaneously (what some people refer to as synchronous tumors) have a significantly higher risk than tumors that occur on different dates. Generally, this involves maintaining a long-term, close eye and intercepting any alerts as soon as possible is paramount, especially for individuals who already have a greater risk of skin cancer among other cancers (Almasan et al., 2023). Daily factors, such as what we do day by day and the settings we inhabit, add another dimension to the puzzle of risk by combining with intrinsic weaknesses. Excessive sun, for example, puts skin in the direct path of ultraviolet (UV) radiation that can kill cell DNA and ultimately transform normal cells into something even more sinister. Habits like using a tanning bed or failing to cover up at all just contribute to it. Furthermore, being exposed on the job to certain chemicals or even types of radiation yet again increases the risk. Ultimately, the story of every individual is a combination of genes, immune resilience, family cancer history, and the impact of the world around us. Therefore, balancing together screening for internal conditions such as immunosuppression with external threats, including sunlight exposure, is key to pinning down improved prevention, early detection, and smarter management of skin cancers (Figure 9.5).

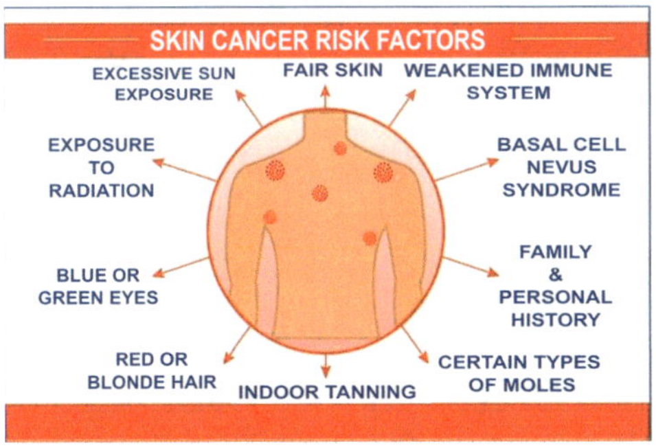

Figure 9.5. Skin cancer risk factors.

Source: Medicover Hospitals. (n.d.). *Skin Cancer: Symptoms, Causes and Treatment.* https://www.medicoverhospitals.in/images/diseases/skin-cancer-causes-risk-factors.webp.

9.2.1. Genetic Predisposition

Genetic characterestics inherited play an enormous part, frequently even larger than those of the environment, in initiating skin cancers and other cancers. Whole genome sequencing now enables researchers to select out finicky gene changes that increase cancer susceptibility, a pattern particularly observed among younger patients. A lot of patients diagnosed at age 25 or younger have these variations that interfere with DNA repair and cell cycle controls. Genes such as TP53, DICER1 and mismatch repair actors (MSH6, MLH1) are more likely to appear, reminding us of how much it matters to maintain our genomic integrity. Other than signaling an increased risk, these alterations also present as clues for early tests and tailor-made treatment plans, which really brings genetic testing to the forefront in oncology (Barnes et al., 2024). Identifying these inherited gene variations sets the stage for discovering how family characteristics can influence skin cancer development. In many cases, these gene errors disrupt DNA repair or disrupt rules of cell cycles, making cells more susceptible to such stimuli as UV light, a known skin cancer trigger. Other research even describes that modifications in genes associated with metabolism and immune response, consider G6PC3 and PRF1—may additionally impact tumor vulnerability by changing how cells manage energy and watch for danger. This broad collection of genetic variations highlights, in the majority of instances, the necessity for comprehensive genomic screening not only for individuals but also for families, opening the door to risk mapping and tailored avoidance measures (Barnes et al., 2024). Apart from these genetic traitfeatures, precision therapies are gradually developing to address cancers driven by one's genetic code. For instance, new treatments that target affected molecular pathways are promising in both blood and solid cancers, an intriguing acknowledgment of the ways genetic discoveries are being translated into new medicines. Even though the majority of the ongoing work focuses on later-life mutations, early-stage trials with drugs such as splicing factor inhibitors indicate that it may become possible in the near future to take advantage of specific genetic weaknesses in cancer cells. In most instances, a patient's native genetic landscape may someday dictate the selection of precision therapies to enhance treatment outcomes, combining our knowledge of hereditary risk with novel treatment strategies and advancing personalized oncology. At times the journey feels slightly ad hoc, but the promise is here unquestionably (Figure 9.6).

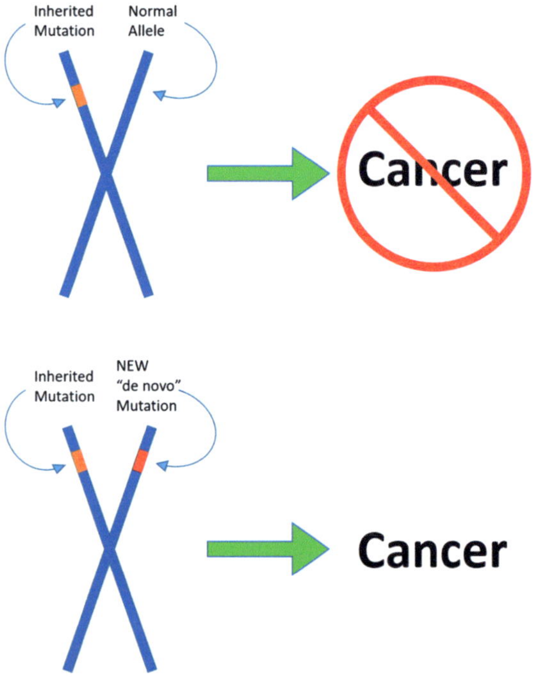

Figure 9.6. The two-hit hypothesis. One germline mutation in a DICER1 allele predisposes the individual to an increased risk for benign and malignant tumors.

Source: Li, Y., Wang, J., & Zhang, X. (2018). The role of tumor microenvironment in tumor progression and metastasis. *Cancers, 10*(5), 143.

9.2.2. Environmental Influences

Skin tumors do not erupt from our DNA alone; they arise from a sloppy combination of inherited characterestics and the stuff that is going on around us. Sunlight's ultraviolet rays head the pack, burrowing directly into our DNA and prodding mutations within our skin cells. In a sense, continuous exposure does more than turn switches on in melanocytes—it disrupts our body's local defense system, making it all too simple for bad changes to catch hold. And it is not just the sun; chemicals you run up against on the job, in pollution, or even via common lifestyle options can supply this process with an added boost, adding to tumor threats. If you take a look at conditions like melanoma or skin cancers, what you find is that these are not merely diseases based on internal genetic mutations but are also about the way the external world prompts our cells to engage in dangerous activities (Birlea et al., 2018). New advances in molecular medicine have been revealing to us that the harm caused by our environments can often initiate gene mutations, and sometimes even shuffle things around with our chief genetic drivers in ways that appear quite unpredictable. For example, you may discover alterations in significant genes such as KRAS and TP53, which are typically associated with severe problems, even in those that do not appear outright malign, especially if they have been subject to environmental stress over time. This produces a strange, complicated range of genomic changes. Occasionally these mutations are innocuous enough, but with additional stimuli or compromised cell defenses, they may just be enough to tip the scales toward a malignant result. It appears that the environment can be both the first spark and the additional fuel that sustains the fire of tumorigenesis (Adashek et al., 2020). Prevention is not merely a matter of considering sunscreen and UV protection. Yes, public health campaigns pound the point about protecting yourself from the sun, but reducing exposure to industrial pollutants and unpleasant chemicals is also a big deal. The accumulating evidence that benign as well as cancerous skin alterations have some molecular signatures in common even implies that drugs that were first developed to attack cancer can one day be used to control environmentally driven skin conditions. Probing these molecular mechanisms-even if the image is not 100% consistent can create more specific strategies, from medications that suppress deleterious gene signals to tests that more accurately distinguish benign marks from lethal lesions. Ultimately, combining a healthy dose of environmental acuity with the newest molecular understanding provides an expanded blueprints for minimizing skin tumor hazards and enhancing health outcomes (Birlea et al., 2018; Adashek et al., 2020).

9.2.3. Lifestyle Choices

The skin's battle with its surroundings sets the stage for how likely it is to develop tumors. Our daily choices, like soaking up too much sun—can nudge skin cells toward a harmful path. The buildup of UV light, whether from intentional or offhand exposure, ends up causing DNA harm, oxidative stress, and inflammation, all of which stir up cellular changes. Simple steps, such as slapping on sunblock, wearing protective clothing, or avoiding the sun during the day, have been proven time and again to reduce the risk of skin cancer. One area that is gaining increasing attention is autophagy, a form of cellular trash removal and recycling mechanism, which appears to assist cells in dealing with stress from our environment. For the most part, having methods to adjust autophagy could be only one of the mechanisms our lifestyles influence cell survival and tumor initiation (Daniel et al., 2021). So, paying attention to how much UV we receive is relatively important for preventing skin cancer. Exercise and nutrition also enter the equation, influencing the inner workings of the body in ways that can stimulate or repress the growth of tumors. Foods rich in antioxidants such as vitamins C and E, polyphenols, and carotenoids can draw back the effects of outside offenders like UV radiation. For the most part, these nutrients assist in supporting cell repair and reducing oxidative stress, which could stall the tumor's advance. Conversely, a subpar diet and excessive sitting around tend to weaken the immune system, disrupt cell cleanup mechanisms, and lead to inflammation-friendly and cancer-conducive conditions. Although studies of other cancers have been making these connections for years, recent discoveries suggest similar processes are involved with skin tumors, which emphasizes lifestyle adjustments that combine diet and exercise. Informing people about eating well and standing up to walk around complements broader cancer prevention strategies and keeps the skin and its cells healthier (Daniel et al., 2021). It is as if our daily decisions and the molecular activity within our skin are dancing in tandem. There is also the combination of vices such as smoking and binge drinking, which similarly tend to drive skin cancer risk higher. Cigarette smoke delivers unpleasant chemicals that trigger the production of reactive oxygen species, resulting in DNA fiascos and interfering with the smooth operation of autophagy—this interference can assist unscrupulous cells in staying around longer. Similarly, excessive alcohol confuses the body's own defenses and the meticulous fix-up work of cells, layering on further distress. Breast cancer research has consistently demonstrated that altering these modifiable behaviors will alter tumor behavior and patient outcomes, and the same concepts arise when considering skin tumors. To some extent surprisingly, these lifestyle factors tend to get complex together, illustrating well that a comprehensive approach is necessary to eliminate the cumulative cancer burden. Combining lifestyle advice into daily skin care could be an innovative means of turning down cancer threats in tandem with supporting early detection and timely treatment approaches.

9.3. Symptoms and Diagnosis

Skin tumors appear in all sorts of manners. At times you notice them as flat lesions or bumpy nodules with irregular borders and mixed pigmentation – things that under initial impression may appear harmless. Oral melanomas, for instance, are fairly uncommon but may present with localized bleeding, swelling, loose teeth, and slow-healing wounds following dental procedures (Jaifi et al., 2024). When these unusual symptoms show up in typical locations such as the hard palate or following the gums, physicians are usually spoken for at high alert. These signs must be caught early because the unpredictable appearance of skin tumors tends to postpone diagnosis and disturb the prognosis. A prompt clinical evaluation culminating in a biopsy sets the stage for additional testing to determine if there is indeed cause for concern. Diagnosis of skin tumors is largely histopathology-based, which remains the gold standard. Conventional histology provides a close-up view of cells and tissue architecture, but is rather confined in the sense that it reveals only a flat, two-dimensional appearance and requires very accurate sectioning. New imaging stunts, such as X-ray virtual histology with micro-Computed Tomography (μCT), are turning heads with a three-dimensional glimpse into tumor microarchitecture (Saccomano et al., 2024). This assists pathologists in determining how deeply a tumor would likely infiltrate, which is particularly valuable for melanomas or BCC. These technological improvements, in the majority of instances, provide new information regarding tumor depth and structural diversity; both are important when it comes to planning treatment and selecting the most appropriate method of cutting the tissue, all without ruining the sample too badly. It is even more challenging to diagnose skin malignancies since their histological characteristics can differ considerably. For oral melanoma, where you may encounter perplexing patterns and cellular diversity, physicians tend to rely on immunohistochemical markers, such as S100 protein, HMB45, tyrosinase, Melan A, and MITF (Jaifi et al., 2024). The markers are quite significant to distinguish from other pigmented lesions and confirm the melanocytic origin. The combination of examining cell forms and applying focused immunohistochemistry not only increases the confidence in making a diagnosis, but also allows for an estimation of prognosis and informs decisions regarding treatment. Since a number of these cancers act aggressively and have poor survival rates, getting a correct diagnosis as early as one can often makes all the difference in starting effective treatment.

9.3.1. Common Symptoms of Skin Tumors

Skin tumors occasionally appear in forms that may not necessarily raise the alarm at first. You could see some minor mole variation—maybe a change in color, a small size difference, or even a subtle change in texture—often confused with run-of-the-mill skin problems. New lumps or changes in prior marks can include characteristics like asymmetrical shapes, disordered borders, or combinations of colors in one area. Bumpy locations or rounded zones, particularly if they begin demonstrating signs such as ulceration or a slight hemorrhage, may be joined by more threatening possibilities. Most times, these preliminary indicators enable physicians to differentiate cancerous tumors from benign dermatopathies. Curiously, some of these cancers also cause what we might refer to as paraneoplastic skin reactions—skin responses that indirectly indicate internal cancers. Studies (Bešlić et al., 2021) have associated several types of skin irritation such as chronic itch, bullous pemphigoid, or even chronic hives with internal tumors, suggesting the possibility that our skin may be saying more than it appears about what is happening further inside. Although such gross red flags as bleeding or frank sores tend to be thought of as definitive, there are more subtle clues not to be ignored. For example, a persistent itch or focal pain persisting near a suspicious area may, in the vast majority of instances, signal malignant change and indicate that a biopsy might be indicated. It is not unusual, either, to notice unusual hair loss in regions such as the beard or scalp—occurrences that appear anomalous and have been documented in conjunction with certain malignancies, creating further complexity regarding the presentation of skin tumors. Symptoms more similar to eczematous dermatitis or even episodes of vasculitis occasionally surface, showing how one's skin problems and cancers inside might be curiously interrelated; oftentimes, these are resolved skin conditions following proper cancer therapies. All of these syndromes overlapping, when considered in conjunction with one another, can assist in pushing the process toward an earlier intervention and more positive outcomes (Bešlić et al., 2021). In real-life clinical practice, physicians tend to rely on methods such as imaging and microscopic testing in combination with close examination of symptoms to determine what a tumor is. However, it is the initial change in skin, sometimes an itchy red rash, sometimes a firm pigmented nodule, which often initiates the entire diagnostic regimen. This wide range, from BCC and melanoma to those less well-known paraneoplastic skin reactions, reminds us that the skin does not always play by one set of rules. Healthcare practitioners, in general, are aided by keeping these diverse presentations in mind to minimize delays in diagnosis, as early detection significantly influences both treatment success and general prognosis. In brief, taking a holistic view of alterations in color, texture abnormalities, and even broader systemic signs associated with paraneoplastic syndromes is most important to achieve optimal patient outcomes when it comes to treating skin tumors (Bešlić et al., 2021).

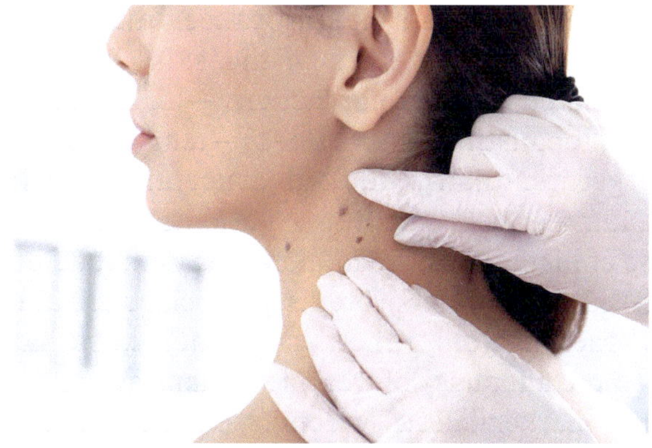

Source: Fibo Health. (n.d.). *Skin Tumors – Comprehensive Care and Treatment in Turkey.* https://fibohealth.com/wp-content/uploads/2024/11/skincancer.jpeg.

9.3.2. Diagnostic Methods

Molecular genetics has truly revolutionized the process of determining complicated cancers—very often providing us with profound insight into where tumors arise and how they develop. Consider, for instance, instances where mediastinal germ cell tumors appear together with acute myeloid leukemia; scientists have, in many instances, employed enhanced exome sequencing to uncover a latent clonal connection between such cancers that may appear unrelated at first glance. In most cases, discovering similar somatic mutations within influential tumor suppressor genes—PTEN, TP53, and others, at frequencies of high variant allele frequency implies that both cancers share a common ancestral clone. This type of genetic insight not only enhances diagnostic accuracy (in general) but also indicates the prevalent biological interaction driving tumor heterogeneity and drug resistance. It would appear to be highly likely that using a similar profiling technique for skin tumors would reveal critical clues for untangling tumor subtypes and predicting clinical outcomes, eventually leading to more targeted treatment plans in dermatologic oncology (Lu et al., 2016). In addition to genomic methods, biochemical markers are likewise gaining prominence when making cancer diagnoses, particularly in cancers of the skin. Proteins associated with tumor activity—for example, Metallopanstimulin-1 (MPS-1)—tend to appear in greater-than-predicted concentrations in squamous cell carcinoma patients. With the use of highly sensitive immunoassays that detect MPS-1 and similar proteins, physicians are able to track not only whether a tumor exists but also the adequacy of treatment plans over time. This marker-based screening, in the majority of instances, is full of potential for detecting cutaneous squamous cell carcinomas at an early stage and monitoring their development, which could well be the key to better patient outcomes. Since skin tumors can be quite heterogeneous, a combination of serum biomarkers with the standard histopathological examination can greatly enhance diagnostic precision and assist with timely therapy decisions (Stack et al., 2004). Despite advances in state-of-the-art approaches, time-tested diagnostic methods such as histopathology and immunohistochemistry remain the foundation for the analysis of skin tumors. When a biopsy is examined microscopically, the observation of cell shapes and patterns—those subtle architectural patterns—remains essential for identifying cancer. In addition, immunohistochemical staining that identifies the presence or absence of specific antigens assists in the narrowing down of tumor subtypes; this is important in distinguishing between benign and malignant lesions, or primary from metastatic tumors. Combining these traditional tests with new molecular diagnostics and blood-borne biomarkers develops a sort of multi-layered strategy that optimizes the total diagnostic yield. In short, this blended strategy not only refines the detection and classification of skin malignancies but also lays the groundwork for gauging prognosis and crafting individualized treatment plans (Figure 9.7).

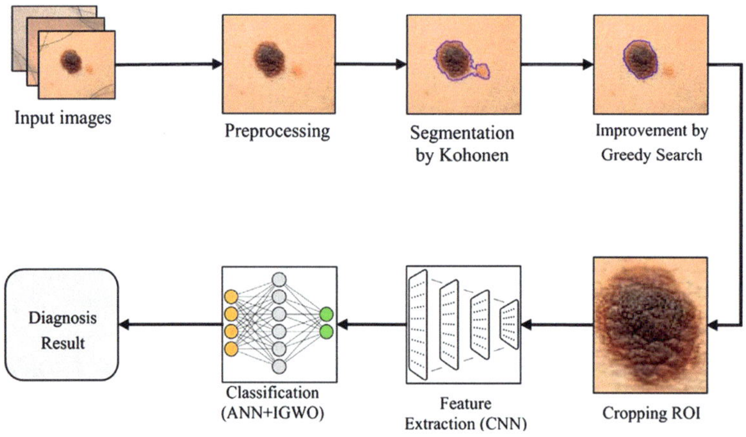

Figure 9.7. The steps of the proposed method for skin cancer diagnosis.

Source: Pal, R., & Mishra, S. (2023). A survey on techniques and steps of computer aided skin cancer diagnosis system. *International Journal of Research and Analytical Reviews, 10*(2).

9.3.3. Importance of Early Detection

Early intervention can significantly enhance the prognosis for skin tumors and cancers. Occasionally, they appear as small, almost imperceptible changes in the skin that many people end up writing off as benign marks. In general, because many of the malignant forms, such as BCC or squamous cell carcinoma, are so aggressive, the earlier they are discovered, the less invasive the treatments may be and the greater the likelihood of complete removal. It is particularly important in sensitive areas like the eyelids, where a delayed diagnosis could cause both functional complications and undesirable cosmetic consequences. Innovative developments in technology in recent years, such as machine learning systems that analyze images and utilize transfer learning, are also enhancing early detection accuracy. For instance, the Disease Prediction System employs models such as ResNet50 and VGG16 to differentiate between hazardous lesions and benign or inflammatory lesions with high accuracy, hence accelerating clinical decisions and enhancing patient care (Maria et al., 2023; Thayalan et al., 2024). Not being reactive does not only reduce the physical burden of skin cancers; it also simplifies the psychological and economic burden of patients. Catching the condition at its initial stages when it is localized tends to result in less complicated interventions and brief hospital stays, which reduces costs. When highly sensitive diagnostic equipment is employed, the risk of misdiagnosis or unnecessary overtreatment becomes very minimal, leaving the quality of life of the patient intact. The random character of skin tumors, particularly in problematic areas such as eyelids, requires that clinicians remain extra vigilant. Since these cancers can be so different in composition and character, thorough screening protocols can avert delays, retard disease development, and prevent metastasis (Maria et al., 2023). In many instances, detection at an early stage forms the foundation for tailored treatments that genuinely suit every patient's individual case. Incorporating state-of-the-art technology into routine dermatological examinations has enhanced our capacity to identify skin tumors and cancers at an early stage. Machine learning algorithms designed from extensive data sets now detect very subtle trends in medical images, allowing doctors to differentiate between malignant and non-malignant conditions with levels we have not witnessed heretofore. Platforms that merge multiple neural network structures, such as EfficientNetB0 and ResNet50, provide new insights into lesion features, which serve to augment diagnostic confidence and minimize human errors (Thayalan et al., 2024). These technologies herald the era of personalized medicine, where detection not only enhances survival but also addresses functional and cosmetic results. Ultimately, applying these new tools to everyday practice promises a future where skin cancer outcomes are radically enhanced through the empowerment of clinicians and patients alike (Figure 9.8).

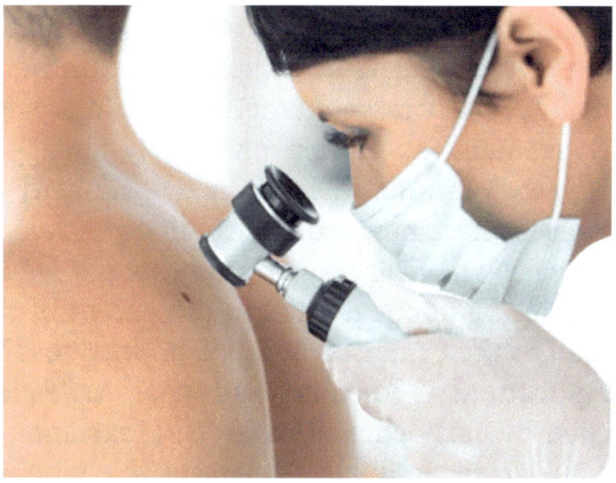

Figure 9.8. Skin cancer screening.

Source: Elite Health and Wellness. (n.d.). Skin cancer screening: What you need to know. *Elite Health and Wellness*. https://www.elitekearney.com/wp-content/uploads/2023/11/skin-cancer-screening-elite-health-and-wellness-kearney-nebraska.png.

9.4. Treatment Options

Skin cancers do not have one-size-fits-all solution. Each case has its own combination; tumor type, cancer stage, and patient characterestics all count. Surgery still is the best bet, particularly for basal cell, squamous cell, and even Merkel cell carcinomas; but surgeons now adjust the strategy to balance eradicating all the bad with preserving essential functions and looks. On sensitive areas such as the head and neck, choices regarding how much to incise or whether to include a parotid or neck dissection are based on the tumor's particular characteristics and risk, typically assisting in limiting the possibility of recurrence. This moves toward individualizing the treatment—combining what we understand about tumor biology with a patient's own specific anatomy, appears to enhance success and overall quality of life. Far beyond the surgeon's scalpel, emerging systemic therapies are shaking things up as well. In instances where cancer has spread locally or even distantly, physicians are relying on immunotherapy and targeted agents as part of an overall strategy. Checkpoint inhibitors and molecularly targeted therapies now provide new avenues for tumors previously shrugged off by conventional means. In the majority of instances, these newer drugs combine with local treatment when surgery or radiotherapy would likely not be adequate due to the extent of the spread of the tumor or because of other health complications. This combination of strategies, backed by early clinical research (Psarianos et al., 2024), is gradually changing the way we approach skin cancer treatment. Radiotherapy, as widespread as it is, is not without its risks, particularly for certain patients. Individuals with germline TP53 mutations (consider Li-Fraumeni syndrome, for example) are at increased risk of developing secondary cancers due to the radiation itself. Recent preclinical suggestions even indicate that the inclusion of metformin in the treatment may benefit; by quietly reprogramming the way cells react to radiation, it seems to nudge injured cells into apoptosis and potentially halt the emergence of new tumors. This new strategy could open doors for individuals who might otherwise be at risk of radiation, highlighting the increasing need to design treatments around genetic signals and precise tumor profiles (Psarianos et al., 2024).

9.4.1. Surgical Interventions

Skin cancers most often require a concerted effort. Surgery tends to be in the lead as far as keeping the cancer in balance is concerned. Sometimes, physicians will attempt to treat it with creams or even with radiation in certain situations, but excising the lesion is still most likely at the top of the list due to it eradicating the tumor completely and allowing professionals to examine the affected tissue. There is a wide range of ways to do it – sometimes a straightforward cut will do, and other times the process may involve more complex work like rebuilding tissue afterward. The choice really comes down to what kind of tumor it is, how big it is, and exactly where it is located. Usually, physicians weigh factors such as the chance of the cancer recurring or loss of function, attempting to weigh those risks against the benefits they anticipate. In most instances, changing concepts borrowed from other aspects of cancer treatment result in each treatment plan being negotiated on the basis of the tumor's behavior and the patient's overall health. When a skin cancer has advanced or infiltrative features, a more extensive procedure may be required to remove everything. This could involve removing some of the surrounding tissues or even deeper structures, which can complicate the operation with more possible complications. Consider head and neck cases – when the tumors infiltrate deeper tissues, surgeons may have to add craniofacial resection to other treatments to keep things in check. There is some indication that a little preliminary psychiatric intervention before and after surgery can help mitigate the psychological burden (Mukoyamaet al., 2020).). Although these larger operations involve higher risks, sometimes they do offer a real opportunity for long-term survival to appropriately selected patients. Most of the time, the presence of surgeons, oncologists, and psychiatric specialists collaborating is really beneficial in enhancing both the physical and psychological outcomes after surgery. Despite all the new surgical techniques, physicians still have to be vigilant about the increased complexity introduced by donor-related cancers, particularly where transplants are involved. The possibility of transmitting malignancies through donated organs is a major concern, meaning that it is extremely important to screen the donor's history before any transplant procedure taking place (Nalesnik & Ison,2011). Certain tumors are so dangerous that physicians will not even use that organ at all, and others may be usable if the tumor can be removed or if special requirements are fulfilled. With skin cancers, this simply makes even more apparent the necessity for careful, individualized risk assessments. Surgeons need to carefully plan each step so that cancer cells will not spread undesirably. In general, treating skin tumors is changing, surgical approaches are keeping up with broader safety practices in cancer and transplantation to provide patients with the most favorable balance of effective care and safety (Figure 9.9).

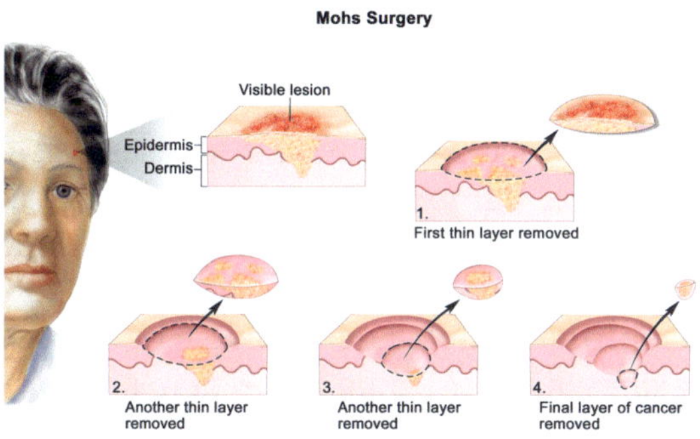

Figure 9.9. Mohn surgery.

Source: National Cancer Institute. (n.d.). *Illustrates Different Types of Skin Cancers*. https://nci-media.cancer.gov/pdq/media/images/599831.jpg.

9.4.2. Radiation Therapy

Cancer therapy has evolved a lot over the years, improving outcomes for patients while minimizing side effects – particularly with skin cancers. Today, employing imaging to assist in radiating treatment is a giant step forward. Consider Image Guided Superficial Radiation Therapy (IGSRT) for instance. This approach marries ancient superficial radiation with high-resolution dermal ultrasound so physicians can finally observe a tumor's margins and depth *in vivo*. Research typically indicates that using IGSRT, tumor control rates exceed 99%, outperforming old traditional radiation techniques as well as some surgeries. Dermatologists, radiation oncologists, and medical physicists all working together have really fine-tuned how treatments are planned and delivered; it is no wonder that IGSRT has become a favorite non-surgical option for early-stage skin cancers, balancing effective treatment with preserving appearance in outpatient clinics (Peyton et al., 2024). Radiation treatment is not just reserved for common skin conditions anymore. While it was previously primarily employed for noncancerous problems, today its primary function is for cancer ; working on issues such as keloids, BCC, and squamous cell carcinoma. Newer methods such as intensity-modulated radiation therapy (IMRT) have, in the majority of instances, made it possible for clinicians to conform the dose exactly around tumor volumes and spare significant amounts of healthy tissue. This is particularly crucial when the cancer is adjacent to sensitive portions of the skin. Nevertheless, despite these advances, skin toxicity from radiation is still a very real clinical challenge, appearing as either acute reactions or more chronic issues that can truly impact a patient's quality of life. Scientists are always looking for ways to learn about and reduce these side effects so that the therapeutic gain and skin health remain more in balance (Kemin et al., 2024). Since skin is anatomically and physiologically fragile under radiation, determining the appropriate treatment regimen requires a delicate, nearly nuanced touch. Radiation damage can be as simple as redness and peeling or as advanced as fibrosis, so avoiding these complications is no easy task for the fighters of skin cancers. Current research continues to emphasize the need to catch things early and take steps to relieve them. In addition, with the development of new systems for radiation delivery and the increased prevalence of team care, patient results have remained visibly improved. Not only does this collaborative approach ensure that doses reach precisely where they are needed but also integrates additional support to maintain an intact look and functionality of the skin. All these continuous developments emphasize that radiation therapy continues to play a central role in the general struggle against skin tumors, finding that adaptive equilibrium between firm treatment outcome and patient-focusing care (Kemin et al., 2024; Peyton et al., 2024) (Figure 9.10).

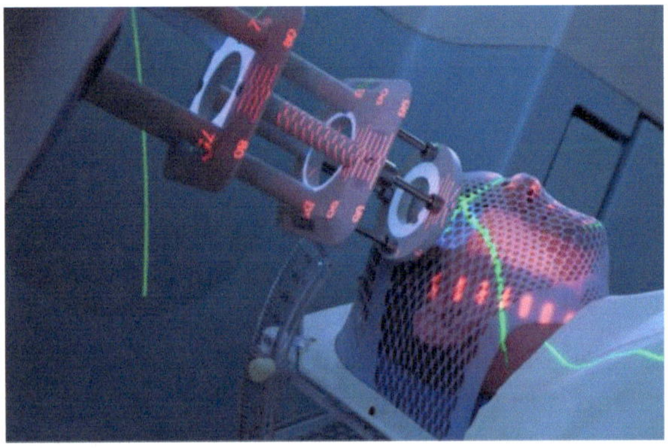

Figure 9.10. Radiation therapy.

Cancer Care Centers of Brevard. (n.d.). *How Radiation Therapy is Used for Skin Cancer Treatment.* https://www.cancercarebrevard.com/uploads/_550x350_crop_center-center_none/how-radiation-therapy-is-used-for-skin-cancer-treatment-brevard-country-oncologists.jpg.

9.4.3. Chemotherapy and Targeted Therapies

Recent advances in the fight against cancer have truly turned things around for individuals struggling with skin tumors and cancers. Surgery remains the first step when the tumor is localized, but as things become more complex , such as in advanced or metastatic cases – chemo and targeted therapy begin to take center stage. Chemo predominantly functions by disrupting the fast proliferation of cancer cells, which serves to reduce the burden of the tumor; however, it appears to also alter the way that our immune system responds. At times, these cell-killing regimens end up altering the ways in which immune cells act so as to assist in eradicating the tumor, but other times they may even make things worse by fostering resistance or recurrence. Wrestling with these combined influences is usually essential for maintaining the disease at bay for as long as possible (Coffelt et al., 2015). A newer take has emerged from targeted therapies that target the tiny molecular characterestics behind tumor development. Use BCC , the most frequent skin cancer , as an illustration; in this case, the issue is often one of an ever-present Hedgehog (Hh) signaling pathway. This continuous signal renders the pathway an ideal target for new medications. Medications such as Vismodegib are created to inhibit the Hh receptor Smoothened (Smo), and they have had fairly good success with those BCC cases that are refractory to surgery. This minimally invasive approach can occasionally save patients the greater cost of extensive surgery. And then there are additional molecules – even repurposed molecules like Itraconazole – that appear to be able to disrupt Hh signaling, promising an increasingly diverse set of weapons for the fight against skin tumors (Cucchi et al., 2012). Despite such encouraging developments, however, there are still challenges. Cancer cells can be recalcitrant – they could be inherently resistant or become increasingly resistant to treatment over time. For example, alterations further along the Hh pathway, including mutations in Gli transcription factors, may weaken the impact of drugs targeting Smo, which in most instances has encouraged researchers to look at next-generation therapies. Others suggest that by pairing targeted drugs with immune modulators or other pathway inhibitors, resistance can be overcome and the overall antitumor effect increased. There are also current clinical trials now experimenting with different combinations , such as PI3K inhibitors in combination with retinoids – hoping to further refine these therapies. At the end of the day, a deeper look into the molecular culprits behind skin tumors, in addition to a clearer understanding of the role of the immune system, is crucial to making therapies more durable and less toxic, ultimately resulting in better patient outcomes (Cucchi et al., 2012; Coffelt et al., 2015) (Figure 9.11).

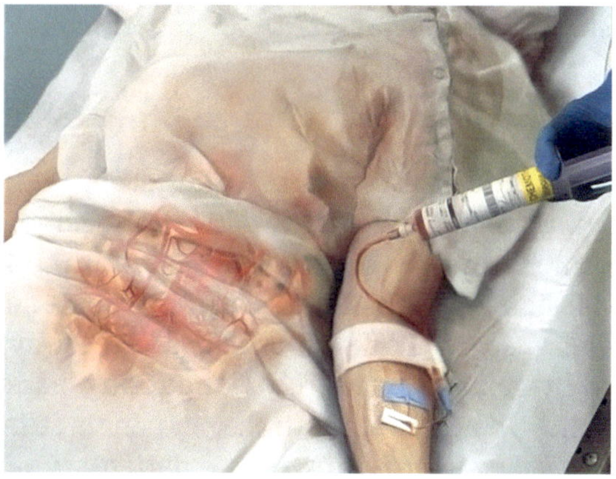

Figure 9.11. Chemotherapy to treat cancer.

Source: StoryMD. (n.d.). *Illustrates Different Types of Skin Cancers* https://cdn.storymd.com/optimized/PqEk3kH1o2/original.jpg.

9.5. Prevention Strategies

Genes are a large factor in who may develop skin tumors early, so preventing that risk requires prevention that suits the individual. Take the case of Xeroderma pigmentosum (XP), for instance, a genetic disorder in which the DNA repair simply is not good enough. People with XP turn out much more sun-sensitive, usually developing basal cell or squamous cell carcinomas at an astonishingly young age. An early diagnosis allows physicians to get a headstart on aggressive sun protection measures, frequent skin exams, and even some genetic counseling. All these interventions, collectively, slow down the growth of the tumor and indicate how prevention can work differently (Aftab et al., 2025). Viral infections have also been gaining attention, particularly those associated with human papillomavirus (HPV). Scientists have observed that some beta papillomavirus types appear in the history of cutaneous squamous cell carcinoma—very different from the mucosal HPV types responsible for anogenital and oropharyngeal cancers. The vaccines available to us primarily address those mucosal types, so they do not address beta HPV at all, which really complicates full prevention coverage. Since beta HPV is commonly acquired in childhood and since immunocompromised individuals are even more vulnerable, novel vaccination approaches are being investigated. There are some possibilities suggested by animal models, although no human-licensed vaccine, whether prophylactic or therapeutic, has yet been developed. The concept of vaccination in the majority of situations appears encouraging but remains more of a hoped-for ideal in the battle against HPV-related skin cancers (Meyer & Stockfleth, 2024). In addition to genetic and viral hazards, day-to-day precautions continue to be the mainstay of reducing skin tumor occurrences. Basic measures such as applying high-SPF sunscreens, dressing protectively, and altering behavior to avoid excessive exposure to UV are generally recommended. Public health campaigns that increase awareness of such risk factors and promote early screening for abnormal skin moles are also crucial. Regular surveillance for any unusual spots entails faster doctor's visits, which can significantly lessen the pain and danger associated with skin cancers. Also, combining these preventive routines with our increased understanding of genetic and viral influences appears to sharpen our overall tactics. Lifestyle adjustments, early detection, and new medical concepts holds the greatest hope for lightening the burden of skin tumors.

9.5.1. Sun Protection Measures

UV light does a lot more than simply make us tan – it has a significant role in initiating skin tumors and other problems. Our skin is exposed to harm over a period from the UV, and although things like BCC, squamous cell carcinoma, and melanoma result from a combination of pesky gene activity and other environmental pieces, the sunbeam remains the direct trigger most of the time. Sun protection is not merely a suggestion; it is front and center when it comes to preventing skin cancers. A broad-spectrum sunscreen, for instance, provides a barrier against UVA and UVB rays, and research tends to highlight that regular, diligent use can prevent DNA damage from getting out of hand and turning into cancer (Brockman, 2020). This treatment, in the majority of instances, complements treatments such as Mohs surgery by reducing the likelihood of new lesions developing while otherwise promoting overall skin well-being (Brockman et al., 2020). Protective clothing is another important contributor here – it is not just the lotion. Clothing with high UV Protection Factor values will block UV light well without reapplication every couple of hours, something that, let us be honest, can be inconvenient with sunscreen. This protection is particularly suitable for people who have fair skin or a family history of skin cancer. Additionally, sun-protective clothing tends to cover up those small areas that individuals may overlook when applying sunscreen, providing one more level of protection against cumulative UV damage that can cause tumors (Sieniawska et al., 2024). Incorporating these measures into one's daily routines will decelerate photoaging and ward off premalignant lesions, emphasizing the general importance of combining various types of protection. How we act in the sun also makes a big difference. All things considered, attempting to steer clear of the hottest hours of the day ; approximately 10 AM through 4 PM. , can significantly reduce both short-term burns and long-term skin damage. Public health campaigns tend to encourage us to look at the UV index and learn why it is so important to protect our skin. When good habits are combined with routine sunscreen applications and appropriate clothing, the outcome is a more even strategy against exposure to UV. All of these steps not only cut down on the danger of skin tumors; they also cut down on the need for invasive treatments such as Mohs surgery (Brockman, 2020; Sieniawska et al., 2024). In short, proper sun protection is a necessity in our constant struggle to combat the ever-increasing incidence of skin malignancies.

9.5.2. Regular Skin Examinations

Early diagnosis truly makes a difference when treating skin tumors—it can determine a patient's treatment and prognosis. A little variation in a skin lesion may sometimes signal that something is amiss, so regular skin checks are the way to go. Physicians, by merely conducting hands-on and visual examinations, can sometimes identify strange features that patients would not notice on their own. How a lesion feels and appears—its shape, size, and rate at which it is changing, is telling. Frequent skin checks, in most instances, catch things early enough to avoid more complicated issues. This type of vigilant practicality is comparable with what occurs in screening for other organs, illustrating that being vigilant indeed pays dividends (Bhosale et al., 2023). Even beyond a physician's gut, emerging technology has assisted in enhancing these skin screenings. Consider dermoscopy, for instance; it allows professionals to look beneath the surface in manners that allow it to become simpler to distinguish between an innocuous mark and one that is of concern. When regular skin exams are combined with devices such as imaging, risk sorting becomes much more apparent and unnecessary biopsies diminish. In addition, on these visits, patients are taught to watch for themselves, seeing if an area begins to look or feel different. Similar to how imaging revolutionized breast cancer screening with mammography, including these additional tools with skin examination provides more holistic and team-based methodology for identifying malignancies early (Pachana et al., 2024). Consequently, these methods expand on what the clinician can detect and assist in monitoring individuals who might be at higher risk. However, even with such advantages, frequent skin checks are not without challenges. Problems such as access, proper awareness generation, and adherence to advised check-up intervals prove to be challenging. Variations in skin type and age also result in skin tumors not impacting all individuals similarly, meaning screening frequently must be adjusted accordingly. Strides to standardize guidelines for exams and further educate providers are assisting in increasing quality in a variety of settings. Public campaigns, somewhat similar to those in mammography programs for breast cancer, are promoting more frequent skin examinations to bridge the gaps in participation and increase public enthusiasm (Bhosale et al., 2023; Pachana et al., 2024). All these practices, when taken together, emphasize that routine skin examination is an integral component of prevention and early intervention in skin cancer (Figure 9.12).

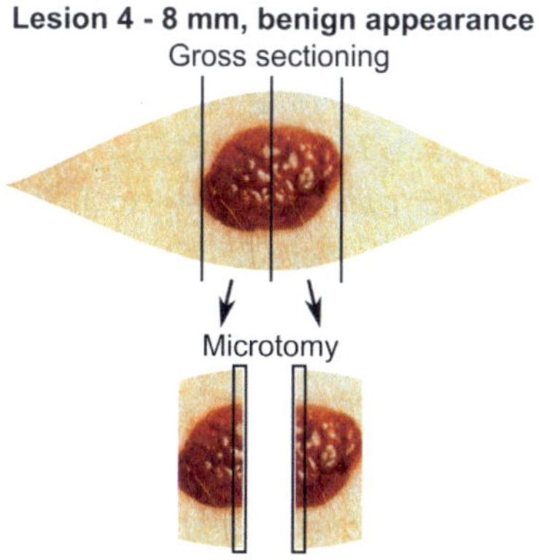

Figure 9.12. Skin examination.

Source: By Mikael Häggström, M.D. Author info- Reusing images- Conflicts of interest:NoneMikael Häggström, M.D. - editOwn workSource imagesNormal mole. Public DomainSuperficial basal cell carcinoma. Public DomainReferencesHandläggning av hudprover – provtagningsanvisningar, utskärningsprinciper och snittning (Handling of skin samples - sampling instructions, cutting principles and incision. Swedish Society of Pathology.- For number of slices and coverage of lesions, depending on size. Monica Dahlgren, Janne Malina, Anna Måsbäck, Otto Ljungberg. Stora utskärningen. KVAST (Swedish Society of Pathology). Retrieved on 2019-09-26.- For slices towards the pointy ends to determine radicality, which can be parallel to the slices through the lesions (shown), or as longitudinal slices that go through each pointy end.Dermatopathology Grossing Guidelines. University of California, Los Angeles. Retrieved on 2019-10-23.- For microtomy of the most central side at the lesion(2003). "The principles of mohs micrographic surgery for cutaneous neoplasia". Ochsner J 5 (2): 22–33. PMID 22826680. PMC: 3399331.- With a "standard histologic examination" that, in addition to the lesion, only includes one section from each side along the longest diameter of the specimen.- It also shows an example of circular coverage, with equal coverage distance in all four directions.- The entire specimen may be submitted if the risk of malignancy is high., CC0, https://commons.wikimedia.org/w/index.php?curid=83306495

9.5.3. Public Awareness Campaigns

Battling skin tumors is quite difficult because so many individuals just do not have the information and engagement required. Many people ignore the initial signs of skin cancers, consider BCC, squamous cell carcinoma (SCC) or melanoma, and low awareness does just that: slow down diagnosis, resulting in poorer outcomes. It requires widespread, occasionally haphazard public awareness campaigns that blend prevention advice with advice on early detection, emphasizing that rapid medical screenings count. These are not campaigns about distributing facts, but nudging frequent skin checks and encouraging a discussion with a dermatologist if something looks amiss. Matching new technology with targeted messaging gives these campaigns a boost, so it is a good thing that we are still refining our methods as we proceed. The adoption of artificial intelligence (AI) in these campaigns is yielding some definite hope for both the identification of skin cancer and educating everyone about it. For example, there is a mobile app that utilizes AI, which allows individuals to conduct self-checks—it is programmed to draw big crowds while highlighting possible skin malignancy threats (Uskova et al., 2024). The device passed more than 500,000 images and even married demographic information to provide a straightforward, binary opinion regarding whether or not a lesion is concerning. Its affordability and simplicity of access nicely supplement conventional health measures, driving individuals toward earlier visits to dermatologists. All these technology-supported steps appear to emphasize how central technology is becoming in equipping individuals with actual, actionable information. Nevertheless, despite these advantages, there are challenges for campaigns against skin tumors, particularly in identifying new danger signs for health and gaining enough public consensus for intervention policies. Current polls indicate that the majority of individuals remain unaware of new threats, such as some substances that cause excessive skin ulcers for drug abusers (Olivia et al., 2025). And apart from this, support for measures addressing these problems remains quite low, so we must clarify the risks and initiate broader community action. When campaign efforts adapt to various backgrounds and even previous drug use histories, they more effectively resonate, creating a crowd that is not only more well-informed but also more engaged. Ultimately, consistent—if at times flawed—public education is still essential to diminishing skin cancer damage and generating backing for efficient prevention and treatment practices.

9.6. Current Research and Advances

Breakthroughs in skin cancer diagnosis have fueled a revolution toward employing machine-assisted techniques for identifying issues early and enhancing treatment outcomes. Traditionally, physicians relied heavily on biopsies and more intuitive pathology examination, which, admit it or not, would sometimes differ quite significantly—but nowadays, innovative computer-assisted tools are giving them a shakeup. Consider machine-aided skin cancer diagnosis (MASCD) systems, for instance; they rely on quantifiable information and sophisticated imaging methods, and that generally equates to diagnoses being more accurate and consistent. As melanoma and non-melanoma diagnoses increase globally, these advancements really count, as making the diagnosis accurately is paramount to patient care and can reduce the risk of fatal outcomes.

Continuous research continues to blend findings from biology with computational approaches to identify malignant lesions at an earlier stage, which in turn increases the opportunities for effective treatment (Meshram et al., 2022). There has been a more explicit examination of the genetic pieces involved in some of those uncommon, yet aggressive, skin cancers, a discovery that is unveiling new therapeutic avenues. Scientists investigating adenoid cystic carcinoma—yes, that cancer most commonly referred to in cases of the salivary gland—have suggested that some genetic abnormalities, such as the MYB-NFIB fusion and alterations in essential transcription factors, may also appear along with aggressive skin tumors. Okay, these biomarkers do not appear in all instances, but overall, learning about their involvement in the development of tumors could make it possible for more targeted therapies. This genetic perspective is gradually altering the way we approach and treat these cancers, holding out hope for improved risk evaluation and outright new approaches to treatment (Wysocki et al., 2016). Although we are progressing on both molecular and technological levels when it comes to identifying and treating skin tumors, much still remains between us and routine clinical application. Skin tumors are so diverse, in their genetic constituency as in how they conduct themselves on the skin surface, which disentangling all the causative threads still poses a formidable challenge. And, honestly, merging these high-tech diagnostic tools with old trusted routines is not easy; diligent tests for accuracy, cost, and, yes, availability is essential. Scientists, doctors, and computer specialists are finally banding together, even if it means wading through some challenging intersections, to accelerate the creation of good screening tools and focused treatments. As the work proceeds, the goal is to improve patient outcomes by detecting cancers earlier, personalizing treatments to the case, and, hopefully, lowering the overall burden of these cancers.

9.6.1. Innovations in Treatment

Treatment of skin cancer has taken a new direction. Radiation therapy is no longer all about zapping away tumors with wide X-rays. Nowadays, proton therapy appears as a targeted solution that, in the majority of instances, is more effective on tumor cells and leaves the surrounding healthy skin alone – an important consideration with how the anatomy of the skin is both superficial and strangely convoluted. IMRT and IGRT now appear in the picture as well, allowing physicians to customize the dose in a manner that addresses irregular tumor forms and reduces the side-effects characteristic of earlier radiation techniques (Collins, 2017). These breakthroughs seem to represent a step in the direction of safer and more customized care that really enhances patient results and general quality of life. Newer approaches in immunosuppressive therapy are also charting new avenues, particularly when it comes to skin cancers that are associated with transplants or involve complicated immune involvement. Physicians are trying out adjustments in dosing regimens with agents such as tacrolimus and sirolimus in order to decrease complications, but maintaining graft survival intact in the process—this strategy is sort of coming into its own for immune-associated skin cancers as well (Reyes et al., 2005).

Too much immunosuppression risks infections and even secondary cancers, whereas too little might not keep the disease at bay, so finding that balance is crucial. It is a reminder, generally speaking, of how important tailoring the treatment to each patient's needs can be, even if it sometimes comes with a few hiccups in execution. In looking at the larger picture, these technological breakthroughs are becoming part of the greater drive for precision medicine in treating cancer. Molecular diagnosis now assists in identifying tumor subtypes and mutations more distinctly, which in turn directs the combination of targeted treatments, radiation, and immunosuppressive adjustments. Checkpoint inhibitors and other immune therapies that are tailored to skin cancer catch this sea change well by administering a kind of stimulus to the body so that it can fight the cancer and leaving the normal tissues largely alone. Essentially, the combination of precise radiation, intelligent immune modulation, and targeted molecular drugs is changing how we treat skin tumors, resulting in improved survival chances and less burden of side effects. Continued research, as emphasized by Reyes et al. (2005) and Collins. (2017), continues to be the mainstay in extending these gains to more patients, and that is something worth noting (Figure 9.13).

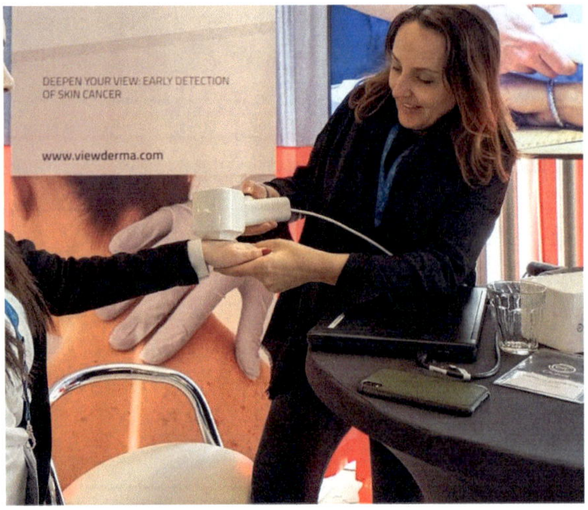

Figure 9.13. Ultra-early detection of skin cancer using multispectral camera and AI algorithms.

Source: Brainport Eindhoven. (n.d.). *Innovation Day Benelux.* https://brainporteindhoven.com/fileadmin/_processed_/2/4/csm_Eindhoven.InnovationDay-1280x640_7eb150e420.jpg.

9.6.2. Genetic Research and Implications

It has truly gone deeper into our understanding of tumor biology, particularly skin cancers. Researchers have learned that processes such as DNA methylation and slight variations in histone structures can fine-tune gene expression without physically rewriting the DNA code. At times, these alterations silence the very genes that have protective functions for cells, and at other times turn on genes that get tumors moving. In the majority of instances, by unwinding this complex interaction, scientists are able to identify patterns that recur – biomarkers that suggest early diagnosis and even prognosis. Attacking these epigenetic errors could pave the way for therapies that are more targeted and effective, a consideration that highlights why continued epigenetic research is vital to streamlining our clinical approaches and improving patient outcomes (Rehman et al., 2025). Genetic mutations, it turns out, do not stop at twisting epigenetics. Errors in RNA splicing—when the normal process of cutting and rejoining RNA goes off track—have also gathered interest for their role in oncogenesis. Mutations in genes that normally wedded together precise splicing factors often result in messy RNA processing, leading to proteins that just do not function right, thereby nudging cells toward malignancy. Scientists are already experimenting with new chemicals that attack these broken pathways. Take one inhibitor, for example; although still in the research stage, it is demonstrating encouraging trends in blood cancers by regulating splicing regulation, and this could very well translate to addressing similar splicing defects in skin cancer. This entire trajectory emphasizes the way genetic studies can assist in the design of therapies that target extremely precise tumor defects, reducing toxicity and increasing rates of success (Yokoyama et al., 2024). Translating these genetic findings into real-world patient care is about considering the bigger picture—the tug and pull between gene alterations and a tumor's local environment. Epigenetic modifications and splicing mistakes do not work in isolation. They tend to combine with other signaling pathways that promote tumor growth or help the cancer evade immune surveillance. By untangling these shadowy networks, scientists are starting to identify combination therapies that target multiple of these cancerous pathways simultaneously. This wider, occasionally chaotic perspective provides clinicians with the opportunity to tailor treatments to the individual genetic and epigenetic profile of each tumor, paving the way for what many refer to as precision medicine in skin cancers. Eventually, combining these genetic leads with therapy regimens holds a great deal of promise for reducing both the disease and mortality associated with skin cancers, and it confirms the importance of maintaining molecular research (Rehman et al., 2025; Yokoyama et al., 2024).

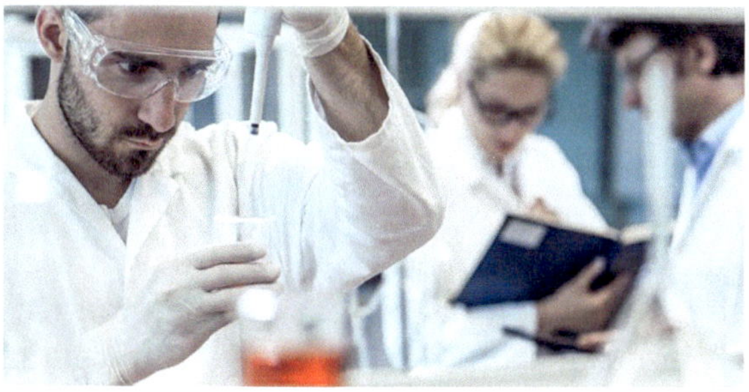

Source: Sanjeri. (2016). *Scientists Working in the Laboratory.* https://medicinehealth.leeds.ac.uk/images/resized/750x375-0-0-1-80-iStock_597645726_800x400.jpg.

9.6.3. Future Directions in Skin Cancer Studies

Advancements in molecular methods have now opened up a new avenue towards skin tumor understanding – single-cell RNA sequencing (scRNA-seq) is proving to be a true game-changer. Researchers can now excavate the tumor microenvironment with an unprecedented level of detail; they discover various groups of cells and even glimpse the nature of how these cells interact in order to power tumor growth and enable it to evade the immune system. In most instances, unearthing these clandestine maneuvers provides new insights into tumor heterogeneity, a problem long creating difficulties for effective therapy. This type of fine-grained profiling has the ability to disrupt established systems of classification and pave the way for new targets of therapy, potentially enhancing personalized medicine. In skin cancers such as BCC, squamous cell carcinoma, and melanoma, which are steadily increasing, integrating scRNA-seq into the clinical and research environments appears quite critical for creating more specific therapies that address tumor complexity (Feng et al., 2025). Immunotherapy, however, has transformed our way of treating skin cancers – particularly through immune checkpoint inhibitors (ICIs), which have revolutionized treatment paradigms. Despite their triumph, patients continue to struggle with resistance and persistent disease progression, emphasizing the establishment of new approaches to augment or complement existing immunotherapies. Oncolytic viruses, such as *talimogene laherparepvec* (T-VEC), have been gaining more and more interest for their capacity to destroy tumors directly while igniting a more general systemic immune reaction. The FDA approval of T-VEC in melanoma attests to their potential, but trials combining these viruses with ICIs have yielded equivocal results—toward the messy intricacies of realizing a real immunologic synergy. Additional investigation of the best ways to administer these viruses, why resistance arises, and how to optimize combination regimens is an important step towards bridging the existing gap in immunotherapy in skin cancer treatment (Nassief et al., 2024). In the future, the convergence of cutting-edge molecular tools with new-generation immunotherapies will redefine the future of skin cancer research. There is unmistakable movement towards individualized strategies that integrate extensive tumor profiling with sharp read of the individual patient's immune landscape, which broadly holds the promise of better treatment accuracy and efficacy. Meanwhile, widening research on the tumor microenvironment's role in therapeutic resistance might open the door to more complex intervention approaches. At the same time, progress in oncolytic virotherapy is worthy of even greater scrutiny, particularly when combined with next-generation agents and potentially used against tumors other than melanoma, thereby expanding its utility to other skin cancers. It will be important to address the shortcomings that have been observed in current clinical trials and take advantage of novel biotechnologies to improve survival rates and quality of life in skin tumor patients and advance research to an increasingly active, integrated treatment model (Feng et al., 2025; Nassief et al., 2024).

CLOSER LOOK

Tumor Suppressor Genes

Tumor suppressor genes are healthy genes that have an important role in controlling cell growth and stopping abnormal cell division, which might result in cancer. They are like "brakes" on cell growth to prevent cells from growing too rapidly and to trigger programmed cell death (apoptosis) in damaged or aged cells. If these genes are deformed or turned off, the "brakes" of the cell are let off, resulting in out-of-control cell growth and possibly tumoration.

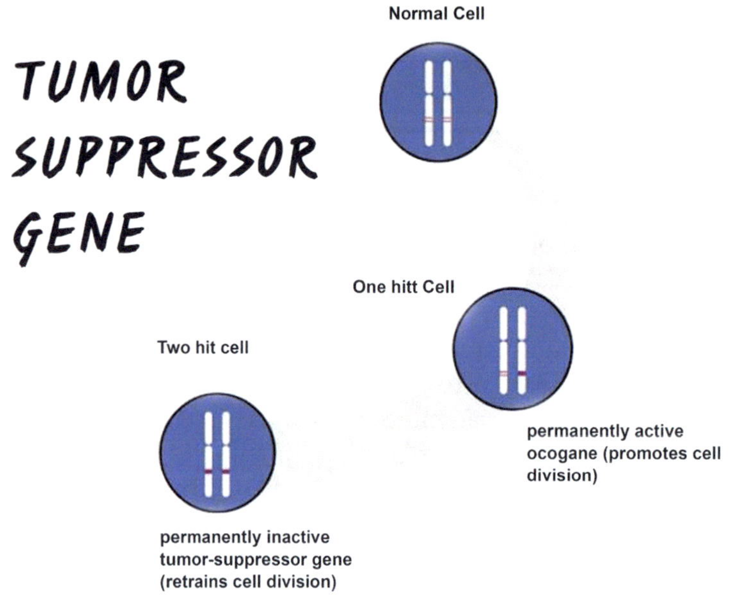

Source: Freepik. (n.d.). *Tumor Suppressor Gene: Gene that Regulates Cell Growth and Division. When Mutated, It Can Lose Its Ability to Control Cell Growth, Contributing to Cancer Development.* https://img.freepik.com/premium-vector/tumor-suppressor-gene-gene-that-regulates-cell-growth-division-when-mutated-can-lose-its-ability-control-cell-growth-contributing-cancer-development_37925-5802.jpg.

- **Functions of Tumor Suppressor Genes:**
  - **Cell Cycle Regulation:** Tumor suppressor genes regulate the cell cycle so that cells divide when they should divide and also with the correct amount of DNA.
  - **Inhibiting Cell Growth:** They prevent cells from growing and dividing too rapidly, which can lead to uncontrolled cell proliferation.
  - **Inducing Apoptosis:** They cause programmed cell death (apoptosis) to destroy damaged or defective cells.
  - **DNA Repair:** Certain tumor suppressor genes are associated with DNA repair processes, which correct DNA errors and prevent them from becoming mutations.

- **Examples of Tumor Suppressor Genes:**
  - **TP53 (p53):** This gene is involved in the regulation of the cell cycle and the induction of apoptosis. TP53 mutations occur in most cancers.
  - **RB (Retinoblastoma):** This is a gene that is responsible for regulating cell cycle progression. RB mutations are linked to retinoblastoma as well as other cancers.
  - **BRCA1 and BRCA2:** Both of these genes play a role in DNA repair and cell cycle regulation. BRCA1 and BRCA2 mutations predispose to breast and ovarian cancer.

SUMMARY

Clinical progress has truly revolutionized the way we manage skin tumors and associated cancers now. For instance, excision of recalcitrant scalp carcinomas now requires extremely cautious slicing accompanied by certain reconstruction techniques. In most cases, research indicates that split-thickness skin grafts do better than full-thickness skin grafts when applied to skull regions treated with burr; this indicates a more dependable procedure following the removal of a tumor. A tactile exam to test how far the tumor adheres is still useful, but occasionally imaging is required for larger lesions to ensure nothing is left behind. These methods all serve to ensure clean margins and reduce the risk of recurrence, ultimately improving patient outcomes. It would appear evident that the combination of surgical innovation and sound clinical acumen is essential when treating malignant skin tumors (Al-Aswad et al., 2024). Taking a step back to the larger context of malignancy diagnosis, advances in genetic and molecular testing are gradually altering the way we evaluate tumor risk and detect early warning signs of dysfunction. The recent surge of high-throughput sequencing has, in the majority of instances, brought with it an opportunity for an expanded examination of myeloid neoplasms with germline predisposition, a challenge that strangely parallels what we face in skin tumors, where genetic hints increasingly inform prognosis. Nevertheless, securing germline variants depends significantly on obtaining uncontaminated samples of tissue, something that can be difficult in reality. In certain cases, other sampling such as hair follicle biopsies have already started to act as useful substitutes for conventional skin biopsies when it comes to genetic testing, particularly where problems arise from treatment such as stem cell transplantation. These emerging techniques demonstrate how molecular diagnostics can marry with routine cancer evaluations and lead to a future of even more tailored management of skin cancers (Perani et al., 2023). Ultimately, combining surgical accuracy, meticulous pathological examination, and contemporary molecular testing makes for a pretty good system for managing skin tumors and cancers. Recent research, in the majority of instances, emphasizes how surgeons, pathologists, and geneticists must more closely work together to enhance both diagnostic precision and treatment success. The combined strategy enables treatment plans that accommodate both the tumor's behavior as well as the patient's genetic characterestics, advancing the standard of care a little further. As more research is done, new technologies will refine early detection, enhance margin analysis and further advance reconstructive methods, all in hopes of minimizing post-surgery complications. Ultimately, the constant change in diagnostic and treatment procedures is paramount to ensuring better survival rates and a better quality of life for patients struggling with cutaneous malignancies.

Signaling pathways involved in skin cancer development kind of dance in a complex, unforeseeable manner. Ras and Notch, two significant pathways which otherwise direct cell conduct—may lose their way in the process of tumor growth. For instance, when Notch1 falls out of sync (as opposed to Notch2), skin tumors appear to receive a kickstart. And then there is the puzzling appearance of PDX1 in suprabasal keratinocytes and peaking during wound repair, suggesting, in the majority of instances, a function in cell differentiation of the skin not on our minds until now. All this sloppy evidence leads us to suspect the complicated web of molecular contacts driving skin cancers and that adjusting these signals may tip the balance in tumor growth and advancement (Barbara et al., 2010). It truly illustrates why closer examination of the functions of individual receptors is necessary for better treatment of skin cancer. BCC is, undoubtedly, the most prevalent form of skin cancer, and it comes with a myriad of clinical and economic nightmares around the globe. Surgery may remove local lesions but tends to be followed by visible scars – not what one wants, particularly when further advanced or metastatic BCC appears, necessitating other tactics because patients are prone to grow new tumors down the road. Almost all cases have some wayward Hh signaling, with the Smo receptor being particularly prominent. With drugs such as Vismodegib being approved and others ; consider off-label utilization of Itraconazole and Vitamin D3 in development, there is an evident movement toward treatments targeting this molecular pathway. Scientists are now, in general, attempting to bypass resistance to drugs and balance combination regimens in order to enhance patient outcomes (Cucchi et al., 2012). If you take a step back and collate these findings, you have a pretty messy picture of skin tumor biology. Ras, Notch, and Hh—each playing its own idiosyncratic role—impinge on tumor initiation, cell differentiation, and subsequent progression. Observing how Notch1's behavior contrasts with that of Notch2 provides a new twist to our vision of epidermal cancer (Mazur et a;., 2010). Concurrently, the exclusive dependence of BCC on Hh signaling has opened doors to treatments that go beyond the classic surgery-first protocol. As researchers continue to unravel these molecular enigmas and perfect targeted therapy, there is guarded hope that more effective and minimally invasive solutions are in the offing. All this truly highlights the necessity of combining molecular understanding with clinical practice to address the general load of skin cancers (Mazur et al., 2010; Cucchi et al., 2012).

KEY TERMS FROM THIS CHAPTER

- Aggressive growth
- Basal cell carcinomas
- Cancer-associated fibroblasts
- Cd+ t cells
- Chemo
- Immunohistochemistry
- Immunotherapies
- Microenvironment
- Natural killer t cells
- Neurofibromatosis type
- Pre-cancerous lesions
- Precision therapies
- Radiation
- Skin tumor development
- Squamous cell carcinomas
- Tumors

REFERENCES

1. Adashek, J. J., Kato, S., Lippman, S. M., & Kurzrock, R. (2020). The paradox of cancer genes in non-malignant conditions: implications for precision medicine. Genome medicine, 12(1), 16. https://doi.org/10.1186/s13073-020-0714-yAftab, K., Maqsood, S., & Yaqoob, N. (2025). Skin tumors in pediatric patients with xeroderma pigmentosum: A case series. Indian Journal of Medical and Paediatric Oncology. Ind J Med Paediatr Oncol 2025;46:99–103 https://www.semanticscholar.org/paper/fcb9200ee299956b620eccd3ad44e298fe0aa475 (accessed on 12 May 2025).
2. Al-Aswad, F., Al-Hassani, F., Fernandez-Diaz, O., & Al Naser, M. (2024). Management of immobile scalp skin tumors and analysis of skin graft survival on burred calvaria. Plastic and Reconstructive Surgery Global Open, 12. https://www.semanticscholar.org/paper/03c66cb0b61ab6710a7b44aadd921529344d971e (accessed on 12 May 2025).
3. Almasan, I., & Piciu, D. (2023). Triple primary malignancies: Tumor associations, survival, and clinicopathological analysis: A 25-year single-institution experience. Healthcare, 11. https://www.semanticscholar.org/paper/28f881325a116e754086f2e064067219b8d38779 (accessed on 12 May 2025).
4. Bešlić, I., Krišto, M., Lugović-Mihić, L., Novak-Bilić, et al. (2021). Mogu li se na koži odraziti malignomi unutarnjih organa? Dokazi iz kliničkih slučajeva. https://core.ac.uk/download/493043780.pdf.
5. Bhosale, S. J. , Janugade, H. B., & Kanase, V. V. (2023). Evaluation of breast disease using triple assessment test with ultrasonography as the fourth component. Vol. 44 No. S1 (2023): Microbial Diversity and Disease Management: The Interface Between Animals and People . https://doi.org/10.53555/jaz.v44iS1.896
6. Birlea, S., Bosenberg, M. W., Box, N. F., Brash, et al. (2018). Frontiers in pigment cell and melanoma research. http://arxiv.org/abs/1808.01869 (accessed on 12 May 2025).
7. Blanco, R., Rengifo, E., Rengifo, C. E., Cedeño, M., Frómeta, M., & Carr, A. (2011). Immunohistochemical Reactivity of the 14F7 Monoclonal Antibody Raised against N-Glycolyl GM3 Ganglioside in Some Benign and Malignant Skin Neoplasms. ISRN dermatology, 2011, 848909. https://doi.org/10.5402/2011/848909.
8. Bray, F., Laversanne, M., Sung, H., Ferlay, J., Siegel, R. L., Soerjomataram, I., & Jemal, A. (2024). Global cancer statistics 2022: GLOBOCAN estimates of incidence and mortality worldwide for 36 cancers in 185 countries. CA: A Cancer Journal for Clinicians, 74, 229–263. https://doi.org/10.3322/caac.21834.
9. Brockman, Andrew M., ""Skin Cancer Types and the Effectiveness of Mohs Surgery Against Them"" (2020). Honors Theses. 722. https://encompass.eku.edu/honors_theses/722 (accessed on 12 May 2025).
10. Browne, I., Weadick, C., Duffy, A., Jones, H. I., Doig, R. K., Bradley, E., Bell, N., Nagda, et al. (2021). Assessing the impact of anti-PD-1/PD-L1 inhibitors on cancer care health and budget in Ireland. Journal of Clinical Oncology, 39. https://www.semanticscholar.org/paper/d13982e3363133ce7d3b007914278ba7b7e8c991 (accessed on 12 May 2025).
11. Collins, Cielle, "Radiation Therapy Medical Physics Review – Delivery, Interactions, Safety, Feasibility, and Head to Head Comparisons of the Leading

Radiation Therapy Techniques" (2017). Honors Theses and Capstones. 377. https://scholars.unh.edu/honors/377 (accessed on 12 May 2025).

12. Cucchi, D., Occhione, M. A., Gulino, A., & De Smaele, E. (2012). Hedgehog signaling pathway and its targets for treatment in basal cell carcinoma. Journal of experimental pharmacology, 4, 173–185. https://doi.org/10.2147/JEP.S28553(accessed on 12 May 2025).

13. David James Barnes, Bea Storer-Prescott, Aditi Vedi, Claire Palles; Abstra*ct PR001: Inheri*ted *ge*netic variants in known cancer predisposition genes: A survey of the largest European cohort of patients under the age of 25 with whole genome sequencing data. Cancer Res 1 September 2024; 84 (17_Supplement): PR0*01. https://d*oi.org/10.1158/1538-7445.PEDIATRIC24-PR001(accessed on 12 May 2025).

14. E. Thayalan, A. Arumugavel, S. Ganeshan, M. Dalaxshan, H. Fernando and K. Rajapakse, "Web Application to predict Skin Disease: An Approach Using Deep Learning Algorithm," 2024 International Congress on Human-Comput*er Interaction, Optimization and Robotic* Applications (HORA), Istanbul, Turkiye, 2024, pp. 1-6, doi: 10.1109/HORA61326.2024.10550492.(accessed on 12 May 2025).

15. Feng, Y., Liu, L., Hu, C., Su*n, J., Yin, M.*, & Li, X. (2025). Advances and applications of single-cell RNA sequencing in deciphering the tumor microenvironment of malignant skin tumors. Eurasian Journal of Medicine and Oncology. https://www.semanticscholar.org/paper/c806552e713787b83ea0933cd31a52d109ce5cf9 (accessed on 12 *May 2025).*

*16. Forsthuber, A., Asch*enbrenner, B., Korosec, A., Jacob, T., Annusver, K., Krajic, N., Kholodniuk, D., et al. (2024). Cancer-associated fibroblast subtypes modulate the tumor-immune microenvironment and are associated with skin cancer malignancy. Nature Communications, 15. https://www.semanticscholar.org/paper/ccd27*13b0c663df0e2e3bdf2c0d5d4c1*8aaa48b4 (accessed on 12 May 2025).

17. Golan, Olivia K. PhD; Liu, Weiwei PhD; Taylor, Bruce PhD. Public Xylazine Awareness and Support for Policies and Initiatives to Address the Xylazine Threat among US Adults. Journal *of Addiction Medicine ():10.1097/ADM.*0000000000001431, January 16, 2025. | DOI: 10.1097/ADM.0000000000001431(accessed on 12 May 2025).

18. Gong, W., Zhou, J., Hou, Y., Zhang, J., He, P., & Yu, Q. (2024). The causal relationship between immune cells mediating FIT3L, CCL4, OSM, and skin-derived deteriorated tumors. Skin Research and Technology, 30. https://www.semanticscholar.org/paper/fa3df06cdb3e64c1db9516c5dc16d6eda1455cec (accessed on 12 May 2025).

19. Hardy, N., Vegivinti, C. T. R., Mehta, M., Thurnham, J., Mebane, A., Pederson, J. M., Tarchand, R., Shivakumar, J., Olaniran, P., Gadodia, R., Ganguly, A., Kelagere, Y., Nallabolu, R. R., Gaddam, M., K*eesari, P. R., Pulakurthi, Y. S., Reddy, R.*, Kallmes, K., & Musunuru, T. N. (2023). Mortality of COVID-19 in patients with hematological malignancies versus solid tumors: a systematic literature review and meta-analysis. Clinical and experi*mental medicine, 23(6), 1945–1959. https://doi.org/10.1007/s10238-023-01*004-5(accessed on 12 May 2025).

20. Harris, P. M., Farberg, A. S., Hopkins, J., Ma, L., Serure, D., Robbins, B., Osborne, C., et al. (2024). The state of the art of image guided superficial radiation therapy treatment of non-melanoma skin cancer in outpatient dermatology clinics in the United Sta*tes and review of the literature. Oncolog*y and Therapy, 13, 31–48. https://www.semanticscholar.org/paper/db3903ec7be105ead1461c3286e9120ee9bd33fc (accessed on 12 May 2025).

21. Jaifi, A., Hattab, M., Bennaoui, Y., Mourabit, F., Maidame, S., Ghazoui, H., Aziz, Z., et al. (2024). A rare case of gingivomaxillary melanoma: Case report and systematic review. Scholars Journal of Medical Case Reports. h*ttps://www.semanticschola*r.org/paper/ef1308939a00a8a3c5bab0f18cb291309c6094cc (accessed on 12 May 2025).

22. Karner, C., Anders, I., Vejzović, D., Szkandera, J., Scheipl, S., Deutsch, A., Weiss, L., et al. (2023). Targeting epigenetic features in clear cell sarcomas based on patient-derived cell lines. Journal of Translational Medicine, 21. https://www.semanticscholar.org/paper/951cd2981f22c8737f97b3e34f76fba8f4b0d3c9 (accessed on 12 May 2025).

23. Klionsky, D. J., Petroni, G., Amaravadi, R. K., Baehrecke, E. H., Ballabio, A., Boya, P., Bravo-San Pedro, J. M., et al. (2021). Autophagy in major human diseases. The EMBO Journal*, 40. https://doi.org/10.15252/e*mbj.2021108863.

24. Li, K., & Yin, R. (2024). A critical review of the progress in prevention and treatment of radiation-induced skin damage. Frontiers in Oncology, 14. https://www.semanticscholar.org/paper/16a3e8dfae61bd390100b602063a1438a960a418 Kemin, L., & Rutie, Y. (2024). A critical review of the progress in prevention and treatment of radiation-induced skin damage. Frontiers in oncology, *14, 139*5778. https://doi.org/10.3389/fonc.2024.1395778(accessed on 12 May 2025).

25. Lu, C., Riedell, P., Miller, C. A., Hagemann, I. S., Westervelt, P., Ozenberger, B. A., O'Laughlin, M., Magrini, V., Demeter, R. T., Duncavage, E. J., Griffith, M., Griffith, O. L., & Wartman, L. D. (2016). A common founding clone with TP53 and PTEN mutations gives rise to a concurrent germ cell tumor and acute megakaryoblastic leukemia. Cold Spring Harbor molecular case studies, 2(1), a000687. https://doi.*org/10.1101/mcs.a000687 (accessed* on 12 May 2025).

26. Luna, A., Merino, M. E., Alberdi, C. G., Abba, M. C., Segal-Eiras, A., & Croce, M. V. (2013). MUCI positive cutaneous metastasis with transepidermal elimination from a breast carcinoma. International medical case reports journal, 6, 81–84. https://doi.org/10.2147/IMCRJ.S52614 (accessed on 12 May 2025).

27. Mazur, P. K., Grüner, B. M., Nakhai, H., Sipos, B., Zimber-Stro*bl, U., Strobl, L. J., R*adtke, F., Schmid, R. M., & Siveke, J. T. (2010). Identification of epidermal Pdx1 expression discloses different roles of Notch1 and Notch2 in murine Kras(G12D)-induced skin carcinogenesis in vivo. PloS *one, 5(10), e13578.* https://doi.org/10.1371/journal.pone.0013578

28. Meshram, A. A. ., & Abhimanyu Dutonde, A. G. . (2022). A Review of Skin Melanoma Detection Based on Machine Learning. International Journal of New Practices in Management and Engineering, 11(01), 15–23. https:*//doi.org/10.17762/ijnpme.v11i01.145*

29. *Meye*r, T., & Stockfleth, E. (2024). Treatment and Prevention of HPV-Associated Skin Tumors by HPV Vaccination. Vaccines, 12(12), 1439. https://doi.org/10.3390/vaccines12121439(accessed on 12 May 2025).

30. Michael R. Migden, Wanxing Chai-Ho, Gregory A. Daniels, Theresa Medina, Trisha M. Wise-Draper, Meenal Kheterpal, Jennifer C. Tang, Sherrif F. Ibrahim, Diana Bolotin, Claire Verschraegen, Nathalie C. Zeitouni, Katy K. Tsai, Laxminarasimha Donthireddy, Praveen K. Bommareddy, Jeannie W. Hou, Walter Hong, Diwakar Davar; Abstract CT003: Initial results from an open-label phase 1b/2 study of RP1 oncolytic immunotherapy *in solid organ transplant recipients* with advanced cutaneous malignancies (ARTACUS). Cancer Res 1 April 2024; 84 (7_Supplement): CT003. https://doi.org/10.1158/1538-7445.AM2024-CT003(accessed on 12 May 2025).

31. Mukoyama, N., Nishio, N., Kimura, H., Kishi, S., Tokura, T., Kimura, H., Hiramatsu, M., Maruo, T., Tsuzuki, H., Fujii, M., Iwami, K., Takanari, K., Kamei, Y., Ozaki, N., Sone, M., & Fujimoto, Y. (2020). Prospective Evaluation of Health-Related Quality of Life in Patients Undergoing Anterolateral Craniofacial Resection with Orbital Exenteration. *Journal of neurological surgery*. Part B, Skull base, 81(5), 585–593. https://doi.org/10.1055/s-0039-1694010

32. Nalesnik M, Ison M. Organ transplantation from deceased donors with cancer: is it safe?. Open Access Surgery. 2011;4:11-20 https://doi.org/10.2147/OAS.S14720 (accessed on 12 May 2025).

33. Nassief, G., Anaeme, A., Moussa, K., Chen, D., & Ansstas, G. (2024). Where are we now with oncolytic viruses in melanoma and nonmelanoma skin malignancies? Pharmaceuticals, 17. https://www.semanticscholar.org/paper/7d47fddceef624e6d1c81bf9bc89531639b25819 (accessed on 12 May 2025).

34. Nipunika Somatilaka, Laasya Madana, Ali Sadek, Renee M. McKay, Lu Q. Le; Abstract 5170: STING inflames NF1 malignancies for immunotherapy. Cancer Res 1 April 2023; 83 (7_Supplement): 5170. https://doi.org/10.1158/1538-7445.AM2023-5170(accessed on 12 May 2025).

35. Pachana, M., Piersiak, M., Sawczuk, H., Tomasiewicz, A., Zabierowski, J., Kukuła, P., ... Ziomek, M. (2024). Mammography In Breast Cancer Screening – Current Knowledge, Challenges, The Impact of Artificial Intelligence, And Effectiveness With A Focus On Poland. Quality in Sport, 31, 55967. https://doi.org/10.12775/QS.2024.31.55967 (accessed on 12 May 2025).

36. Pamela Psarianos, Nicholas Fischer, David Malkin; Abstract 1124: Prevention of radiation-induced malignancies in Li-Fraumeni syndrome. Cancer Res 15 March 2024; 84 (6_Supplement): 1124. https://doi.org/10.1158/1538-7445.AM2024-1124(accessed on 12 May 2025).

37. Perani, A., Bourthoumieu, S., Rizzo, D., Chauzeix, J., Dauriat, B., Turlure, P., Girault, S., et al. (2023). Hereditary predisposition to malignant myeloid hemopathies: Caution in use of saliva and guideline based on our experience. Frontiers in Oncology, 13. https://www.semanticscholar.org/paper/cd9578c36bd6f845cd1a4043cb80e081738e0a81 (accessed on 12 May 2025).

38. Rampinelli, V., Pinacoli, A., & Piazza, C. (2024). Head and neck nonmelanoma skin cancers: Surgical management and debated issues. Current Opinion in Otolaryngology & Head and Neck Surgery, 32, 62–70. https://www.semanticscholar.org/paper/9d94b9c774a95078ebf8c0bb9e22496d54215184 (accessed on 12 May 2025).

39. Reyes, J., Mazariegos, G. V., Abu-Elmagd, K., Macedo, C., Bond, G. J., Murase, N., Peters, J., Sindhi, R., & Starzl, T. E. (2005). Intestinal transplantation under tacrolimus monotherapy after perioperative lymphoid depletion with rabbit anti-thymocyte globulin (thymoglobulin). American journal of transplantation : official journal of the American Society of Transplantation and the American Society of Transplant Surgeons, 5(6), 1430–1436. https://doi.org/10.1111/j.1600-6143.2005.00874.x

40. Saccomano, G., Pinamonti, M., Longo, E., Marcuzzo, T., Tromba, G., Dreossi, D., & Brun, F. (2024). The potential of x-ray virtual histology in the diagnosis of skin tumors. Skin research and technology : official journal of International Society for Bioengineering and the Skin (ISBS) [and] International Society for Digital Imaging of Skin (ISDIS) [and] International Society for Skin Imaging (ISSI), 30(10), e13801. https://doi.org/10.1111/srt.13801(accessed on 12 May 2025).

41. Satsuk *A.V., Solopova G.G., Ploskireva A.A., Akimkin V.G., Novichkov*a G.A. The significance of risk factors for acquiring hepatitis B and C virus infections in children with oncological and hematological diseases and immunodeficiencies. Health Risk Analysis, 2024, no. 1, pp. 100–110. DOI: 10.21668/health.risk/2024.1.10.eng(accessed on 12 May 2025).

42. Shen, B., Cen, Z., Tan, M., Song, C., Wu, X., Wang, J., & Huang, M. (2022). Curre*nt Status of Malignant Tumors after Organ Transplan*tation. BioMed research international, 2022, 5852451. https://doi.org/10.1155/2022/5852451 (Retraction published Biomed Res Int. 2024 Mar 20;2024:9879310. doi: 10.1155/2024/9879310.)Siegel, R. L., Giaquinto, A. N., & Jemal, A. (2024). Cancer statistics, *2024. CA: A Cancer Journal for Clinicians, 74, 12–49. https://doi.org/10.3322/caac.21820.*

*43. Shirley Maria D' Souza, K. Kamalaksha Shenoy, Purnima S. Rao. Spectrum of eyelid malignancies at a tertiary care hospital in coastal Ind*ia. Biomedicine: 2022; 42(6): 1376-1379(accessed on 12 May 2025).

44. Sieniawska, D., Proszowska, P., Madoń, M., Kotowicz, Z., Orzeł, A., Pich-Czekierda, A., & Sieniawska, J. (2024). Ultraviolet-Protective Clothing and Sunscreen: Sun-Protection for Healthy Skin. Journal of Education, Health and Sport, 71, 51237. https://doi.org/10.12775/JEHS.2024.71.51237(accessed on 12 May 2025).

45. Stack, B. C., Jr, Hollenbeak, C. S., Lee, C. M., Dunphy, F. R., Lowe, V. J., & Hamilton, P. D. (2004). Metallopanstimulin as a marker for head and neck cancer. World journal of surgical onco*logy, 2, 45. https://doi.org/*10.*118*6/1477-7819-2-45

46. Steinberg, I., Huland, D. M., Vermesh, O., Frostig, H., Tummers, W. S., & Gambhir, S. S. (2019). Photoacoustic clinical imaging. Photoacoustics, 14, 77–98. https://doi.org/10.1016/j.pacs.2019.05.001.

47. Ur Rehman, S., Abdullah, M., Khan, Z. K., & Shurovi, M. (2025). The role of DNA methylation and histone modifications in the pathogenesis of hematological malignancies and solid cancers: mechanisms, clinical implications, a*nd therape*utic potential. Asian Journal of Medical and Biological Research, 11(2), 23–36. https://doi.org/10.3329/ajmbr.v11i2.79668(accessed on 12 May 2025).

48. Uskova, K., Garanina, O. E., Ukharov, A., Klemenova, I., Gamayunov, S. V., Mironycheva, A., D*ardyk, V. I., et a*l. (2024). Artificial intelligence as a tool for population screening of skin tumors. Effective Pharmacotherapy. https://www.semanticscholar.org/paper/01638418d257580d8779de6819487bc74a01dde0 (accessed on 12 May 2025).

49. Wyso*cki, P. T., Izumchenko, E., Meir, J., Ha, P. K., Sidransky, D., & Brait, M. (2016). Adenoid cystic carc*inoma: emerging role of translocations and gene fusions. Oncotarget, 7(40), 66239–66254. https://doi.org/10.18632/oncotarget.11288

50. Yale-New Haven Hospital. (2009). Yale-New Haven Magazine, Fall 2009. https://core.ac.uk/download/571283440.pdf.

51. Yokoyama, H., Fukuhara, N., Ando, K., Iida, H., Yamau*chi, T., Fukuhara, S., Izu*tsu, K., et al. (2024). Abstract CT115: A first-in-human phase I study of CTX-712 in patients with advanced, relapsed or refractory malignant tumors (CTX-712-CL-01 study): Efficacy and safety in a hematologic malignancies cohort. Cancer Research. https://www.semanticscholar.org/paper/d727edb8237a03b16c87411012a94204aaf5b0e6 (accessed on 12 May 2025).

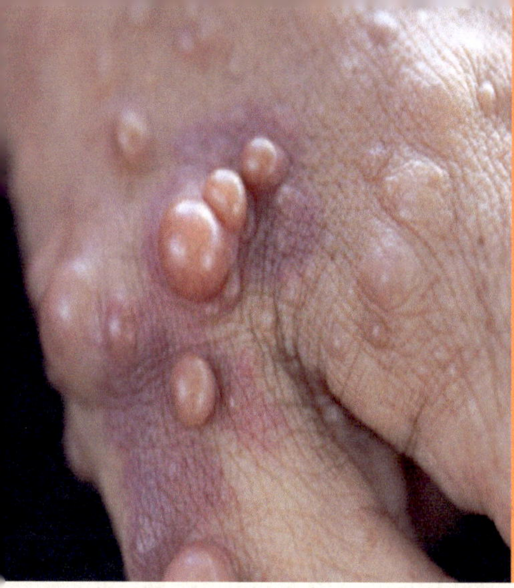

Chapter 10
VESICULOBULLOUS DISEASES

Contents

Introduction

The skin is the body's most effective barrier against environmental insults, protecting inner tissues from infection, physical trauma, and desiccation. Once the barrier is compromised by disease processes, it can manifest in a variety of dermatological presentations that are often difficult to diagnose and manage appropriately. Among the dermatological manifestations of such compromise are the vesiculobullous diseases, which manifest with the formation of vesicles or bullae fluid blisters found on the skin and mucous membranes. These conditions form a broad category of autoimmune, infectious, and genetic disorders, each with unique pathogenetic mechanisms and clinical courses. Acute recognition and clear diagnosis of vesiculobullous diseases are important because they may cause considerable morbidity and require complex treatment. The clinical spectrum of vesiculobullous diseases would be adequately explored if their etiologies and manifestations are explored in detail. Infectious pathogens, including viruses and bacteria, can cause vesiculobullous lesions with unusual characteristics, making diagnosis and treatment more challenging. For example, unusual hand-foot-and-mouth disease has presented with vesiculobullous eruptions that are most commonly found on sites like the buttocks, feet, and hands, and can be accompanied by purpuric lesions and limited oral involvement. These presentations reinforce the heterogeneity and complexity of vesiculobullous diseases and emphasize the modulating influence of co-infections, e.g., streptococcal infections, on the clinical presentation and treatment strategy (Horishna & Pavlyshyn, 2020). Delay in the recognition of such presentations hampers effective control, highlighting the need for ongoing clinical alertness. In addition to cutaneous manifestations, vesiculobullous diseases have systemic significance with rare but serious complications such as ocular involvement. Recent observational data suggest emerging links between selected viral infections manifesting with vesiculobullous skin rashes and ocular disorders like central serous retinopathy, which can have a permanent visual impact. Although the number of case reports is increasing to better depict these complications, standard guidelines for prevention or management remain poorly developed. This knowledge gap requires focused study to improve knowledge of these diseases as occupational exposures, especially in high-exposure environments like childcare (Horishna & Pavlyshyn, 2020). Successful multidisciplinary approaches will be paramount to improve outcomes and reduce the burden of these multifactorial dermatological diseases.

Definition of Vesiculobullous Diseases

The skin, being the body's largest organ, acts as an essential barrier against environmental insults. If this barrier capacity is lost, several pathological expressions follow, among which are vesiculobullous diseases. These are conditions that include the appearance of vesicles and bullae, small to large blisters containing fluid, on the skin and mucous membranes. Vesicles are described as blisters less than 5 millimeters, whereas bullae are more extensive, usually causing extreme discomfort and danger of secondary infection. Pathogenesis of the lesions most commonly involves cellular adhesion disruption or direct epidermal or basement membrane damage, leading to fluid collection. This category of diseases includes both infectious and autoimmune etiologies, indicative of the intricacy behind skin integrity and immune homeostasis. Grasping the clinical and histopathological characteristics of vesiculobullous disorders is critical for proper diagnosis and treatment. For example, certain diseases like hand, foot, and mouth disease (HFMD), whose etiology is mainly viral, manifest in atypical forms with vesiculobullous lesions, particularly in adult patients. Coxsackievirus A6 has recently been recognized as a major causative agent of atypical HFMD, identified through sophisticated molecular methods like real-time polymerase chain reaction and immunohistochemistry. These observations highlight the importance of including both clinical and laboratory information in order to define vesiculobullous diseases correctly. Further, correct identification of the etiological agent aids in prognostication and optimizing treatment strategies that reduce the severity of the disease and avoid complications (Barrera et al., 2011). Vesiculobullous diseases can also be linked with systemic diseases, indicating underlying immunological derangements or infection processes. For instance, in the setting of the COVID-19 pandemic, a subgroup of patients had cutaneous expression in the form of vesiculobullous eruptions. These cutaneous lesions were varied in morphology and associated, at times, with the severity of the disease. The occurrence of certain types of rash such as chilblain-like lesions generally was associated with less severe outcomes, whereas others such as acro-ischemia, which may present as bullous lesions, were associated with increased severity of systemic illness and risk of mortality. Hence, the distribution and nature of vesiculobullous lesions in systemic infections can be of significant clue not just for diagnosis but also for the disease course. This systemic connection emphasizes the need to observe vesiculobullous diseases in a holistic clinical context (Holmes et al., 2022) (Figure 10.1).

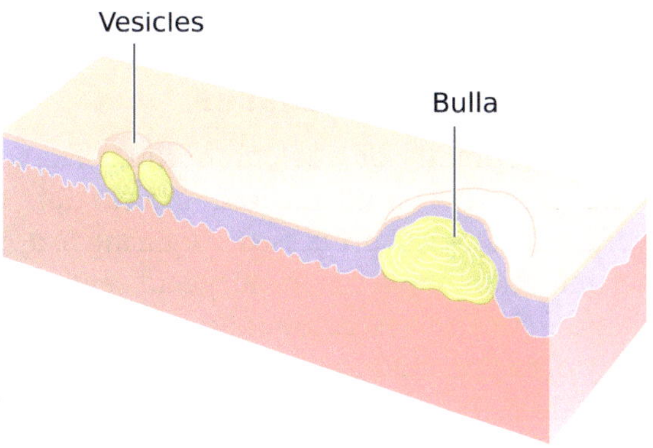

Figure 10.1. Vesicles and bulla.

Source: OpenStax. (n.d.). *Diagram Showing Vesicles and Bulla. Wikimedia Commons.* https://upload.wikimedia.org/wikipedia/commons/thumb/f/fd/Vesicles_and_Bulla.svg/1024px-Vesicles_and_Bulla.svg.png.

10.1. Classification of Vesiculobullous Diseases

The nosology of vesiculobullous diseases entails an complex familiarity with their pathophysiological basis, which is composed of layers of skin involvement. The disorders are predominantly divided into intraepidermal and subepidermal entities, according to the level of blister formation. Intraepidermal vesiculobullous diseases, like pemphigus vulgaris, occur secondary to acantholysis of the epidermis, which produces blisters that easily break. In contrast, subepidermal disorders such as bullous pemphigoid show separation at the dermoepidermal junction, with stronger bullae that are less likely to rupture. Histopathological diagnosis continues to be crucial in differentiating these conditions, supported by immunofluorescence studies identifying characteristic deposition patterns of antibodies. This subclassification not only helps in diagnosis but also determines prognosis and therapy, highlighting the importance of accurate disease categorization among this heterogeneous population.

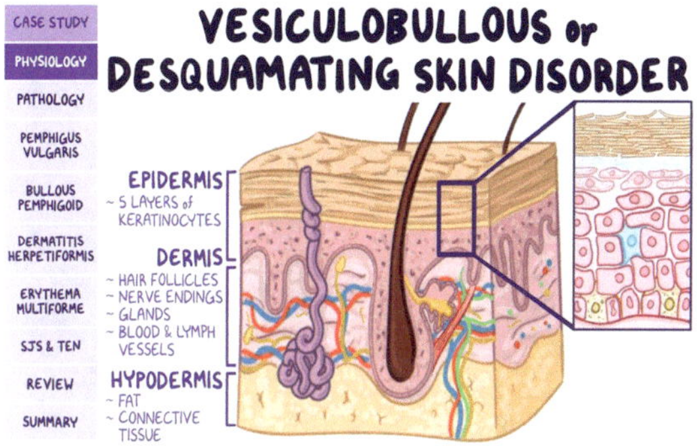

Figure 10.2. Vesiculobullous diseases.

Source: Smith, J. (2023). *Diagram Illustrating Data Flow in Osmose IT System.*

At the center of vesiculobullous disease classification is the determination of their immunological basis. Autoimmune blistering disorders are a large subclass wherein antibodies are directed against structural proteins that are responsible for epidermal cohesion or dermoepidermal adhesion. Pemphigus forms entail autoantibodies against desmogleins of desmosomes, causing interference in cell-to-cell adhesion of the epidermis. By contrast, pemphigoid conditions involve antibodies against hemidesmosomal constituents like BP180 and BP230, which are responsible for attaching the epidermis to the basement membrane. There are also inherited types, such as epidermolysis bullosa, characterized by categorization according to genetic abnormalities in keratins or collagen, representing an alternate pathogenic paradigm. Knowledge of these molecular targets makes it possible to design specific diagnostic tests and opens the door to precision medicine treatments in treating vesiculobullous diseases. Outside of immunological and genetic categorization, the natural history and clinical presentation further narrow the vesiculobullous disease categorization. Sudden, acute blister progression with mucosal involvement characterizes pemphigus vulgaris, necessitating aggressive immunosuppression (Figure 10.2).

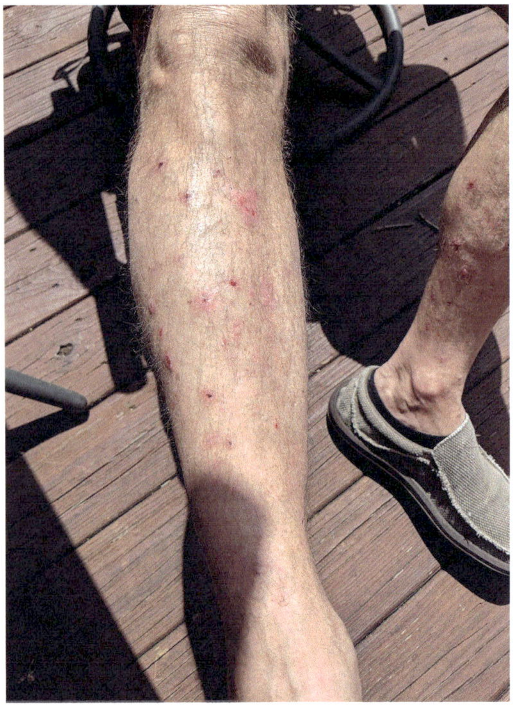

Figure 10.3. Bullous pemphigoid.

Source: By Jubward - Own work, CC BY-SA 4.0, https://commons.wikimedia.org/w/index.php?curid=70038371

In comparison, bullous pemphigoid typically occurs as a chronic, pruritic eruption in mostly the elderly. Subtypes such as dermatitis herpetiformis are associated with gluten sensitivity, introducing an environmental element to the classification scheme. The subtle differences between these entities require detailed clinical assessment in conjunction with laboratory investigations. These multi-dimensional classification schemes enhance diagnostic precision and direct treatment stratification, underpinning the complexity of vesiculobullous disease and its treatment (Draibe et al., 2024; Jacovas et al., 2025) (Figure 10.3).

10.1.1. Primary vs. Secondary Vesiculobullous Diseases

The development of vesiculobullous lesions in the skin is a multifaceted interaction of several pathological processes, requiring proper discrimination between primary and secondary causes. Primary vesiculobullous diseases are mainly distinguished by intrinsic immunological or genetic defects directed against the structural elements of the skin, resulting in blistering. These conditions, including pemphigoid and linear IgA disease, are characterized by autoimmune responses to the basement membrane zone or hemidesmosomal antigens with subepithelial blistering. They typically present with mucous membrane onset followed by the development of cutaneous surfaces and pose a clinical dilemma because of their chronic and relapsing nature. Diagnostic verification is mainly based on biopsy and immunofluorescence analyses that illustrate characteristic immune deposits, which are necessary for the differentiation of these primary autoimmune blistering diseases from other causes (Arvind et al., 2020). Prompt identification is important in order to accomplish successful therapy to avoid progression and systemic complications. Secondary vesiculobullous diseases, on the other hand, occur as skin manifestations secondary to systemic or infectious disorders. These diseases are not caused by autoimmune processes but usually are manifestations of cutaneous reaction secondary to infections, drugs, or malignancies. For example, *Staphylococcus aureus* bacteremia may cause generalized skin blistering owing to underlying septicemia and inflammation, stressing the need to look for the underlying causes different from primary autoimmune disorders. The secondary vesiculobullous diseases are characterized by resolution of lesions on treatment of the primary systemic disease, which underlines the value of extended patient evaluation outside the formal dermatologic examination (Fabio et al., 2011). The secondary nature also mandates a multidisciplinary strategy involving infectious disease care and supportive dermatologic care to achieve optimal outcomes in the patient. Clinical and pathological differences between primary and secondary vesiculobullous diseases apply also to therapeutic and prognostic factors. Primary autoimmune blistering disorders usually call for immunosuppressive treatments targeting aberrant immune responses, whereas secondary vesiculobullous diseases require therapy to address the underlying systemic or infectious cause. The subepithelial nature of primary vesiculobullous lesions, as evidenced by immunostaining methods, directs dermatologists in developing therapy approaches according to the immune target engaged (Arvind et al., 2020). On the other hand, inability to recognize a secondary cause, i.e., bacterial sepsis, might lead to incorrect treatment and unwanted outcomes, as these lesions might be erroneously diagnosed as primary dermatosis (Fabio et al., 2011). Finally, separation of these two groups is crucial for proper diagnosis, specific treatment, and better prognostic evaluation in patients with vesiculobullous skin diseases (Figure 10.4).

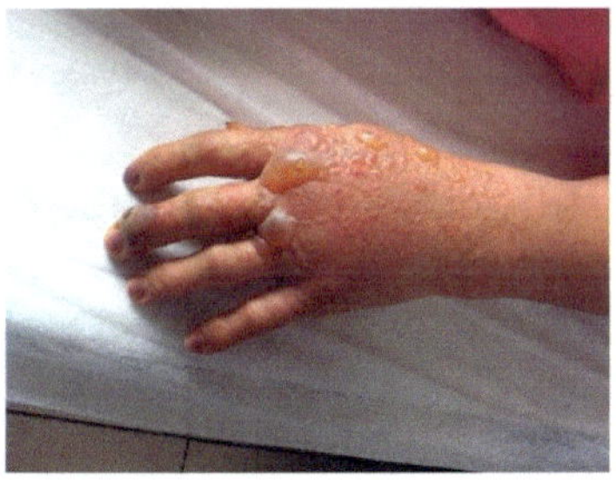

Figure 10.4. Vesiculobullous lesions, the first day of admission.

Source: Alian, S., Ahangarkani, F., & Arabsheybani, S. (2015). A Case of Orf Disease Complicated with Erythema Multiforme and Bullous Pemphigoid-Like Eruptions. *Case reports in infectious diseases, 2015*, 105484. https://doi.org/10.1155/2015/105484

10.1.2. Inherited vs. Acquired Conditions

The nuance of vesiculobullous skin diseases lies in their varied etiology, which can be broadly defined as inherited and acquired conditions. While inherited types usually arise due to mutations within genes that code for structural epidermal or basement membrane proteins, acquired types usually follow an external insult or autoimmune phenomenon. The hereditary variants can occur early in life and take a chronic course because of disruptions in skin integrity, causing blistering with minor trauma. On the other hand, acquired vesiculobullous disease typically occurs later and can include immune responses that are induced by drugs, infection, or exposure to environmental toxins. An understanding of these differences is most important in precise diagnosis and treatment planning, as inherited disorders need genetic counseling and supportive therapy, whereas acquired diseases may be amenable to immunosuppressive treatments. This differentiation also underscores the importance of complete clinical assessment and proper laboratory work in treating these disorders efficiently. Environmental and chemical exposures play a relatively underemphasized role in causing or worsening acquired vesiculobullous diseases. Some toxins and chemicals can interfere with cellular metabolism or immune regulation, thus triggering blistering skin disease. Disturbance in biochemical pathways such as heme biosynthesis, for example, can present with cutaneous manifestations that mimic vesiculobullous lesions in some porphyrias. These are either inherited or acquired through exposure to industrial chemicals such as metals and halogenated hydrocarbons, exemplifying the interaction of genetic susceptibility and environmental factors in disease causation. These cases highlight the need for a thorough occupational and environmental history in patients with vesiculobullous symptoms. Although hypotheses regarding chemical exposures and acquired conditions have been proposed, pathophysiologic mechanisms are as yet unclear and require investigation and laboratory evaluation is required to exclude mimicking disorders (Anderson et al., 1997).

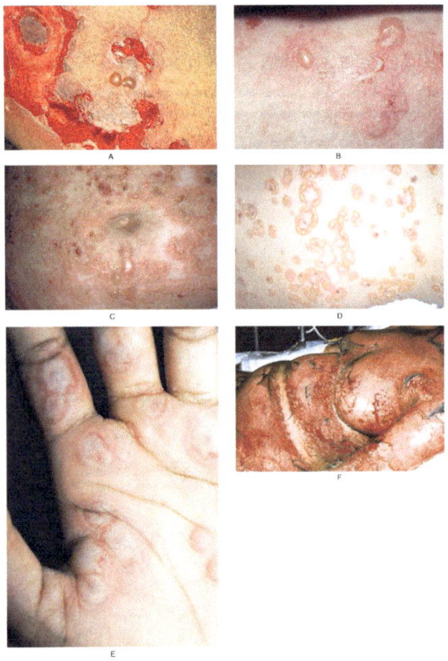

Figure 10.5. Acquired bullous skin disease.

Source: Alian, S., Ahangarkani, F., & Arabsheybani, S. (2015). A Case of Orf Disease Complicated with Erythema Multiforme and Bullous Pemphigoid-Like Eruptions. *Case reports in infectious diseases, 2015*, 105484. https://doi.org/10.1155/2015/105484.

Clinical assessment is crucial in differentiating inherited vesiculobullous diseases from acquired conditions, especially by careful physical and oral examination. Because the oral mucosa usually mirrors mucosal involvement in vesiculobullous disease, a thorough examination of this site is vital no matter what the initial complaint. Identification of small lesions like vesicles, erosions, or erythema in the mouth can facilitate diagnostic certainty, particularly since some inherited diseases may manifest with mucosal fragility. In addition, extraoral examination such as examination for lymphadenopathy, facial asymmetry, and nerve function testing supplement the diagnostic process. Careful observation of lesion features; size, color, texture, and tenderness—perpetuates precise discrimination between inherited genetic disorders and acquired immune-mediated or chemically mediated diseases. The synthesis of careful clinical observation and history in a patient enables an efficient diagnostic approach essential for the management of vesiculobullous diseases (Burgess et al., 2017) (Figure 10.5).

10.1.3. Common Types of Vesiculobullous Diseases

Among the many dermatological conditions, vesiculobullous diseases are a group of disorders with complicated pathogenesis involving formation of blisters or bullae in the skin and mucous membrane. Pathogenesis typically involves autoimmune destruction of targeted structural components of the skin proteins leading to formation of fluid-filled lesions. Diagnostically, a combination of clinical assessment and histopathology with immunological investigation is essential in distinguishing these diseases because of similarity of presentations. For instance, pemphigus vulgaris is the most common vesiculobullous disease seen in clinical practice and normally presents with intraepidermal blisters and mucosal involvement. Its recognition is necessary not only due to its morbidity but also because therapy protocols are markedly different from others of vesiculobullous diseases. Early diagnosis and treatment greatly enhance patient outcomes in these frequently chronic and recurrent diseases (Atla et al., 2019). Variety of vesiculobullous conditions differ in their immunofluorescence and histopathological patterns, which are extremely useful in diagnosis and treatment. Pemphigus foliaceus, another autoimmune bullous disease, only involves the superficial epiderm, forming more superficial bullae than pemphigus vulgaris. Bullous pemphigoid, on the other hand, involves subepidermal blistering and is typically observed in geriatric populations. It has clinical overlaps with epidermolysis bullosa acquisita, a disease characterized only by direct immunofluorescence (DIF) methods, highlighting the necessity for these diagnostic modalities.

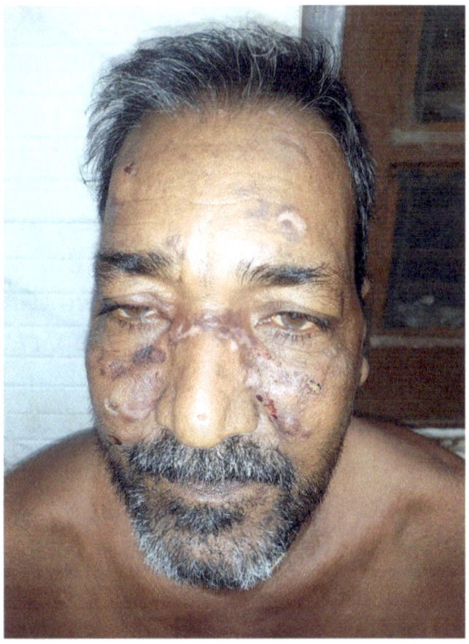

Figure 10.6. Pemphigus vulgaris on face.

Source: Mohammad2018. (2018). Pemphigus vulgaris. *Wikimedia Commons.* https://upload.wikimedia.org/wikipedia/commons/thumb/8/87/Pemphigus_vulgaris.jpg/800px-Pemphigus_vulgaris.jpg.

Distinguishing these subtypes is important because their prognosis and treatment significantly differ; while pemphigus diseases may need systemic immunosuppressants, bullous pemphigoid frequently responds to corticosteroids. These differences point out the intricacy of vesiculobullous disease and the requirement of careful clinical and laboratory correlation (Atla et al., 2019). Although cutaneous presentation is salient, vesiculobullous disease also presents diagnostic difficulty when involving mucosal membranes, such as within the oral cavity. Oral ulcers, as in the case of pemphigus vulgaris, can be confused with other ulcerative conditions owing to similar overlapping clinical characteristics such as duration, multiplicity, and etiology. Systemic diagnosis is important, given that oral ulcers may be secondary to trauma, infections, systemic diseases, or malignancies. Diagnoses depend on proper clinical history supplemented by special investigations, permitting clinicians to rule out other etiologies and direct attention toward vesiculobullous pathology. Awareness of oral manifestations of vesiculobullous diseases contributes to timely identification and necessitates proper treatment so as to avoid morbidity due to delayed intervention (Figure 10.6).

10.2. Pathophysiology

The complex interaction between structural components of skin and the immune system plays an important role in the pathophysiology of vesiculobullous disorders. These diseases are defined by the development of vesicles and bullae on the basis of impaired integrity of the epidermis or the dermoepidermal junction. Autoantibodies to structural proteins responsible for cell adhesion, for example, desmogleins in pemphigus or basement membrane antigens in bullous pemphigoid, interfere with cellular cohesion.

This immunologic attack triggers separation of the epidermal layers, resulting in water accumulation and blistering. Immunity is both cellular and humoral and enhances tissue injury through inflammatory cell recruitment and release of proteolytic enzymes. Such mechanisms are a sign of the disease process's complexity, in which autoimmunity and inflammation meet to yield the classical vesiculobullous lesions, underscoring the vital balance between immune surveillance and skin integrity in pathology. In addition, the action of cytotoxic T lymphocytes becomes a central feature of vesiculobullous disease pathogenesis. Studies show that in infectious disease conditions, such as *Mycoplasma pneumoniae*-associated erythema multiforme, clonal proliferation of $CD4^{+}CD8^{+}$ double-positive cytotoxic marker-positive T cells directly cause keratinocyte apoptosis and blisters.

This novel subset of T cells infilters into lesion sites, causing specific killing of epidermal cells and contributing to mucocutaneous disease. The dynamic traffic and tenacity of these cells within pathologic tissues highlight the adaptive immune systems role beyond mechanisms involving antibodies. Thus, cell-mediated cytotoxicity adds to autoantibody impact, yielding a sophisticated appreciation for vesiculobullous disease pathophysiology that includes both humoral and cellular immune dysregulation (Volkers et al., 2021). In more severe systemic infections associated with vesiculobullous presentations, the pathophysiological landscape broadens to involve extensive immune activation and tissue damage. As an example, infections with chikungunya virus have been linked with life-threatening consequences manifesting as intense skin involvement and severe immune responses. Histopathologic findings demonstrate viral antigen distribution within mesenchymal and mononuclear cells, where ensuing inflammation and tissue edema are responsible for blister formation and necrosis. Immune-mediated vascular leakage and hemorrhage also add to skin damage, with systemic inflammatory processes potentially causing septic shock. This demonstrates ways in which infectious causes may induce or exacerbate vesiculobullous disease by direct viral cytopathology and aberrant host responses. The comprehension of these processes is crucial in understanding the multifactorial characteristics of vesiculobullous disease in clinical and scientific applications (Bhatnagar et al., 2021).

10.2.1. Mechanisms of Blister Formation

The complex structure of the skin is important to ensure its integrity and defend the underlying tissues. Disturbance in this complicated arrangement results in blister development, a characteristic of vesiculobullous diseases. Blisters develop when there is separation at multiple levels within the skin layers, commonly between the epidermis and dermis or within the epidermal layers alone. This separation is due to disruption of cellular adhesion molecules or mechanical trauma. Vesicles and bullae clinically present as fluid-filled sacs, indicating the accumulation of serum or cellular debris in areas where cells have lost contact. The specific area and character of this separation are critical to the classification of vesiculobullous diseases and informing diagnostic and treatment approaches, highlighting the need for knowledge of the pathogenic mechanisms for optimal clinical management (Patel et al., 2023).

Autoimmune mechanisms are pivotal to the pathogenesis of most vesiculobullous diseases, most notably pemphigus and bullous pemphigoid. In pemphigus, autoantibodies are directed to desmosomal cadherins, i.e., desmoglein 1 and 3, responsible for intercellular adhesion within the epidermis. Binding of these antibodies induces enzymatic activity leading to disruption of the desmosomes in a process referred to as acantholysis, with resulting loss of cohesion among keratinocytes and intraepidermal blister formation. The site of these blisters, usually suprabasilar in pemphigus vulgaris, is dependent on the particular desmoglein being targeted. This process demonstrates the process of a targeted immune response against adhesion molecules being directly translated into the clinical feature of skin lesions (Busch et al., 1991). The molecular explanation of autoimmune interference illuminates the process of possible targeted therapy. By comparison, subepidermal blistering disorders such as bullous pemphigoid are characterized by autoantibody-mediated basement membrane zone disruption, a distinct process for blister formation.

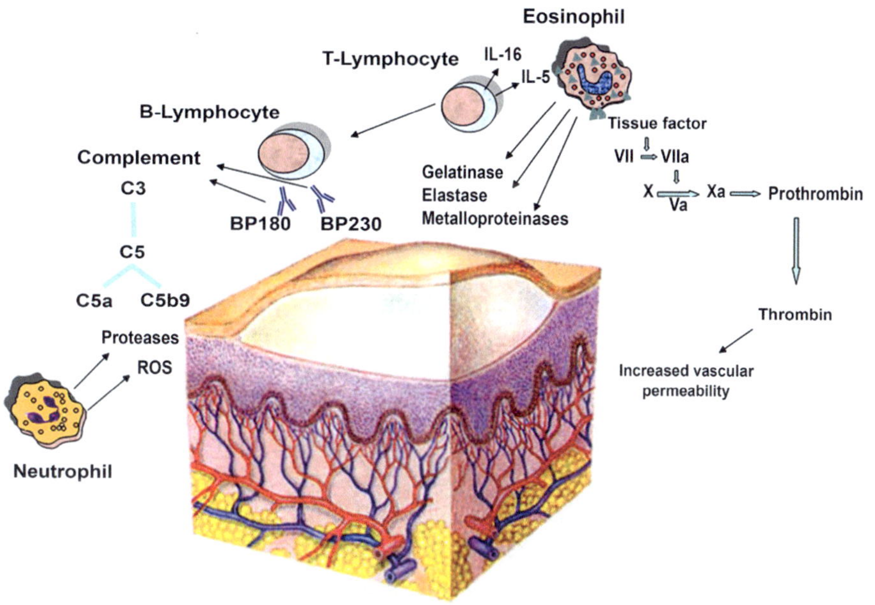

Figure 10.7. Pathomechanisms of the blister formation in bullous pemphigoid including the involvement of coagulation activation.

Source: Cugno M, Borghi A, Garcovich S and Marzano AV (2019) Coagulation and Skin Autoimmunity. Front. Immunol. 10:1407. doi: 10.3389/fimmu.2019.01407

In this condition, autoantibodies against hemidesmosomal proteins holding the epidermis in place to the dermis, e.g., BP180 and BP230, cause blistering. These antibodies bind, activate complement and inflammatory cells, and initiate enzymatic destruction and separation at the dermoepidermal junction. Blisters formed are generally tense and subepidermal due to the more profound plane of cleavage. This variation in level of blister formation significantly influences both clinical presentation and histopathological classification of vesiculobullous conditions. These mechanistic differences highlight the need for a precise histopathological and immunological evaluation to guide appropriate therapy (Patel et al., 2023) (Figure 10.7).

10.2.2. Role of the Immune System

The complex interaction of the skin with the immune system is vital for the preservation of integrity and reaction to environmental abuses. Vesiculobullous disorders, which are associated with blistering, usually develop as a consequence of immune dysregulation with autoantibody targeting of structural elements of the skin. The ensuing disruption in cell adhesion molecules results in vesicle and bulla formation. The pathogenic process involves a fine balance between innate immune reactions and adaptive immunity, with T and B lymphocytes playing the key role in mediating specific autoantibody production. Immune cells like macrophages and dendritic cells play a role not only in antigen presentation but also in cytokine release, which adds to tissue inflammation and damage. In understanding such immune pathways, one can apply that knowledge in the development of targeted therapies that modulate the immune response and restore skin barrier function. In vesiculobullous conditions such as pemphigus and bullous pemphigoid, innate immune components such as Langerhans cells and keratinocytes act as initiators and multipliers of disease pathology. These cells are equipped with pattern recognition receptors that can recognize pathogen-associated molecular patterns or signals of damage, initiating inflammatory cascades. Dysregulation of these receptors leads to chronic inflammation and autoimmunity, upsetting the fine balance of the epidermal-dermal junction. The roles of Toll-like receptors and NOD-like receptors in skin inflammation serve to emphasize the importance of innate immunity to these diseases. Inhibition of these innate immune pathways may provide new therapeutic opportunities, as with other inflammatory skin diseases. This serves to emphasize the need for an expanded knowledge of innate immune receptor functions in vesiculobullous skin diseases (Svitich et al., 2024). Outside of localized cutaneous effects, systemic immune dysfunction and aging can affect the severity and course of vesiculobullous disease. Immune regulation changes that occur with aging make individuals more susceptible to chronic inflammatory and autoimmune processes. Abnormalities in mechanisms of immune tolerance enable the development of pathogenic autoantibodies, which are key drivers of vesiculobullous disease. Moreover, disruption of skin barrier function is aggravated by an aging immune system's reduced ability to resolve inflammation and repair tissue damage. The interactions between immune senescence, chronic inflammation, and tissue degeneration demonstrate a multisystem engagement underlying the pathogenesis of such diseases. Such understanding is necessary for the formulation of age-specific immunomodulatory therapies targeting both immune dysregulation and skin pathology (Bendig et al., 2024).

10.2.3. Genetic Factors Influencing Disease Development

The mechanisms of immune response complexity are important for the pathogenesis of vesiculobullous skin diseases, with genetic vulnerabilities usually determining disease initiation and development. Genetic differences in genes that control immune tolerance and antibody production may induce abnormal immune function, leading to the formation of autoantibodies against structural elements of the skin and mucous membranes. These autoantibodies interfere with cell adhesion, which causes characteristic blistering in vesiculobullous conditions. For instance, in benign mucous membrane pemphigoid, an autoimmune disease, genetic influences play a role in creating pathogenic autoantibodies against basement membrane constituents, causing subepithelial blistering and serious clinical manifestations such as ocular scarring and mucosal damage (Ojha & Yadav, 2020). Elucidation of the genetic basis for immune dysregulation is critical for the formulation of targeted therapeutic interventions and enhanced disease control in such affected patients. Besides autoimmune-mediated vesiculobullous disease, infectious causes also demonstrate the interfolding of genetic susceptibility and disease manifestations. Genetic predispositions could influence host susceptibility to viral infections with vesiculobullous manifestations, such as hand, foot, and mouth disease caused by Coxsackievirus A6.

This viral infection has unusual and serious presentations in specific populations, with molecular testing showing viral presence and correlating with clinical severity (Barrera et al., 2011). Host genetics most probably control immune response effectiveness and viral clearance, affecting the severity of vesiculobullous lesions. Consequently, the host genetic background can therefore influence viral pathogenesis, extent of immune activation, and resulting skin involvement, underlining the need for personalized methods in the diagnosis and management of infectious vesiculobullous diseases. In addition, susceptibility to and severity of the disease also extend beyond genes coding for immune responses to structural skin proteins that vary in their coding sequences. Gene mutations or polymorphisms in genes that encode basement membrane zone proteins or desmosomal proteins can undermine skin integrity, with susceptibility to blistering under autoimmune or infectious injury. This structural susceptibility coupled with immunogenetic mechanisms comprises a sophisticated etiologic paradigm for vesiculobullous diseases, in which both genetic and acquired factors intersect. Clarification of these genetic contributions allows clinicians to predict disease course more accurately, individualize treatments, and potentially prevent disease onset in individuals at increased risk. Advances in genetic research therefore promise to improve diagnostic criteria and therapeutic effectiveness in vesiculobullous skin diseases.

10.3. Clinical Presentation

The clinical presentation of vesiculobullous skin diseases is varied, with a tendency to pose diagnostic difficulties owing to the similarity of symptoms and lesion morphology. Patients usually complain of the sudden onset of vesicles or bullae, sometimes associated with erythema, pruritus, or pain. The lesions are filled with fluid and range in size and distribution, often involving areas of friction or trauma, including the trunk, limbs, or mucous membranes. The course of these lesions may vary from transient vesicles to tense bullae that burst, resulting in erosions and possible secondary infection. Heterogeneity in presentation requires thoughtful clinical assessment since various dermatoses present similarly despite differing etiology and prognosis. Identification of such patterns as the site, size, and course of the lesions is important in making an initial diagnosis and in directing future histopathological examination for proof (Kumar et al., 2022). Age and gender distribution also characterize the clinical picture of vesiculobullous diseases. It has been established in studies that the diseases tend to affect middle-aged adults and present most frequently during the fourth to fifth decades of life. The minor predominance of either sex will differ based on the disease entity, but overall observations reflect small differences in rates. Furthermore, the site of involvement may give valuable hints; for example, pemphigus vulgaris frequently has mucosal involvement in addition to cutaneous lesions, while bullous pemphigoid involves predominantly the elderly with extensive tense bullae on the trunk and extremities. These demographic elements combined with clinical data support a more focused diagnosis in the handling of vesiculobullous eruptions (Patel et al., 2023). An effective clinic assessment also involves assessing systemic symptoms that might accompany skin lesions, considering that certain vesiculobullous diseases carry important morbidity and, in some instances, mortality. Patients will sometimes present with fever, malaise, or secondary infections from compromised skin barriers that underscore the systemic burden and recognize dermatological manifestations. The occurrence of such signs will usually parallel disease severity and require intervention to avoid complications. Chronicity and local recurrence pattern also differentiate autoimmune from infectious or medication-induced vesiculobullous diseases. In general, an extensive clinical presentation involving morphology of the lesions, patient population, and systemic presence is crucial for definitive diagnosis and best treatment planning in vesiculobullous dermatoses (Kumar et al., 2022; Patel et al., 2023) (Figure 10.8).

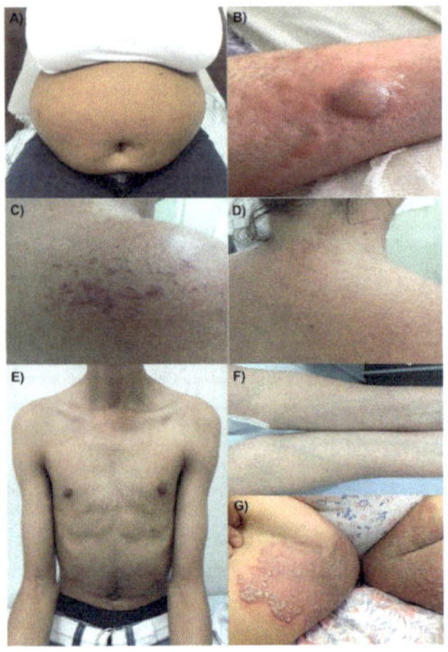

Figure 10.8. Cutaneous clinical manifestations of patients during the acute phase of CHIKV infections: (A) Case 2: urticaria; (B) Case 3: vesiculobullous lesion; (C) Case 4: minor vesiculobullous lesions; (D) Case 4: erythema; (E) Case 7; and (F) Case 8: diffuse papular erythematous rash; and (G) Case 9: vesiculopustular lesions, erythema, and scaling.

Source: Benjamanukul, S., Chansaenroj, J., Chirathaworn, C. *et al.* Atypical skin manifestation in severe acute chikungunya infection in a pregnant woman: a case report. *J Med Case Reports* **16**, 5 (2022). https://doi.org/10.1186/s13256-021-03197-3.

10.3.1. Common Symptoms and Signs

The reaction of the skin to vesiculobullous diseases usually appears in the form of a characteristic constellation of signs and symptoms that are most important to clinical assessment and prompt diagnosis. The patients usually present with severe itching, burning, or pain before lesions appear, which is an indication of the inflammatory condition. A characteristic of these diseases is the occurrence of vesicles and bullae—fluid-containing blisters of different sizes, which erupt suddenly on normal or erythematous skin. These lesions tend to rupture easily, resulting in erosions and ensuing crusting, setting the patient up for secondary infection. Physical examination may also uncover associated erythema and swelling, indicative of active inflammation. In a few instances, systemic manifestations like fever or malaise accompany the cutaneous presentation, pointing to the disease's effect on areas beyond the skin itself, which requires a complete clinical strategy. Although vesicles and bullae constitute the defining clinical feature of these conditions, knowledge of their distribution and course improves diagnostic reliability. Such lesions have a propensity to localize in zones subjected to pressure, friction, or trauma, such as the trunk, limbs, or mucosal surfaces, contributing to patient discomfort and making therapeutic management challenging. Outside of blister development, erythematous macules and purpuric spots can occur together, indicating vascular involvement and immune complex deposition in the dermis, such as in atypical presentations of vesiculobullous infections (Horishna & Pavlyshyn, 2020). The course of the lesions is variable, from self-limited eruptions to chronic, recurrent eruptions resulting in extensive damage to the skin and scarring. Identification of these patterns is critical, as they direct differential diagnosis between autoimmune, infectious, and genetic vesiculobullous diseases. Moreover, chronic systemic diseases commonly co-exist with vesiculobullous skin lesions, that affect symptomatology and complicate management. For example, elderly diabetic patients commonly present with pruritus, eczema, and fungal infections, which can mask or aggravate the classical presentation of vesiculobullous lesions (Dhumale & Khyalappa, 2016). Poor hygiene and immunocompromised statuses also exacerbate the risk of secondary infection and delayed healing. These findings highlight the need for a detailed history and systemic assessment upon presenting with vesiculobullous eruptions, especially in elderly groups in whom several co-morbidities influence the clinical presentation. As such, the interactions between cutaneous manifestations and systemic cofactors are integral components of pathology and therapeutic approaches to vesiculobullous disease.

10.3.2. Variability in Presentation Among Different Diseases

The cutaneous vesiculobullous diseases have marked variability in clinical presentations that makes diagnosis and management challenging. The disorders cover a broad spectrum of presentations ranging from focal blistering to generalized erosions, which mirror varied underlying pathophysiology. This is further modulated by the age of onset, intensity of the immune response, and histopathological characteristics, which tend to overlap across conditions. For example, some vesiculobullous lesions can be confused with infectious or inflammatory dermatoses, highlighting the importance of histopathological proof for a proper diagnosis. This diagnostic dilemma is reflected in the fact that clinical presentation alone cannot distinguish between conditions like pemphigus vulgaris and other bullous conditions with certainty. Combined analyses by pathologists and dermatologists are thus essential in recognizing disease-specific patterns amidst conflating clinical and histological presentation (Kumar et al., 2022). In addition, the underlying etiology of vesiculobullous diseases is a factor for their heterogeneity. In most instances, autoimmune mechanisms are predominant, but triggers and related systemic conditions differ widely. Paraneoplastic pemphigus, for instance, emphasizes the association between neoplastic disorders and vesiculobullous skin disease. Paraneoplastic pemphigus tends to present in the form of an overwhelming vesiculobullous eruption in the presence of underlying tumors like thymomas. Clinical presentation in these instances may occur prior to the diagnosis of the neoplasm, reflecting the potential for cutaneous manifestations to be significant diagnostic pointers to underlying systemic pathology. The difference between idiopathic and paraneoplastic pemphigus highlights the intricacy of immune-mediated vesiculobullous disease and emphasizes the necessity of complete patient assessment (Bobbio et al., 2008). Along with etiologic factors, demographic and geographical factors control the clinical spectrum of vesiculobullous diseases. Epidemiological research shows variations in disease prevalence and presentation between populations that can be due to genetic susceptibility, environmental exposures, and infectious agents prevalent in a region. A study of non-neoplastic skin diseases proved that vesiculobullous lesions comprised a large percentage of biopsied diseases, with differences in prevalence attributable to age, gender, and regional disease patterns. Pemphigus vulgaris, for example, is still the most common vesiculobullous condition in some regions, while other diseases such as bullous pemphigoid are more common in other locations. Knowledge of these epidemiological distinctions is critical for the clinicians to make effective diagnostic suspicions and management strategies in heterogeneous patient populations (Kumar et al., 2022).

10.3.3. Diagnostic Criteria for Vesiculobullous Diseases

Correct diagnosis of vesiculobullous diseases is crucial because they share overlapping clinical presentations but have distinct underlying pathologies. They generally come in the form of blisters or bullae that will also present similarly to many conditions, and based on this, clinical evaluation is not enough for final diagnosis. Histopathological examination is an essential technique in this regard. Biopsy specimens stained with hematoxylin and eosin show characteristic patterns; e.g., the differentiation between intraepidermal and subepidermal blistering may lead to individual vesiculobullous disorders. In an investigation comparing different vesiculobullous lesions, pemphigus vulgaris and pemphigus foliaceus were characterized mainly on the basis of intraepidermal bullae, while bullous pemphigoid was characterized by subepidermal blisters. These morphological variations are crucial for the initiation of accurate treatment regimens and the optimization of patient outcomes, pointing to the critical function of histopathology in diagnostic processes (Patel et al., 2023). Outside of histopathology, DIF is now a crucial ancillary aid to diagnose vesiculobullous diseases. DIF entails the use of fluorescent antibodies to identify in situ immune deposits, representing immunopathological proof to add to histological evidence. This method is especially important in separating disorders with similar microscopic appearances, for example, bullous pemphigoid and epidermolysis bullosa acquisita, that could have identical subepidermal blistering patterns.

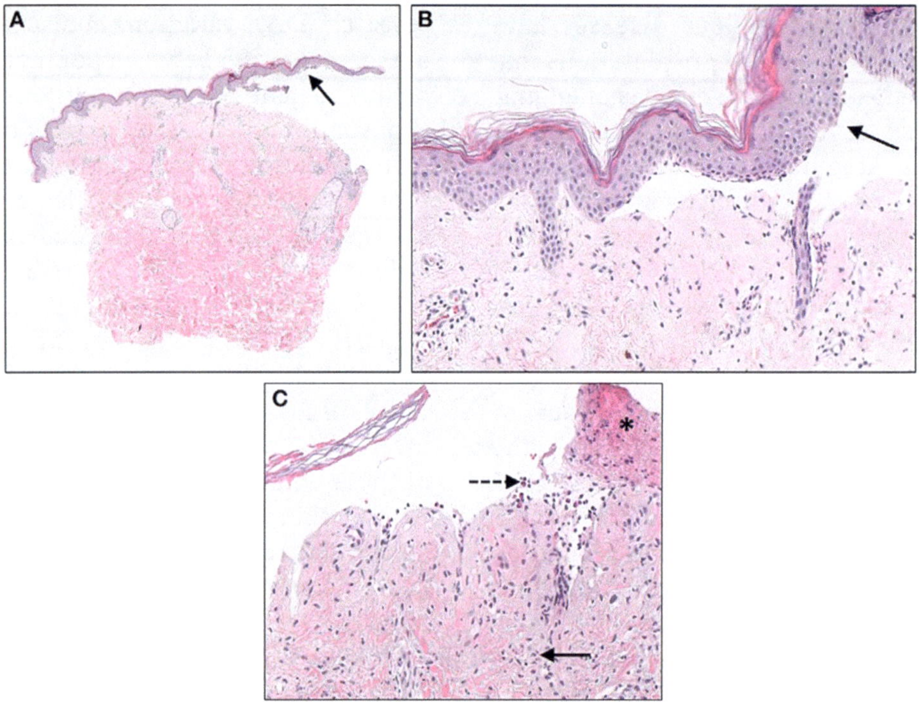

Figure 10.9. Micrograph of bullous pemphigoid. Subepidermal blistering [solid arrows in (A, B)] and influx of inflammatory cells including eosinophils and neutrophils in the dermis [solid arrow (C)] and blister cavity [dashed arrows (C)]. In (C) also deposition of fibrin is noted (asterisks).

Source: Giang J, Seelen MAJ, van Doorn MBA, Rissmann R, Prens EP and Damman J (2018) Complement Activation in Inflammatory Skin Diseases. Front. Immunol. 9:639. doi: 10.3389/fimmu.2018.00639

One study proved that 80% of vesiculobullous cases had DIF positivity, which helped produce an improved clinico-pathologic correlation in about three-fourths of the examined cases. Hence, association of DIF with histopathology improves diagnostic sensitivity, allowing clinicians to individualize treatment based on the particular immunopathogenic processes at play (Atla et al., 2019). The diagnostic criteria for vesiculobullous disorders thus include an integrated multi-modal approach that combines clinical assessment, histopathological examination, and immunofluorescence investigations. Although clinical presentation offers provisional hints, the subtle histological patterns like degree of blister formation and accompanying cellular infiltrations sharpen differential diagnoses. Immunofluorescence then provides a confirmatory level where characteristic deposition patterns of immunoglobulins and complement proteins, which are pathognomonic for different autoimmune bullous diseases, are identified. Like this multifaceted diagnostic approach not only enables early and accurate diagnosis, it also guides therapeutic interventions that prevent morbidity and mortality. With research advancing, the combination of these approaches continues to be the foundation of the success in vesiculobullous skin diseases (Atla et al., 2019; Patel et al., 2023) (Figure 10.9).

10.4. Diagnostic Methods

Correct diagnosis of vesiculobullous diseases involves a multidisciplinary strategy that integrates clinical assessment with specialized laboratory methods. Clinical variability tends to make first impressions complicated, and confirmation by diagnostic procedures is often needed. Punch skin biopsy still remains the gold standard technique with tissue samples available for detailed histopathological examination. Through this method, pathologists can determine the relevant morphological characteristics like the site of blister formation and the type of inflammatory infiltrates. In addition, the incorporation of DIF on peri-lesional skin biopsy also enhances diagnostic sensitivity by demonstrating characteristic immune complex deposits. It has been found that DIF is highly sensitive in detecting complement proteins, such as C3c, and immunoglobulins, which facilitates differentiation between autoimmune vesiculobullous disorders such as pemphigus vulgaris and bullous pemphigoid (Ali et al., 2021). Therefore, the synthesis of histopathology and immunopathology offers a strong basis for diagnosis. Histopathologic study of vesiculobullous lesions not only substantiates the clinical presumption but also allows classification into different subtypes according to specific microscopic features. For instance, intraepidermal and subepidermal patterns of blistering are important discriminators for different vesiculobullous dermatoses. Intraepidermal bullae are usually seen in pemphigus vulgaris, while subepidermal blistering is typical for bullous pemphigoid (Patel et al., 2023). The dependence on hematoxylin and eosin-stained sections allows pathologists to notice microscopic changes like acantholysis, inflammatory cell infiltrates, and basal cell degeneration which are crucial for diagnosis. Clinical correlation maximizes the interpretive significance of such findings to avoid the misapplication of histopathology as a solitary tool and instead make it part of a holistic diagnostic protocol. As a result, a combined histopathological and clinical strategy remains key to maximum patient management. Histology and immunofluorescence are bedrock, yet the diagnosis for vesiculobullous diseases needs also to account for patient demographics and lesion distribution in order to properly contextualize lab data. Patterns of age-related prevalence and lesion localization frequently yield additional clues that limit differential diagnoses. For example, patients in advanced age will most commonly present with bullous pemphigoid, while others of younger age may present with other autoimmune or genetic variants (Ali et al., 2021). In addition, generalized or localized distribution of lesions carries therapeutic and prognostic significance, highlighting the necessity of comprehensive clinical history. In a few instances, sequential biopsies of lesional and peri-lesional skin are needed to document the dynamic pathological range and patterns of immune deposition properly. This holistic diagnostic approach is intended to minimize morbidity and mortality related to these complex diseases by informing specific and prompt interventions (Ali et al., 2021; Patel et al., 2023).

10.4.1. Clinical Examination Techniques

Correct diagnosis of vesiculobullous skin diseases depends on careful clinical examination methods, which yield critical preliminary information prior to definitive investigations. The procedure starts with a thorough visual survey, documenting the morphology, distribution, and evolution of the lesions. These factors enable intraepidermal versus subepidermal blistering to be differentiated, which is important since such differentiation determines future management approaches. Tactile inspection may disclose the tenderness or induration of lesions, giving clues to underlying inflammatory processes. In addition, eliciting the Nikolsky sign, which consists of applying gentle lateral pressure to apparently uninvolved skin to inspect for development of new blisters, is still an important bedside test to implicate conditions such as pemphigus vulgaris. This clinical insight is especially important as vesiculobullous disorders tend to have overlapping presentations, which call for a detailed understanding of lesion attributes to make an accurate diagnosis as well as therapeutic intervention (Patel et al., 2023). Along with cutaneous examination, oral mucosal examination is also a core component of clinical evaluation, particularly since vesiculobullous disorders can often involve mucous membranes. The oral cavity examination should be done in a systematic manner, tending to find early or concurrent lesions not seen on the surface of the skin or even missed. With appropriate light and instruments such as tongue depressors, clinicians evaluate for vesicles, erosions, or white plaques that can guide both the severity and extent of the disease. Since oral mucosal manifestations are closely related to dermatological manifestations, they not only increase diagnostic certainty but also direct biopsy site selection for histopathology. Identification of oral involvement is crucial for the prediction and treatment of the condition, reinforcing the importance of standard oral cavity examination within dermatology practice (Suliman et al., 2011). Advanced clinical diagnostic methods go beyond morphology and distribution to encompass special diagnostic maneuvers like Tzanck smear and DIF, usually done simultaneously with physical examination. Though direct biopsy is the yardstick for true diagnosis, Tzanck smear is a quick, minimally invasive bedside test that detects acantholytic cells in conditions such as pemphigus, facilitating early detection. DIF augments clinical findings through the localization of immune deposits within the epidermal or basement membrane zones, thus enhancing diagnostic specificity. Clinicians have to synthesize these methods with patient history and lesion examination, recognizing that vesiculobullous diseases present with broad age and demographic variability. Hence, an orderly, layered process of clinical examination supports precise diagnosis, facilitating directed, effective treatment that enhances patient outcomes (Suliman et al., 2011; Patel et al., 2023).

10.4.2. Laboratory Tests and Skin Biopsies

Proper diagnosis of vesiculobullous diseases largely depends on meticulous laboratory testing and histopathological analysis via skin biopsies. Most of these diseases, involving blistering, tend to be confused with infectious or neoplastic processes. Laboratory testing gives valuable information, such as immunofluorescence testing for detection of autoantibodies and direct markers of disease activity. While routine laboratory examination can encompass cultures of biopsy specimens to rule out infectious causes, it is microscopic examination of skin sections that usually clinches the diagnosis by demonstrating characteristic patterns of epidermal or dermal cleavage. It facilitates differentiation between intraepidermal and subepidermal blistering diseases and directs therapeutic maneuvers accordingly. Microbiological testing integrated with histopathology, especially in doubtful cases, improves diagnostic precision and maximizes patient benefit (Miller et al., 2024). Although routine histopathological examination is unavoidable, the function of laboratory investigation goes beyond standard microscopy. New methods like direct and in DIF, enzyme-linked immunosorbent assays (ELISA), and immunoblotting offer essential information about circulating antibodies and their antigen targets. These serological investigations supplement the biopsy results to make it possible to make a more specific diagnosis of vesiculobullous diseases such as pemphigus vulgaris and bullous pemphigoid. Skin biopsy sampling also requires precise technique to maintain tissue architecture and antigenicity for use in immunofluorescence assays. The biopsy should ideally be obtained from perilesional, non-ulcerated skin to maximize diagnostic yield. Laboratories also need to handle specimens properly to preserve viability, with rigid fixation and transportation protocols, allowing for consistent interpretation and minimizing false negatives. Integration of laboratory and clinical information continues to be essential to precise disease delineation (Miller et al., 2024). Where infectious diseases have a simulating pattern of vesiculobullous diseases, the laboratory and biopsy results are increasingly important in distinguishing etiologies. For example, overlapping clinical morphologies of tropical infections like mycetoma may complicate vesiculobullous lesion diagnosis. Retrospective studies underscore the need for correlating histopathology with microbiological cultures in identifying pathogenic fungal or bacterial organisms precisely. Negligent or lacking microbiological assessment results in delayed or missed diagnosis with potential aggravation of the patient's prognosis. Increased laboratory capacity, such as the capability to conduct special stains and culture methods on biopsy material, is crucial to separate infectious mimickers from autoimmune blistering diseases. This makes the need for increased clinical suspicion and bolstered diagnostic infrastructure, especially in endemic regions, important for improving disease prognosis through early, directed therapy (Figure 10.10).

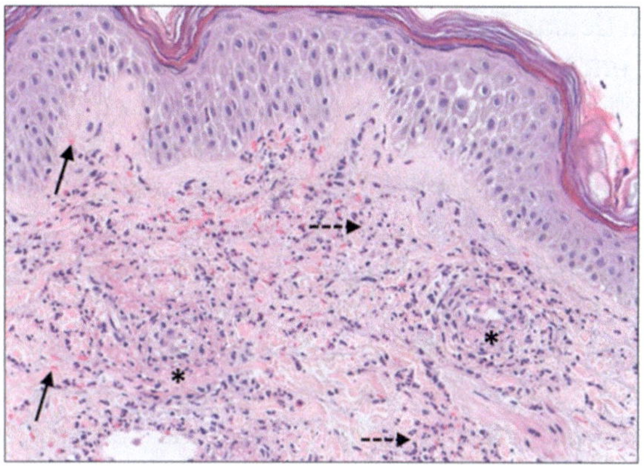

Figure 10.10. Small vessel leucocytoclastic vasculitis. The section shows all features of leucocytoclastic vasculitis. A mixed inflammatory cell population surrounding the postcapillary venules of the superficial dermis. The infiltrate consists of neutrophils with nuclear dust (dashed arrows) and shows high affinity for the vessels. Features of vascular injury are shown including fibrinoid necrosis (asterisks) and erytrocyt extravasation (solid arrows). *Source*: Giang J, Seelen MAJ, van Doorn MBA, Rissmann R, Prens EP and Damman J (2018) Complement Activation in Inflammatory Skin Diseases. Front. Immunol. 9:639. doi: 10.3389/fimmu.2018.00639

10.4.3. Imaging Studies and Their Relevance

In the clinical diagnosis of vesiculobullous skin diseases, imaging studies provide an adjunctive function that is in addition to histopathological and immunological studies. While these diseases initially present with cutaneous and mucosal manifestations, imaging can provide clues to deeper tissue involvement, especially when systemic involvement or secondary infections are suspected. For example, ultrasound and magnetic resonance imaging (MRI) may demonstrate the severity of subcutaneous edema, inflammatory soft tissue, or abscess, which are not necessarily evident on examination. Therefore, imaging aids in a greater determination of disease severity and helps direct therapeutic maneuvers, particularly in complex cases. The subtle use of imaging has the ability to separate superficial vesiculobullous conditions from those affecting deeper anatomic structures, thus affecting prognosis and management plans. Additionally, application of imaging modalities is most appropriate in vesiculobullous disease when mucous membrane involvement is seen and there are apprehensions of airway compromise or involvement of internal organs. For instance, computed tomography (CT) scans can assess oropharyngeal and respiratory tract involvement in conditions like pemphigus vulgaris, with extensive mucosal blistering potentially causing airway compromise. This diagnostic method allows for early intervention, which is vital to avoid life-threatening complications. Furthermore, imaging can be critical in revealing associated systemic manifestations like interstitial lung disease or esophageal strictures, which might not be clinically apparent. In this regard, imaging examinations guarantee that treatment regimens reach beyond cutaneous lesions to treat systemic sequelae in a complete manner. Even with the main reliance on clinical and laboratory assessment, the expanding role of imaging in vesiculobullous diseases represents a multidisciplinary strategy to diagnosis and treatment. New imaging modalities, such as high-resolution ultrasound and non-invasive optical imaging, hold promise for early detection and monitoring of therapeutic response, thus reducing invasive interventions. These developments are consistent with infectious disease preparedness guidelines' recommendations for overall disease surveillance and control strategies, but for other pathologies (Barrera et al., 2011). Correlating imaging results with serological and histopathological findings improves diagnostic performance, enables personalized therapy, and ultimately enhances patient outcomes in skin vesiculobullous diseases.

10.5. Treatment Options

The treatment of vesiculobullous skin diseases must be tailored to the pathophysiology of the condition as well as to the side effects of therapy. Conventional management consists of systemic corticosteroids and immunosuppression to suppress inflammation and forestall disease progression. These carry a price of serious adverse effects, and therefore, there has been a push for investigation into other modalities that can provide efficacy with superior safety. New technologies for dermatologic therapy, for example, the application of focused ultrasound technologies, illustrate this change. In particular, hyperthermic 20 MHz high intensity focused ultrasound (HIFU) has been seen to be promising by triggering immunological activation without widespread tissue necrosis, offering a less harmful alternative than traditional therapies such as cryotherapy. It has been shown to be clinically effective in inflammatory dermatoses and has the potential for use in vesiculobullous diseases where immune modulation is essential (Calik et al., 2024). In addition to immunomodulation, symptomatic management in vesiculobullous disease usually mirrors that used in other complex dermatoses involving hyperhidrosis or inflammation. For instance, advancements in hyperhidrosis treatment focus on a stepped strategy, starting with topical agents and progressing to more aggressive procedures depending on severity and patient response. Topical therapy, such as aluminum salts, offers first-line relief of symptoms with minimal systemic involvement. For intractable conditions, botulinum toxin injections provide site-specific suppression of sweat gland activity, with fewer systemic side effects prevalent in oral anticholinergics. Surgical treatments are still an option for refractory severe cases but pose a greater risk profile (Pawlak et al., 2024). These multilayered treatments emphasize the need for individually tailored treatment plans to disease severity and patient-specific considerations, a lesson that has significant implications for vesiculobullous disease management. Combining cutting-edge technologies with proven treatment protocols promises to improve vesiculobullous skin disease treatment outcomes. Numerical modeling research assessing HIFU shows its ability to produce localized hyperthermia that initiates immune responses without extending to extensive skin necrosis, different from the more destructive cryotherapy tissue injury. Such lessened collateral damage can be translated into enhanced healing and reduced post-procedure complications like scarring or pigmentary alterations, important factors considering the chronicity and high frequency of relapse of vesiculobullous diseases (Calik et al., 2024). In addition, emphasis on non-invasive or minimally invasive modalities is consistent with rising demand for therapies that maximize patient quality of life. Multimodal treatment regimens combining these new technologies with traditional immunosuppressants may redefine standard of care, justifying additional clinical evaluation to support efficacy and safety profiles in this challenging set of skin conditions.

10.5.1. Topical Therapies and Their Applications

Successful control of vesiculobullous diseases typically requires localized therapy to avoid systemic side effects while providing high drug levels to involved sites. Topical treatments, especially corticosteroids, are commonly used to inhibit inflammatory processes within sites of blistering and associated decrease in disease severity and symptom. Intralesional corticosteroid injection (ICSI) is a prime example of one of these options, which provides effective anti-inflammatory effects by localizing the drug within lesions. This method has proved to be superior to traditional topical steroids in causing localized immunosuppression with less systemic side effects. It has been shown that triamcinolone, which is widely applied steroid in ICSI, has increased efficacy in the treatment of inflammatory and immunologic lesions, rendering it very useful in dermatologic practice. Additionally, the mild and transient nature of the side effects even more supports its use as a first-line therapeutic agent in carefully selected cases (Gholizadeh et al., 2020). These benefits highlight the central position of targeted topical therapy in the management of complicated vesiculobullous diseases. In combination with corticosteroids, there are other topical drugs with important roles in treating vesiculobullous diseases, frequently employed in an adjuvant capacity to treat symptom relief and repair the barrier. Barrier repair mixtures and emollients play a critical role in reducing blistering-induced epidermal disruption, transepidermal water loss, and re-epithelialization. Their routine use can help prevent secondary infection and reduce patient discomfort, improving quality of life. Photochemotherapy, including PUVA (psoralen plus UVA), although more frequently systemic or semi-topical, is another essential modality for refractory cases by balancing immune responses in the skin. Notwithstanding few large-scale randomized controlled trials, clinical practice and smaller trials have shown PUVA to be effective for chronic hand eczema and associated vesiculobullous lesions, suggesting its promise as a therapeutic intervention after topical corticosteroids (Guttmann et al., 2008). The inclusion of such treatments is testimony to the increasing knowledge of skin barrier physiology and immunologic modulation in disease control. In addition to topical corticosteroids and photochemotherapies, the choice and combination of topical therapy in vesiculobullous disorders should be determined by disease severity, site of lesions, and patient-specific characteristics in order to achieve maximal benefit and avoid unwarranted adverse effects. Combination treatments, as corticosteroids in combination with soothing agents or antimicrobial preparations, can treat multifaceted pathologies such as inflammation, pruritus, and infection risk. Importantly, intralesional delivery of anesthetic agents may be used in conjunction with this mode of therapy without exacerbating patient pain, maximizing tolerability of treatment upon administration (Gholizadeh et al., 2020). Further, adherence to therapeutic algorithms, which detail the initial use of topical corticosteroids prior to progression to phototherapy or systemic therapy, preserves an evidence-based, stepwise treatment approach individualized to specific disease refractory states. This is especially critical in the management of chronic relapsing diseases where avoidance of long-term systemic corticosteroid use is ideal. Together, these observations demonstrate the subtle use of topical treatments in vesiculobullous disease, with efficacy balanced against patient safety and improved quality of life (Figure 10.11).

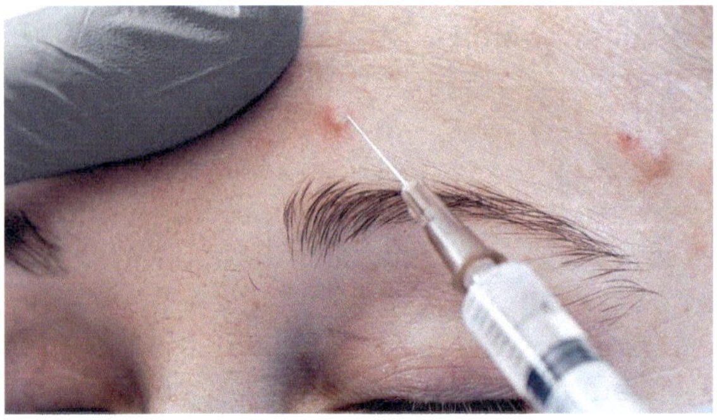

Figure 10.11. Intralesional corticosteroid injection (ICSI).

Source: Premier Clinic. (2020). *Intralesion Corticosteroid Injection.* https://premier-clinic.com/wp-content/uploads/2020/08/Intralesion-Corticosteroid-Injection-01-768x427.jpg.

10.5.2. Systemic Treatments and Their Effectiveness

The management of vesiculobullous diseases of the skin often necessitates systemic therapies due to the widespread and severe nature of these conditions. Immunosuppressive agents such as corticosteroids, azathioprine, and mycophenolate mofetil have long been the cornerstone of treatment, aiming to reduce inflammation and autoantibody production. Systemic corticosteroids are most effective at quickly suppressing acute disease flares through immunosuppression but are limited by severe adverse effects on long-term use, such as osteoporosis, diabetes, and increased risk of infections. Thus, these drugs are often used with steroid-sparing agents to promote sustained remission on reduced steroid doses. Newer developments have brought about biologics that act on specific immune mechanisms, providing more specific interventions with potentially better safety profiles. In light of these alternatives, the interindividual variability in response and the chronicity of vesiculobullous diseases emphasize the imperative for individualized treatment regimens and regular follow-up to evaluate therapeutic success as well as side effects (Annessi et al., 2015). The efficacy of systemic treatments in vesiculobullous disorders is usually assessed based on their capacity to induce and sustain remission of disease, suppress relapse, and decrease treatment-related complications. Evidence suggests that systemic corticosteroids produce an aggressive initial response but long-term dependence results in morbidity that may exceed benefits. The steroid-sparing drugs azathioprine or cyclophosphamide are useful adjuncts, usually allowing tapering of corticosteroids while controlling disease activity. More recently, biologic agents such as rituximab have shown remarkable efficacy in resistant cases by selectively targeting B cells, thus directly treating the underlying autoimmune pathology. ICSI also have also been promising, especially in localized disease, by the administration of high doses to the involved areas with minimal systemic absorption and side effects (Gholizadeh et al., 2020). However, the variability in vesiculobullous diseases necessitates disease-specific treatment strategies based on severity, distribution, and comorbidities of the patient to maximize outcomes. Despite the progress with systemic therapies, long-term management remains problematic and finding a balance between efficacy and safety in vesiculobullous diseases. Although systemic corticosteroids and immunosuppressants provide wide-ranging immune suppression, undesirable side effects lead to compromises in patient quality of life. Targeted therapies like biologics have arguably revolutionized the treatment paradigm, focusing on precision medicine to maximize efficacy while preventing systemic toxicity. Ongoing clinical trials are testing additional agents, such as T-cell modulators and new monoclonal antibodies, to increase rates of sustained disease remission. Nonetheless, frequent relapses reflect the multifactorial nature of immune dysregulation in such conditions. Moreover, patient compliance and vigilant clinical observation are pivotal determinants of success with treatments. Therefore, combining systemic treatment with supportive care and individually tailored care plans continues to be the key to effective and safe control of vesiculobullous skin diseases (Annessi et al., 2015; Gholizadeh et al., 2020) (Figure 10.12).

Treatment outcomes	Rituximab	Omalizumab	Dupilumab
Patients, n (%)	122 (100.0)	53 (100.0)	36 (100.0)
Resolution outcomes, n (%)			
Complete remission	86 (70.5)	36 (67.9)	24 (66.7)
Partial remission	29 (23.8)	11 (20.8)	7 (19.4)
No remission	6 (4.9)	6 (11.3)	5 (13.9)
Deterioration	1 (0.8)	0 (0.0)	0 (0.00)
Time to remission, months			
Mean	5.7	6.6	4.5
Range	1.0-13.0	0.5-15.0	1.0-15.0
NR, n (%)	48 (39.3)	17 (32.1)	11 (30.6)
BP recurrence, n (%)			
Yes	25 (20.5)	3 (5.7)	2 (5.6)
No	86 (70.5)	42 (79.2)	26 (72.2)
NR	4 (3.3)	2 (3.8)	3 (8.3)
Adverse events, n (%)			
None	73 (59.8)	34 (64.2)	30 (83.3)
Death	11 (9.0)	1 (1.9)	0 (0.0)
Infection	8 (6.6)	0 (0.0)	0 (0.0)
Altered mental status	4 (3.3)	0 (0.0)	0 (0.0)
Anemia	2 (1.6)	0 (0.0)	0 (0.0)
Tachycardia	1 (0.8)	0 (0.0)	0 (0.0)
Compression fracture	1 (0.8)	0 (0.0)	0 (0.0)
Prostate cancer	1 (0.8)	0 (0.0)	0 (0.0)
Metastatic breast cancer	1 (0.8)	0 (0.0)	0 (0.0)
Mucoepidermoid carcinoma	1 (0.8)	0 (0.0)	0 (0.0)
Dyspnea	1 (0.8)	0 (0.0)	0 (0.0)
Thrombocytopenia	0 (0.0)	1 (1.9)	0 (0.0)
NR	19 (15.6)	17 (32.1)	6 (16.7)

BP, bullous pemphigoid; NR, not reported; N/A, not applicable.

Figure 10.12. Bullous pemphigoid treatment algorithm.

Source: Cao P, Xu W and Zhang L (2022) Rituximab, Omalizumab, and Dupilumab Treatment Outcomes in Bullous Pemphigoid: A Systematic Review. Front. Immunol. 13:928621. doi: 10.3389/fimmu.2022.928621

10.5.3. Emerging Therapies and Research Developments

New developments in the pathophysiology of vesiculobullous diseases have fueled efforts to identify new therapeutic approaches that transcend traditional immunosuppressive therapies. One such area is the repurposing of drugs through the application of genomic and transcriptomic research.

For instance, combining gene expression with quantitative trait loci has allowed for the development of sophisticated molecular networks that implicate important pathways in disease pathogenesis. This systems biology strategy has enabled the discovery of candidates such as vitamin D analogues, retinoids, and immunomodulatory drugs that have the potential to provide alternative or adjunctive therapeutic value for conditions like vesicular hand eczema, an intractable subtype of vesiculobullous disease (Rosenberg et al., 2024). Such drug repurposing strategies seek to meet previously unmet clinical needs by targeting molecular mechanisms more selectively, which may have enhanced efficacy and safety profiles over conventional treatment modalities. Concurrently, drug repurposing is advancing alongside research into the genetic causes of related neurological and systemic signs and symptoms of vesiculobullous diseases. In the last few years, next-generation sequencing technology has revealed mutations in genes for kinesin motor proteins like KIF4A and KIF5C that are vital for intracellular transport as well as synaptic function. Dysfunction in these genes is associated with changed neuronal excitability and intellectual disability, demonstrating the multisystem, complex nature of the autoimmune blistering disease, which presents with occasional neurological complications. Functional testing in neuronal models reinforces the promise of the development of targeted therapies that correct synaptic imbalances, offering a conceptual model for prospective therapies that could alter disease progression at the molecular level, independent of the management of cutaneous symptoms. Along with genetic and pharmacologic innovations, novel biologic treatments are being recognized as realistic possibilities for intractable vesiculobullous diseases. Monoclonal antibodies against specific immune mediators that participate in the autoimmune cascade are yielding promising results in clinical trials, providing the possibility for targeted immune modulation with reduced side effects. In addition, investigations into gene editing and RNA-based technologies have the transformative power of correcting pathogenic mutations that confer susceptibility to blistering disease development. This intersection of molecular biology, immunology, and pharmacogenomics represents an evolving paradigm shift toward personalized medicine in dermatology. Further integration of such multidisciplinary research findings will be critical to maximizing the treatment effects and optimizing patients' quality of life with vesiculobullous diseases (Rosenberg et al., 2024).

10.6. Complications and Prognosis

The course of vesiculobullous skin diseases can be complicated by both local and systemic complications that markedly influence the outcome of patients. Secondary bacterial infections are usually seen as a consequence of disruption of the skin barrier, which may cause cellulitis and sepsis. In addition, prolonged erosion and blistering predispose to fluid and electrolyte imbalance, resulting in dehydration and renal insufficiency in advanced cases. Psychological distress also often complicates the prognosis, with chronic pain and disfigurement affecting quality of life. Some autoimmune vesiculobullous conditions, like pemphigus vulgaris, can have mucosal involvement, and this can have complications such as dysphagia or compromise of the airway. These together emphasize the need for early diagnosis and multi-factorial management plans that not only address the underlying pathology but also predict and prevent such complications to enhance long-term outcomes in patients so affected. Neurological involvement, although less frequent, is a significant complication of some vesiculobullous diseases and can play an important role in determining the prognosis. For instance, herpes zoster ophthalmicus, a vesiculobullous condition, may lead to cranial nerve palsies, for instance, lateral rectus palsy with symptoms of diplopia and compromised ocular motility. Although this is usually a transient and self-limiting complication, antiviral treatment is necessary to avoid sight-threatening effects and additional neurological injury. If such presentations are not identified early, then irreversible deficits can follow, emphasizing the need for careful clinical examination and cognizance of possible neurological sequelae. Therefore, knowledge of these neural complications helps the clinician better provide focused treatment as well as enhance the overall outcome for patients afflicted with vesiculobullous conditions (Yalcinbayir et al., 2011). Recent data suggest a prognostic value of cutaneous lesions in systemic diseases with vesiculobullous presentation, particularly in the case of viral infections like COVID-19. Cutaneous symptoms can be extremely variable and may vary with some morphologies being associated with the severity and prognosis of the disease. Chilblain-like lesions, for example, occur in young patients and correlate with less severe disease not requiring hospitalization. On the other hand, acral ischemia and livedo reticularis strongly correlate with worse outcomes, such as higher intensive care admission and mortality. These results imply that vesiculobullous skin lesions could be clinical markers for systemic disease prognosis and possibly be used to inform risk stratification and treatment. Skin manifestations in vesiculobullous disease, therefore, go beyond local disease, providing prognostically important insight into associated systemic conditions (Holmes et al., 2022).

10.6.1. Potential Complications Associated with Vesiculobullous Diseases

The clinical presentation of vesiculobullous diseases goes beyond cutaneous manifestations, usually followed with severe systemic complications that challenge diagnosis and management. The disease mainly involves the epidermis and dermal layers, disrupting the skin barrier to different extents. Such a disruption greatly predisposes to secondary infections, worsening the patient's condition and causative morbidity. For example, rupture of bullae offers an entry point for bacterial and fungal colonization, increasing the risk of cellulitis and sepsis. Also, the ongoing loss of skin integrity often ultimately leads to fluid and electrolyte imbalance, particularly in generalized conditions such as pemphigus vulgaris. These systemic derangements not only increase hospital stays but also complicate management approaches, and thus underscore the importance of early detection and treatment. Histopathological analysis continues to play a crucial role in the diagnosis and prevention of undesirable outcomes for such diseases (Patel et al., 2023). Vesiculobullous disease complications go beyond infectious mechanisms to include relevant immunological and inflammatory sequelae. Scarring, pigmentary changes, and contractures restrictive of mobility and function may follow chronic inflammation of the affected areas of the skin. Certain autoimmune blistering diseases are compounded by mucosal involvement, which may be life-threatening in blocking pertinent anatomical structures like the oral cavity and respiratory tract. Such mucosal impairment tends to complicate alimentation and respiration, thus elevating morbidity and impacting quality of life. Systemic immune dysregulation induced by such diseases can also induce other autoimmune manifestations or exacerbate established disease. Knowledge of the immunopathogenesis and surveillance of patients for such complications are critical to individualizing broad treatment regimens and minimizing morbidity (Patel et al., 2023). Although most vesiculobullous diseases mainly involve the skin, unusual presentations can lead to delays in diagnosis and complicate clinical courses. For instance, atypical distribution of the lesions or co-infections can mask the underlying pathology, as in the uncommon manifestations of hand-foot-and-mouth disease with widespread vesiculobullous eruptions and streptococcal co-infection. Atypical instances could present with purpuric lesions and limited mucosal involvement, necessitating early identification and treatment to avoid advancement to systemic manifestation. Prompt hospitalization and directed therapy in these situations have proven to lead to quick recovery and good clinical outcomes, emphasizing the need for awareness of rare modes of disease presentation and complications.

10.6.2. Long-Term Prognosis for Patients

The chronicity of vesiculobullous diseases normally poses a multifaceted course of treatment for patients whose long-term prognosis largely depends on early detection and the success of therapeutic management. Most of these diseases, especially autoimmune conditions such as pemphigus vulgaris, necessitate ongoing immunosuppressive therapy to sustain remission and avert relapse. Improved outcomes have resulted from advances in corticosteroid and immunomodulatory therapies, but patients are still vulnerable to disease and treatment complications. The ongoing immune insult against keratinocytes weakens the skin and mucous membranes, predisposing them to infection and scarring. Vigilance and multidisciplinary care are crucial to track disease activity and prevent complications. Thus, the prognosis depends not just on biological considerations but also on adherence to treatment by the patients and regular medical monitoring (Indupuru et al., 2015). In patients who are old or have comorbid conditions, the prognosis is worse because of the additional factor of polypharmacy and increased risk of drug-related adverse effects. The treatment of vesiculobullous diseases in these populations requires a fine balance between disease activity control and avoiding iatrogenic damage. Chronic corticosteroid therapy, while being useful in suppressing inflammation, is fraught with potential hazards such as osteoporosis, diabetes, and susceptibility to infections. More than one drug for associated conditions also makes the therapeutic environment difficult, potentially worsening the skin lesions or making recovery troublesome. Close observation and individualized treatment modifications provide a route to enhancing the quality of life for these needy patients, but prognosis frequently hinges on meticulous interdisciplinary planning and strict follow-up (Bennani-Ziatni et al., 2015).

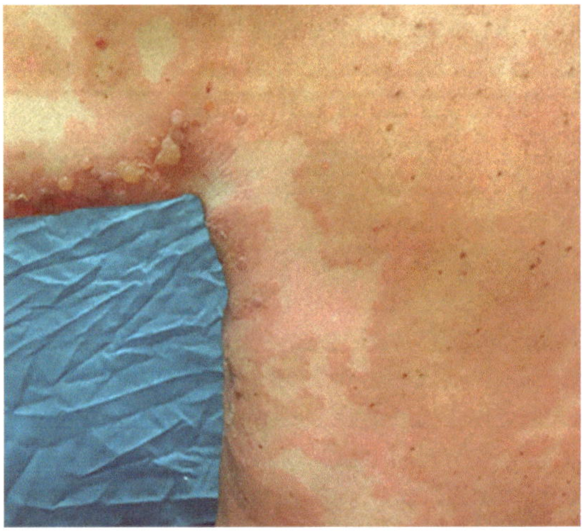

Figure 10.13. Clinical pictures of chronic bullous pemphigoid.

Source: Tedeschi, A., Asero, R., Marzano, A. V., & Cugno, M. (2015). Clinical pictures of chronic urticaria and bullous pemphigoid. In Activation of blood coagulation in two prototypic autoimmune skin diseases: A possible link with thrombotic risk. *Clinical and Experimental Immunology, 181*(3), 384–389.

Even with advances in therapy, the psychological component of vesiculobullous disease also plays a key part in long-term prognosis since chronic symptoms and cutaneous manifestations impact mental well-being and social functioning. Patients often face repeated flare-ups interfering with normal routines and causing emotional distress, leading to poorer adherence to treatment plans. The incorporation of psychosocial intervention along with medical management thus assumes a crucial role in supporting resilience and facilitating long-term remission. In addition, novel therapies directed at unique immune mechanisms provide exciting avenues for the attainment of more long-lasting control of disease activity at reduced side effects. With advancing research, targeted treatment plans that consider both the psychosocial and biological aspects will be critical to improving the overall prognosis of patients with these difficult dermatological diseases (Bennani-Ziatni et al., 2015; Indupuru et al., 2015) (Figure 10.13).

10.6.3. Impact on Quality of Life

The occurrence of vesiculobullous diseases significantly changes the daily life of patients, usually in terms of extreme physical discomfort and mental distress. These skin and mucous membrane diseases, which involve blistering and erosions, interfere with normal activities like eating, speech, and mobility. The pain and pruritus of these lesions may also cause insomnia and fatigue, which contribute to a general decline in well-being. In addition, the uncontrollable and recurrent tendency of autoimmune vesiculobullous diseases puts a chronic psychological strain. The need for frequent medical consultations and invasive diagnostic tests contributes to patient anxiety. The quality of life, therefore, is not only compromised by the somatic symptoms but also secondary to the cumulative psychological and lifestyle effects that these diseases place on individuals (Adityan et al., 2007). Social interaction and self-image are also significantly impacted by vesiculobullous diseases, leading to lower quality of life. Evident lesions, especially on body parts or oral mucosa, may cause stigmatization as well as social isolation. Patients tend to feel embarrassed and reduced self-esteem because of the disfiguring nature of the disease. This social isolation can amplify feelings of depression and anxiety, thus aggravating the psychological burden. Treatment courses, often extended and involving immunosuppressive treatments, have their own complications that further diminish satisfaction with life. Chronicity and symptom severity demand multifaceted management strategies that treat not just the physical but emotional and social aspects of health as well (Adityan et al., 2007). Oral manifestations, frequent in subepithelial vesiculobullous diseases, also pose problems that significantly affect the quality of patient life. Painful erosions of the oral cavity compromise nutrition as eating becomes painful and uncomfortable, resulting in weight loss and malnutrition in more advanced cases. The lesions also predispose to secondary infections, adding to morbidity. Prompt diagnosis and treatment, particularly by the use of immunofluorescence methods, are important in averting evolution to widespread cutaneous involvement, thereby preventing greater systemic burdens. Maximizing therapy approaches that focus on lesion control and symptom relief directly corresponds to enhancement in daily functioning and psychosocial well-being, highlighting the need for integrated care models for the patients.

CLOSER LOOK

DERMAL-EPIDERMAL JUNCTION (DEJ)

The DEJ is the site through which the dermis and epidermis layers of skin intersect, serving as a structural and functional link between the two. It is a highly specialized region tasked with attaching the epidermis to the dermis, supporting it, and controlling interactions between the two layers.

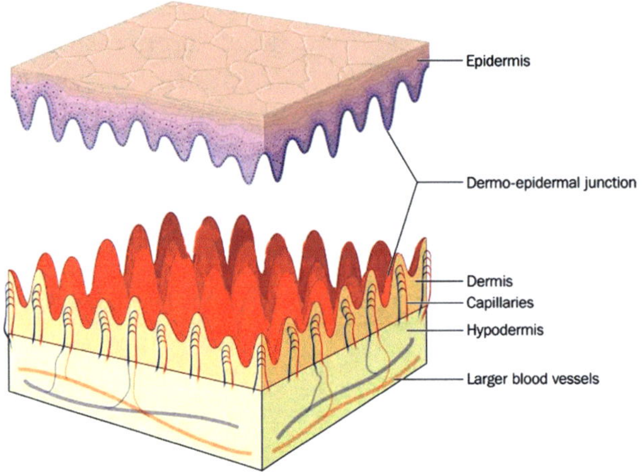

Source: Legger. (n.d.). Skin epidermal dermal junction showing dermo capillaries & deeper blood vessels. Dreamstime. https://thumbs.dreamstime.com/b/skin-epidermal-dermal-junction-showing-dermo-capillaries-deeper-blood-vessels-created-adobe-illustrator-contains-52603496.jpg.

- **Structure and Components**:
  - **Basement Membrane:** The DEJ is a basement membrane, a unique extracellular matrix that lies between the epidermis and dermis.
  - **Hemidesmosomes:** Basal keratinocytes (cells that line the base of the epidermis) bind to the basement membrane by way of hemidesmosomes, which are specialized cell adhesion molecules.
  - **Anchoring Fibrils:** Anchoring fibrils connect the basement membrane to the dermis and consist of type VII collagen.
  - **Other Structures:** In addition to these structures, DEJ contains other structures such as lamina lucida, lamina densa, and sub-basal lamina.
- **Functions:**
  - **Structural Support:** The DEJ offers mechanical support to the epidermis, enabling the skin to resist stress and remain intact.
  - **Cell Adhesion:** It ensures adhesion of the epidermal cells (keratinocytes) to the underlying dermis so that they will not become detached.
  - **Permeability Barrier:** The DEJ is a barrier to the movement of some cells and

molecules between the epidermis and dermis and ensures the skin barrier is maintained intact.

- **Signal Transduction:** It involves signal transduction, affecting cell behavior and differentiation in the dermis and epidermis.
- **Communication:** The DEJ mediates communication and interactions between fibroblasts, keratinocytes, and melanocytes, and is involved in the complex processes of skin development and function.

- **Clinical Significance:**
  - **Age-Related Changes:** As age advances, the DEJ may change, such as a loss of proteins and collagen, which can result in a flattened appearance and decreased surface area.
  - **Skin Disorders:** Disturbances of the DEJ can be related to several skin disorders, including bullous diseases (blistering skin diseases).

SUMMARY

The diagnosis and treatment of vesiculobullous skin diseases are a challenge because they have varied clinical presentations and shared histopathology. Even with improved diagnostic methods, precise identification may require a combination of clinical investigation, histopathology, and immunofluorescence tests. As illustrated by recent research, histopathological evaluation alone can distinguish some entities such as pemphigus vulgaris and pemphigus foliaceus but DIF is still essential for documenting diagnoses and separating diseases that share identical histological appearances, including bullous pemphigoid and epidermolysis bullosa acquisita (Atla et al., 2019). This multi-faceted system not only contributes to enhanced diagnostic accuracy but also directs proper therapeutic planning, ultimately optimizing patient outcomes by reducing morbidity and mortality related to these conditions. In addition, the systemic nature and common involvement of mucosal surfaces in numerous vesiculobullous disorders underscore the need for a complete patient assessment. Investigations have highlighted the common association between oral mucosal lesions and patients experiencing dermatologic vesiculobullous diseases, with their prevalence in some demographic and behavioral parameters (Suliman et al., 2011). This highlights the significance of oral mucosa examination by routine during dermatologic diagnosis to avoid missing mucosal involvement and related consequences. Understanding the interconnection between systemic disease, lifestyle, and mucocutaneous manifestations opens the door to more comprehensive care paradigms. This holistic worldview is essential for managing the entire gamut of disease burden and enhancing quality of life in impacted patients. In conclusion, vesiculobullous skin diseases need careful diagnostic workups that blend clinical observation, histopathology, and immunofluorescence to successfully classify them. The incorporation of such diagnostic tools enables focused treatment strategies that can counteract the severity of disease and minimize undesirable outcomes. Further, the identification of the predominant oral mucosal involvement in association with skin features necessitates multidisciplinary interaction between dermatologists and dental professionals to enable comprehensive patient evaluation and management (Suliman et al., 2011; Atla et al., 2019). Finally, ongoing investigation and clinical awareness are essential in further establishing diagnostic standards, optimizing therapeutic regimens, and confronting the multifaceted issues of vesiculobullous patients for the best health results.

Progress in the pathogenesis of vesiculobullous dermatoses has emphasized the complexity and heterogeneity of these disorders. At their core is the abnormality of cellular adhesion within the epidermis or dermoepidermal junction with resultant characteristic vesicle and bullae formation. Ongoing research emphasizes the key role of autoimmune processes, specifically autoantibody profiles, in disease classification and prognosis, facilitating an individualized therapeutic approach. The clinical range varies from focal blistering to disseminated, life-threatening disease, and requires early and precise diagnosis. Advances in immunopathologic methods, such as direct and in DIF, have enhanced diagnostic specificity. At the same time, therapy has evolved toward selective immunomodulation with the aim of reducing disease activity with minimal systemic side effects, a reflection of an appreciation of the subtleties of immunogenetics and molecular mechanisms. These findings cumulatively guide improved outcomes and highlight the necessity for ongoing research to further refine management protocols (Leclair, 2023). Socioeconomic and geographical influences have a subtle impact on the clinical presentation and management of vesiculobullous diseases, emphasizing the significance of context in the provision of healthcare. Differences in disease prevalence, availability of specialized services, and treatment adherence have the potential to profoundly shape patient outcomes. Research on healthcare use shows inequalities associated with socioeconomic status, impacting early diagnosis and treatment, which is most important in diseases that have rapid course and complication rates. Mapping healthcare resources geographically shows deficiencies in specialist presence, especially in areas short of resources, leading to recourse to primary care or alternative medical practices, which are likely to cause delays in proper treatment. Interventions to enhance patient education, access to healthcare, and combining of traditional and contemporary medical practice could strengthen disease management systems. An understanding of these systemic factors is critical to modifying public health policies and resource utilization to maximize the care of vesiculobullous disease patients (Magrabi et al., 2001). The integration of clinical, immunological, and epidemiological information provides a global view of vesiculobullous diseases but also highlights areas needing more investigation. Genetic susceptibility and environmental stimuli interact in disease initiation and progression, but their exact mechanisms need further research. Existing therapy regimens, although successful in most instances, are linked to excessive morbidity from chronic immunosuppression, highlighting the necessity for less toxic, more specific therapies. Additionally, the psychosocial burden of such disfiguring diseases necessitates multidisciplinary management involving psychological counseling in addition to medical therapy. Economic studies have shown high healthcare expenditures and the impact on the patient and healthcare systems, particularly in areas where disease prevalence overlaps with lower socioeconomic levels. The solution to these complex problems lies in future research improving diagnostic accuracy, broadening therapeutic choices, and optimizing equity of healthcare delivery to minimize morbidity and mortality from vesiculobullous diseases (Magrabi et al., 2001; Leclair, 2023).

KEY TERMS FROM THIS CHAPTER

- Autoimmune bullous disease
- Bacterial sepsis
- Blister
- Bullous lesions
- Bullous pemphigoid
- Cellular metabolism
- Chilblain-like lesions
- Covid- pandemic
- Dermatitis herpetiformis
- Dermoepidermal junction
- Direct immunofluorescence
- Etiology
- Hemidesmosomal antigens
- Immune homeostasis
- Immune regulation
- Immunofluorescence
- Linear iga disease
- Lymphadenopathy

REFERENCES

1. Adityan, S. (2007). A clinicopathological study of autoimmune vesiculobullous diseases. https://core.ac.uk/download/235664077.pdf (accessed on 12 May 2025).
2. Ali, J., Islam, S., Ali, S. M., Yaqeen, S. R., Aslam, A., Khan, Q. U. A., Malik, U. A., Irfan, M., Naqvi, H., & Hashmi, A. A. (2021). Morphological Spectrum of Vesiculobullous Skin Lesions: An Institutional Perspective. Cureus, 13(5), e15330. https://doi.org/10.7759/cureus.15330(accessed on 12 May 2025).
3. Ali, R. W., Johannessen, A. C., Salman, H., Suliman, et al. (2011). Oral m*ucosal* lesions in skin diseased patients attending a dermatologic clinic: A cross-sectional study in Sudan. https://core.ac.uk/download/pdf/8625298.pdf. Suliman, N. M., Astrøm, A. N., Ali, R. W., Salman, H., & Johannessen, A. C. (2011). Oral mucosal lesions in skin diseased patients attending a dermatologic clinic: a cross-sectional study in Sudan. BMC oral health, 11, 24. https://doi.org/10.1186/1472-6831-11-24
4. Al Magrabi, & Aldean, K. S. (2001). Geographical aspects of health and use of primary health ca*re services in* Jeddah, South Arabia. Thesis; 10.48730/nm7m-nt49https://core.ac.uk/download/571222661.pdf (accessed on 12 May 2025).
5. Alvi, U., Fatima, Y., Khan, M., Taylor, et al. (2018). Central serous retinopathy and hand-foot-mouth disease: Coincidence or causation? https://core.ac.uk/download/303788163.pdf (accessed on 12 May 2025).
6. Alwadaani, H., Kashif, M., Khurshid, Z., Minhas, et al. (2019). Oral ulcers presentation in systemic diseases: An update. https://core.ac.uk/download/275664568.pdf (accessed on 12 May 2025).
7. Anderson, K. E., Bissell, D. M., Bloomer, J. R., Daniell, et al. (1997). Environmental chemical exposures and disturbances of heme synthesis. https://core.ac.uk/download/pdf/3962918.pdf.
8. Annessi, G., Boccaletti, V., Cortelazzi, C., Di Nuzzo, et al. (2015). Calcipotriol/betamethasone dipropionate ointment compared with tacrolimus ointment for the treatment of erosive pustular dermatosis of the scalp: A split-lesion comparison. https://core.ac.uk/download/217779193.pdf (accessed on 12 May 2025).
9. Arvind, M., & Abhinaya, L. M. (2020). Immune mediated sub-epithelial blistering disorders: Case series. https://core.ac.uk/download/613011468.pdf (accessed on 12 May 2025).
10. Atla, B., Kumar, S. S., Patnala, G. P., Priyanka, et al. (2019). Clinical, histopathological and immunofluorescent study of vesicobullous lesions of skin. https://core.ac.uk/download/539913287.pdf (accessed on 12 May 2025).
11. Ba, W., Bienek, M., de Brouwer, A., Haas, et al. (2010). Oral long-term complications of allogeneic haematopoietic stem cell transplantation. https://core.ac.uk/download/41234085.pdf (accessed on 12 May 2025).
12. Barrera, Roberto et al. (2011). Preparedness and response for Chikungunya virus introduction in the A*mericas.*
13. *Bendig, J., Frank, A., & Re*ichmann, H. (2024). Aging and Parkinson's disease: A complex interplay of vulnerable neurons, the immune system and the blood-brain barrier. Ageing and Neurodegenerative Diseases. https://www.semanticscholar.org/paper/9ed7808b7b35e21bfccc7db1459edf3534b7806e (accessed on 12 May 2025).

14. Bennani-Ziatni, M., Bennis, N., El M'barki Kadiri, R., Mesfioui, et al. (2015). Difficulty in managing polypharmacy in the elderly: Case report and review of the literature. https://core.ac.uk/download/pdf/82709955.pdf.

15. Bhatnagar, J., Blau, D., Bollweg, B., Fischer, et al. (2021). Clinical characteristics, histopathology, and tissue immunolocalization of Chikungunya virus antigen in fatal cases. https://core.ac.uk/download/617036044.pdf.

16. Bobbio, A., Camisa, C., Proby, C., Tsilikas, C., Asteriou, C., Paliouras, D., Winkler, D. T., et al. (2008). Paraneoplastic pemphigus regression after thymoma resection. https://core.ac.uk/download/pdf/8171878.pdf.

17. Burgess, J., Eisen, D., Lynch, D. P., Nordlund, et al. (2017). *Oral examination. https://core.ac.uk/download/213072873.pdf (accessed on 12 May 2025).*

18. *Busch, D. S., & Takayama, A.* K. *(*1991). Pemphigus: An autoimmune complex in dogs and cats. https://core.ac.uk/download/38907930.pdf.

19. Calik, J., Zawada, T., Sauer, N., & Bove, T. (2024). High intensity focused ultrasound (20 MHz) and cryotherapy as therapeutic options for granuloma annulare and other inflammatory skin conditions. Dermatology and Therapy, 14, 1189–1210. https://www.semanticscholar.org/paper/cf9d1c2a1b9f380e11383a1b0bab590b02d11b6a (accessed on 12 May 2025).

20. Denison, A. M., Bhatnagar, J., Jahan-Tigh, R. R., Fair, P., & Hale, G. L. (2021). Detecti*on of coxsackievirus A6 in* formalin-fixed, paraffin-embedded skin biopsy specimens using immunohistochemistry and real-time reverse-transcriptase PCR. J Clin Virol Plus, 1(1, 2). https://core.ac.uk/download/619628499.pdf (accessed on 12 May 2025).

21. Dhumale, S. B., & Khyalappa, R. (2016). Study of cutaneous manif*estations in geriatrics. Internatio*nal *J*ournal of Research in Medical Sciences, 4(5), 1343–1346. https://doi.org/10.18203/2320-6012.ijrms20160988 (accessed on 12 May 2025).

22. Draibe, J., Marco, H., Ibernon, M., Agraz, I., Arcal, C., Barros, X., Cabrera, V., et al. (20*24). Diagnosis and trea*tment of renal ANCA vasculitis: A summary of the consensus document of the Catalan Group for the Study of Glomerular Diseases (GLOMCAT). Journal of Clinical Medicine, 13. https://www.semanticscholar.org/paper/f64076604455fc0b4c144c241686e7cf73ceabbeb (accessed on 12 May 2025).

23. Fabio, G., Carrabba, M., Mellace, L., *Hu, C., Spagnoli, D.*, & Cappellini, M. D. (2011). Metastatic Spreading of Community Acquired Staphylococcus aureus Bacteraemia. Case reports in infectious diseases, 2011, 234018. https:*//doi.org/10.1155/2011/234018*

*24. Gholizadeh, N., Sadrzad*eh-Afshar, M. S., & Sheykhbahaei, N. (2020). Intralesional corticosteroid injection as an effective treatment method for oral lesions: A meta-analysis. Braz. J. Pharm. Sci. 56 • 2020 • https://doi.org/10.1590/s2175-97902019000418077

25. Guttmann, O. (2008). Hand eczema. https://core.ac.uk/download/11030085.pdf (accessed on 12 May 2025).

26. Holmes, Z., *Courtney, A., Lincoln, M., & Wel*ler, R. (2022). Rash morphology as a predictor of COVID-19 severity: A systematic review of the cutaneous manifestations of COVID-19. Skin health and disease, 2(3), e120. https://doi.org/10.1002/ski2.120 (accessed on 12 May 2025).

27. Indupuru, K., K. L., Keerthana, M., Sowjanya, C., et al. (2015). Oral pemphigus: A case report. https://core.ac.uk/download/235919920.pdf.

28. Jacovas, V. C., Zelnick, M., McNulty, S., Ross, J. E., Khurana, N., Pan, X., Nieto, A., et al. (2025). The ClinGen Severe Combined Immuno*deficiency Disease Variant C*uration Expert Panel: Specifications for classification of variants in ADA, DCLRE1C, IL2RG, IL7R, JAK3, RAG1, and RAG2. medRxiv: The Preprint Server for Health Sciences. https://www.semanticscholar.org/paper/7e8cbf346ae48a00cac2f5c425e9d5ccdddaf304 (accessed on 12 May 2025).

29. Leclair, Valérie (2023). Risk factors and outcomes in inflammatory myopathies. Karolinska Institutet. Thesis. https://hdl.handle.net/10616/48573 (accessed on 12 May 2025).

30. Mathew, T. (2007). A validation of ELISA test for detection of desmoglein 1 & 3 antibodies as a diagnostic test of pemphigus. htt*ps://core.ac.uk/download/235664148.pdf (accessed* on 12 May 2025).

31. Miller, J. M., Binnicker, M., Campbell, S., Carroll, K. C., Chapin, K. C., Gonzalez, M. D., Harrington, A., et al. (2024). Guide to utilization of the microbiology laboratory for diagnosis of infectious diseases: 2024 update by the Infectious Diseases Society of America (IDSA) and the American Society for Microbiology (ASM). Clinic*al Infectious* Diseases: An Official Publication of the Infectious Diseases Society of America. https://www.semanticscholar.org/paper/510d403fc246070b044950a3ccba623e6e8177a3 (accessed on 12 May 2025).

32. Ojha, N., & Yadav, O. P. (2020). Benign mucous membrane pemphigoid: A case report. ISSN: 2456-8090 (online) DOI: https://doi.org/10.26440/IHRJ/0402.05333(accessed on 12 May 2025).

33. Patel, K., Vasudha Bhagat, Jahanvi Vyas, & Prashant Patel. (2023). Histomorphological study of vesiculobullous lesions of skin: a study of 66 cases at tertiary care center. International Journal of Research in Medical Sciences, 11(2), 606–610. https://doi.org/10.18203/2320-6012.ijrms20230172(accessed on 12 May 2025).

34. Pavlyshyn, H., & Horishna, I. (2020). Atypical case of hand, foot and mouth disease (envirovir*al exanthem) from clinical practice. Case report; https://doi.org/10.13112/PC.2020.7*

*35. Pawlak, I., Pe*rkowska, K., Kaźmierczak, A., Izdebska, W., Sornek, P., Borkowska, A., Kiełb, A., et al. (2024). Variety of therapeutic approaches to primary hyperhidrosis (HH) and botulinum toxin priority over other treatment options in this condition: A review. Quality in Sport. https://www.semanticscholar.org/paper/1dbf0cd4572760cb4bc9154bca371d8522b5d840 (accessed on 12 May 2025).

36. Rosenberg, F. M., Kamali, Z., Voorberg, A. N., Oude Munnink, T. H., van der Most, P. J., Snieder, H., Vaez, A., & Schuttelaar, M. L. A. (2024). Transcriptomics- and Genomics-Guided Drug Repurposing for the Treatment of Vesicular Hand Eczema. Pharmaceutics, 16(4), 476. https://doi.org/10.3390/pharmaceutics16040476 (accessed on 12 May 2025).

37. Shah, MOR & Uddin, MN & Khan, M.s & Khondker, Lubna. (2013). Efficacy of Low Dose Low Molecular Weight Heparin in the Treatment of Cutaneous Lichen Planu*s. Journal of Ar*med Forces Medical College Bangladesh. 9. 2-7. (accessed on 12 May 2025).

38. Svitich O.A., Yazkova O.S., Bystritskaya E.P., Olisova O.Y. Role of innate immune receptors in the psoriasis development // Russian Journal of Skin and Venereal Diseases. - 2024. - Vol. 27. - N. 5. - P. 538-547. doi: 10.17816/dv634427

39. Vibhuti Kumar, Anita Sharan, Sunita Poriya, Sonia kundu. Clinico-Histopathological Correlation of Non-NeoplasticDermatological Lesions. Int J Med Res Rev [Internet]. 2022Mar.6 [cited 2025Jun.13];10(1):24-0. Available from: https://ijmrr.medresearch.in/index.php/ijmrr/article/view/1351 (accessed on 12 May 2025).

40. Volkers, S. M., Meisel, C., Terhorst-Molawi, D., Burbach, G. J., Schürmann, D., Suttorp, N., & Sander, L. E. (2021). Clonal expansion of CD4+CD8+ T cells in an adult patient with Mycoplasma pneumoniae-associated Erythema multiforme majus. Allergy, asthma, and clinical immunology : official journal of the Canadian Society of Allergy and Clinical Immunology, 17(1), 17. https://doi.org/10.1186/s13223-021-00520-x

41. Yalcinbayir, O., Yildiz, M., Gunduz, G. U., & Gelisken, O. (2011). *Herpes zoster ophthalmicus and lateral rectus palsy in* an elderly patient. Case reports in ophthalmology, 2(3), 333–337. https://doi.org/10.1159/000334236

42. Zeeshan, M., Fatima, S., Farooqi, J., Jabeen, K., Ahmed, A., Haq, A., Arif, M. O., et al. (2022). Reporting of mycetoma cases from skin and soft tissue biopsies over a period of ten years: A single center report and literature review from *Pakistan. PLoS Neglected Tropical D*iseases, 16. https://www.semanticscholar.org/paper/d0b4e9822b30cb9c85851dd7ef4bd1f07599a34c (accessed on 12 May 2025).

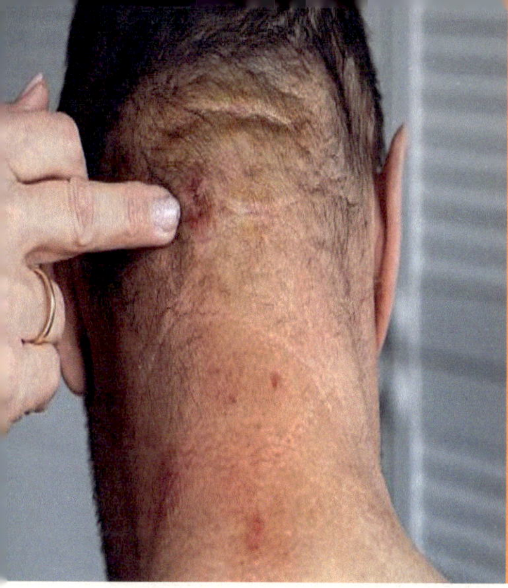

Chapter 11

URTICARIA AND DRUG REACTIONS

Contents

Introduction

Side effects from drugs continue to present a formidable challenge in day-to-day clinical practice. They manifest in dermatologic reactions in many forms that can throw a spanner into therapy by inducing uneasiness, therapy breaks, and occasionally even hospital visits. Hives or urticaria tend to strike swiftly and can become quite bad at times, quite often leading to immediate medical attention. It is essential to understand which drugs are causing these skin reactions and how they manifest in patients so that treatment can be safer and more effective. Seeing the way these reactions appear across various groups provides physicians with a lead time for recognizing risks and making changes, which is why sound reporting and analysis of drug-induced skin conditions are so vital (Packiaseeli, 2024). When it comes to children, particularly newborns, things just get even more complicated. Newborns are usually not included in most clinical trials, and news on their adverse reactions is sparse. Their bodies process drugs differently than older children and adults, so they are more susceptible to problems like hives. Although many drugs are administered in neonatal intensive care units, spontaneous reporting of such adverse events is still quite lean—leaving us with a rather incomplete picture of drug safety in this vulnerable population. Increased monitoring and targeted surveillance systems are the most important strategies to be able to better understand and deal with drug-induced allergic reactions in neonates (Pernille et al., 2024). Skin reactions due to drugs have a wide spectrum, but hives usually result in being among the most frequent presentations. Reviewing reports across different populations, physicians have observed that antibiotics, particularly fluoroquinolones and cephalosporins, often end up being the offending agents for such allergic cutaneous reactions. In general, this type of knowledge makes it apparent why it is so crucial that clinicians know which drugs are prone to causing problems and when these reactions typically happen. With this knowledge, not only do repeat episodes get avoided but also in deciding on antimicrobial therapies that reduce the risk of eliciting hives or other dermatologic conditions (Packiaseeli, 2024).

Definition of Urticaria

At other times, skin transformations will indicate an underlying immune response that is not at first evident. Hives, also called urticaria informally, are those annoying, raised bumps that come on suddenly when fluid accumulates under the skin. They tend to resolve in 24 hours without trace but they may recur at random times based on the cause and the individual's sensitivity. Essentially, this occurs due to the release of histamine and other substances by mast cells in the skin, making the blood vessels leak slightly and resulting in localized swelling. This entire phenomenon lies at the center of most allergic reactions even when a drug is involved because occasionally it is the immune system overreacting or, conversely, mast cells releasing substances on their own. Most times, it is knowing this big picture that counts, particularly when things such as other medications can trigger or exacerbate the reaction (Bellanti et al., 2015). Peeling back a little further, hives do not only describe the condition—they are also an early warning sign when a person may be struggling with a medication. For example, ubiquitous analgesics such as NSAIDs are frequently held responsible for causing hives, either by an appropriate immune-mediated mechanism or what may appear to be a pseudoallergic reaction. This combination of variables renders it significant, in general, to determine whether a reaction is part of an extended cross-sensitivity to a variety of drugs or merely a single reaction to one drug. Some patient populations, such as children with pre-existing atopic tendencies, appear to be especially susceptible to hives from NSAIDs, highlighting the necessity for a thorough, often lengthy, clinical workup and testing (Bellanti et al., 2015).

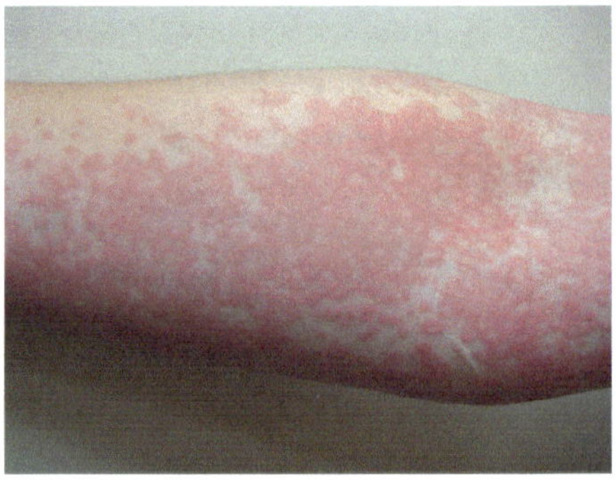

Figure 11.1. Hives on the arm.

Source: James Heilman, M.D. (2010). *Erythema Multiforme Minor on Arm.* https://upload.wikimedia.org/wikipedia/commons/thumb/6/63/EMminor2010.JPG/800px-EMminor2010.JPG.

And then there are the less common scenarios, such as when breastfeeding mothers develop hives. In these instances, changing hormones and a unique immune environment appear to be at work, indicating that not all reactions are from a traditional allergen. In such cases, the postpartum hormonal fluctuations, like a decrease in progesterone's typical soothing effect on mast cells, may be a factor in the attack. Though studies on such cases are still quite limited, such instances contribute to expanding our knowledge about urticaria by demonstrating that many factors may come into play. This knowledge encourages clinicians to scrutinize patient histories carefully when balancing the alternatives between simply alleviating symptoms and choosing whether to continue a drug treatment in the face of risks (Figure 11.1).

Overview of Drug Reactions

Adverse drug reactions usually introduce an unexpected wrench into patient care. They can manifest themselves as anything from a slight drowsiness or nausea to more alarming symptoms such as unusual liver tests or a sudden drop in blood pressure. In hives, it is particularly critical to determine how frequently these reactions occur and how they manifest themselves so treatment can be modified on the fly. Certain studies note that combining H1 antihistamines, as opposed to using one drug by itself, may be more effective and even result in fewer side effects. This concept, drug conflicts and how each patient responds to medication, simply cannot be dismissed. More often than not, if an individual does have an adverse effect, the effects usually subside when the offending drug is discontinued, which makes it so important to monitor patients closely while under treatment (Luo et al., 2024). Reactions to medications are not always obvious signs such as hives; they can cascade throughout the entire system due to how a medication operates and unique characteristics of each individual. Consider central nervous system stimulants like methylphenidate, which you typically find prescribed for attention-deficit/hyperactivity disorder—these can induce reactions that require close monitoring in clinical environments. In general, these unanticipated responses remind us that each individual may respond differently, compelling clinicians to balance benefits versus risks at all times. It also implies that doctors and pharmacists must be working together, providing patient-specific guidance, and offering insights to make better-informed decisions. Such collaboration, although it may appear loose at times, is critical in addressing the messy reality of drug interactions (Heerfordt et al., 2024). Knowing about drug reactions during hives therapy requires examining both the sunny and not-so-bright aspects of the available medications. Urticaria presents in multiple forms and patients may react in unforeseen fashions to antihistamines, so a reliance on good evidence, from randomized trials to meticulous case reports, is indispensable. Current reviews generally indicate that combination antihistamine therapies can produce benefits while maintaining side effects at acceptable levels. However, it is a good idea for clinicians to remain vigilant because although severe side effects may occur relatively infrequently, they can be fairly serious when they do. Systematically examining both a drug's effectiveness and monitoring for any adverse signs makes it much easier to make changes to treatment plans for patients with chronic hives, ultimately improving patient care as a whole (Luo et al., 2024).

Importance of Understanding the Relationship Between Urticaria and Drug Reactions

Controlling sudden drug reactions is not so much a matter of adhering to guidelines—it is a matter of understanding the relationship between a medication and a response from the skin. When hives (urticaria) appear, those brief raised areas with severe itching are an early warning that the body is not particularly pleased with a drug. Identifying these symptoms quickly is crucial, as failing to do so may allow the reaction to develop into a more serious systemic problem. There is a complicated mix of immune mechanisms and other non-immune variables in play here, which tend to make it difficult to anticipate whether or when the wheals will recur. In the majority of instances, physicians must understand the particular ways various drugs induce these reactions so that they may alter treatment regimens in the moment, providing for safety in patients and adherence to therapy (Zhu et al., 2024). NSAIDs have a strange knack for being involved in these affairs. These ubiquitous painkillers, though they exist in numerous chemical forms, all tend to block COX-1 similarly, and that commonality frequently leads to the production of hives or even angioedema. Curiously, epidemiologic studies indicate that females are more frequently affected and that significant differences in the presentation of chronic urticaria between different groups of individuals exist. Such complexity is that, in general, physicians are better off categorizing patients according to risk level. Such sorting directs them toward less risky alternatives such as selective COX-2 inhibitors or even paracetamol, which appear less likely to induce unfavorable skin reactions (Myasnikova et al., 2024). It is messy, but it goes a long way to reducing recurrence and enhancing overall therapeutic outcomes. When it comes to personalizing treatments, realizing the various safety profiles of drugs does make a large impact. Consider some antiviral drugs such as tenofovir alafenamide compared with tenofovir disoproxil fumarate—each has its own pattern of cutaneous side effects, so a close reading of the nuances is essential on prescription. This is particularly relevant in populations such as pregnant women, where an adverse drug reaction could impact not only the individual but also the baby. In all but a few cases, being aware of these fine distinctions allows clinicians to more accurately forecast and even mitigate potential skin issues. The combination of drug safety information with what is observed on a patient's skin is a good method to navigate the difficult path of urticaria and drug reactions (Zhu et al., 2024).

11.1. Types of Urticaria

Urticaria presents in a multitude of different forms, and considering how drugs could possibly trigger it, the specifics do count. Acute instances, which typically persist for fewer than six weeks, tend to occur due to recognizable triggers such as certain medications. There is also the chronic variety that persists longer than six weeks and sometimes appears to have no discernible pattern. Occasionally, you even notice subtypes like the ones caused by physical factors—pressure, cold, or heat, or autoimmune ones where the body's own antibodies interfere with mast cells, causing those maddening red welts. Identifying these differences is crucial because drug reactions can trigger any flavor of urticaria, so treatments and monitoring plans must be carefully adjusted. When drugs are responsible for hives, the scenario gets even more complicated. Sudden hypersensitivity, usually an IgE-mediated response—may result in immediate hives following drug administration. While this is happening, non-immune mechanisms also come into play; some medications, like fluoroquinolones, activate mast cells directly, increasing the complexity further (Hanan et al., 2025). These are very commonly used antibiotics in most instances and are recognized for a significant incidence of adverse reactions that at times appear to be linked to neurological or immune mechanisms. Therefore, staying focused on the particular patterns through which drug-induced urticaria manifests is important; it can quite significantly change the way we treat it. New cancer therapies, such as targeted therapies and immunotherapies, are also causing interesting challenges regarding skin-related side effects such as a wide range of hives.

These new drugs tend to produce urticaria patterns that are not quite what we would expect with conventional chemotherapy, likely due to the fact that they manipulate the immune system in some other way. Scientists, in the majority of situations, have constructed models that take into account factors such as patient age and immune cell types in addition to laboratory findings in order to better grasp how to predict these cutaneous reactions (Zhang et al., 2025). With treatments becoming increasingly varied, the precise type of urticaria must be nailed down, even if it sometimes seems a little untidy, so that every patient can be given the optimal treatment (Figure 11.2).

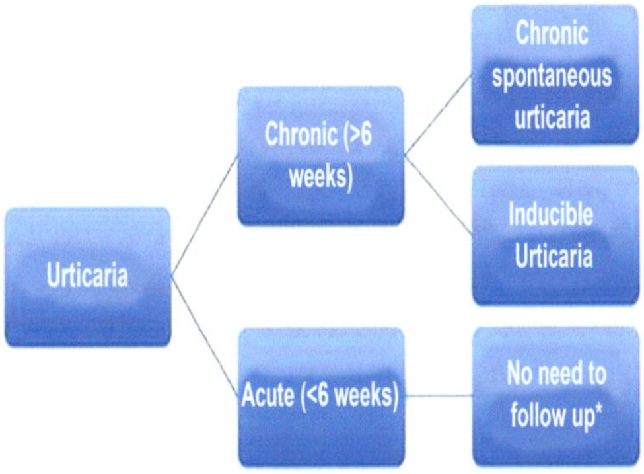

Figure 11.2. Classification of urticaria.

Source: HealthXchange.sg. (n.d.). *Classification of Urticaria,* https://www.healthxchange.sg/sites/hexassets/Assets/head-neck/classification-of-urticaria-table.jpg.

11.1.1. Acute Urticaria

Occasionally itchy, red welts suddenly erupt and complicate diagnosis—children in particular can be difficult. In clinical practice, acute hives arise rapidly, disappearing within hours but sometimes recurring over a period of days. There is a combination of reasons behind these attacks, ranging from infection and food reactions to drug reactions. Understanding what triggers these attacks is fairly significant in that it prevents future recurrences and makes patients safer. Most of the time, an antihistamine is all that is needed, but corticosteroids may be indicated when it becomes more recalcitrant. It also assists to speak with patients and their families regarding allergens and how unpredictable idiopathic situations can be; a little knowledge eases concern. These are concepts from a combination of some recent research done on children who have acute hives (Barros et al., 2024). Once drug-induced hives appear, things become somewhat more complex. A reaction appearing like common hives may on occasion indicate the issue is more systemic in nature. For example, drug reaction with eosinophilia and systemic symptoms, better known as DRESS syndrome, though rare, shows just how severe a drug-triggered allergy might become. Its progress often sees fever, a widespread rash, and even some internal organs getting involved, which means treatment has to be prompt and forceful. Even with the use of immunosuppressive techniques such as corticosteroids, certain patients will have additional problems including opportunistic infection, putting a twist in the treatment process. Finding a balance between needing to soothe the immune overdrive yet avoiding suppressing it too much is, in all honesty, a challenging task. Such cases going awry really point out how vital it is to remain very vigilant and catch complications in their early stages (Zhou et al., 2024). Considering the way immune responses, drug exposure, and individual characterestics all blend together, managing drug-induced hives is not something that one individual can do in isolation. It is well beyond simply examining a rash in diagnosis—often including careful history and laboratory studies when systemic pathology is suspected. Avoidance of the causative drug is paramount, though physicians must be prepared to intensify therapy if things deteriorate. Studies indicate that the causes of acute hives are highly varied, so individualized treatment strategies are essential in order to prevent undesirable outcomes. Combining sound patient education with regular monitoring seems to enhance overall health outcomes and minimizes complications from both regular hives as well as drug-related hives. This detailed plan, as backed by current evidence, promotes more knowledgeable decisions in actual clinical situations (Barros et al., 2024; Zhou et al., 2024) (Figure 11.3).

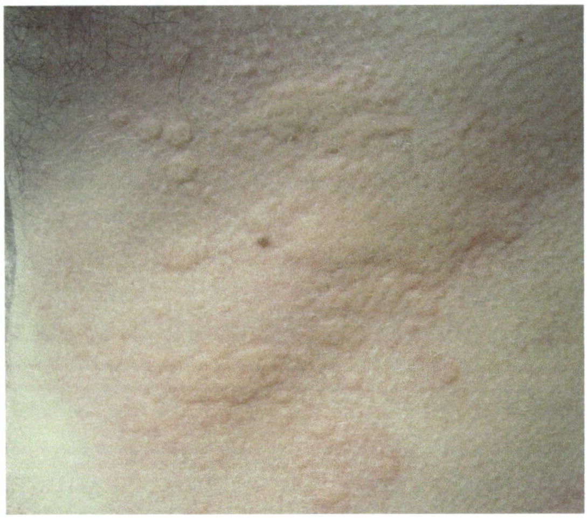

Figure 11.3. Acute urticaria.

Source: By James Heilman, MD - Own work, CC BY-SA 3.0, https://commons.wikimedia.org/w/index.php?curid=11508979

11.1.2. Chronic Urticaria

Chronic skin problems can make it quite difficult to determine a diagnosis and treatment, particularly when sudden welts and swelling begin appearing out of nowhere. Chronic urticaria, for example, persists, usually for more than six weeks, with these repeated episodes that are not always caused by something obvious. In most cases, this is not like the temporary flare of acute urticaria; it is more elusive, sometimes associated with the body's own mistakes or to reactions to medications. The issue goes well beyond mere physical distress—it disrupts general well-being and everyday routines. Determining why these attacks occur is central to selecting the proper sort of aid, and physicians are often left to unravel whether what they observe is actual chronic urticaria or perhaps a reaction to some drug. This overlap necessitates precise, occasionally uneven, clinical evaluations to maintain the symptoms at bay and avoid further attacks. Drug reactions also contribute significantly to rendering chronic urticaria a true challenge. Nonsteroidal anti-inflammatory drugs (NSAIDs) are oftentimes accused; they have the potential to induce a variety of skin responses that are not always predictable. Oftentimes There is just a general deterioration of the condition, sometimes it is just a matter of single episodes of wheals or swelling, and sometimes it is a reaction to a particular NSAID. Identifying these reactions is truly critical for making the proper treatment plan, especially since the degree to which various NSAIDs cross-react can be completely random. Normally, the treatment begins with a thorough examination of the patient's history, and even sometimes by doctors' use of oral provocation tests. The principle behind this is the elimination of exposure to the offending drug while sometimes attempting selective COX-2 inhibitors as a safer option. Notably, in some instances, aspirin desensitization procedures have proven effective, showing how the delicate balancing act of drug consumption and the body's reactions can be effectively managed (Woessner et al., 2015). When dealing with chronic urticaria in general, an expansive and individualized approach is required, one that not only calms symptoms but addresses the underlying source of the triggers. Generally speaking, the non-sedating oral antihistamines are the first choice in most patients, with good control, although there are certainly situations where they simply do not work. For those more difficult cases, newer biological agents such as omalizumab have truly revolutionized management by directly addressing IgE-mediated pathways. Despite these advances, cost and access continue to be barriers for many. Meanwhile, clinicians need to remain vigilant for any drugs that could be provoking the condition—scrutinizing a patient's existing therapy often constitutes an important step. In the end, adapting the therapy to suit each patient's individual profile generally produces improved results and, by and large, a better general quality of life (Aquilina et al., 2016) (Figure 11.4).

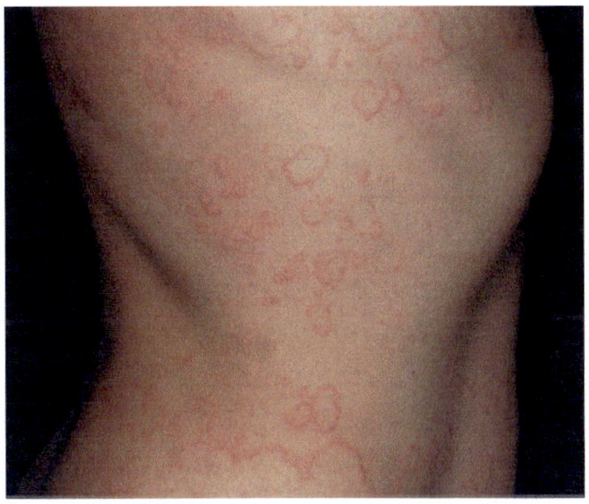

Figure 11.4. Typical presentation of chronic spontaneous urticaria.

Source: U.S. National Institutes of Health. (n.d.). *Chronic Spontaneous Urticaria*. Wikimedia Commons. https://upload.wikimedia.org/wikipedia/commons/thumb/0/0d/Chronic_spontaneous_urticaria.jpg/800px-Chronic_spontaneous_urticaria.jpg.

11.1.3. Physical Urticaria

Urticaria may appear due to a multitude of reasons, and occasionally it is the physical type that utterly shocks you. Certain inducers such as pressure, changes in temperature, sun exposure, or even slight vibration may trigger the skin to respond—mast cells cause histamine to be released immediately. This is not your typical IgE allergic response; rather, an immediate physical shock triggers the entire process, creating a distinct difference in how one feels. Activities of daily living can suddenly awaken these symptoms, disrupting quality of life significantly. A meticulous, sometimes hands-on examination with some controlled tests is instrumental in identifying physical urticaria, given that the image may get fuzzy when drug reactions intervene (Aquilina et al., 2016). This type of urticaria is typically treated according to the overall game plan for hives, but with modifications. Physicians often begin with second-generation, non-sedating H1-antihistamines since these are generally effective without many side effects. The dose is often increased in many cases — sometimes even four times the normal — when patients continue to have flare-ups. For those who nevertheless experience little relief, alternative options such as H2-antihistamines, leukotriene receptor antagonists, or even immune suppressants such as cyclosporine A enter the scene after risk-benefit balancing. This stepwise process truly highlights how critical it is to individualize care since physical triggers might persist even when the medications appear to work. Combining avoidance of triggers with appropriate medication makes up a central component of minimizing the total symptom burden (Chow, 2012). It can sometimes become even more complicated when urticaria that is physical combines with drug-induced reactions. On occasion, drugs administered to address hives, or even medications for entirely unrelated afflictions—may instead ironically push the condition along by forcing out histamine in an indiscriminate manner or modulating immune interactions. That is why it is crucial for the doctor to get to the bottom of a patient's drug history; even the slightest mistake could result in confusion between a medication-induced hump and a physical trigger, or vice versa. Because physical urticaria tends to stick around in the long term, regular follow-up and honest discussions about avoiding triggers or not forgetting to take meds become the norm. There is also been some recent hype over new biological treatments such as omalizumab for those especially resistant cases, even if, in the majority of cases, cost may be a factor. Comprehension of these shared mechanisms is crucial to achieving the proper balance when treating both drug-induced and physical types of urticaria (Chow, 2012; Aquilina et al., 2016) (Figure 11.5).

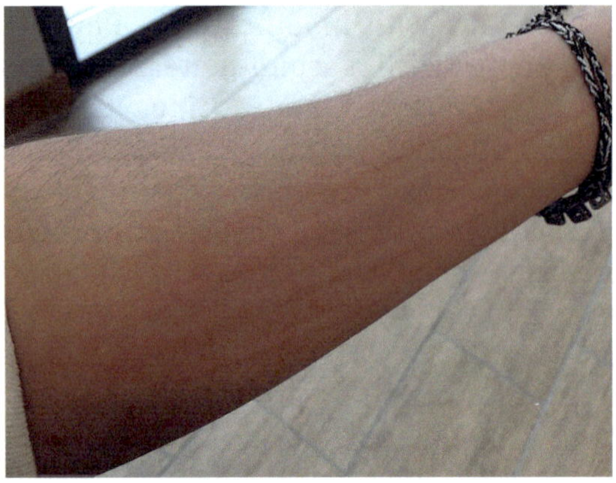

Figure 11.5. Physical urticaria, more specifically dermatographism.

Source: Daniele, B. (2019). *Physical Urticaria on Forearm*. Wikimedia Commons.

11.2. Mechanisms of Urticaria

Mast cells trigger urticaria by releasing mediators that initiate itchy, swollen bumps—those memorable wheals. They are largely responsible for whether or not the reaction is allergic, because when they degranulate, they release histamine, prostaglandins, leukotrienes, and proteases. Surprisingly, not all mast cell responses take the traditional allergic pathway. Some people exhibit symptoms of mast cell activation syndromes (MCAS) even when there are no apparent markers of mastocytosis and no visible allergen to be found. In general, these syndromes are diagnosed by seeing periodic flare-ups that correlate with quantifiable increases in such things as serum tryptase, with symptoms resolving after medication that targets mediators. This difference is pretty important for understanding drug-induced urticaria because it suggests that certain medications might trigger mast cell activity through non-IgE routes, making diagnosis and treatment a bit more challenging (Valent et al., 2012). Often, you will see that IgE is deeply involved, especially in cases linked to drug allergies. IgE molecules bind to high-affinity receptors on mast cells and basophils, so when an antigen appears, the mediator release is super-quick. This unambiguously defined pathway has directed the development of treatments such as anti-IgE monoclonal antibodies—drugs that decrease mast cell sensitivity and maintain the mediator release in check. For instance, omalizumab has proved useful in chronic spontaneous urticaria (CSU) and chronic inducible urticaria (CINDU), especially when conventional therapies simply do not work. By turning down the level of circulating IgE, the treatment breaks the allergic chain reaction, highlighting IgE's central position in drug-induced urticarial reactions despite the very specific cellular pathways differing from patient to patient (Ertaş, 2017).

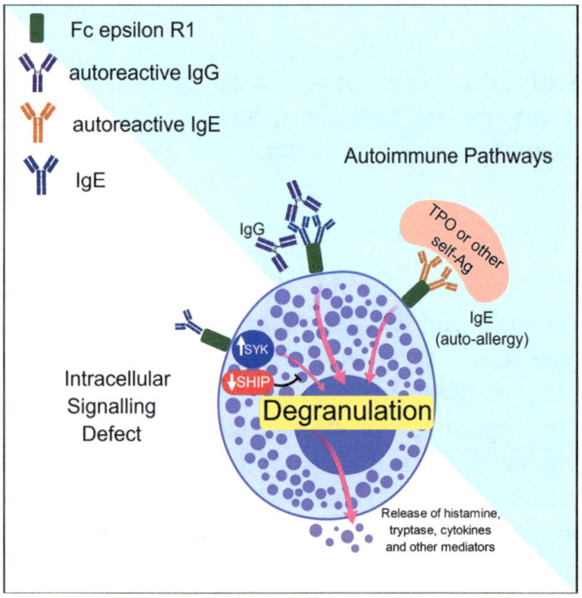

Figure 11.6. Model of the mechanisms underlying chronic urticaria.

Source: Bracken SJ, Abraham S and MacLeod AS (2019) Autoimmune Theories of Chronic Spontaneous Urticaria. Front. Immunol. 10:627. doi: 10.3389/fimmu.2019.00627

It truly does make a difference to understand the numerous ways drug reactions can trigger urticaria if we are to have improved results. In addition to the IgE pathway, certain drugs immediately induce mast cells or basophils to release their granules, or they may act on receptors without any association with IgE, releasing mediators to increase vascular permeability and inflammation. This sloppy mix of pathways makes it essential to pinpoint a definitive diagnosis and tailor treatment regimens—because aiming at one molecular pathway, such as with anti-IgE therapies, is not always the optimal solution. Further studies into precisely how mast cells become activated and release their mediators in drug-induced urticaria will assist us in untangling the numerous subtypes and refining our treatment approaches (Valent et al., 2012; Ertaş, 2017) (Figure 11.6).

11.2.1. Histamine Release and Its Effects

Allergic reactions and drug allergies initiate a series of chemical messages—histamine, in the majority of instances, is a key player. When your body is exposed to a stimulus, mast cells and basophils suddenly release their contents, releasing histamine into surrounding tissues. The surge activates alterations such as leaky, dilated vessels, which bring about the characteristic symptoms of hives—redness and swelling. You can easily observe how wheals develop and itching sets in, highlighting the quick effect of histamine. It works by bonding with H1 receptors on cell linings and nerves, only fueling inflammation and pain further. In general, understanding this process helps elucidate why some reactions to drugs create skin problems, so treatments targeting histamine pathways are truly significant (Camelo-Nunes et al., 2006). After release, histamine's impact can extend beyond the skin. For example, when it binds to H1 receptors, smooth muscles can contract, occasionally leading to bronchoconstriction and respiratory distress in affected people. Furthermore, histamine's action on sensory nerves will produce a highly severe itch—yet another hives hallmark. These responses not only contribute to patient distress but also emphasize the necessity of antihistamines in alleviating symptoms. The newer, second-generation blockers primarily act on peripheral receptors, a development that results in them usually staying away from heavy effects on the brain and typically having fewer drowsy side effects. Nevertheless, even with these developments, the general intricacy of histamine's function necessitates researchers continuing to find improved treatment strategies (Camelo-Nunes et al., 2006).

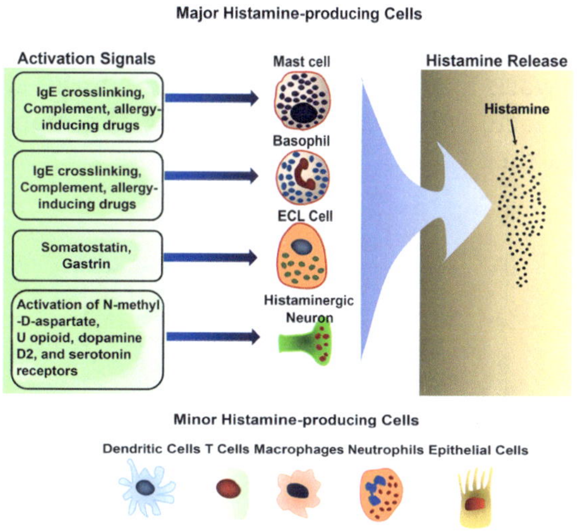

Figure 11.7. Histamine-producing cells and stimuli that trigger histamine release.

Source: Nagata, M., & Hirai, Y. (2018). *Histamine-Producing Cells and Stimuli That Trigger Histamine Release.*

Histamine's activity is seldom one-dimensional. It leaps into action during immediate allergic reactions and also appears to propel the long-term inflammation characteristic of chronic hives. New findings tend to indicate overall that histamine has the ability to modify the immune response by calling in other inflammatory cells and intensifying cytokine release, so the response could snowball after the initiating stimulus. Drug-induced hives may not be simply a simple spasm of histamine but instead an entangled dance of immune signals that histamine fuels further. As such, an even-handed clinical response, one that combines antihistamine therapy with a judicious search for causative factors, is most frequently required. In the end, a profound, if sometimes flawed, comprehension of histamine's varied functions directs clinicians to better manage allergic skin reactions (Figure 11.7).

11.2.2. Role of Mast Cells in Urticaria

Mast cells become the center of attention when urticaria hits. They reside in the skin and can respond in a split second to a combination of stimuli—be it usual allergens or even drug molecules. When all goes wrong, these cells degranulate, releasing histamine along with a whole range of other inflammation messages that relax the walls of the blood vessels and result in swelling. This response not only initiates those sudden bumps and itchiness but also sends other immune cells into the fray. More recent research has started to unravel how mast cells communicate with T cells and cytokines; for instance, embryonic-stem-cell-derived mesenchymal cells can dial back mast cell bursts by engaging TGF-β pathways, opening up new avenues for treatment (Hyun et al., 2023). Mast cells are not solely for immediate flare-ups, either. They operate a fairly sophisticated internal network that keeps them humming in the skin environment. One key player here is KIT, a stem cell factor (SCF)-activated receptor that appears nearly indispensable for the cells' maintenance. And then

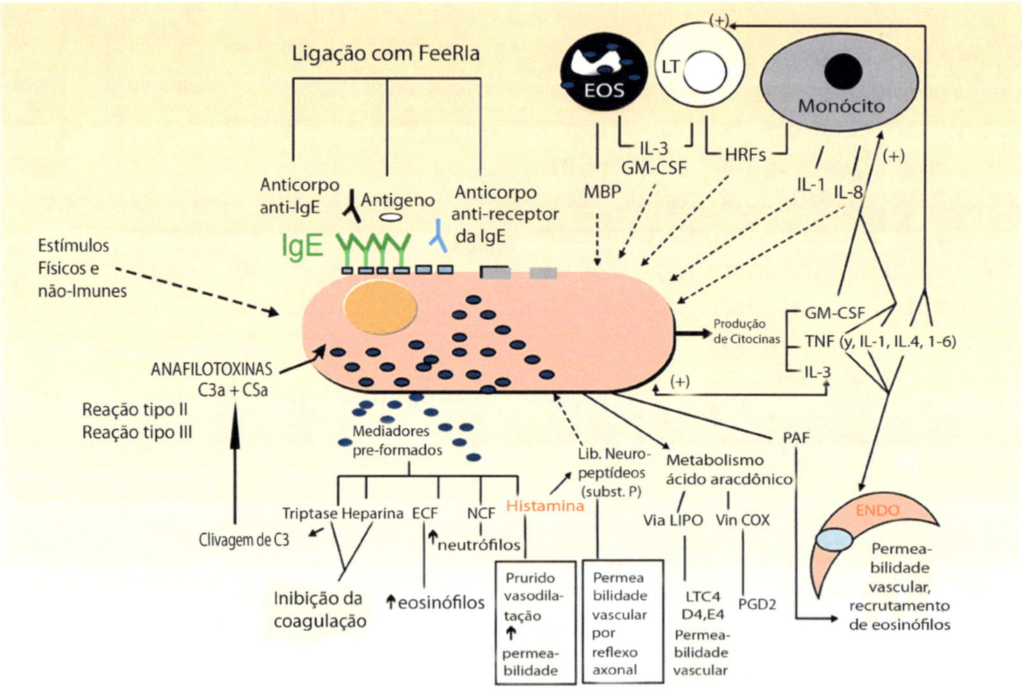

Figure 11.8. Mast cell stimulation in urticaria and subsequent events.

Source: Criado, P. R. (2015). *Mast Cell Stimulation in Urticaria and Subsequent Events*. ResearchGate.

There is the cAMP response element binding protein (CREB), which works in tandem with KIT in a kind of back-and-forth loop. And if CREB gets tripped up, KIT levels decrease, and downstream effectors such as ERK1/2, AKT, and STAT5 (all of which are crucial to cell survival and growth) lose their capacity. For the most part, CREB is not just a transcriptional regulator; it is the foundation of global mast cell well-being. Any glitching here can disrupt the skin's mast cell numerals and could even impact how severe or protracted urticaria becomes (Gürkan et al., 2023).

Occasionally the image becomes even more complicated, particularly with drug-induced urticaria. When mast cells collide with drug allergens or even tiny haptens, they secrete mediators that trigger the classical rash. At the same time, mesenchymal stem cells exhibit an immunomodulatory capability by suppressing mast cell degranulation via TGF-β, adding another complication to the tale. This interaction suggests that, through the application of targeted stem cell therapies, we could potentially mitigate the inflammation driven by mast cells sufficiently to alleviate symptoms. Mast cells, in the context of the larger immune environment, reveals exciting paths for future treatment of drug-induced urticaria, combining our understanding of cell biology with new ideas for therapy (Hyun et al., 2023) (Figure 11.8).

11.2.3. Immune System Involvement

Immune reactions play a significant role in how drug reactions sometimes are responsible for the scratchy, swollen skin we know as urticaria. When a drug or some of its metabolites are "marked" by our immune system as intruders, a complex chain of events follows – cells begin to communicate with each other in ways that pull on antibody chains and cell defenses. Mast cells and basophils rapidly enter the action, releasing histamine and other chemical messengers that ignite the characteristic red, swollen welts. T-cell activity, too, plays a role, particularly when the reaction does not appear for some time; cytokine surges here tend to bring on more swelling and even tissue injury. Not everyone reacts the same way, largely because our genes and what we are exposed to in the environment mix things up in unpredictable measures. In most cases, grasping these immune traitfeatures is key for a proper diagnosis and effective treatment – a fact that becomes even more crucial when these reactions muddle pediatric cases (Caffarelli et al., 2018). Examining how kids handle drug hypersensitivity, the scene is far from simple. Clinicians commonly rely on provocation tests, in which they reintroduce the offending drug in small amounts carefully to simulate a natural immune arousal. The tests take a glimpse of both the body's instantaneous IgE-mediated pop and delayed, T-cell dependent responses – a range that informs us better regarding immunologic memory and how reaction thresholds may differ. Today's laboratory tests can fall short at times with low sensitivity, so assembling these provocation protocols effectively means assembling a better, more informative test, even if the pieces do not always fall neatly into place (Caffarelli et al., 2018). It really is all about an entangled interaction between our genes, our environment, and how our immune systems misbehave. Genetic characterestics, such as variations that alter immune receptor functions or cytokine production—can tilt the scales toward an enhanced response, whereas common environmental exposures may set the bar for such reactions low. These confluences of influences remind us that diagnosis or treatment of a reaction is not one-size-fits-all but must be adjusted to different backgrounds. With research whittling down these complex immune hints, a brighter future for novel methods of desensitizing or modulating responses becomes increasingly possible. Targeting the specific immune pathways in the majority of instances not only might prevent undesired urticarial exacerbations but also result in improved outcomes, even for the more susceptible pediatric populations (Burns, 2019).

11.3. Common Drug-Induced Urticaria

Drug allergy is a valid concern in clinics. Hives, for instance, frequently erupt as a manifestation that something is amiss in a drug response. As a general rule, the body responds through a complicated interplay of immune messages and other mechanisms that induce a spurt of histamine and similar chemicals—this in turn introduces those fleeting bumps and some swelling. In kids in particular, beta-lactam antibiotics, non-beta-lactam antibiotics and NSAIDs are most likely to be the culprits. Because laboratory tests often fail to see the complete picture, physicians usually have to fall back on drug provocation tests (DPTs) that gradually raise doses in order to identify the culprit and find safe substitutes (Caffarelli et al., 2018). All this process, in the majority of circumstances, underscores how vital accurate testing is when it comes to drug-induced skin problems. Treating drug-induced hives can be a puzzle to solve. These reactions appear in such a varied fashion, sometimes suddenly and others persist, it is difficult to discern whether or not to attribute to a drug. That brief rash, with its itchy welts and, at times, life-threatening swelling that can impact respiration, can make a patient quite uncomfortable. In general, the first step is withdrawing the offending medication and soothing symptoms with oral antihistamines, which provide relief by binding to the histamine receptors causing the rash. For other patients, however, if antihistamines simply are not sufficient, more recently developed options such as omalizumab, albeit more expensive—have entered the mix with promising results (Aquilina et al., 2016).

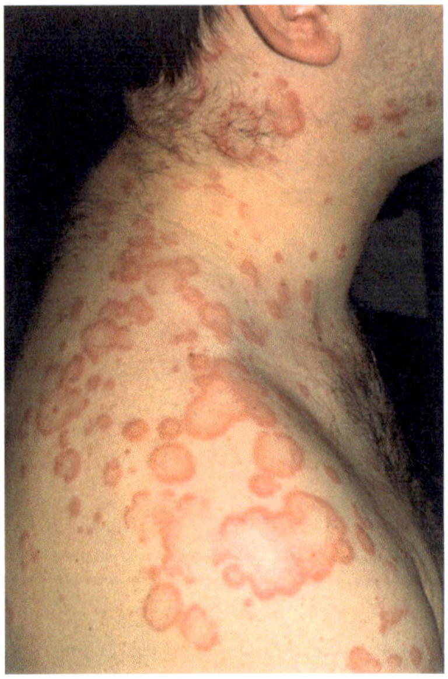

Figure 11.9. Illustration of drug-induced urticaria.

Source: Clinical Advisor. (2018). *Urticaria with widespread Wheals on Upper Body.* https://www.clinicaladvisor.com/wp-content/uploads/sites/11/2018/12/urticaria0310_wheals_90990.jpg.

More often than not, comparing all these treatments is the most effective way to gain the optimal outcome. The reality is, drug-induced hives are all over the map, so each case often demands its own mix of testing and treatment. Patient factors, like age and how severe or quickly a reaction appears—play a huge role here. Kids, for instance, generally follow stricter protocols because they are more likely to react to common drugs such as antibiotics and NSAIDs. Apart from quitting the offending drug, much of the strategy is educating patients on what drugs to steer clear of and what alternatives could work for them. Continued research into exactly how these allergies trigger has consistently refined our testing protocols and treatment approaches. This multi-faceted strategy—integrating identification, avoidance, and evidence-based treatments—operates to address both the clinical issues and daily disruptions associated with drug-induced hives (Aquilina et al., 2016; Caffarelli et al., 2018) (Figure 11.9).

11.3.1. Antibiotics and Their Association with Urticaria

Drug allergic reactions are sometimes simply unpredictable. A patient may present with hives on some occasions, and it is difficult to determine precisely why. These rashes are often not the result of the chemicals acting on the drugs but of the immune system reacting to them—leaving clinicians to deal with a tricky problem. Frequently, antibiotics are involved, with beta-lactam drugs strangely enough being the most common perpetrators. The body might respond in an instant, creating tiny, itchy welts that complicate the decision to treat, especially when a patient has to continue taking antimicrobial drugs. For the majority of instances, understanding how these immune reactions trigger hives is paramount for physicians as they weigh the advantages of a medication and the risk of hypersensitivity (De Castro et al., 2018). Results from a number of studies in general target antibiotics as major culprits of adverse skin reactions. Out of one study involving more than 300 patients exhibiting drug-induced skin conditions, close to 60% ultimately developed sudden hives—preceded by fixed eruptions and maculopapular rashes. These figures, in most situations, vividly illustrate the clinical burden that hives caused by antibiotics bear. Interestingly, there is a remarkable pattern—women are more impacted, suggesting that intrinsic biological mechanisms could be at work here. Such findings are extremely important for informing individualized treatment regimens and optimizing patient outcomes in the case of hives induced by antibiotics (Farshchian et al., 2015). Confronting challenges in the diagnosis and treatment of hives induced by antibiotics requires a rather wide-ranging approach, one that merges learning from genetics and immunology research. While we have made some strides in tracing genetic clues linked to these allergies, plenty of underlying mechanisms still escape a clear explanation, which in most instances complicates efforts to predict or prevent a reaction. And because these allergic reactions are not based on the quantity of a drug administered, physicians usually have to rely on thorough patient histories, careful monitoring of symptoms, and on occasion even skin tests to differentiate between real allergic reactions and the others. Marrying new molecular knowledge with some old-fashioned clinical acumen can, for the most part, hone diagnoses, steer safer prescribing, and reduce nasty allergic reactions, ultimately helping to ensure patients remain safe when they need their antibiotics (De Castro et al., 2018).

11.3.2. Non-Steroidal Anti-Inflammatory Drugs (NSAIDs)

Drug-induced urticaria is not cut and dried; it makes us consider drugs that are widely used. Consider NSAIDs, for instance; these are frequently the offending agents in allergic skin manifestations. They exert their effects by inhibiting cyclooxygenase enzymes, which reduce prostaglandin synthesis and also incorporate anti-inflammatory, analgesic, and antipyretic advantages. But ironically, that same mechanism may also evoke hypersensitivity in certain individuals, occasionally provoking acute hives or even exacerbating established spontaneous urticaria. Adjustments in how arachidonic acid is processed also appear to have a role, disturbing the natural equilibrium of inflammatory mediators, which then pushes mast cells into spilling out histamine. Grasping this puzzle-like combination of reasons is relatively critical for clinicians, particularly as the resultant immune responses are not very clear and tend to blur definitions when it comes to diagnosis and treatment. Wider concerns regarding drug safety also remind us that NSAIDs do not act the same on all people. Genetic characterestics are involved here—pharmacogenetics steps in when determining why some individuals develop side effects such as hives. For example, small variations in enzymes such as CYP2C9 can fine-tune the metabolism of drugs such as ibuprofen and celecoxib, causing variations in blood levels and potentially increasing the risk for an urticarial reaction. On top of that, interactions with other transport proteins and metabolic enzymes introduce another level of unpredictability.

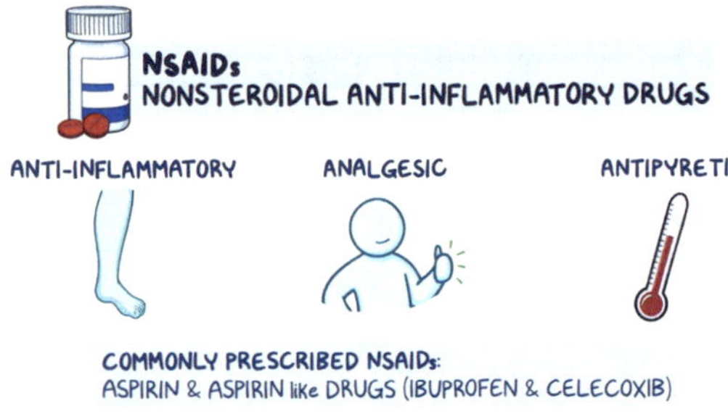

Figure 11.10. Non-steroidal anti-inflammatory drugs (NSAIDs).

Source: Osmosis. (n.d.). *NSAIDs – Nonsteroidal Anti-Inflammatory Drugs: Effects and Examples.* https://www.osmosis.org/_next/image?url=https%3A%2F%2Fd16qt3wv6xm098.cloudfront.net%2FiYLvKJHST8GSLtxF3ToTeGQ8Rnm76IJG%2F_.jpg&w=3840&q=75

Typically, stronger studies are required to disentangle these interactions and identify safer use of NSAIDs in patients at risk for skin reactions (Zobdeh et al., 2022). In the meantime, while earlier concerns suggested that NSAIDs could exacerbate some infections or inflammatory issues, recent comprehensive reviews have demonstrated that these medications do not necessarily drive patients into serious systemic conditions. Observational evidence even indicates that when NSAIDs are taken during episodes of inflammation, it does not necessarily mean a worse fate or an increased number of hives. This more recent evidence tips its hat towards recent clinical guidelines, supporting the use of NSAIDs when necessary—of course, with careful monitoring of those who are at risk. This more distinct image aids physicians in prescribing these drugs more assuredly, reserving them as an asset in therapy while remaining vigilant to potential urticarial side effects (Kushner et al., 2022) (Figure 11.10).

11.3.3. Opioids and Their Potential Reactions

Controlling pain with opioids always raises difficult questions since medications have so many different responses. Everybody knows these analgesics are prescribed widely for pain management, but sometimes they cause undesirable effects such as hives. Hives, in contrast with common side effects, appear due to the immune system of the body, and that can complicate the entire course of treatment. It is not always obvious; a response can just appear to be a non-immune histamine release or some indistinct reaction. Determining whether it is an allergy has much to do with investigating the history of a patient and employing one's clinical intuition, as the symptoms are often indistinguishable from other drug sensitivities. In situations where opioids are pretty much a must-have, telling apart a real allergic reaction from ordinary side effects becomes key to keeping patients safe without cutting off effective drugs.

Things get even murkier when you consider that many opioid allergies are based on what patients remember, which is not always spot on. Patients will often remember these reactions vaguely or incompletely, so it is difficult to pinpoint whether an immune reaction underlies the hives. A few hospital studies have suggested that much of what has been reported as allergies are probably not supported by solid data one would think necessary for hypersensitivity—it may simply be side effects or even simply unrelated skin problems. This type of confusion can pressure physicians into skipping opioids that do work and requiring them to select lesser substitutes that could have larger risks. Prescribers and pharmacists, in the majority of instances, must take more time to collect thorough allergy histories and verify these statements using clinical judgment and additional testing so that pain management does not unnecessarily rule out opioids (Grant, 2015).

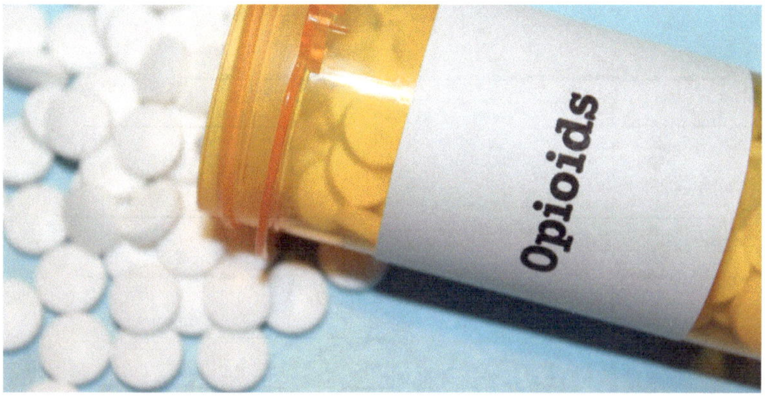

Source: Oasis Rehab. (2024). *Opioid Medication Bottle with Spilled Tablets.* https://cdn.rehabfiles.com/sites/oasisrehab/wp-content/uploads/2024/10/OR-opioid-addiction%20%281%29.svg.

When patients present with hives following exposure to opioids, having a unit that includes the allergy specialists can make a big difference. The procedure tends to require tests, occasionally *in vitro*, occasionally even controlled oral challenges, to pin down just what is occurring. Drug allergy is usually diagnosed firmly only when there is clear evidence of an immune response, distinguishing it from reactions due to non-immune mechanisms.

This type of clarity assists in guiding the decision to whether a patient should not take the drug at all, attempt a desensitization method, or have other treatment options in place. Although anesthesiologists and surgeons encounter these problems more frequently in the perioperative setting, consultation with allergists can enhance the precision of differentiating opioid-induced hives from other hypersensitive reactions, which overall contributes to enhanced patient safety and treatment results (Vicovan et al., 2019).

11.4. Diagnosis of Drug-Induced Urticaria

Drug-induced urticaria is diagnosed less with ticking off a checklist of symptoms and more with having to combine a good patient history with targeted tests. For example, recording when skin reactions strike following drug use and marking any previous instances of hypersensitivity is important. More often than not, this sort of meticulous history suggests something is amiss—maybe with drugs such as NSAIDs—but in most situations, it is not with a history alone. Confirmatory testing turns out to be important because it can be rather difficult to separate out a drug reaction from other skin conditions or even idiopathic rashes. Indeed, identifying the various flavors of NSAID-related reactions—be it NSAID-exacerbated cutaneous disease, the more typical urticaria/angioedema cases (NIUA), or even a reaction simply related to one particular drug, a informs both diagnosis and what follows (Woessner et al., 2015).

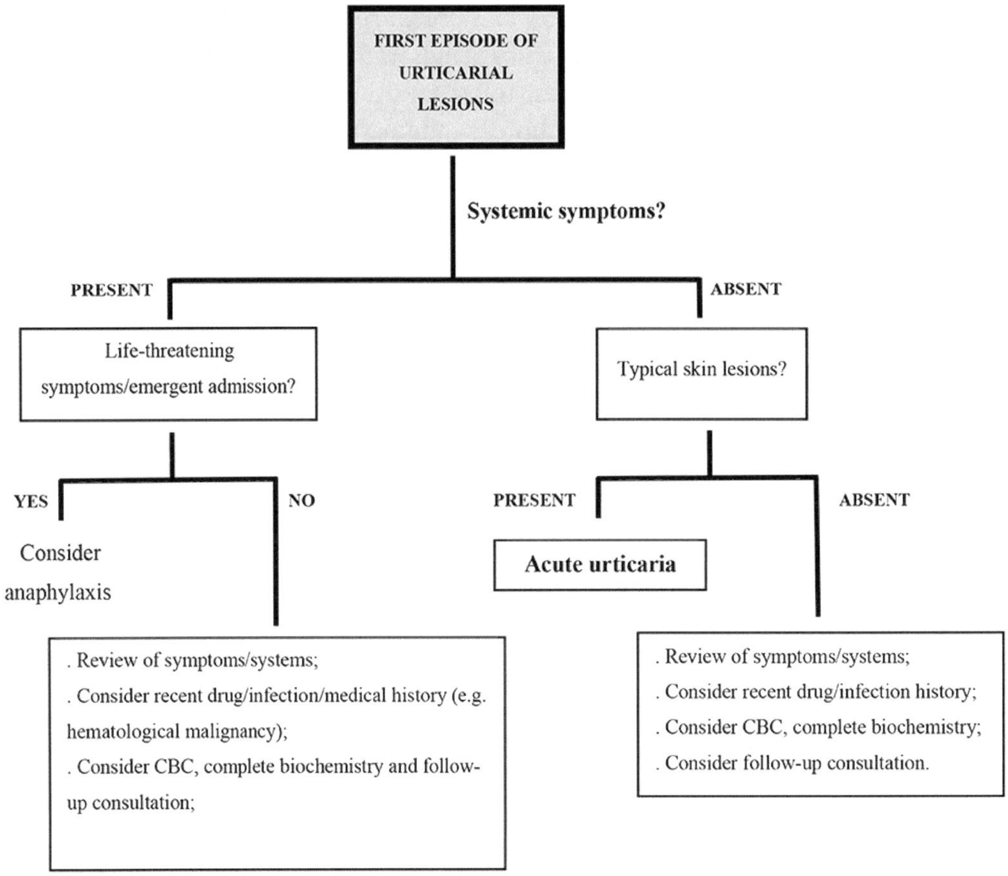

Figure 11.11. Recommended diagnosis algorithm for urticaria.

Source: Matos AL, Figueiredo C and Gonçalo M (2022) Differential Diagnosis of Urticarial Lesions. Front. Allergy 3:808543. doi: 10.3389/falgy.2022.808543

Lab tests for these reactions have not been entirely conclusive, particularly in children. In general, the gold standard is still the DPT, with the offending drug administered in gradually increasing doses under close conditions with a view to establishing the association and assessing drug tolerance.

This technique is all the more necessary in children and adolescents who tend to react to familiar offenders such as beta-lactam antibiotics and NSAIDs. DPT protocols will change depending on the specific pharmacology of each drug and the rate at which a reaction appears, so the testing is typically very individualized to make it safe and diagnostically beneficial. Pediatric allergy guidelines, for instance, emphasize careful watching during these tests and remind us that DPT test results contribute significantly to subsequent clinical decisions (Caffarelli et al., 2018).

Despite the DPT being a definitive measure, it is not risk-free, particularly for individuals with a history of severe or even life-threatening reactions. Practitioners have to weigh the benefits against the potential risks before they decide to go ahead. If an oral challenge simply is not safe to attempt, alternative approaches such as skin testing or *in vitro* assays may be employed, but their sensitivity and specificity can differ quite significantly.

It is also useful to know how cross-reactivity occurs between similar drugs; for instance, patients with NIUA will usually react to multiple NSAIDs, and hence selective cyclooxygenase-2 inhibitors are a frequently used safer alternative. Clinical presentation plus results from provocation testing and a clear understanding of drug pharmacology appear to be the most subtle approach for the optimal benefit of the patient (Woessner et al., 2015) (Figure 11.11).

11.4.1. Clinical History and Patient Interviews

Discovering if a person's response is urticaria or merely an effect of a drug depends on truly discussing with the patient. Physicians usually hear most regarding the case while inquiring about when and how it initially began. Taking a precise conversation regarding those moments can clarify whether a problem is an actual allergic reaction or merely a non-immunological reaction. Omitting or missing out on information in these consultations can result in patients being inappropriately labeled as allergic, thus potentially restricting their treatment unnecessarily. A thesis (Grant, 2015) mentioned that few of the drug reaction reports gave a description of symptoms that match a true allergy, so it is evident that obtaining a good patient history is important in assessing urticaria associated with drug use—it provides a background for additional testing and planning. Systematic patient interviews indeed enhance the validity of the histories physicians use for drug-induced urticaria and other adverse reactions. By asking sharp questions regarding when the issue arose, how bad it was, and precisely what occurred, healthcare professionals can more accurately determine whether an allergic process is occurring. In general, what patients give as an allergy could simply be common side effects and not an immune reaction at all, and this subtlety tends to get lost unless questioned. Some of the pharmacovigilance work has found that these self-reports can tend to be quite subjective or imprecise (Grant, 2015). In effect, these discussions serve to confirm or lay to rest the possibility of a drug allergy and avoid unnecessarily avoiding medicines that might be safe. Beyond merely pinning down allergies, simply hearing a patient out can capture and deal with all manner of bad drug reactions. Careful analyses of what occurs during a reaction tend to reveal patterns, for example, with drug classes like NSAIDs or antibiotics, which are themselves known to cause skin problems. For example, an observational study of the treatments for blood pressure revealed differing rates of adverse reaction by drug class, which implies that treatments may have to be tailored depending on patients' risk factors and histories. The same principle holds for urticaria patients; a properly documented patient history not only directs an accurate diagnosis but also influences risk determinations and individualized treatment protocols. A detailed patient history obtained through open discussions provides the basis for improved drug-induced urticaria management.

11.4.2. Skin Tests and Their Relevance

Identifying what triggers drug-induced urticaria truly does matter if we are working towards successful treatment and prevention of future reactions. Skin tests are helpful by allowing physicians to safely induce or identify these sensitivity attacks under medical control. They do this by exposing the skin to the actual drug or components, so you can tell whether the body's immune messages, such as those suggesting an allergy,are appearing. This approach provides tangible hints, distinguishing immune-mediated reactions from those that are not, and encourages clinicians to choose safer replacement drugs. Naturally, the accuracy of the tests does vary; it can change depending on the drug as well as the type of urticaria, which does tend to require standard practice and a little added precaution when interpreting to avoid misdiagnoses or unnecessary avoidance. Drug skin testing itself is not a cut-and-dry procedure; it is more of a combination of various methods—prick tests, intradermal tests, and patch tests—each directed at various types of allergies and clinical situations. By standard recommendation, it is better to conduct these tests several weeks after the eruption in the skin has fully resolved so that false negatives do not creep in and the patient remains safe. The usual practice involves employing different concentrations of the suspected drug, either pure or in commercially available strengths, and then testing the reaction of the skin immediately and after a lapse.

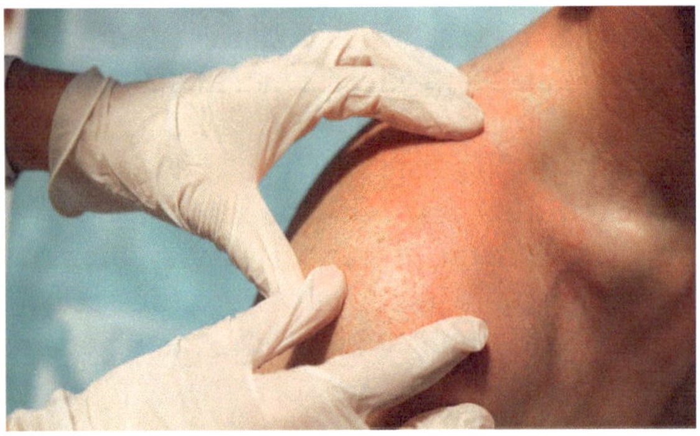

Figure 11.12. Skin test for drug-induced urticaria.

Source: Healthgrades. (n.d.). *Close-up of a Shoulder Rash Being Examined by a Healthcare Professional.* https://www.grxstatic.com/4f3rgqwzdznj/18uwruYkfW9LLF2pYvpTJO/4ca55097f0ba97970b37cb90d9aaa176/closeup_man_shoulder_rash_1327181307.jpg?format=pjpg&auto=webp&width=704.

In urticaria, sequential prick tests with modification of dose are particularly expensive, whereas patch tests reveal slower, delayed sensitivity, particularly if there is eczema or evidence of contact urticaria present. This judicious, step-by-step procedure truly enhances diagnostic precision and ultimately facilitates individualized patient care based on comprehensive clinical histories and reflective drug immutability assessments (Barbaud et al., 2001). Skin tests are also invaluable when it comes to separating contact urticaria, a type of localized response that begins when the skin or mucosal surfaces come directly into contact with topical medications or excipients.

This condition is unpredictable, and you may just see a small wheal or bump one time, but then the next time it could build up to angioedema or even anaphylaxis. The immune mechanisms involved may be IgE-mediated, or they could be non-immune pathways, so an extensive skin test analysis is usually required to truly identify the culprit. This is particularly crucial in the workplace or with frequent mucosal exposure, as it can both prevent chronic conditions or more serious allergic attacks. It is generally in most instances that knowing and applying skin tests properly sets the foundation for not just a proper diagnosis but for prudent measures in avoidance and risk management, keeping severe reactions at bay (Gameiro et al., 2016) (Figure 11.12).

11.4.3. Differential Diagnosis Considerations

Accurate diagnosis is key to hives caused by drug reactions. Several conditions can present similarly, so physicians have to get down to specifics, such as exactly how soon after taking a medication the symptoms occurred. For instance, consider NSAIDs like ibuprofen; in most instances, an immediate allergic reaction appears all at once in the form of hives and may even be accompanied by swelling or, in the most severe cases, anaphylaxis. It is crucial to nail down if these signs are an isolated problem or part of a larger landscape. Reactions to ibuprofen can be messy, as at times the reaction is a particular immune reaction and at others it is more of a non-immunological cross-reaction; this subtlety guides treatment decisions well (Blanca-Lopez et al., 2024). A good history—inquiring about previous exposure and tolerance, and testing for reactions to even chemically distinct NSAIDs—can tip clinicians off regarding cross-reactivity dangers and determine whether the drug ought to be discontinued in the future. Occasionally, however, it is not the drug that is the issue. Clinicians also need to consider blood disorders such as mastocytosis, a clonal disorder of mast cells that can simulate drug reactions by producing flushing, pruritus, and hives secondary to an accumulation of mediators. As a general rule, mastocytosis patients may experience reactions that are precipitated by a particular event, as well as spontaneous allergic events; triggers may be an insect sting (e.g., from Hymenoptera) or even medications such as antibiotics or NSAIDs. The true test is distinguishing between whether the skin reactions are from mast cell activation or indeed an allergy to drugs—misdiagnosing this can result in unnecessarily eliminating beneficial medications. Clinical history, testing in the lab, and sometimes even biopsy enter into the picture here, assisting in the tailoring of the management so that symptoms are kept at bay without too much collateral damage (Giannetti et al., 2024). A strong understanding of mastocytosis is crucial when compiling the complete picture of chronic or recurring hives. There are also causes not drug-related that can confuse the diagnosis. Occasionally, viral diseases, autoimmune conditions, or even so-called idiopathic hives present in a manner that appears very much like drug-induced reactions, and there is a danger of depending on timing only. In the majority of instances, DPTs and skin tests can resolve uncertainty, particularly when history is not clear-cut or when multiple drugs have been used. Ibuprofen, for example, frequently appears in these situations due to common usage and the broad range of reactions it can cause (Blanca-Lopez et al., 2024). By piecing together data from clinical examinations, laboratory tests, and occasionally even histopathological analysis, doctors can improve distinguishing drug-induced hives from those of other etiologies. This cautious and sometimes imprecise strategy minimizes misdiagnosis and leads the way to safer, more effective therapy as a whole.

11.5. Treatment Options

Treating drug-triggered hives often puts doctors in a bind—they must tackle the primary illness while keeping the allergic flare-ups in check. If the go-to medicine starts causing reactions like urticaria, the first step is typically to just stop it. But sometimes, alternatives are not available, especially when you are dealing with a life-saving drug—so protocols like drug desensitization step in. For most situations, the strategy involves gradually reintroducing the drug in increasing doses to allow the body to adapt without setting off the fuse for an enormous allergic reaction. This is especially handy when life-saving therapies, such as GLP-1 receptor agonists for type 2 diabetes, have already demonstrated a background of hypersensitivity with no space for alternatives. Current research generally indicates that these increasing dose protocols allow the patients to maintain necessary treatments even after an initial reaction (Yeğit et al., 2023). Apart from desensitization, alleviating the physical symptoms then takes center stage in controlling these allergic attacks. Antihistamines, which are H1 receptor blockers, are generally the primary weapon in soothing the itch and inflammation; occasionally, a brief course of corticosteroids is prescribed if the symptoms are persistent or particularly obstinate. Remember, however, that these medications primarily just even out the symptoms without concerning the immune system's global sensitivity to the medication. When patients respond to drugs essential to their treatment, such as iron chelators in hemochromatosis, most clinicians have adopted desensitization protocols with encouraging, though not flawless, outcomes. Rapid escalation of dose, for example, has even enabled continuation of deferasirox therapy in the face of prior episodes of hives and angioedema (Hinojosa et al., 2023). Another vital component is ongoing patient monitoring and education. Immediately following a desensitization procedure, patients must be closely monitored for any delayed flare or recurrence of hives, sometimes necessitating adjustments in the treatment regimen. An interdisciplinary team of allergists, dermatologists, and other prescribing physicians will usually be able to customize the entire approach to an individual's situation. For the most part, if patients can learn to identify early signs of hypersensitivity, early interventions can keep things from going awry into full-blown complications such as anaphylaxis. As these desensitization techniques change, their incorporation into routine care may redefine the management of drug reactions, particularly among individuals with limited other choices, and allow treatments to continue while, on the whole, minimizing side effects and ensuring patient safety (Hinojosa et al., 2023; Yeğit et al., 2023).

11.5.1. Antihistamines and Their Effectiveness

Management of urticaria, particularly when medication initiates it, typically comes down to getting clever with antihistamines. They act by inhibiting those H1 receptors – yes, the ones driving the itch and the characteristic bumps – and that makes a big difference in relieving the symptoms. The majority of clinical recommendations refer to second-generation H1 blockers, which, in general, are safer and less likely to make you drowsy than the older varieties. Occasionally, when the normal dose is not quite getting the job done, increasing the dose to somewhere around four times may facilitate things. Naturally, raising the dose is not something done on a whim; it requires looking closely at how effective it is compared to any potential side effects, emphasizing that each instance of urticaria is unique (Chow, 2012). When the usual routine and even quadrupled dosing of second-generation H1 antihistamines leaves a patient hanging, physicians may try shaking things up with additional therapy. They can throw in some H2 blockers, add a leukotriene receptor antagonist, or even introduce immunosuppressants such as cyclosporine A. These added extras target other areas in the inflammatory process that may be responsible for chronic urticaria, providing a multi-pronged approach. Even so, the choice of a second-line treatment is balancing benefits, expenses, and any undesirable reactions – it is not necessarily so black and white as it first appears, but it does cope with the erratic manner that drug reactions can present in urticaria (Chow, 2012). International and US guidelines largely concur in one respect: second-generation H1 antihistamines are at the center of the care of chronic urticaria.

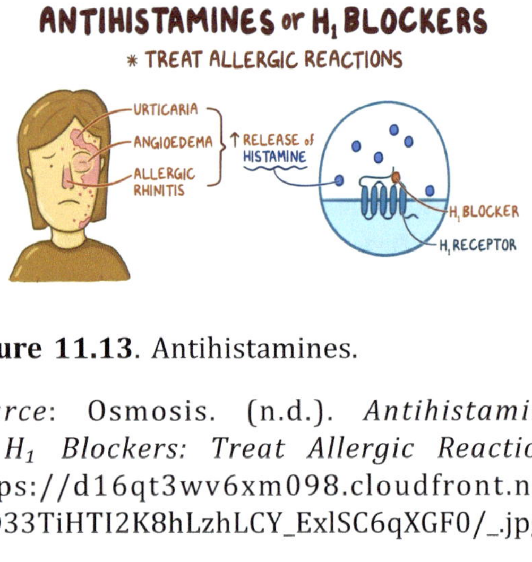

Figure 11.13. Antihistamines.

Source: Osmosis. (n.d.). *Antihistamines or H_1 Blockers: Treat Allergic Reactions.* https://d16qt3wv6xm098.cloudfront.net/QtD33TiHTI2K8hLzhLCY_ExlSC6qXGF0/_.jpg.

Most patients who visit specialists have attempted antihistamines first, so in a way it confirms their central part. Although the diagnostics and tests may vary from physician to physician, incrementing the treatment step by step is a widespread practice that could make symptoms subside and even reduce expenses. For most, adherence to these guidelines not only enhances care but also makes certain that any other therapies are implemented at the appropriate time. Briefly stated, knowledge of how these antihistamines function within this blended paradigm is crucial for clinicians managing drug-induced urticaria (Figure 11.13).

11.5.2. Corticosteroids for Severe Cases

Recognizing skin reactions is not always straightforward. Sometimes, a quick look at a patient's skin might hide the fact that what seems like typical hives can be another issue entirely. Acute hives can oddly resemble conditions like erythema multiforme or even urticarial vasculitis – a twist that shows up even more in kids, whose skin often behaves unpredictably. A solid check-up, which digs into a detailed history and a thorough physical exam, helps decide exactly which tests to run and what treatment steps to take. Getting this right means that severe cases, especially those tied to drug reactions, get prompt care (even if that care sometimes involves systemic corticosteroids to quell strong inflammation (Guerrier et al., 2011). Everyone knows corticosteroids are champion inflammation fighters, yet they can sometimes throw a curveball. It sounds ironic, but there are recorded cases where these drugs, especially forms charged with a succinate group—spark immediate allergic reactions. In these rare, tricky moments, doctors end up relying on a mix of skin tests, basophil activation checks, and carefully observed challenge trials to figure out if the medicine is, in fact, causing harm. Figuring out which corticosteroid alternatives are safe is a must for clinicians trying to ease severe hives or drug-related rashes without inadvertently worsening the allergy (Walker et al., 2011). Balancing treatment benefits against potential side effects means that corticosteroid use needs to be fine-tuned for each patient. When extensive skin involvement or widespread symptoms push the need for systemic treatment, doctors must also weigh the risk of an allergic response to these meds. Sometimes, a little extra testing to check if a patient can manage a nonsuccinylated option can preserve the desired anti-inflammatory effect without upping the allergy odds. At the end of the day, keeping a close, sometimes even imperfect, watch over patient reactions is key to moving forward safely – a reminder of just how nuanced the use of these treatments can be (Walker et al., 2011).

11.5.3. Avoidance Strategies for Known Triggers

Treating hives due to drug reactions simply means finding out what is triggering it. If a person is left with an allergic flare or an episode of urticaria, they usually require a comprehensive allergy workup to identify the offending agent. Once you know the offending agent, the best course of action is to avoid it. This may involve taking a close, hard eye on the drug list and history of a patient to eliminate the culprit drugs, and it tends to include discussing how some classes of drugs may have similar trigger properties.

Consider, for example, certain antibiotics such as penicillins or even nonsteroidal anti-inflammatory drugs; these tend to trigger these reactions, so alternate therapies often come into play. It also assists in reminding patients how to read labels and identify sneaky allergens masked in over-the-counter medications or supplements. The incorporation of a specialist, as well as a care plan that is truly tailored to the person, can increase the extent to which someone adheres to avoiding triggers, ultimately reducing flare-ups and overall quality of life (Burks et al., 2011). It is not just the pills, either; daily environments and physical conditions can trigger or aggravate urticaria, too. Many people with chronic hives report being more sensitive to rapid changes in temperature, pressure, or even stress, and these can combine with drug reactions to make an issue. That is why it is reasonable to address both the medications and these external forces. They may be instructed to avoid certain physical stimuli, maintain soft skin, and come up with ways to relax—perhaps a little exercise, possibly some casual psychological counseling. Oftentimes, additional complicating factors such as some kind of minor infection or other illness may exacerbate the reactions, so routine examinations and rapid treatment of any new disease become very critical. This wide-ranging avoidance strategy reduces the incidence of symptom flares, ultimately that minimizes the necessity for additional medication and more effectively maintains the disease under control (Banerji et al., 2011). Perhaps most important is assembling an action plan that is specifically designed for the patient, one that increases sensitivity, encompasses an emergency plan, and involves constant medical support. Individuals who have experienced severe hives or even anaphylaxis are usually provided with epinephrine auto-injectors in case of sudden exposure to any trigger, reminding us that speed is essential in halting a hazardous reaction in its tracks (Burks et al., 2011).

Being in regular, open communication with physicians, either primary care providers or specialists in allergy, assists everyone in maintaining the avoidance plan up-to-date as new information is revealed. And in those long-standing instances where it is all but impossible to avoid each and every trigger, supplementing with some preventive therapies can keep the symptoms in control. Regularly monitoring what specifically triggers the reactions over time allows for avoidance plans to remain flexible and effective, highlighting how drug-related problems and urticaria really are an evolving, ongoing process (Banerji et al., 2011).

11.6. Prevention Strategies

Prevention of drug reaction hives begins with truly knowing the patient's history and what could place them at risk. Even before they write out any prescription, doctors have to thoroughly examine previous drug allergies and sometimes select alternative meds so that the possibility of a negative reaction is minimized. Patients are encouraged—nearly as if a reminder, is asked to inform their care providers at the first sign of rash or discomfort, as early detection of these symptoms can reduce both the severity and subsequent complications of such drug reactions. Individualizing these prevention strategies for each individual by tracking their age, health history, and even where they reside is consistent with today's emphasis on tailored care. Maintaining accurate records and freely discussing with the healthcare team a patient's allergy status continues to be an essential process in preventing hives and other problems from surfacing (Guntapalle et al., 2025). These approaches together create a more secure treatment area that supports patient safety. In addition to examining every case on its own, there is an entire system operating—pharmacovigilance, which provides an extra layer of safety in preventing severe allergic reactions such as hives. National databases and more ad-hoc reporting networks strive to identify dangerous drugs and susceptible populations ahead of time, allowing healthcare professionals to act before matters become bad. Information usually indicates that characteristics like being older, male, having a history of drug allergies, or even residing in specific locations will usually intensify the severity of the reaction (Sittiphan et al., 2025). Leveraging this information with the use of technology such as electronic prescribing and risk ranking technologies, clinicians can adjust medication schedules in advance. Regular monitoring also pushes guidelines into even better form, steering the decision away from drugs that are more likely to induce allergies. In most instances, combining these findings into routine practice increases the overall protection against drug-induced hives. It is not all on one person's shoulders managing these risks proves to be a team effort between physicians, drugstore pharmacists and, naturally, the patients themselves. Education sessions for health professionals serve to emphasize the do's and do nots of how exposure to drugs could result in hives, making it simpler to identify the initial warning signs and brainstorm a speedy solution. In the meantime, good, straightforward safety information provided to patients tends to keep them adhering to treatments and reporting something does not feel right to someone. Pharmacists, who review patients' med lists on a regular basis, can catch potential interactions, or even the occasions where one medication could have a bad reaction to another, and recommend alternatives that seem safer. Numerous centers now even require allergy tests in instances classified as high risk, along with judicious dose adjustments and frequent check-ups, all emphasizing the need for on-going risk management. Individuals, as a group, are thus issued a series of occasional meandering but functional steps toward the creation of a sort of general framework to reduce both how frequently and how severely drug-induced hives appear, ultimately leading to greater patient outcomes and a safer standard of care (Guntapalle et al., 2025; Sittiphan et al., 2025).

11.6.1. Patient Education on Drug Allergies

Patient education is key to successfully managing drug allergies. Rather than adhering to a rigid checklist, sound counsel reduces the likelihood of unwanted reactions. If individuals are taught about the dangers associated with particular drugs, such as NSAIDs, which occasionally cause hives—they can identify early warning signs better and notify medical personnel promptly, which in the majority of instances leads to prompt treatment and decreases major flare-ups. Tailored counseling—in which a medical practitioner not only describes why adhering to the drug regimen is important but also what could occur if an allergy is left untreated—frequently enhances a patient's adherence to therapy, particularly in the case of chronic diseases that involve prolonged and complex regimens (Kaur et al., 2025). A properly managed debate on drug allergies does not only reduce the risks; it also opens doors for improved outcomes. Educating patients regarding the complicated nature of drug hypersensitivity is not an easy job. The immune system tends to respond unpredictably, and the triggers are quite diverse. Take NSAIDs, for instance: they induce a variety of responses, sometimes selective, sometimes cross-intolerant. Patients must understand these subtleties so they do not unwittingly take a medication that might make their condition worse. Because accurate tests for drug-induced hives are routinely questionable, or sometimes even unavailable—the emphasis must fall, instead, on meticulous history-taking and vigilant symptom observation. In the majority of scenarios, encouraging patients to report any suspicious signs aids healthcare professionals determine the proper kind of reaction and adjust therapy accordingly (Miniello et al., 2023). Ultimately, the discussion needs to reach beyond mere awareness, leading patients to treatment regimens written uniquely for them. Having an informal yet systematic approach to patient counseling in routine practice has obvious advantages for the prevention of mishaps as well as the management of allergic reactions.

Research, for the most part, reveals that a hands-on education method reduces unnecessary drug reactions and enhances how well patients adhere to their medication—this holds in particular for individuals in vulnerable categories, such as people on anti-tubercular treatment (Kaur et al., 2025). Health workers should emphasize the importance of adhering to substitute prescriptions and avoiding established allergens, as well as reminding patients to return for follow-up visits that reevaluate if the treatment is effective. Patients, on their part, should be encouraged to bring their allergy information with them—so that any physician they encounter is aware of the situation, and this little gesture could make a big difference. Such forward-looking, even slightly imperfect, educational initiatives not only empower patients but also instill a spirit of collaboration in addressing drug allergies and reducing the risk of hives and associated problems.

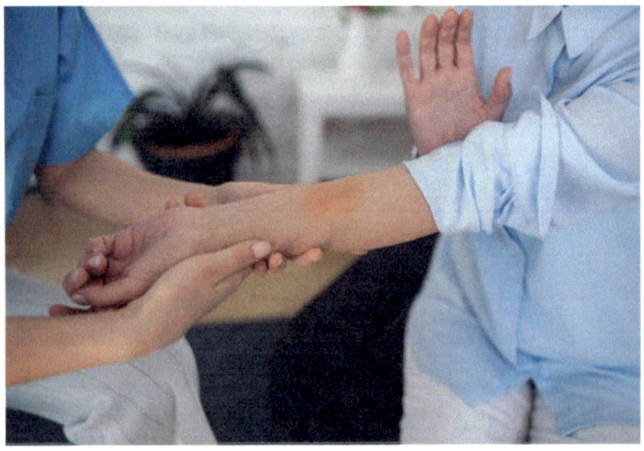

Source: iStock. (2022). *Medical Staff Treating a Skin Condition.* https://media.istockphoto.com/id/1390339324/photo/medical-staff-treating-a-skin-condition.jpg?s=612x612&w=0&k=20&c=bf70UK4yZBWVIPQLiM_pQUcW8LhogpgXjzB5KaUVrJU=.

11.6.2. Importance of Medical History Documentation

Too often, sound clinical decisions depend on knowing the whole, fully documented patient history—it is not only about tidy files on a shelf. When a person displays evidence of a drug reaction such as hives, taking a close account of prior use of medicines, known allergy, and timing of previous reactions can reveal dodgy patterns immediately. For the most part, if hives crop up shortly after the medication is administered, immediate access to these records prevents clinicians from repeating dangerous errors and guides them toward safer alternatives. In most instances, such precise logs also end up being input into broader checks for safety, providing valuable leads for assessing drug risk in large datasets (Dubrall et al., 2020). Briefly, these histories are essential for directed care, but they are also important for overall patient welfare. In the settings of hospitals, particularly the larger teaching institutions—the habit of documenting even minor details comes a long way. Research typically indicates that departments that monitor closely each morsel of a patient's history are more likely to detect more adverse drug reactions, such as unanticipated skin problems, and can respond faster to them (Sangeetha et al., 2017). At other times, the pattern of reporting assists in identifying which drug is likely the culprit, and although the procedure is somewhat of a repetition, it also provides a rough estimate of how serious a reaction may potentially be. This cycle of writing down notes, checking through them, and then acting upon them appears to eventually cut down on repeat errors while keeping health teams in the loop about new safety issues. In general, when hospitals commit careful, if sometimes flawed, documentation, patient safety is automatically enhanced. Beyond immediate care, proper records of medical histories also support larger studies and regulatory measures to minimize drug-induced hives and associated reactions. By collecting a broad range of patient histories, researchers are able to identify trends, such as which age ranges or types of medications (e.g., antibiotics or NSAIDs) are most likely to be associated with these problems (Dubrall et al., 2020). In most instances, identifying such trends is based on the type of detail that only proper record-keeping can ensure, and such information tends to be applied to changing prescribing guidelines and enhancing drug safety alerts (Sangeetha et al., 2017). It is also important to mention that if the patients notice that their data is well-documented, this can lead to more informed consent and collaborative decision-making. Despite a few minor documentation errors, maintaining complete histories is an important element of a complete plan to control drug reactions such as urticaria efficiently.

11.6.3. Role of Healthcare Providers in Prevention

Healthcare practitioners have a key role in preventing allergic hives and drug reactions, even from the beginning. Practitioners research a patient's history, investigating not only medical history but also genetic indicators and past exposure to medications that could nudge an individual toward a reaction. Sometimes just a simple discussion of typical environmental stimuli and allergens alerts patients to pay attention to early warning signs and seek treatment more quickly. This strategy not only reduces the extent to which such reactions occur but also allows for tailored treatment protocols that consider potential allergies, ultimately minimizing hospitalizations and expense (Burns, 2019). In daily practice, creating a prevention habit is the first step to safeguarding those most vulnerable. Close observation of patients' responses to drugs is another vital component of the equation. Most often, monitoring side effects in clinics will disclose patterns that compel practitioners to reconsider what drugs they prescribe. Retrospective evidence has indicated that skin problems will appear most frequently with antibiotics, NSAIDs, and even certain blood pressure medications (Rathinam et al., 2018). By improving adverse drug reaction reporting systems, healthcare teams can rapidly identify warning signs, sometimes even avoiding high-risk medications entirely. By this type of close monitoring, patient safety is enhanced while real-world information informs changing, evidence-based guidelines throughout diverse clinical environments. In addition to being keen diagnosticians and observant monitors of drug action, clinicians need to also excel in patient education and collaboration between specialties. Educating on why it is critical to adhere to a prescribed regimen, recognizing the early signs of an allergy, and avoiding known allergens puts patients in charge of their own care. When pharmacists, allergists, and primary care physicians work together, they can better evaluate risks and create coordinated plans, particularly for children, where heredity and daily exposures combine in unpredictable ways (Burns, 2019). Ultimately, by taking on these preventative roles in their entirety, healthcare professionals decrease how frequently and how severely drug-induced allergic reactions happen, opening the way to safer results in a variety of patient populations.

CLOSER LOOK

Urticarial Vasculitis

Urticarial vasculitis is an uncommon skin disease with long-lasting urticarial lesions on the skin, on microscopic examination, having evidence of leukocytoclastic vasculitis, an inflammation of small blood vessels. It is different from ordinary urticaria (hives) in that the skin lesions persist for more than 24 hours and leave a bruise-like effect.

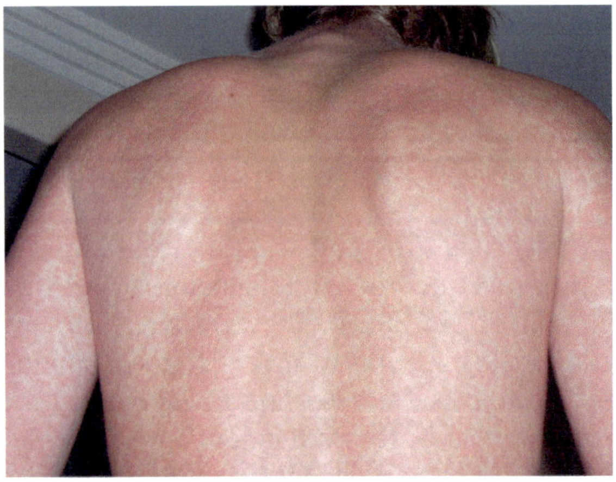

Source: By Rashy100 at English Wikipedia - Transferred from en.wikipedia to Commons., Public Domain, https://commons.wikimedia.org/w/index.php?curid=11362712

- **Mechanism**

Antibodies are typically induced against foreign proteins, like those produced by a virus that is replicating or an invading bacterium. Viruses or bacteria with antibodies opsonized or "adherent" to them mark them out for other immune cells to destroy.

Antibodies against self-proteins are referred to as autoantibodies, and do not occur in healthy patients. Autoantibodies may be applied to detect certain illnesses.

- **C1q:** C1q is a constituent part in the complement pathway – a complex series of protein-protein interactions, leading up to an immune response against a wide range of pathogens. The anti-C1q autoantibodies in hypocomplemententemic urticarial vasculitis patients activate C1q, leading to the activation of the whole complement pathway. As a result, the levels of all the complement proteins decrease.
- **Impaired Classical Complement Pathway:** The complement pathway consists of several subset pathways: the lectin/mannose pathway, the alternative pathway, and the classical pathway. All these converge into the formation of a C3 convertase, which catalyzes C3 to its constitutive components (better elaborated here – classical complement pathway).

In short, the key function of C1q in the pathway is its significance as the initial protein to initiate the complement cascade (which culminates in the killing of the invading bacteria or virus), and its capacity to bridge the two significant arms of the immune system - the innate immune system: a general defense system; and the adaptive immune system: the powerful immune response with the ability to remember past infections, enabling rapid response against recurring infections, i.e., individuals with a normal immune system do not keep getting the same cold or same type of flu over and over again.

- **Diagnosis:** An uncommon autoimmune condition with recurrent urticaria (nettle rash), initially reported in the 1970s. No paradigm for the syndrome etiology and severity of progression is established. Diagnosis is established with the presence of at least two of the following conditions: venalities on skin biopsy, arthritis, ocular inflammation, abdominal pain or positive C1q antibodies to immune complexes. It is this last category, anti-C1q antibodies, that all HUV patients test positive for. In vitro tests and mouse models of the disease have not fully established the connection between these antibodies and the disease, despite the connection being so strong. (Neupane & Rai, 2017)

SUMMARY

Looking at the multiple ways that urticaria appears following drug exposures is really a reminder that it is important to know both how the body works and the specifics of how a drug was administered. Immune reactions and drug precipitants are prone to commingle in complex patterns, so physicians are frequently forced to take a general view, particularly when more than one medicine is involved. It only becomes more complicated when hives are caused by infections, idiopathic reasons, or drug reactions; in many such instances, a thorough examination of the patient's history and some reliable diagnostic tests are important. Recent research has even indicated that dermatological problems like hives are not only prevalent, but they could indicate more critical issues elsewhere, placing additional emphasis on treatment options. A prudent and comprehensive diagnostic strategy can assist in avoiding the adverse effects of drug hypersensitivities and enhance patient safety across diverse environments (Gökhan al., 2024). The pharmacology of drug responses is continuously evolving, requiring treatment strategies to be revised periodically, particularly when novel therapies and more than one drug are concerned. Combining various approaches, including constant vigilance (pharmacovigilance) with tailored, patient-specific therapy may reduce the frequency of such annoying hives, as well as how severe they become. In most cases, resorting to alternative or complementary treatments is promising too; these practices may alleviate the inflammatory and oxidative stress pathways that arise in allergic reactions. A few of these additional treatments have been combined with the old standbys in small studies, and they may help balance the immune response and reduce side effects, so they are a field of study worth exploring further and applying to practice (Bhalerao et al., 2023). Putting it all together what we do about drug-induced urticaria reveals that early detection and an individually tailored approach really are important. Identifying suspect drugs early, and not being afraid to take them away or replace them—still stands as a bedrock of good patient care. New diagnostic methods, whether molecular or immunological, can also contribute by providing more accurate cause-and-effect clues, which in most instances means improved outcomes. There is much still to learn about the multifaceted biology behind these reactions and the markers that could anticipate who is at greater risk, in general. And providing more insight to healthcare professionals about the numerous skin conditions associated with drug allergies might alleviate the burden overall. All the evidence to date pushes us toward patient-centeredness, wherein optimizing treatment efficacy alongside reducing risks achieves safer medication therapy (Bhalerao et al., 2023; Gökhan et al., 2024).

Drug-induced hives can get downright ugly; uncovering what is happening takes a keen eye on both symptoms and the body's underlying responses. Mast cells are at center stage here; when they erupt and release all sorts of chemicals, you have got the characteristic itchy bumps. In current times, many clinicians call this MCAS, and that serves to distinguish primary from secondary or causeless issues. The term MCAS stands for Mast Cell Activation Syndrome. In the majority of instances, physicians monitor for the typical symptoms, fleeting flashes in markers such as tryptase and histamine, and observe if treatment targeted against these mediators works. Identification of these indicators, even though they appear in a variety of forms, can differentiate true mast cell–associated hives from those conditions that simply appear to be the real thing—thus avoiding misdiagnosis and inappropriate treatment. This type of strategy not only informs doctors in the face of suspected drug-induced urticaria but also leans investigation toward new targets in mast cell biology (Valent et al., 2012). On a general level, such understanding opens up to more tailored treatment and improved predictions regarding outcomes. In trying to combat drug-induced urticaria, exploring receptor interaction at the molecular level has effectively turned the focus around. Recent computer docking research, for instance, indicates that some natural substances bind well to histamine receptors, which are big players in initiating such reactions. Consider the herbal mixture called Kuppaimeni Choornam—employed in alternative medicine for many years—it seems to block the human histamine H1 receptor in a promising way. Interestingly, certain plant components such as beta-sitosterol, apigenin, and kaempferol appear to bind more strongly to these receptors compared to conventional antihistamines such as cetirizine. These findings point toward the possibility that bioactive compounds present in natural remedies may modulate receptor function in a manner that quiets the symptoms. For the most part, this molecular logic is used to promote the concept of integrating herbal therapy into practice patterns, but additional laboratory research and clinical trials certainly are necessary (Gayatri et al., 2019). Combining what we observe in the clinic with what molecular research tells us results in a general approach to the treatment of drug-induced hives. Identifying the distinctive patterns of mast cell activation allows practitioners to refine treatment, and molecular docking experiments help guide the synthesis of more selective and potent antihistaminic agents. By bridging these various disciplines, medical professionals can gain a better understanding of why patients respond so variably, particularly with the inherent variability of urticaria and the way drugs interact in each individual. In general, ongoing investigation of mast cell stimuli and histamine receptor antagonists should further define diagnosis and treatment. This dual approach encourages a more scientifically oriented and specific approach to treating drug-induced hives, ultimately resulting in improved patient care, and paving the way for new pharmacologic alternatives (Valent et al., 2012; Gayatri et al., 2019).

KEY TERMS FROM THIS CHAPTER

- Antibiotics
- Aspirin desensitization
- Chronic inducible urticaria
- Drug administration
- Mast cell activation
- Ubiquitous analgesics
- Anti-ige monoclonal antibodies
- Attention-deficit
- Chronic spontaneous urticaria
- Drug-induced allergic reactions
- Mast cells
- Urticaria
- Pseudoallergic reaction
- Hyperactivity disorder
- Dress syndrome
- Hypersensitivity
- Neonates

REFERENCES

1. Aguilar Hinojosa, N. K., & Figueroa Saavedra, E. I. (2023). Desensibilización a deferasirox en una paciente con hemocromatosis. Reporte d*e un caso. Revista Alergia* Mexico, 70(4), 159–162. https://doi.org/10.1007/dbb99923276da5b25ad173a636ecbc2b1ad4ce16.
2. Aquilina, S. (2016). Urticaria: Diagnosis and Management. https://core.ac.uk/download/83020050.pdf.
3. Bal, G., Schneikert, J., Li, Z., Franke, K., Tripathi, S. R., Zuberbier, T., & Babina, M. (2023). CREB is indispensable to KIT function in human skin mast cells, a positive feedback loop between CREB and KIT orchestrates skin mast cell fate. Cells, 13. https://doi.org/10.1007/b6bf8c8596f2c153703f50ef5b10ebb4133d277*c.*
4. *Banerji, A., Kanani, A., Kaplan, A. P., Grat*tan, C. E., Weldon, D. R., Frigas, E., Vena, G. A., et al. (2011). Urticaria and angioedema. https://core.ac.uk/download/pdf/8661846.pdf.
5. Barbaud, A., Gonçalo, M., Bruynzeel, D., Bircher, A., & European Society of Contact Dermatitis (2001). Guidelines for performing skin tests with drugs in the investigation of *cutaneous adverse drug reactions. Conta*ct dermatitis, 45(6), 321–328. https://doi.org/10.1034/j.1600-0536.2001.450601.x(accessed on 12 May 2025).
6. Beck, L. A., Bernstein, J. A., & Maurer, M. (2017). A Review *of International Rec*om*m*endations for the Diagnosis and Management of Chronic Urticaria. Acta dermato-venereologica, 97(2), 149–158. https://doi.org/10.2340/00015555-2496(accessed on 12 May 2025).
7. Bellanti, J., & Settipane, R. (2015). *Children at risk: Conditions which can increase th*e occurrence of allergic disease. Journal of Allergy, 36, 329–331. ht*tps://doi.org/10.1007/4ef4fd2db0d053* a034720ffa280e5b4fed1e10c9.
8. Bhalerao, S., Joshi, A. A., Khadke, S., & Sathiyanarayan, A. (*2023).* Anti-obesity effects of Triphala at biochemical and molecular level in high-fat diet-induced obese rats. Pharmacogn*osy Magazine,* 2**0(**30–42). https://doi.org/10.4103/pm.pm_118_23.
9. Blanca-Lopez, N., Agúndez, J., Fernández, J., García-Martín, E., & Blanca, M. (2024). Ibuprofen and other arylpropionics: The relevance in immediate hypersensitivity drug reactions. International Archives of Allergy and Immunology. https://doi.org/10.1007/8aa5959af941e61c65d65db*51f15353d*50bdc2d3.
10. Burks, A., Muraro, A., Brown, A. F., Terr, A. I., Ellis, A. K., Stark, B. J., Canadian Society of Allergy and Clinical Immunology, et al. (2011). Anaphylaxis. • This act*ivity is an Accredited Gr*oup Learning Activity (Section 1) as defined by the Maintenance of Certification Program of the Royal College of Physicians and Surgeons of Canada and approved by Canadian Society of Allergy and Clinical Immunology. https://core.ac.uk/download/pdf/8661843*.pdf.*
11. *Burns, H. (20*19*).* The Development of Hypersensitivity Reactions in The Pediatric Population: A Review. A Senior Thesis submitted in partial fulfillment of the requirements for graduation in the Honors Program Liberty University Spring 2019. https://core.ac.*uk/download/213464303.pdf* (acc*essed on 12 May 2025).
12. Byskov, P. K., Baden, C. S., Andersen, J. T., Jimenez-Solem, E., Olsen, R. H., Gade, C., & Lausten-Thomsen, U. (2024). Adverse drug reactions in neonates: A brief analysis of t*he FDA adverse event* reporting system. Frontiers in Pharmacology, 15. https://doi.org/10.3389/fphar.2024.987401.

13. Caffarelli, C., Franceschini, F., Caimmi, D. et al. SIAIP position paper: provocation challenge to antibiotics and non-steroidal anti-inflammatory drugs in ch*ildren. Ital J Pediatr 44,* 147 (2018). https://doi.org/10.1186/s13052-018-0589-3 (accessed on 12 May 2025).

14. Camelo-Nunes, I. C. (2006). New Antihistamines: A Critical View. https://core.ac.uk/download/37706676.pdf.

15. Chow S. K. (2012). Management of chronic *urticaria in Asia: 2010 AADV consensus guidelin*es. Asia Pacific allergy, 2(2), 149–160. https://doi.org/10.5415/apallergy.2012.2.2.149

16. de Sá, J. B., de Sá Santos, J. G., & de Sá, V. C. (2024). Acute urticaria in children. Health and Society. https://doi.org/10.*1007/e1ac*1826972fe8720dd8026d0fffa66b6554b192.

17. Dias de Castro, E., Carolino, F., Ribeiro, L., & Cernadas, J. R. (2018). Overview of Drug Allergy: From Immunogenetic Basis to Practice. Acta medica portuguesa, 31(10), 581–588. https://doi.org/10.20344/amp.10092 (accessed on 12 May 2025).

18. Dubrall, D. (2020). Analyses of Spontan*eous Adverse Drug Reaction Databases Using Descriptive and Inferential Statistics.* https://core.ac.uk/download/618184549.pdf.

19. Ertaş, R. (2017). Anti IgE Therapy in Chronic Urticaria. InTech. doi: 10.5772/68015 (accessed on 12 May 2025).

20. Farshchian, M., Ansar, A., Zamanian, A., Rahmatpour-Rokni, G., Kimyai-Asadi, A., & Farshchian, M. (2015). Drug-induced skin reactions: a 2-year study. Clinical, cosmetic and investigational dermatology, 8, 53–56. https://doi.org/10.2147/CCID.S75849

21. G., H., Rathinam, J., *A., P., & R., D. (2018). A r*etrospective analysis of adverse drug reactions reported at a tertiary ca*re hospital in South India. Interna*tional Journal of Basic & Clinical Pharmacology, 7(7), 1257–1262. https://doi.org/10.18203/2319-2003.ijbcp20182423 (accessed on 12 May 2025).

22. Gameiro, A., Gonçalo, M., Gouveia, M., *Ramos, et al. (2016).* Urti*c*ária de contacto induzida por fármacos. https://core.ac.uk/download/322632189.pdf (accessed on 12 May 2025).

23. Gayatri, R., Vinayak, S., & Elansekaran, S. (2019). MOLECULAR DOCKING STUDIES OF SIDDHA HERBAL FORMULATION KUPPAIMENI CHOORNAM ON HUMAN HISTAMINE RECEPTOR (3RZE*) . International Journal* of Ayurveda and Pharma Research, 7(3), 11-19. Retrieved from https://ijapr.in/index.php/ijapr/article/view/1158 (accessed on 12 May 2025).

24. Giannetti, M., Nicoloro-SantaBarbara, J., Godwin, G., Middle*sworth, J., Espeland, A., Douvas, J. L., & Ca*stells, M. (2024). Challenges in drug and hymenoptera venom hypersensitivity diagnosis and management in mastocytosis. Diagnostics, 1*4. https://doi.org*/10.1007/0bc645cfaa62b47ec40e484ea887a5bced2ce408.

25. Grant, E. (2015). Validity and accura*cy of self-reported drug allergies. Nelson Mandela Metropolitan University; http://hdl.handle.net/1*0948/3295

26. Guerrier, G., Daronat, J. M., & Deltour, R. (2011). Unusual presentation of acute annular urticaria: a case report. Case reports in dermatological medicine, 2011, 604390. https://doi.org/10.1155/2011/604390

27. Guntapalle, J. B., Gore, A. B., Rathod, N. D., Paratkar, G. M., Patil, K. K., & Sagar, A. G. (2025). Drug-induced diseases: A comprehensive review of classification, risk factors, and prevention strategies. International Journal of Advanced Research in Science, Communication and Technology. https://doi.org/10.1007/a5276257bf1f8b7869e06ad976159b2db94c7f64.

28. Heerfordt, I. M., & Horwitz, H. (2024). Frequently asked questions about adverse drug reactions of methylphenidate. Adverse Drug Reaction Bulletin, 345, 1339–1342. https://doi.org/10.1007/ef2596828cdfe7f7ba53fe9b265dfcaadf920a6d.

29. Hyun, S. Y., Kim, E. Y., Kang, M., Park, J. W., Hong, K. S., Chung, H. M., Cho*i, W., et al. (*2023). Embryonic-stem-cell-derived mesenchymal stem cells relieve experimental contact urticaria by regulating the functions of mast cells and T cells. Scientific Reports, 13. https://doi.org/10.1038/s41598-023-34049-3.

30. Kaur, J., Gupta, T., Saini, A., Khosla, P. P., Rani, N., & Verma, I. (2025). Adverse drug reaction of antitubercular drugs and impact of patient counselling on compliance in tuberculosis patients: A *prospective study. Current Drug Therapy. https://doi.org/10.1007/97a1c6cefffe1f84c3*7915324a87d6e3deae54eb.

31. Kaya G, Dizman D, Su Küçük Ö. Dermatological manifestations, and drug-induced reactions in COVID-19 patients: an observational study from İstanbul, Turkiye. J H*ealth Sci Med / JHSM. September 202*4;7(5):555-563. doi:10.32322/jhsm.1508495Kushner, P., McCarberg, B., Grange, L., Kolosov, A., Lihic Haveric, A., Zucal, V., Petruschke, R., et al. (2022). The use of non-steroidal anti-inflammatory drugs (NSAIDs) in COVID-19. NPJ Primary Care Respiratory Medicine, 32. https://doi.org/10.1007/90a923a67bdd13c5aad5749c09ff2f18d*641eebe.*

32. Luo, M., Shen, K., Dong, X., Zhang, W., & Tang, F. (2024). Efficacy and safety of combinations of H1 antihistamines in the treatment of urticaria: A scoping review. Indian Journal of Dermatology, Venereology and Leprology. https://doi.org/10.1007/3a5fe4c7439cc5a86530ae47c051939c0172f3b1.

33. Masferrer, E., Martin-Ezquerra, G., Martínez-Escala, E., Pujol, R. M., & Giménez-Arnau, A. (2011). Eosinophilic panniculitis triggered by intramuscular penicillin and occupational setting. Allergy, 66(3), 436–437. https://doi.org/10.1111/j.1398-9995.2010.024*90.x(accessed on 12* May 2025).

34. Miniello, A., Casella, R., Loverre, T., Aloia, D., Di Bona, D., & Nettis, E. (2023). An update on nonsteroidal anti-inflammatory drug-induced urticaria. Endocrine, Metabolic & Immune Disorders Drug Targets. https://www.semanticscholar.org/paper/d99c8fd38369234bdfa001fd59401a3a0378cd56 (accessed on 12 May 2025).

35. Myasnikova, T. N., Nekrasova, T., Romanova, T. S., Smirnov, V., & Latysheva, T. (2024). Cross-hypersensitivity reactions to non-steroidal anti-inflammatory drugs, *manifested as urticaria and/or angioedem*a, anaphylaxis. Russian Journal of Allergy. https://doi.org/10.18821/2221-7220-2024-31-2-78-85.

36. Neupane, G. P., & Rai, M. (2017). Adverse drug reaction profile and prescription pattern of antihypertensive drug monotherapy at tertiary *care hospital Nepalgunj, Nepal. International Journal of* Basic & Clinical Pharmacology, 7(1), 75–79. https://doi.org/10.18203/2319-2003.ijbcp20175678

37. Packiaseeli, S. P. (2024). A retrospective analysis of reported cutaneous adverse drug reactions in a tertiary care teaching hospital. Asian Journal of Pharmaceuti*cal and Cli*nical Research. https://doi.org/10.1007/911cfd77b0d4d73b0269e6f56464d82f4ea416e1.

38. SANGEETHA RAJA*, JAMUNA RANI R, KALA P. (2017). Pattern of adverse drug reactions in a tertiary care teaching hospital: A cross-sectional study. Asian J Pharm Cl*in Res, Vol 10, Issue 3, 2017, 170-173. https://cor*e.ac.uk/download/477852549.pdf (accessed on 12 May 2025).

39. Sittiphan, S., Lim, A., Khurram, H., Dureh, N., & Dittakan, K. (2025). Epidemiology of reported serious adverse drug reactions due to anti-infectives using nationwide database of Thailand. PLOS One, 20. https://doi.org/10.1371/journal.pone.0270012.
40. Valent, P., Akin, C., *Arock, M., Brockow, K., Bu*tterfield, J. H., Carter, M. C., Castells, M., Escribano, L., Hartmann, K., Lieberman, P., Nedoszytko, B., Orfao, A., Schwartz, L. B., Sotlar, K., Sperr, W. R., Triggiani, M., Valenta, R., Horny, H. P., & Metcalfe, D. D. (20*12). Definitions, criteria and global classification* of *m*ast cell disorders with special reference to mast cell activation syndromes: a consensus proposal. International archives of allergy and immunology, 157(3), 215–225. https://doi.org/10.1159/000328*760Alshareef, H. M., Alenzi, K., Albalawi, B. R., Al*anazi, R., Albalawi, N., Alasoufi, W., Alqifari, S., et al. (2025). Comparative analysis of adverse drug reactions associated with fluoroquinolones and other antibiotics: A retrospective pharmacovigilance study. Drug, H*ealthcare and Patient Safety, 17, 51–62. https://doi. o*rg/10.1007/e18f913222eae1de5b3e5c595486a590621ba716.
41. Vicovan, A. G., Veres, L., Cucu, A., Turliuc, D., & Ghiciuc, C. M. (2019). Nonsteroidal anti-inflammatory drugs-induced hypersensitivity reactions: Algorithm for the diagno*stic and management. Romanian Neurosurgery, 33(4*), *41*1–416. https://doi.org/10.33962/roneuro-2019-066 (accessed on 12 May 2025).
42. Vykhrystenka, L. R., & Yanchanka, U. V. (2008). Handbook of clinical allergology. Core. Retrieved from: https://core.ac.uk/download/80149814.pdf (accessed on 12 May 2025).
43. Walker, A. I., *Räwer, H. C.*, Sieber, W., & Przybilla, B. (2011). Immediate-type hypersensitivity to succinylated corticosteroids. International archives of *all*ergy and immunology, 155(1), 86–92. https://doi.org/10.1159/000318678 (accessed on 12 May 2025).
44. Woessner, K., Kowalski, M. L., & Sanak, M. (2015). Approaches to the diagnosis and management of patients with a history of nonsteroidal anti-inflammatory drug-related urticaria and a*ngioedema. Journal of* Allergy, 36, 329–331. https://doi.org/10.1007/90a923a67bdd13c5aad5749c09ff2f18d641eebe.
45. Yeğit, O. O., Sarıbeyliler, G., Karadağ, P., Demir, S., Gül, N., Ünal, D., Gelincik Akkor, A. (2023). The first successful desensitization protocol in exenatide allergy: A ca*se report. Allergy, Asthma, and Clinical Immunology: Official Journal of the Canadian Society of Allergy and Clinical Imm*unology, 19. https://doi.org/10.1007/3ed72693f58feae9a688740bbf4f8866ec083f2e.
46. Zhang, Z., Zhu, M., & Jiang, W. (2025). Risk factors analysis of cutaneous adverse drug reactions caused by targeted therapy and immunotherapy drugs for oncology and establishment of a predict*ion model. Clinical and Translational* Science, 18. https://doi.org/10.1111/cts.13458.
47. Zhou, C., Li, J., Zhou, F., Huang, L., Liu, X., & Li, H. (2024). Fat*al case of Pneumocysti*s jirovecii pneumonia (PJP) during treatment for drug rash with eosinophilia and systemic symptoms (DRESS) *syndrome. Infection and Drug Res*istance, 17, 153–159. https://www.semanticscholar.org/paper/ad274b49408210476cd149f37a11cae8a9563d3d (accessed on 12 May 2025).
48. Zhu, M., Jia, L., Wang, Y., Zhang, Y., & Lv, S. (2024). Comparative evaluation of adverse drug reactions for tenofovir alafenamide and tenofovir disoproxil fumarate using the FAERS Database: A disproportionality *analysis. Expert Opinion on* Drug Safety. https://doi.org/10.1007/c06f389681f788b9d22f7b2fbaefcfa3a5991763.

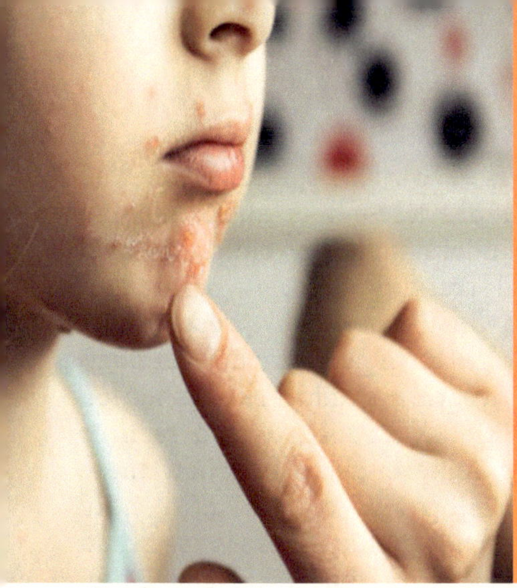

Chapter 12

PEDIATRIC DERMATOLOGY

Contents

Introduction

Pediatric dermatology is a specialty characterized as much by the innate characterestics of children's skin as by the variety of conditions they encounter. Children's skin develops and evolves—its particular composition can turn an otherwise innocuous rash into a big deal and a chronic inflammatory disorder into a true enigma. In the majority of cases, as the skin ages, its reaction to therapy and general disease behavior develops new complexities that add additional hurdles to diagnosis, therapy, and even long-term prognoses. When skin issues strike, it is not only the child who suffers; families are affected too, making a strong argument for early, targeted intervention to alleviate both short-term distress and any residual concerns. Taking a closer look, comprehending how skin disease appears in children is essential to defining pediatric dermatology as a distinct specialty of medicine. As a general rule, the forces in operation there—everything from genetics, immune responses, and infections to environmental stimuli—do not reflect those in play in adults, tending to produce a pretty random picture. Differences in rates of disease and presentations appear within various ethnic groups, geographic locations, and socioeconomic strata, so that not all cases can be put into an organized box. Medical histories and large population epidemiological investigations, including those found in extensive medical data banks, assist in filling out this complex puzzle (Schmidt et al., 2019). Recent advances in molecular biology and immunology have, in most instances, cast new light on what causes pediatric skin problems. This advancement holds out the promise of treatments more precisely targeted—shaped almost on a case-by-case basis to each child's genetic legacy and physical characteristics. Global health issues of late have also served as a reminder that body-wide infections can suddenly cause skin issues, prompting physicians to balance carefully the need to combat infection and protect the skin. Such information highlights the importance of a combination of specialties, a multidisciplinary model that further integrates pediatric dermatology into the larger healthcare system to effectively address new threats (Salamanna et al., 2020). Finally, consistent commitment to hands-on research and continued training continues to be totally crucial to enhancing pediatric dermatology's overall impact and long-term viability.

Definition of Pediatric Dermatology

Pediatric dermatology is not your run-of-the-mill skin care—it is where skin science intersects with kids' medicine in a pretty surprising way. Skin problems in babies, children, and adolescents do not play by the adult rules, so physicians here have to be well-versed in how the skin develops and evolves. For most children, a child's skin is not merely a smaller equivalent of an adult's; it requires its own diagnostic tests and treatment protocols that take into consideration both the body's physical developments and the more delicate, at times fragile, psychological aspect. Most clinicians, for instance, plunge into interdisciplinary training that combines dermatologic expertise with pediatric understanding, a combination that really gets them ready for dealing with these special challenges (University of Nebraska Medical Center, 1976). This specialty is not all about clinical practice—it is about moving forward our understanding of children's skin problems and treating them in ways that correspond to their true-world presentation. When we hear the term pediatric dermatology, we know that treating a child's skin condition is more than simply dealing with a rash or spot; it means going in-depth into how these conditions develop and change as a child ages. The specialty encompasses a broad spectrum of issues, ranging from congenital characterestics and inflammatory issues to infections and even those occasional genetic disorders that sometimes appear at the start of life. For example, mastocytosis, where there is an abnormal accumulation of mast cells primarily in the skin, illustrates how at times a skin issue is an indication of something more systemic in nature (Heide, 2009).

Typically, initial skin signs in children will point to underlying, underlying health conditions, so these physicians are instrumental in early diagnosis and overall management, combining clinical dermatology and pediatric skills into a smooth if occasionally erratic, treatment. As pediatric dermatology continues to evolve, it evolves in step with new medical knowledge and treatments specifically designed for children. Treatment of skin disorders in young patients is not as simple since medications and treatments can act extremely differently in a developing body, influencing growth and well-being. This requires not only strong clinical skills but also a keen focus on research and evidence-based practices that advocate for a more sophisticated approach to care. The commitment to innovation appears in the structure of academic programs and clinical protocols, establishing a solid foundation without sacrificing flexibility (University of Nebraska Medical Center, 1976). At the end of the day, pediatric dermatology is all about solving, treating, and even preventing skin conditions in children through a mix of varied expertise, continuous learning, and a dedication to addressing the unique needs of an age group.

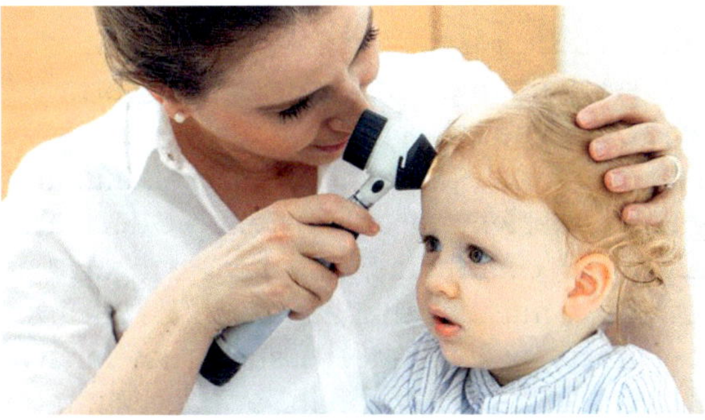

Source: MedStar Health. (n.d.). *Pediatric Dermatology Examination.* https://medstarhealth-delivery.sitecorecontenthub.cloud/api/public/content/services%2FPediatric-Dermatology?v=608fa78e.

Importance of Skin Health in Children

Kids' skin is our body's first line of defense—it protects us from the daily onslaught of environmental toxins such as germs and allergens. In children, this layer is still in development; it is softer and more permeable than skin in adults and therefore more susceptible to letting irritants invade and causing afflictions like eczema, infection or even dermatitis. Healthy skin, therefore, is not merely about keeping out outside dangers—it keeps the body's temperature even, too, and aids the senses necessary for optimal growth. Most of the time, catching skin problems early will prevent long-term issues and bring about a greater quality of life in general. Several pediatric care specialists now emphasize prevention by instructing caregivers in simple skin care procedures and employing treatment regimens that suit individual children's special needs. Such an approach tends to reduce both rapid and prolonged skin damage while supporting overall wellness in young children (Marilyn et al., 2022).

New studies, in most instances, also suggest an association between certain genetic disorders and skin alterations. Syndromes such as Down syndrome and tuberous sclerosis complex frequently present with characteristic skin features that can be early warning signs, not only of skin problems but sometimes of underlying, more systemic pathology as well. Children with these conditions might have difficulty with a compromised immune system and increased infection risk in addition to other developmental challenges. Pediatric dermatologists in most cases collaborate with experts in other areas to take care of both the primary skin issues and any additional complications that arise. Newly released guidelines and consensus statements provide physicians with a basis for monitoring these signs, assuring a balanced care plan (Marilyn et al., 2022). Skin problems in children can also strike them emotionally and socially, frequently in ways that may not be immediately apparent. Issues such as noticeable psoriasis, atopic dermatitis (AD), or even large birthmarks can make children feel stigmatized or embarrassed, impacting their self-image and social interaction. Pediatric dermatology is thus not simply about curing the skin, but typically entails a wider, biopsychosocial intervention that combines medical treatment with counseling, family guidance and support systems. Simple measures like proper hygiene, regular sun protection and allergen avoidance become major steps towards long-term skin well-being. In addition, novel noninvasive diagnostic tests and directed treatments are poised to make care more straightforward to adhere to and effective, ultimately enhancing both physical and emotional well-being in these young patients (Marilyn et al., 2022).

Overview of Common Pediatric Skin Conditions

Children present with skin conditions that are not exactly the same as in adults. Dermatitis, for example, is a serious business ; it encompasses many forms, such as atopic, contact, and seborrheic, which all have their own appearance but all demonstrate kinds of inflammation. Environmental factors, a not-yet-mature immune system, and genes all contribute, which is why these problems crop up so frequently in children.

Physicians must be alert, catching even the slightest variations so that treatment arrives in a timely fashion. And when signs begin to mingle with signs of infections or other skin diseases, it certainly merits a more thorough, vigilant examination. Skin infection is also a significant issue. Fungal and bacterial conditions such as impetigo typically appear when the natural barrier of the skin is breached or the immune system is not quite up to it. These infections can escalate into other issues if treated immediately. Fungal infections, for instance, most often strike in some climates or seasons and often develop patterns that may be confused with eczema or psoriasis. Impetigo, being super contagious, needs swift intervention to reduce its spread in children. In the majority of cases, being aware of the environmental and epidemiological factors involved helps significantly in organizing effective care (Hebert et al., 2023).

Psoriasis in children, while not as prevalent as dermatitis or infections, presents its own difficulties. Its symptoms can readily masquerade as eczema or other inflammatory dermatoses, so it may go unnoticed during a routine examination. Nevertheless, early detection is important because this condition is not merely skin-deep; it can cause actual physical pain and even affect a child's mood. Many times, psoriasis in children is accompanied by joint disease and psychiatric issues, so sometimes a team of specialists is required. Most of the time, providing primary care physicians with a holistic picture of what to detect truly makes a difference in outcomes (Hebert et al., 2023).

12.1. Common Pediatric Skin Conditions

Children's skin issues can be quite mysterious because the symptoms appear in a variety of ways. One time it is a fleeting rash that resolves on its own; other times, persistent inflammation signals underlying problems. Atopic dermatitis (AD), viral exanthems, and acne vulgaris are common conditions that appear in practice, and these are not just skin-deep issues. They can truly impact a child's quality of life, even precipitating social and emotional issues. Recognizing them early is vital because what appears to be a common rash may be indicating infections or system problems. Medical students, for instance, tend to struggle with determining when that added dermatologist input is required, leaving a training gap which requires filling (Adel et al., 2025). Treating these skin problems involves more than simply relieving the symptoms. Physicians must find a balance between providing immediate relief and protecting the sensitive nature of children's skin. Consider the example of eczema: children might require daily maintenance with moisturizers, intermittent use of steroid creams, and monitoring for triggers. At the same time, infections such as impetigo or molluscum contagiosum need appropriate antimicrobial treatment along with hygiene to assist in preventing them from spreading. It is also worth remembering that physical skin problems can get into a child's head, so some reassurance will come a long way. Even though this combination may seem to be a no-brainer, it is crying out for collaboration in which general practitioners and specialists share responsibilities—serving as the first bridge until complete referral to a dermatologist becomes the appropriate option (Adel et al., 2025). How future healthcare professionals manage these dermatological issues can make all the difference. Recent evidence indicates that med students tend to have a good understanding of relatively common pediatric skin problems and their complications, but most would benefit from a better sense of when to refer out to a specialist (Adel et al., 2025). That fine line between treating something you can in primary care and something that requires additional expertise is thin but enormously critical, because it can mean the difference between prompt treatment and delay or even over-treatment. Problems such as congenital melanocytic nevi or psoriasis almost always require the attention of a dermatologist due to long-term risk. Therefore, adjusting medical training to hone decision-making abilities in pediatric dermatology is crucial. More concentrated training and a dash of good old-fashioned intuition will allow clinicians to better counsel families so that children receive the proper care at precisely the right time.

12.1.1. Eczema and Its Prevalence

Chronic skin conditions in children manifest themselves in so many different forms, largely due to genes, the environment, and the immune system's response. Eczema, for instance, is a widespread skin condition that disrupts a child's daily comfort and even overwhelms our healthcare system. Worldwide figures tend towards approximately 15% to 30% of children being affected with eczema, although these figures can trend upwards or downwards based on heredity and other allergic conditions. Children with a history of eczema in their families tend to have very dry skin and have a greater chance of flare-ups, particularly if there are other allergic conditions involved. All of this collectively reminds us that eczema is not a single-track disorder—it is an intertwined combination that requires timely attention and treatment (Yazeed et al., 2025). Contemporary genetic research has now started unveiling how filaggrin gene mutations contribute to pediatric AD. Filaggrin is a critical protein for maintaining the skin's barrier, and when its ability is compromised—due to genetic errors—it also appears to lay the foundation for early, persistent, and frequently more challenging cases of eczema. Studies of Indian children with AD have even identified some novel filaggrin mutations not found in other ethnic populations. While these genetic abnormalities tend to bring with them a greater family link and greater immunoglobulin E levels, there is still a somewhat nebulous pattern between the gene alterations and the condition, at least in part due to the fact that most research has limited numbers. This very much emphasizes the heterogenous genetic underpinning of eczema and largely necessitates larger and more diverse studies in the near future (Somasundaram et al., 2025). On top of that, how prevalent eczema is in children appears to oscillate with local and environmental influences, with socioeconomic and climatic information having their say.

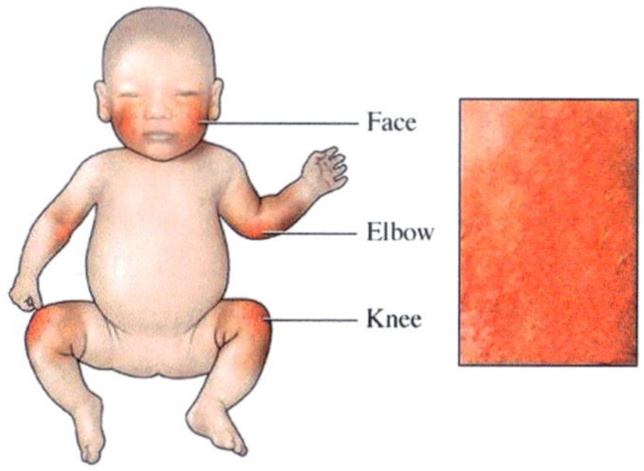

Figure 12.1. Eczema in children.

Source: Kaiser Permanente. (n.d.). *Infant Eczema.* https://mydoctor.kaiserpermanente.org/mas/Images/Infant%20Eczema_tcm88-737739.jpg.

Certain studies suggest that there is an association between dry skin or numerous allergies and an increased likelihood of the onset of eczema, especially when children access treatment later—often because they have less knowledge or lesser access to health centers. This delay can compound the condition, necessitating the roll-out of public health measures that intercept the problem early, particularly in resource-constrained settings. By tackling the things, we can modify and offering useful tips on skin care and allergy management, healthcare practitioners could ease the burden and enhance the health outcomes for these children (Yazeed et al., 2025) (Figure 12.1).

12.1.2. Acne in Adolescents

Teenage years are crazy, a period in which hormones flip and the body undergo changes that can trigger annoying skin problems like acne. Excessive oil production, changes in skin cell turnover, and even annoying bacteria all seem to combine and ignite inflammation. In most instances, learning about these origins benefits treatments that not only resolve the bumps but also reduce the mental burden of having them. Recently, physicians have been combining old, trusted creams with new, innovative concepts. Consider cold atmospheric plasma (CAP) therapy, for instance; it is proved to be effective and cost-saving when treating mild-to-moderate acne in children (Korotkiy, 2024). All of this comes back to a landscape where teen acne care is always in motion. When it comes to the treatment, newer skin treatments are combining multiple ingredients to attack acne from multiple fronts at once. A standout example is a fixed-dose triple-combo gel—stuffed with clindamycin phosphate, adapalene, and benzoyl peroxide, which is making waves as a game-changer option. Clinical trials also tend to indicate that this gel decreases inflammatory and noninflammatory lesions with the understanding that young skin may be particularly sensitive. Teens achieve clear or almost clear skin in over half the cases after approximately 12 weeks (Eichenfield et al., 2024). Occasionally, a little bit of pain at the site of application appears, but the side effects themselves are normally mild or moderate; this minor discomfort tends to make overall treatment stickiness better. This approach embodies a move toward therapies that balance both strength and sensitive care. Affordability and quality of life matter a great deal today when selecting acne treatments for teenagers.

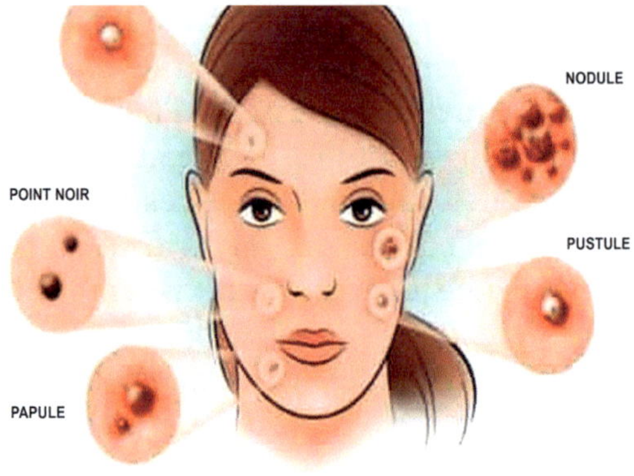

Figure 12.2. Acne in adolescence.

Source: LM Natura. (2021). *Types of Acne Lesions*. https://www.lm-natura.com/wp-content/uploads/2021/09/acne-adolescent-1-1.jpg.

Research tends to reveal that combining CAP with standard topical remedies provides improved results, reducing side effects and aiding in maintaining costs at a minimum (Korotkiy, 2024). Maintaining the skin's built-in defense mechanism, such as a balanced pH level and an adequate amount of moisture, appears to enhance the efficacy of the treatment and how well patients tolerate it, which works far more in favor of keeping them compliant. In addition, given that acne can strike self-esteem with a vengeance and awaken social anxiety, it is obvious that treatments must address more than one level. By combining cutting-edge alternatives with thoroughly tested combination regimens, pediatric dermatology is slowly attacking the complex layers of teen acne, doing more than promoting clear skin but also more resilient emotional well-being (Figure 12.2).

12.1.3. Psoriasis and Its Impact on Children

Chronic skin issues in children—psoriasis, say—present their own challenges. Children who have severe scalp problems frequently struggle with constant itching, actual pain, and a considerable amount of stress that disrupts their daily lives. Healing is not merely about clearing away symptoms; it is about making it safe for developing bodies too. Recent clinical practice, for instance, considered the combination of calcipotriene with betamethasone dipropionate in a topically applied suspension and determined that scalp psoriasis in adolescents improved significantly.

The therapy was largely effective, with only a few individual cases experiencing mild adrenal suppression and very few adverse side effects, something that necessitates some vigilance but still indicates the safety of the therapy. Individuals have also registered fewer instances of severe itching, so the treatment addresses both the outward symptoms and the discomfort, a success for child-centered skin care (Eichenfield et al., 2014). This advancement foretells of even more tailored treatments that address not only the skin itself but also the emotional burden psoriasis can impose. General practitioners usually become the first ones children with skin problems visit, particularly with such disorders as psoriasis. Recently, there has been a feeling that skin disorders receive insufficient attention in medical education, with many general practitioners feeling slightly ill-equipped as a result. This shortfall sometimes results in delays or suboptimal treatment, and this only perpetuates the issue in the long run. When you take a look at the way family physicians are dealing with these topics right now, you see on the one hand the difficulties they are having diagnosing and addressing these conditions and on the other opportunities to improve.

By identifying where the loopholes in their working knowledge are, researchers have made some quite important points about improving frontline care. Most times, increasing education and training in family medicine would be faster, and better care for children who are suffering from psoriasis and other everyday skin issues (Khalid et al., 2023). Psoriasis in children extends far beyond the rash on the skin—it can strike directly at a child's self-esteem and social life. When lesions occur, they tend to bring a combination of unwanted attention, social embarrassment, and decreased self-esteem, which may even extend into school achievement and interpersonal relationships. Top that with the fact that psoriasis is an ongoing problem that necessitates ongoing care, and you have a recipe for added stress, not only for the children but also for their families. With all these layers involved, it is no wonder that the treatment of pediatric psoriasis must also involve some emotional and social assistance in addition to the standard medical aid.

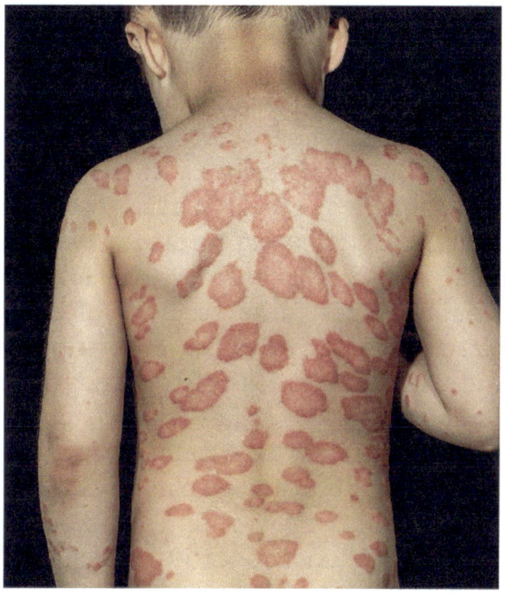

Figure 12.3. Plaque psoriasis on the back of a 4-year-old boy.

Source: Alajlan, A. M. (2021). *Plaque Psoriasis on the Back of a 4-Year-Old Boy*. ResearchGate.

The knowledge of how prevalent it is, what exactly children experience, and with which treatments can they be helped is the way to design the care plans that address the physical and the emotional aspects of the problem. As studies continue, the multidisciplinary approach seems the most promising method to mitigate the overall effect of psoriasis on the lives of children, repeating the call for the use of pediatric dermatological care that considers the big picture (Figure 12.3).

12.2. Diagnosis in Pediatric Dermatology

It is not the same as diagnosing adults. Children's skin conditions come in less predictable forms because their immune systems and development just do not function in the same way. Symptoms can change rapidly at times, so physicians combine a good physical exam with lab work and imaging. Consider Metaiodobenzylguanidine (MIBG) scintigraphy, for instance, it has been a true game-changer in identifying neuroblastoma, a relatively common tumor outside of the brain that may present with skin symptoms, by pinpointing exactly where the tumor resides and determining its stage (Otmane et al., 2025). High-tech together with old-school check-ups enhances the accuracy of treating children with unexplained or complicated skin issues. Teamwork is also making ripples in pedidermatology. It has become common for many centers to establish integrated rheumatology/dermatology clinics (RDCs) that allow specialists to iron out complex cases together. At institutions such as the UCSF Benioff Children's Hospital, such clinics usually have clearer diagnoses – most patients have their first diagnosis validated while those obscure cases end up getting more clarity (Jessica et al., 2024). In the majority of instances, such joint clinics hasten judgments regarding systemic therapy, skin biopsies, or other imaging studies, all the while providing residents an opportunity to learn on the run. It is an earthy solution that truly addresses the filthy reality of diagnosing skin conditions in children. Precision in pediatric dermatology is a combination of good observation and additional tests. You begin with a good physical and history, but then you may require a skin biopsy or additional imaging to differentiate between conditions that appear very similar or to see if other areas of the body are affected. For example, apart from fixing some skin-associated tumors, MIBG scintigraphy usually assists in tracking the progress of treatment over time, thereby allowing clinicians to adjust plans whenever necessary (Otmane et al., 2025). Indeed, according to some pediatric RDCs, approximately one-third of ambiguous or serious cases ultimately require both imaging and biopsy as part of the work-up (Jessica et al., 2024). This multi-layered, at times redundant approach mirrors the diverse nature of pediatric dermatology and encourages diagnostic routes that blend good old-fashioned clinical acumen with current technology.

12.2.1. Clinical Examination Techniques

A good diagnosis of children's skin conditions begins with a very specific, hands-on methodology – physicians gently look at and even explore the skin with a dermoscope to detect every tiny detail. Kids express curiosity about skin problems in quite nonspecific ways, so practitioners need to be adaptable and patient, not overwhelming the experience for them. You might notice details like color, size, or how a spot is spread out – these can oddly steer the diagnostic process. Take alopecia areata for example, patchy hair loss paired with bits of keratin debris can hint at an autoimmune problem (Wydya et al., 2024). Plus, using a dermoscope (which is non-invasive) can help pick up tiny clues like yellow or black dots that often signal specific conditions. These techniques in combination is likely to improve the diagnosis accuracy while keeping the child calmer. When dealing with small patients, the approach must be modified to suit their age and temperament. Children, particularly the younger ones, might find the standard clinical procedures a little too scary, so the doctors typically mix it up a bit – sometimes employing the distraction method or getting a caregiver to assist in making it more comfortable. Clinicians tend to trust their eyes for picking out the distinctive patterns in lesions before they even consider invasive procedures. For example, in the case of pilomatricomas, a consideration of both clinical presentation and a dermoscopic examination frequently provides sufficient clues. In most – about 80% in some studies – lesions present with nodular, variegated colors that strongly indicate pilomatricoma (Chessa et al., 2024).

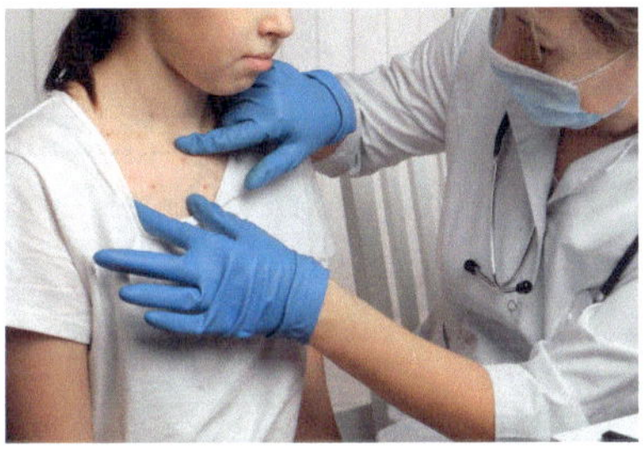

Figure 12.4. Performing clinical examination.

Source: istockphoto. (2022). *Doctor Checking Skin of Sick Girl Kid with Red Rash Being Examined at the Physician.* https://media.istockphoto.com/id/1429059636/photo/doctor-checking-skin-of-sick-girl-kid-with-red-rash-being-examined-at-the-physician-allergic.jpg?s=612x612&w=0&k=20&c=mG0HzPPF0fRVY0EIae9MSGmcY8LQuK_CSCi3GnuP56Q=.

This sort of balance between being thorough and avoiding procedure really demonstrates the art in pediatric dermatology. Other than the physical inspection, having a proper record is essential. High-quality photographs and dermoscopic shots do not just act as a baseline but also as checkpoints to observe whether a situation continues to improve or deteriorate along the way. Physicians may even employ trichoscopy, particularly when confronted with hair problems such as in alopecia areata, to examine follicle specifics that a bare eye may overlook (Wydya et al., 2024). Although the majority of cases are resolved by these less invasive measures, occasionally an unusual presentation necessitates a biopsy – approximately 20% of pilomatricoma cases need this additional step where dermoscopy is not able to give the whole picture (Chessa et al., 2024). Close visual examination with contemporary imaging, and intervening with histology where necessary ; guarantees optimal care is provided, even if the process at times drifts from the immaculately systematic (Figure 12.4).

12.2.2. Importance of Patient History

Kids with skin complaints are not simply bringing forward an outward issue – more times than not, the real story is the whole history behind the problem. And in most instances, you discover that a child's skin problem has an underlying layer: systemic or inherited issues that only reveal themselves when you look deeper into their background. It is not uncommon to find that certain cancer therapies for young patients have inherent, unpredictable skin side effects that, in turn, disrupt treatment habits and quality of life. Without a thorough list of previous diagnoses, medications, and prior skin issues, even seasoned practitioners may be left without crucial information on which to base a tailor-made skincare regimen. There is often a disconnect between what families remember and what is documented on medical charts — a disconnect that truly highlights why good history-taking is so critical. Briefly, having the entire history sets the stage for safer and better care (Meyer& Stockfleth, 2024). Occasionally, the value of this rich history becomes even more apparent, particularly in syndromic illness in which the skin appearance is merely a small piece of a larger puzzle. For example, an illness such as SHORT syndrome does not simply appear with some overt symptom but instead a combination of features , including notable skin changes, such as acanthosis nigricans. With these hints picked up on, and close observation of how a child is growing, any endocrine characterestics, and their heredity, physicians are usually able to nail both a correct diagnosis and the appropriate treatment strategy. In this context, a comprehensive patient history enables clinicians to view skin problems as being part of systemic enigmas, leading them to select interventions like hormonal or metabolic treatments. Without that information, there is more chance for misdiagnosis or delayed treatment, and that can end up harming the child's progress and quality of life (Osman et al., 2024). Furthermore, maintaining precise records and taking a critical look at a child's history is what really drives pediatric skin care and education to progress. Careful, well-maintained historical information not only refines treatment for each person but also helps the study of illness patterns and how diseases react to treatment — especially in those unusual or genetically complicated situations. For kids getting these exact treatments, remembering previous skin reactions along with any other ailments aids physicians in forming more preventive management, even including some preventive skin care guidelines. In addition, once patients and their families are informed about the child's individual history, adherence is enhanced and side effects fall off, underlining a more integrative understanding of care. Finally, integrating an extensive history in daily practice refines diagnostic precision, individualizes treatment, and increases educational efforts — making it an integral aspect of pediatric dermatology practice (Meyer et al., 2024).

12.2.3. Use of Diagnostic Tools and Tests

Diagnosing skin disease in children usually involves a little more than just a quick glance. Oftentimes, the standard examination fails to pick up on all of it because lesions can be uncharacteristic or evolve over time, sometimes resembling adult patterns. Physicians are forced to incorporate the use of tests such as dermoscopy, skin biopsies, blood work, and even microbiologic cultures to get a closer look at what is really happening. For instance, once localized scleroderma is in the pipeline, testing Borrelia serology and for extractable nuclear antigens (ENA) can subtly guide clinicians toward a stronger diagnosis and appropriate treatment regimen. Nevertheless, many practitioners lean heavily on their first impressions since these conditions appear so infrequently, and obviously this drives the necessity to mix in additional diagnostic testing to enhance accuracy and results (Hidv et al., 2018).

Today advances in imaging and lab methods have truly taken it to the next level for detecting inflammatory and autoimmune skin conditions in kids. Non-invasive technologies such as dermoscopy allow experts to take a real-time glance at structures of the skin, reducing the necessity for more invasive biopsies. Laboratory testing—serological panels and tests on inflammatory markers—sorts out conditions that appear too alike on the surface, like AD and cutaneous lupus. Accurate testing is really a necessity, as early treatment halts disease advancement and reduces long-term impacts. All the same, standardized protocols for all these tests remain quite different across regions, which in most instances indicates the necessity of more evidence-based protocols specifically for the pediatric population (Alam et al., 2018). A timely and accurate diagnosis is very important in the management of skin disorders in children, particularly in those rare instances where the symptoms may be insidious or even slightly misleading. Collecting a wide variety of diagnostic information, from lab tests to skin biopsies, not only supports clinical suspicions but also directs treatment choices along the way. Too often, however, not all practitioners adhere to recommended diagnostic guidelines strictly, which can result in undue delays in adequate management. Enhancing education on utilizing these tools and collaborating with referral centers can seriously enhance accuracy and treatment efficacy in managing rare pediatric skin diseases. The integration of these diagnostic tools into daily practice serves to improve the level of care and contribute to improved outcomes in young patients with skin disease (Alam et al., 2018; Hidv et al., 2018) (Figure 12.5).

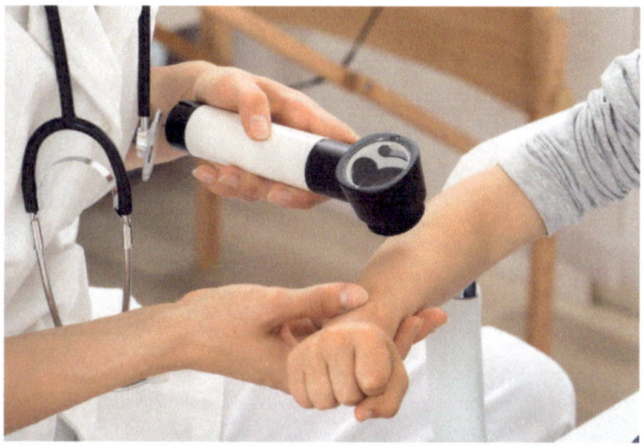

Figure 12.5. Diagnosing skin issues in kids using dermoscopy.

Source: Sri Krishna Hospitals. (2024). *Pediatric Dermatology Examination.* https://srikrishnahospitals.co.in/wp-content/uploads/sites/22/2024/08/Pediatric-Dermatology.png.

12.3. Treatment Options

Children's skin problems are not treated by medication alone. You absolutely must couple the proper drugs with open discussions with families regarding what to do, particularly with conditions like tinea capitis. This frequent fungal issue—if you do not identify precisely what it is—can set you on a misguided treatment course. Doctors typically rely on systemic antifungals, and terbinafine usually emerges victorious against culprits such as Trichophyton. But it is not simply a matter of writing prescriptions; ensuring that young patients adhere to their regimens and that families learn about good hygiene and controlling their environment is crucial to preventing reinfection and resistance to drugs. And then, of course, There is the emotional aspect of things—persistent or perceptible skin issues can have a real effect on a child's spirit, so a good diagnosis and follow-up go far in preventing trouble (Aditya et al., 2024). When behavioral skin disorders like skin picking disorder are concerned, the strategy is even more challenging. It is not solely a matter of the skin or the brain; physicians are now tasked with balancing both. Children demonstrating such behaviors from an early age need clinicians who can identify the problem and differentiate it from other dermatological conditions, avoiding treatments that may be unnecessary. In many cases, therapies such as cognitive-behavioral therapy assist in reducing the habit, and medications are reserved for when things simply do not get better. More recent work even suggests employing skin barrier interventions that are designed to reduce tissue harm and facilitate healing. Describing how, while skin picking can be a long-term issue, it is nevertheless not out of control really puts everyone's mind at rest and keeps everyone on the same page with the treatment protocol—testimony that a team effort is very best (Michael et al., 2022). Emerging treatment approaches in pediatric skin treatment are leading us toward more tailored plans. Gone is the single-size-fits-all approach; physicians now take into account the child's age, the severity of the condition, and even their emotional and social history. Improved laboratory techniques, such as enhanced fungal cultures and more accurate microscope work, are helping to select treatments that target the job and reduce unwanted side effects. On top of that, prevention strategies such as community education and lifestyle adjustments are turning out to be crucial in reducing both the spread and relapse of infection, especially with infectious conditions such as dermatophytosis. It is becoming increasingly evident that quality care equals interprofessional collaboration; by integrating doctors, families, and even public health teams, we treat not only the clinic consultation but also the social determinants of health. In general terms, this holistic approach demonstrates the way in which the specialty of pediatric dermatology is transforming into an entity that addresses both short-term requirements and long-term health (Aditya et al., 2024).

12.3.1. Topical Therapies and Their Applications

Frequently, topical solutions prove helpful when dealing with children's skin problems, as youngsters are particularly sensitive to drugs that reach all areas of the body.

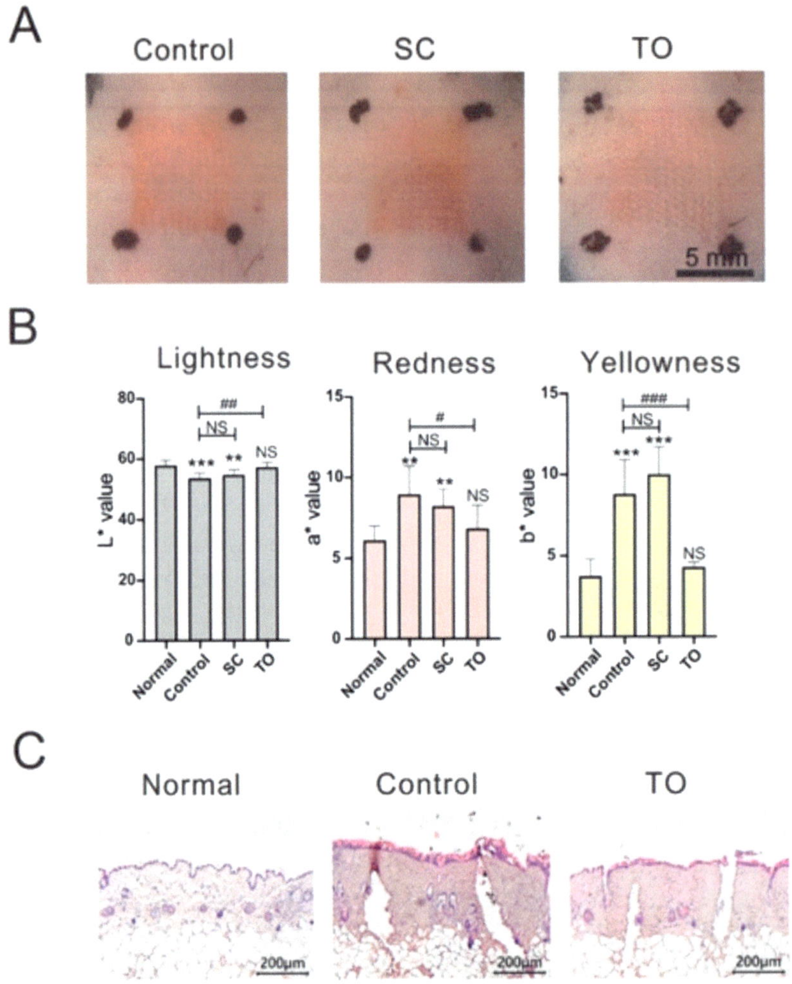

Figure 12.6. Mechanism of topical corticosteroids.

Source: Ou K-L, Wen C-C, Lan C-Y, Chen Y-A, Wang C-H, Wang Y-W. The Optimal Application of Medium Potency Topical Corticosteroids in Preventing Laser-Induced Inflammatory Responses—An Animal Study. *Life*. 2021; 11(4):350. https://doi.org/10.3390/life11040350

Rather than using drugs with systemic actions, these targeted therapies act precisely where they are needed, so professionals rely on agents such as corticosteroids, vitamin D analogs, and calcineurin inhibitors, each tailored to a particular illness or extent of disease. Consider, for instance, teen scalp psoriasis; a combination of calcipotriene and betamethasone dipropionate has been in the main effective by clearing lesions efficiently with minimal side effects. In most instances, this type of customized strategy ensures that it is safe to treat and that adolescent patients adhere to it in the long term (Eichenfield et al., 2014). Topical therapy is not only about the eradication of chronic inflammation; it also has a role in managing precancerous or neoplastic conditions of the skin, even when those are not commonly encountered in children. Managing actinic keratoses in elderly patients, for example, utilizing agents like ingenol mebutate, gives us an idea of how a concentrated, field-directed treatment can be.

Although such uses do not transfer specifically to pediatrics, the concept of targeting atypical skin cells is a common theme in pediatric dermatologic management. On the whole, early diagnosis coupled with the application of effective, well-tolerated topical agents does much to reduce the likelihood that a process becomes invasive. This strategy, in turn, leaves the door open for more exploration and development of treatments that enhance both safety and adherence among younger patients (Skroza et al., 2018). Formulating creams and ointments just for children requires close attention to how they are produced and applied. Kids' skin, usually thinner and of a different barrier function—requires formulations that work effectively and are gentle. For example, a once-daily regimen may minimize treatment burdens and irritation, a function that is particularly beneficial in long-term conditions such as psoriasis. It is often helpful to clearly explain the treatment regimen to the child and the caregiver in order to alleviate concerns regarding side effects and establish reasonable expectations. In the majority of instances, melding these wise, targeted therapies with an understanding of pediatric dermatologic nuances constitutes a comprehensive plan that typically improves both safety and efficacy in taking care of younger skin (Eichenfield et al., 2014; Skroza et al., 2018) (Figure 12.6).

12.3.2. Systemic Treatments for Severe Conditions

Children with rugged skin issues require more than creams. When creams and surface-level treatments fail for large, recalcitrant cases, physicians typically resort to treatments that affect the body as a whole. Consider AD—this prolonged flare sometimes requires drugs that reduce the immune system's reaction since its mechanisms are in disarray. More recently, newer medications such as particular antibodies that target the causing components of the immune system have made a significant impact.

These choices, which aim more precisely and safely, truly hammer home the point that treatment regimens need to suit each kid's individual requirements, weighing pros against potential risks (Lopes et al., 2020). The use of drugs that act systemically has created a new window of hope for children who did not respond to conventional remedies. Considering serious skin conditions in children, particularly uncommon ones like diffuse cutaneous mastocytosis, spotlights that rapid diagnosis and strong, systemic therapies are absolutely crucial. DCM, for short, poses actual peril because it triggers a mast cell and chemical rush, even causing sudden, intense allergic reactions and shocking changes in the skin. With no whole lot of treatment options for children, every option must be chosen methodically to target the underlying mutations while minimizing the symptoms. Recent case histories have even illuminated more about the genetic turns of fate that underpin the condition, allowing for more tailored treatments. These advances not only enhance the prognosis for numerous young patients but also highlight the challenges of managing unusual skin conditions, so a team-based strategy and vigilant ongoing monitoring becomes essential (Otani et al., 2018).

The way of today in pediatric skin care has truly evolved with the increasing involvement of systemic treatments, particularly since immune abnormalities tend to be at the core of serious diseases. Physicians are increasingly employing selective biologics and immunosuppressants to specifically address the damaged immune signals behind conditions like moderate-to-severe AD. For example, a medication such as dupilumab, which inhibits interleukin-4 and interleukin-13 signaling, has worked very well and serves to reduce the need for using more broad-spectrum immunosuppressants. It is also worth noting that stress, allergens, and other daily exposures can exacerbate these skin issues, so an approach that considers the big picture is key. In general, these systemic therapies must be integrated into a larger strategy for long-term stability and improved quality of life for children with severe dermatologic issues (Lopes et al., 2020).

12.3.3. Role of Phototherapy in Pediatric Dermatology

Current advances in children's skin care indicate light therapies have emerged as a convenient option. Phototherapy, employing alternatives such as NB-UVB and UVA1, adjusts the immune system to mitigate chronic inflammation and itching. AD, with its combination of immune dysbalances and external stimuli, is no picnic; too often, regular creams simply are not sufficient. This method, which reduces flare-ups without the severe side effects of systemic medications, can significantly benefit young patients by alleviating physical pain as well as the psychological burden of chronic conditions (Lopes et al., 2020). This non-drug treatment naturally aligns with comprehensive treatment strategies for pediatric skin conditions. Setting phototherapy standards for eczema in children appears quite important today. The global agreement, for the most part, identifies maintaining outcome measurement and follow-up procedures uniform assists. When physicians establish regular check-ups initially and then move to standard reviews, doctors can identify impending problems, such as photo-damage, early. When data collection is coordinated between centers, it is easier to compare studies, and there is a more transparent risk-benefit image (Vermeulen et al., 2019).

By doing so, the strategy not only accentuates clinical decision-making but also enhances international cooperation for improved patient outcomes. One should keep in mind that phototherapy is not an isolated remedy but part of a blended strategy for the treatment of children with moderate-to-severe skin issues. In most cases, such cases require more than one method; clinicians combine topical creams, systemic treatments, and light therapy to address the situation from all sides. Such a combined plan recognizes that triggers vary vastly across patients, and , honestly, responses can be unreliable. Phototherapy frequently takes over when not managed with creams alone and will often reduce dependency on steroids. Ongoing investigations—conducted through registries and clinical studies—continue to refine the balancing act between efficacy and safety. Ultimately, incorporating phototherapy into an individualized treatment plan supports enhanced long-term control and overall results in children presenting with chronic dermatologic issues (LopesVermeulen et al., 2019; Lopes et al., 2020).

12.4. Pediatric Dermatology and Allergies

Children with intractable skin problems tend to bring the entire package of allergy woes with them. AD appears quite frequently in such children's cases, consider persistent inflammation and that terrible itch, which sometimes arises together with asthma or even hay fever. Physicians believe these conditions have some common immune system circuitry, but precisely how skin eruptions and allergens connect is still somewhat of an enigma. Most children with AD have elevated IgE counts, but those figures do not always indicate the full extent of just how bad the condition is, which only complicates matters further when attempting to cure it. Some of the research on allergen-specific immunotherapy (SIT)—treatment that generally works for asthma or rhinitis—has returned with conflicting results for AD, particularly in more challenging cases, pushing us towards treatments that target the skin instead of vaguely interfering with the body's allergy system (Eichenfield et al., 2016). Immunotherapy, however, has some potential to manage IgE-mediated allergies in kids, although its place in pediatric dermatology is not yet cemented. Allergen immunotherapy (AIT) is one of the few methods believed to re-engineer the immune reaction at its core, a property very enticing during childhood when the immune system is more malleable. All that being said, where AD is concerned, the advantages of AIT have been all over the place. Dosages, treatment regimens, and even research methods all vary, which makes it difficult to pin down meaningful results. Regional variation in allergen blends and product availability in most instances only adds to the confusion, further muddying its application in child skincare (Caffarelli et al., 2018). On top of all this, long treatment courses, side effect concerns, and expense can turn it into a real challenge to adhere to therapy. Although avoidance of allergens is typically on the agenda, it infrequently gets AD symptoms in check alone. All this really speaks to the necessity of more balanced treatment regimens, ones that blend sound skin care with wise immune adjustments. Current studies, in the majority of instances, highlight the need for carefully conducted, standardized clinical trials to elucidate the place of AIT in pediatric AD and to facilitate more robust treatment recommendations (Eichenfield et al., 2016; Caffareli et al., 2018) (Figure 12.7).

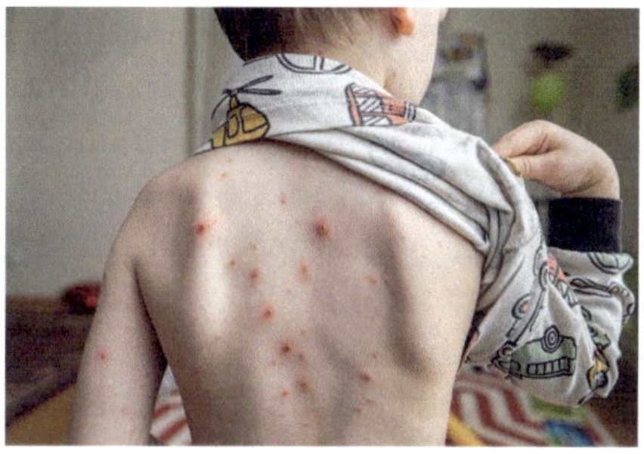

Figure 12.7. Skin allergy.

Source: Westchester Cosmetic Dermatology. (2024). *Pediatric Skin Treatment.* https://www.westchestercosmeticdermatology.com//files/2024/09/pediatric-skin-treatment-1536x1024.jpeg.

12.4.1. Connection Between Skin Conditions and Allergies

Skin microbes and allergies blend in ways not necessarily apparent, particularly in little children. The way a baby is born appears to be quite influential. Babies delivered by C-section, for example, are found in studies to have a different combination of skin pests—often more infections and allergies than babies who are born vaginally. This strange balancing act of microbes may nudge the immune system, making the little ones more susceptible to inflammation and allergies. Further, the day-to-day things, such as if the parent smokes can introduce even more danger for AD in those C-section infants

(Metin & Durmaz, 2023). It all suggests that providing that small microbial community with a good foundation could prevent skin issues and allergies. Clinical trials have been making waves in treating allergic skin conditions such as AD, a challenging disease that is all about itching and recurrent eczema. Rather than resorting to blanket immunosuppressants, physicians now target specific molecular signals that cause the flares. This newer, more specific treatment is a game-changer in children's medicine; timely diagnosis and clever, targeted interventions can decelerate the disease and enhance the quality of life. By exploring the ways the immune system gets tripped up on its own signals, doctors are learning to better contain inflammation, and calm persistent symptoms (Albulaihed et al., 2023). These changes show unmistakably that the management of allergic skin conditions is changing, even if that means dancing a little with a couple of surgical uncertainties along the way. If you compare both atopic and non-AD, you see how genes, environment, and immune reactions all become entwined in children's skin allergy. It is not that just being delivered by C-section brings this about; there are other things, such as a history of allergies in the family or parents smoking, which appear to tip the balance toward atopic symptoms. Surprisingly, children who already have allergies born by C-section sometimes develop fewer infectious skin issues, suggesting an intriguing balance between microbial colonization and immune function. Generally speaking, how well the skin withstands it and how the immune system adapts to functioning appears to be influenced by innate qualities as well as daily exposure. Unraveling these contradictions is the key to developing improved treatments and maybe even preventive measures for pediatric skin allergies (Metin & Durmaz, 2023).

12.4.2. Common Allergic Reactions in Children

Children frequently experience allergic responses that do not fit an organized, textbook pattern. Allergic skin rashes, particularly in individuals with AD, are apt to get complex up with problems such as asthma and sneezing allergy. In many cases, IgE levels are high, but they do not always correlate neatly with how bad the condition becomes—so using them as markers alone is a little deceptive. Most of them. Children's immune reactions tend to vacillate in ways that are described but not completely understood, so they often do not respond to allergy avoidance measures such as simply staying away from allergens. The long-term effectiveness of treatments like SIT is still in the air, due to the variable and conflicting evidence, but especially for children with more extreme symptoms (Eichenfield et al., 2016). Allergen immunotherapy (AIT) has, in the majority of instances, generated a great deal of interest as a potential means to re-direct the immune system in early stages, particularly in IgE-mediated conditions such as allergic rhino-conjunctivitis and even asthma. Nevertheless, in the context of allergic skin conditions like extrinsic AD, its place is more controversial. Scientists tend to grapple with inconsistent results potentially because of varying dosing regimens, non-standardized treatment protocols, and a blend of side effect reports that complicate attempts to lock down exactly how well it works. Ongoing trials do keep things moving, however, with expectations that working these methods further might provide a more consistent method of controlling children's allergic episodes in real life (Caffarelli et al., 2018). At times, it is a matter of understanding that immune reactions in children change with time. Some children may outgrow conditions such as AD spontaneously, while others may end up acquiring new sensitivities or even whole new allergic conditions. This constantly shifting landscape makes clinical decisions a balancing act, with the timing of interventions (such as immunotherapy) needing to balance potential benefits against potential risks and the daily struggle to stay on treatment. With allergies both inherited and inspired by the world around us, after all, we require an approach that is a good fit for the individual, not a one-size-fits-all solution. Combining skin-directed therapies with more general immune therapies – and adjusting them according to the specific circumstances of each child – remains central to achieving optimal results in pediatric allergic disease management (Eichenfield et al., 2016; Caffareli et al., 2018) (Figure 12.8).

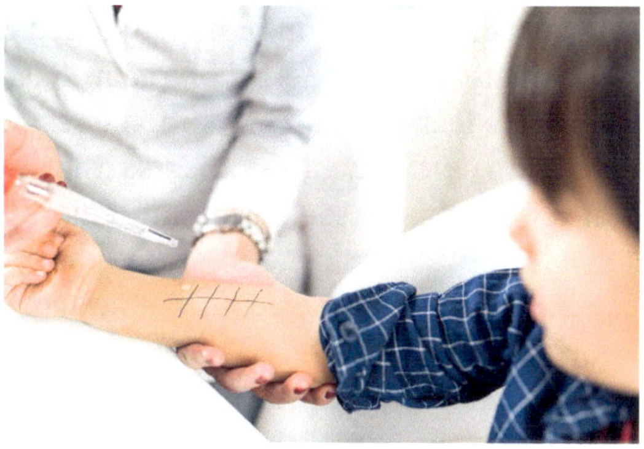

Figure 12.8. Allergy testing for children.

Source: Singapore O&G Ltd. (2022). *Allergy Testing for Children.* https://www.sog.com.sg/wp-content/uploads/2022/04/blog-allergy-testing-for-children-scaled.jpg.

12.4.3. Management of Allergic Skin Disorders

Treating allergic skin conditions in children is not merely a matter of soothing a break-out—it is knowing that there are so many elements at work. AD is one of the more prevalent disorders, influenced both by a child's innate nature and the environment around them. You cannot just work to alleviate the discomfort; you also need to consider how the overall health of the skin impacts daily life. Daily moisturizers repair the skin barrier, and ointments such as topical corticosteroids or even calcineurin inhibitors suppress the inflammation. When it gets more challenging, with severe to moderate cases, physicians resort to systemic immunosuppressants or biologic medications like dupilumab, which target cytokines IL-4 and IL-13. It is also worth noting that the emotional frustration of coping with AD is not imaginary (Lopes et al., 2020), so an integrative plan is essential—no matter how many medications it entails. Determining just how bad a child's skin allergies are requires close observation and an elastic plan. Most specialists today rely on such measures as the SCORAD index to provide an independent assessment of the severity of the disease, and in most instances, this assists in determining the way forward. At other times, even the straightforward process of wet wrap therapy can enhance the efficacy of topical corticosteroids, keeping flare-ups in check. There is tacrolimus ointment employed prophylactically to reduce the number of such recurrences, easing life a little. Although new treatments such as crisaborole are offered now, they typically do not do the trick for the severe ones. And where clarity is not crystal-clear, physicians may take a skin biopsy to eliminate any look-alike conditions. Immunotherapy can be a useful added-on for children with both skin and respiratory allergies, not something to avoid but to augment the primary treatment (Sastre et al., 2020). Despite all these breakthroughs, managing allergic skin diseases in children comes with its own set of difficulties. Conventional methods such as systemic management and light (phototherapy) may not reach all the targets in the case of severe disease, which sets focus on biological therapies that target the Th2 inflammatory process underlying AD. The advent of therapies such as dupilumab, a monoclonal antibody, is a true game-changer, providing safer, long-term management with fewer side effects; but without established tests or biomarkers to determine who is most likely to benefit, making the correct decision can be like trying to complete a puzzle. This lack of trustworthy diagnostics clouds up decision-making and tells us that we have more to do. Evidently, continued study, some trial and error, and willingness to adopt new concepts still are indispensable for refining treatment protocols that work for these children (Sastre et al., 2020).

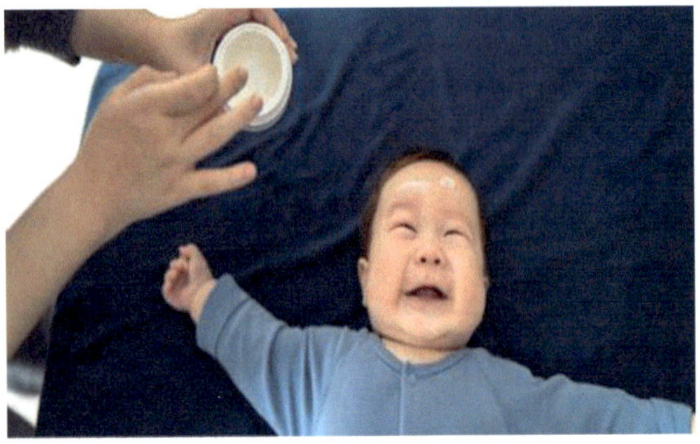

Source: HealthyChildren.org. (n.d.). *Applying Moisturizing Cream to a Baby*. American Academy of Pediatrics. https://www.healthychildren.org/SiteCollectionImagesArticleImages/applying-moisturizing-cream.jpg?RenditionID=3.

12.5. Psychological Impact of Skin Conditions

Children suffering from skin conditions endure much more than simply irritating itchiness. They also grapple with physical irritation due to conditions such as eczema or psoriasis but frequently battle inner emotional and social issues as well. Ongoing itching and discomfort can disrupt daily routines and even sleeping, which—talking broadly—fuels emotional tension. Unexpectedly, what parents tell us about the distress of their children is not always the whole story; research suggests that parents may underrepresent the true itch whilst inadvertently overreport feelings of embarrassment or loneliness (Leahy & Murphy, 2024). It then appears that allowing children to report directly from themselves provides a more accurate impression of the burden that these conditions place, particularly in those formative years of development. Visible skin issues may induce more than mere bodily discomfort; most often, they precipitate social challenges which can have a significant impact on a child's self-esteem.

Some children are so embarrassed about their appearance that they avoid forming friendships, despite parents being prompt to report concerns regarding bullying or ostracism. Strangely, the children themselves may not necessarily sequence out these dilemmas, but merely fear or expectation of being judged can create anxiety and erode self-esteem. Such a cycle—where fear makes it harder to be resilient and leads to withdrawal—indicates that it is crucial to confront these social and emotional issues. More often than not, a care plan with both skin and emotional aftermath in mind is the best for these little ones. Incorporating mental health care into the regimen of skin treatments is fairly important, as well. New concepts such as Mindful Self-Compassion (MSC) have been found to decrease symptoms of depression, anxiety, and stress, increasing self-esteem and quality of life in skin conditions. Although a lot of this work has been conducted with adults, there is a good chance that applying these techniques to children might enable them to develop stronger emotional resilience and coping mechanisms. Dermatologists and mental health professionals collaborating—though not always in a neatly wrapped package—seem to provide a more holistic type of care. This sort of holistic approach could be the answer to providing kids with the comprehensive, individualized assistance they require.

12.5.1. Effects on Self-Esteem and Social Interactions

Children with skin problems tend to struggle with more than a physical level of pain. Public conditions, consider AD as a case in point—can unsettle the inner confidence of a child, sometimes making them shy or even edgy. It is not unusual to witness these kids begin to withdraw from friends and become cranky; in extreme instances, the condition may even prevent them from going to school, where social interaction during the day makes a significant contribution to becoming socially developed. And when you consider it, the harder the skin issue, the more the emotional impact accumulates, and that informs us that addressing both the outer scars and the internal conflict is most important (Goodings et al., 2024).

Adolescence, however, introduces a whole other level of complications. As appearance becomes imbued with additional significance in adolescence, an observable skin disorder has the potential to fuel concerns regarding body image and cause social interactions to become strained. In general, research on inherited skin conditions indicates that even though the stigma may not be immediately apparent, the persistent doubts regarding appearance have the ability to disrupt the way teens feel among others and erode self-esteem. Very frequently, these teenagers worry about how they appear at the moment and worry about the future, sometimes resulting in phases of withdrawal or even falling into depression if one does not take any action (Barke et al., 2016). Viewing the larger picture, managing skin illness in children translates into attending to body and mind. It is not about just blurring the rash; it is about learning about the daily emotional potholes along the way. Frequently, doctors collaborate with dermatologists, mental health professionals, and social service workers to assemble a care plan that feels just right for each child. By providing an environment in which both the body may recover and the spirit may be strengthened, clinicians may reduce the blow to self-esteem and prevent social lives from crashing. Ultimately, this type of total care contributes greatly to improving long-term emotional well-being and overall quality of life for children and their families (Goodings et al., 2024).

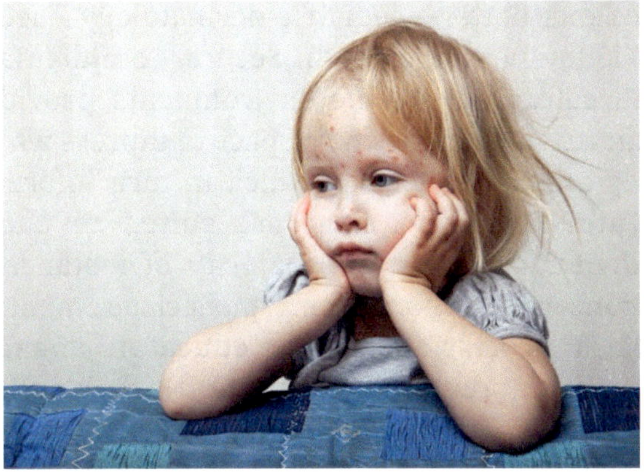

Source: Indian Crest Pediatrics. (2022, June). *Common Skin Problems in Children.* https://www.indiancrestpeds.com/wp-content/uploads/2022/06/Common-Skin-Problems-in-Children.jpg.

12.5.2. Importance of Mental Health Support

Chronic skin conditions in children strike far beyond mere marks on the surface of their bodies—they complicate a whole compounding of social and emotional issues. Children with noticeable disorders typically end up feeling isolated, a sense of stigma that confuses their mental well-being in ways people commonly overlook in routine clinical inspections. Research shows for the most part that when a skin condition is clear and severe, it will cause an inferior quality of life, greater depression and anxiety, and even smaller social circles. It is not sufficient to have a physician merely check off physical signs; the kids' internal struggles deserve attention as well. Identifying these hidden charges can open the door to earlier support, both emotionally and in coping with their skin problems, which might reduce bullying and loneliness (Paller et al., 2024). Creating a network for mental health support in children's skin care involves addressing a complex mix of cultural, environmental, and individual factors. Consider the way some universities demand to increase multicultural self-understanding among personnel so that they can serve overseas students better—pediatric dermatology needs to follow a similar path. Secure, confidential, and culturally specific environments provide children and families with space to express what they are experiencing, which in turn informs treatment options that are suited to each individual case. In the majority of instances, a concerted action among physicians, mental health professionals, and educators makes certain that required care is not a one-size-fits-all answer. Such a combination can combat the deeper social issues associated with chronic skin conditions, enabling young patients to develop resilience and enhance general well-being (Sak et al., 2024). Family members, particularly caregivers, also play an enormous role. Many times, parents are the primary champions and stabilizing influence on their children dealing with these outward conditions. Some research, even though sometimes it presents an incomplete picture, indicates that parents may not always have a complete understanding of the bullying or stigma their children are experiencing, which indicates a genuine need for increased parental leadership. Empowering families with basic coping techniques and straightforward psychosocial information promotes a more favorable home atmosphere, tempering the brutal psychological effect. Such constant, at times faulty, collaboration among clinicians and families is critical to maintaining stigma at bay and enhancing the general management of the disorder (Paller et al., 2024).

12.5.3. Strategies for Coping and Support

Children struggling with severe skin problems require more than medication. Usually, such children are shunned and even blamed, triggering additional anxiety and deterring them from continuing their treatments. Healthcare professionals, for the most part, seek to create a comfortable environment in which children feel at ease talking about their worries, adapted to what they comprehend at their level. Family members getting involved in the care process provides an added dimension of comfort, a form of emotional safety net that makes a difference. Tackling body and feelings simultaneously enhances resilience and self-esteem, demonstrating that a combination of varying expertise is important for maximizing overall outcomes. An example is psychodermatology, an organized field that bridges skin issues with emotions that accompany them. Visible characteristics such as hair loss always carry a high emotional price tag, impacting health regardless of how extreme the affliction appears. Combining a routine skin maintenance routine with regular mental health consultations and counseling catches problems like depression and anxiety early. This means dermatologists must pay attention to indicators of underlying distress and collaborate with mental health professionals.

Even some clinics are experimenting with joint dermatology-psychiatry arrangements, a fairly innovative approach that allows for early, comprehensive support for child patients (Cameron et al., 2021). Including strong support networks and plain education components also brings dramatic improvements. When children and families receive clear, easy-to-grasp information on skin disorders, it reduces anxiety and uncertainty, turning treatment into a collaborative, active process.

Peer groups assist, also—they create a sense of community and reduce that isolation many experiences. Teens, who struggle with things like self-esteem and even concern about impending health, can use a bit more direction (as observed in more comprehensive adolescent oncology strategies that might be applicable to skin clinics as well (Bhatia et al., 2023)). Together, these diverse approaches emphasize that treating skin conditions effectively involves taking care of the entire individual, not merely the visible aspects.

12.6. Preventive Care and Education

Children's skin problems are best addressed early on with a combination of prevention and easy, everyday tips. Parents and caregivers who are taught to pick up on even the slightest whispers of issues, such as the early signs of eczema, tiny patches of psoriasis or a smidge of acne—can really assist in keeping things from deteriorating. Easy-to-write-about points regarding cleaning the skin, observing environmental triggers, and even determining if There is a genetic component to all this can amount to a great deal. For instance, in tuberous sclerosis complex conditions; the newest guidelines tend to favor identifying and monitoring problems immediately so that skin issues along with broader complications do not get out of hand (Northrup et al., 2021).

Routine skin check-ups and down-to-earth advice together go a long way in stopping chronic problems before they fully set in. Education programs aimed at families and healthcare individuals are another big piece of the puzzle. These efforts usually dish out practical tips on dodging allergens, using moisturizers correctly, and catching safe sun exposure—important when dealing with delicate, young skin. At times, such programs loop back to foundational concepts to assist in reducing flare-ups of inflammatory conditions.

They even include genetic counseling, where families are provided advice on how hereditary skin ailments would appear and what they should observe, particularly when there is an indication of cancer risk associated with skin symptoms (Mary et al., 2021). More often than not, this sort of hands-on knowledge sharing makes everyone feel more ready, and it even sometimes generates a team effort when there are several specialists who must contribute. Since kid skin issues tend to alter quite rapidly, making guidelines and tips current is somehow essential. It is all about equilibrium: combining what we realize about genes, day-to-day environment, and the varying phases a child experiences. Physicians, for instance, need to stay abreast of changes in how such things as cortical tubers or even sclerotic bone lesions of some inherited skin diseases are classified so that they are able to identify problems earlier rather than later (Northrup et al., 2021). Concurrently, providing a little extra information through genetic counseling regarding risks, such as those associated with cancer—provides another helpful layer for maintaining close surveillance (Mary et al., 2021). Integrating new knowledge into routine care not only repairs issues as they arise but also maintains an eye towards future issues by emphasizing early intervention and continued learning.

12.6.1. Importance of Skin Care Routines

Children's skin problems are best treated with a consistent, child-friendly regimen. Most afflictions—eczema, in particular—require continuous, diligent care to minimize flare-ups and maintain skin integrity. The psychological impact on children and their families from chronic skin issues makes it apparent that this is not so much about instant solutions. All too frequently, eczema is discounted as something temporary, and so caregivers may overlook the fact that consistent care makes all the difference in reducing symptoms and improving overall health. A regimen that combines frequent moisturizing, gentle washing, and appropriate topical therapy can truly relieve discomfort and prevent abrupt flare-ups. It is also extremely critical to provide caregivers with clear, consistent advice because blended or confusing suggestions may easily ruin the regimen (Teasdale et al., 2020). Most of the time, long-term thinking regarding skin wellness trumps the pursuit of an unattainable remedy. In addition to this, daily regimens for children must address additional skin difficulties that may arise from the use of medical devices. For kids on something like continuous glucose monitors or insulin pumps, skin issues tend to appear precisely where the device is in contact with the skin.

Problems such as contact dermatitis, irregular fat deposits, and so on tend to appear at these areas, making it even more complicated. These rashes and bumps not only add to the discomfort but at times compel families to discontinue device use, then disruptions happen with overall disease control. A regimen that involves swapping device locations, keeping a close watch for soon-to-appear irritation signals, and applying protective barrier creams works significantly in maintaining control (Podwojniak et al., 2024). A small adjustment in the care regimen sometimes makes a tangible difference. Finally, how children are feeling emotionally is as crucial as managing the physical symptoms. Kids with chronic skin conditions tend to feel embarrassed or alienated, and that blow to their self-esteem can impact whether they adhere to treatment programs. A good regimen does not simply regulate body symptoms—it also assists in empowering the child, as well as the child's family, to feel more in control of the situation. Simple, consistent, and straightforward skin care guidance can alleviate confusion and frustration that arises from mixed directions. By doing so, a well-crafted daily schedule serves as a solid foundation for medical care and emotional support for the numerous interwoven difficulties of pediatric patients and their families (Teasdale et al., 2020) (Figure 12.9).

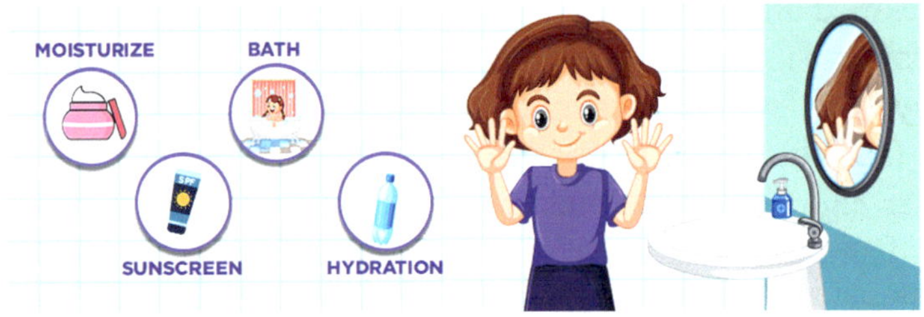

Figure 12.9. Skincare routine for kids.

Source: Bachpan Global. (2024). *Children's Skincare Routine Illustration.* https://www.bachpanglobal.com/blog/wp-content/uploads/2024/01/main.jpg.

12.6.2. Educating Parents About Skin Health

Parents being aware of something about their children's skin problems can make a great difference in catching problems early. Oftentimes, these issues appear with barely visible signs that may be misinterpreted or easily overlooked—this may cause delays in treatment, which, in most instances, creates more problems in the future. By posting daily information about what normal skin signs and symptoms appear like and the danger involved, parents become more prepared to seek assistance before complications arise. Medical education research even suggests that most trainees do not always understand when to refer a child to a dermatologist, which emphasizes the importance of educating not only physicians but also family caregivers (Adel et al., 2025). With a clearer idea of what to be on the lookout for, families can determine whether it is worth making an appointment with a dermatologist or whether they should stick with their primary care physician alone, getting the precise treatment they need while avoiding unnecessary worry. Long-term skin issues in kids bring a whole new level of complexity—not only physically but mentally as well. Such conditions as AD or vitiligo are not only evident on the skin; they often have accompanying social stigma that can erode a child's confidence and well-being. For most children, research indicates a strong correlation between the visibility of the condition, the stigma attached, and ensuing stress (Paller et al., 2024). When parents have a good understanding of these interconnected issues, they are more able to provide genuine support, advocate for their child's needs, and collaborate with healthcare professionals. And then, too, when caregivers realize that bullying and social barriers frequently accompany such conditions, they can intervene with solutions that resolve both the outward signs and inner emotional difficulties, a more holistic approach to childhood skin conditions. On the more applied level, providing parents with explicit guidance on skin care habits, identification of warning signs, and even managing stigma is essential in pediatric dermatology training. Caregiver advice should include maintaining skin cleanliness in terms that suit the child's age and circumstances, observing what may exacerbate the issue, and recognizing when it is truly necessary to involve a specialist (Adel et al., 2025).

Additionally, having a candid conversation about emotional highs and lows and social challenges can help children develop resilience and learn how to cope. Health professionals, in turn, have a vital function in sharing this advice in an uncomplicated, supportive manner, ensuring that parents have the impression that they are a vital component of monitoring their child's skin care. Ultimately, when parents are well-educated and somewhat less stressed out about such matters, treatment adherence is made simpler, the general burden of the condition decreases, and physical and emotional results for the child receive a much-needed boost.

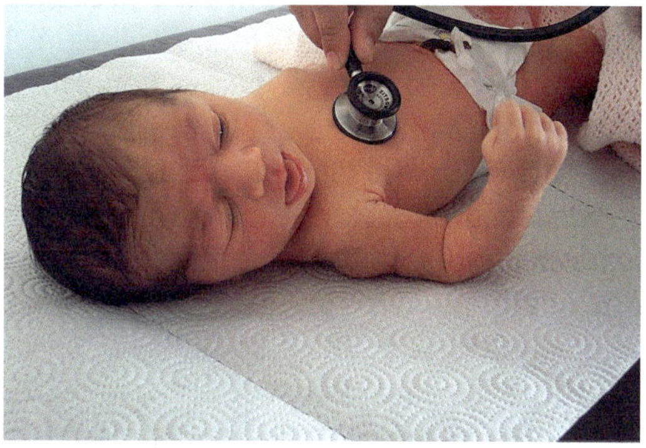

Source: By Nevit Dilmen - Own work, CC BY-SA 3.0, https://commons.wikimedia.org/w/index.php?curid=1428959

12.6.3. Role of Schools in Promoting Skin Health Awareness

Schools can do a great deal about how children learn to look after themselves, particularly in the area of skin care. Children spend most of their day in school, so these environments are an obvious place to casually mention looking after their skin. The process begins with basic advice, such as keeping to a routine, paying attention to small bumps or spots, and seeking assistance early rather than late. Meanwhile, schools have an opportunity to dispel some of those skin disorder myths that can play havoc with a teenager's self-esteem. Education about how the sun can impact the skin, plus basic hygiene and a little about what one should and should not eat, sort of gets integrated into general efforts, such as staying away from acne or sunburn. In general, these continuous programs could result in fewer skin issues when combined with increased awareness of health by the students (Marilyn et al., 2022). But it is not all about the instructions within a classroom. Schools tend to collaborate with specialists, pediatricians, and dermatologiststo keep a close watch. A regular skin screening at school could get early symptoms of conditions such as eczema, acne, or even infection under way before parents and physicians can get in on it quickly. Occasionally, specialists will conduct a workshop that not only brings the children up to speed on what to look for but also provides school nurses and faculty with some practical advice on how to detect any abnormal changes. Schools also draw on the home environment in so far as they encourage parents to come along for a chat or seminar, building something of a three-way system of care that combines professional guidance with day-to-day support (Marilyn et al., 2022). And then there is the curriculum angle. Adding real, evidence-based information about skin health into normal learning appears to be the next sensible step. Consider acne, for example, a rather widespread problem with many teens that can get under their skin. Describing the fundamentals of what happens with it, the various treatment choices, and the small changes one can make in their lifestyle that could help make a big difference. And then, if students learn about intelligent sun protection, which is not simply some fleeting summer phenomenon—it can reduce the chances of something more severe, such as melanoma, later in life. In general, with these types of lessons integrated into the regular rhythm of school life, students begin to understand how important it is to take care of their skin. Ultimately, this strategy, with a little assistance from skin professionals—serves to create a generation that, through a little daily self-care and an understanding of when to seek advice, can avoid both acute and chronic skin issues.

CLOSER LOOK

Cold Atmospheric Plasma (CAP) Therapy

CAP therapy, a technology producing a partially ionized gas at room temperature, holds potential for the treatment of numerous pediatric skin diseases, such as infections, wounds, and inflammatory diseases. Its efficacy can be attributed to the production of reactive oxygen and nitrogen species (RONS) and ultraviolet (UV) radiation, which can be used to fight microbial infections, induce healing in wounds, and possibly suppress the growth of tumor cells. Although further research is being conducted, CAP therapy has proven to be safe and effective in treating disorders such as AD and molluscum contagiosum in pediatric patients.

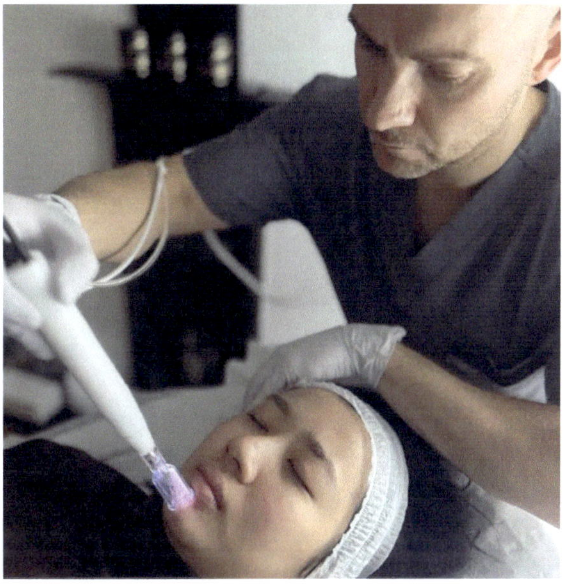

Source: Millward, A. (2024). Cold Atmospheric Plasma Facial Treatment.

- Key Applications of CAP in Pediatric Dermatology
  - Infectious Skin Diseases: CAP has shown antimicrobial activity against bacteria, viruses, and fungi and thus may be used to treat diseases such as molluscum contagiosum and fungal infections.
  - Wound Healing: CAP has the ability to stimulate tissue regeneration and facilitate wound healing, and provide a possible alternative or adjunct to standard wound care for children with chronic wounds or burns.
  - Inflammatory Skin Diseases: CAP has the potential to relieve symptoms of AD, a prevalent inflammatory skin disease among children, by controlling inflammation and minimizing the intensity of lesions.
  - Other Uses: Current research is investigating CAP's use in the treatment of other childhood skin disorders, including actinic keratoses, alopecia (hair loss), and certain skin cancers.

- Safety and Efficacy in Children

Research has indicated that CAP therapy is safe and well tolerated in children, with few side effects noted. More research is required to determine the long-term effects and best parameters for the use of CAP in pediatric dermatology.

- Mechanisms of Action

CAP's therapeutic action is due to various mechanisms, which are:

  - Reactive Oxygen and Nitrogen Species (RONS): These species produced by the plasma can directly harm microorganisms, induce tissue regeneration, and regulate the immune system.
  - Ultraviolet Radiation: The UV radiation of the plasma may be antimicrobial and may induce cell proliferation.
  - Thermal Effects: Although CAP is "cold," it does have some ability to create heat, and this may be part of its therapeutic value.
  - Modulation of Skin Barrier Function: CAP can modulate the skin barrier function by modifying lipid composition and enhancing drug permeability.

SUMMARY

Children with skin conditions require care that brings together various medical specialists and individualized regimens. Today, skin conditions in children appear in unexpected forms, so physicians must be swift and accurate in their diagnoses to avoid complications and enable these children to live healthier. Occasionally, these skin manifestations persist with system-wide issues, complicating treatment. New possibilities—simple medicines targeting particular targets blended with plain changes in routine, are taking center stage. Interestingly, even pediatric migraines have, at times, been linked with such things as nerve inflammation and imbalances in the gut (Khan et al., 2025). Combining various treatments in this way may revolutionize the field, finding that perfect balance between being effective and being safe as kids develop. Getting in on it early is important; not only to alleviate symptoms but also because delaying treatment may put kids on a path to long-term skin issues and anxiety that strikes their self-esteem and makes it more difficult to spend time with friends. Little children can end up having to manage problems that impact social life and general mental health. New evidence tends to follow in the direction of adding tested, non-pharmacologic strategies to standard treatments. Factors such as stress reduction, adjusting the diet, and improved sleep habits may have much to do with soothing inflammatory or allergic skin rashes. These types of integrated steps involve what is proven to work in other pediatric cases where body and mind are engaged in the process, reminding us that child-centered care really matters. For most, combining medical and lifestyle changes can lead the way to improved outcomes and prevent chronic skin issues from getting established. Even with the progress we have seen, diagnosing and handling skin complications that tie into wider health problems still poses a real challenge. Take, for example, infections such as pediatric infective endocarditis – these often give doctors a hard time because their causes vary so much and tests can come back negative (Naguthevar et al., 2025). Skin manifestations associated with underlying infections or congenital diseases require physicians to stay vigilant and frequently collaborate hand in hand by specialty. Upcoming research would likely be best directed toward refining diagnostic techniques and expanding treatment options that suit the individual child's body and immune characterestics. Longitudinal studies can inform us about the natural history of such skin conditions and their association with other diseases, helping us to direct our care more effectively. When new knowledge is blended with treatments developed uniquely for each child, pediatric dermatology will advance, hopefully promoting healthier tomorrows for our children.

Having an understanding of a child's biology is crucial when it comes to addressing skin problems. Physicians will occasionally steal concepts from physical therapy to inform how they treat a young patient's skin issues. Rather than adhering rigidly to symptoms in the skin, they will frequently scan for signs of functional difficulties, leaving the door open to treatment approaches that truly meet each child's individual requirements. Some child dermatologists blend concepts from other disciplines, a tactic that ultimately explains both diagnosis and intervention strategy. Conversing between disciplines and speaking in plain terms can enhance clinical choice and keep families informed in the long run (Cobb et al., 2025). New studies, for example, identify the part played by environmental and sensory factors in a baby's overall development, and that may impact skin conditions as well. Such factors as touch, light, and even balance appear to influence the way an infant's brain and immune system function, which in turn subtly impacts the skin. In general, observing how tactile signals or visual inputs modify immune reactions contributes to fine-tuning treatments to reduce inflammation and fortify the skin barrier. Such a line of thinking pushes care in the direction of considering both internal skin problems and the effects of the environment (Deng et al., 2025). Combining concepts from movement-based tests and the advantages of a stimulating environment provides a layered model that can truly assist in pediatric dermatology. Individualized plans that integrate routine skin examination with testing for motor, cognitive, or sensory development could result in improved outcomes. Pediatric skin experts are frequently urged to collaborate with other child health professionals, employing a combination of classic tests and wider developmental observations. This collaborative, occasionally sound methodology not only addresses what appears on the surface but also uncovers the underlying forces at work, all in the interest of enhancing the lives of young patients and maintaining care focused on the entire family (Cobb et al., 2025; Deng et al., 2025).

KEY TERMS FROM THIS CHAPTER

Adolescents	Babies	Betamethasone dipropionate
Birthmarks	Children	Clinical skills
Down syndrome	Filaggrin	Fixed-dose triple-combo gel
Hygiene	Tuberous sclerosis	Unwanted attention
Pediatric dermatology	Pilomatricomas	Rash
Social embarrassment	Treatments	Trichoscopy

REFERENCES

1. Al-Najjar, *A. M., Al-shameri, A. A., Al-Khateeb, A., Al-Darwani,* A., Al-Boaithi, B., Al-Othmani, M., Jobair, M., et al. (2025). Awareness among 5th–6th year medical students towards referring to appropriate specialist, a dermatologist or a pediatrician, when dealing with common pediatric skin diseases. International Journal of Clinical & Experimental Dermatology. https://doi.org/10.36899/IJCE.*2024.2023.*
2. *Al-Najjar, A.* M., Al-shameri, A. A., Al-Selwi, A. A., Al-Saeedi, M., Al-Khateeb, A., Al-Darwani, A., Al-Boaithi, B., et al. (2025). Awareness among medical students towards referring children with skin diseases whether to a dermatologist or a pediat*rician. I*nternational Journal of Clinical & Experimental Dermatology. https://doi.org/10.36899/IJCE.2024.2016.
3. Alam, M., Murad, A., Andea, A. A., Argenyi, Z., & Armbrect, S. (2018). Appropriate use criteria in dermatopathology: Initial recommendations from the American Society of Dermatopathology. Deep Blue. Retrieved from: http://deepblue.lib.umich.edu/bitstream/2027.42/145218/1/cup13142.pdf (accessed on 12 May 2025).
4. Albulaihed, A. K., Almansour, A. F., Hashim, A., Yaseen, A. K., Aldhafeer, E. S. A., Al Hussain, A. I., Almenyan, M., et al. (2023). Assessment and management of atopic dermatitis in primary care settings. Core. Retrieved from: https://doi.org/10.53555/jaz.v44iS3.1926
5. Alghasham, Yazeed A; Altheyab, Fatimah Yahya; Alkhalifah, Yasir Saleh; Alnadawi, Hadeel Ahmed; Alharbi, Tuqa Yousif; Aloraini, Lina Yousef; Alghaith, Abdullah Mohammed; Almesned, Abdulelah Ahmad; Almutairi, Khaled Ghazzai. Risk factors of eczema among pediatric groups in Qassim region, Saudi Arabia. Saudi Journal for Health Sciences 14(1):p 66-71, Jan–A*pr 2*025. | DOI: 10.4103/sjhs.sjhs_153_24 (accessed on 12 May 2025).
6. Alhuthayli, A. K. A., Almalki, A. S. O., Alharbi, A. S. A., Alneami, A. M., Fadl, A. A., Alsahli, H. M., Ayed Alshammari, H. S., et al. (2023). Pediatric dermatology in family medicine: Common conditions and management strategies. Core. Retrieved from: https://core.ac.uk/download/603897541.pdf.
7. Arasi*, S., Corsello, G., Villani, A. et al. The future outlook o*n allergen immunotherapy in children: 2018 and beyond. Ital J Pediatr 44, 80 (2018). https://doi.org/10.1186/s13052-018-0519-4 (accessed on 12 May 2025).
8. Ashton, R., & Weinstein, M. (2019). Acne vulgaris in the pediatric patient. Pediatrics in Review, 40, 577–589. https://doi.org/10.1542/pir.2018-01*37.*
9. *Barke, J., Coad, J., & Harcourt, D. (2016). The Role of* Appearance in Adolescents' Experiences of Neurofibromatosis Type 1: A Survey of Young People and Parents. Journal of genetic counseling, 25(5), 1054–1062. https://doi.org/10.1007/s10897-016-9944-y (accessed on 12 May 2025).
10. Bhatia, S., Pappo, A. S., Acquazzino, M., Allen-Rhoades, W., Barnett, M., Borinstein, S. C., Casey, R., et al. (2023). Adolescent and young adult (AYA) oncology, version 2.2024, NCCN clinical practice guidelines in oncology. Journal of the National Comprehensive Cancer Network, 21, 851–880. *https://doi.org/10.6004/jnccn.2023.*0040.
11. Bull, M. J., Trotter, T. L., Santoro, S. L., Christensen, C. K., & Grout, R. W. (202*2). He*alth supervision for children and adolescents with Down syndrome. PEDIATRI*CS, 149. https:*//doi.org/10.1542/peds.2022-057010.

12. Chessa, M., Baracca, M. F., Rossi, A. N., Piraccini, B. M., De Pietro, V., Picciola, V. M., Gelmetti, A., et al. (2024). Pilomatricoma: Clinical, dermoscopic findings and management in 55 pediatric patients and concise review of the literature with special emphasis on dermoscopy. Dermatology Practical & Con*ceptual, 14. https://www.semantics*cholar.org/paper/d3565c615a2a5d937f6bd670aa6fc051ff73caa0 (accessed on 12 May 2025).

13. Cobb, Lorene P PT, DPT, EdD, PCS; Shane, Kelly Ann PT, DPT; McGee, Patr*icia Navarro PT, DPT, PC*S; Nesbit, Casey PT, DPT; Brennan, Ellen PT, DPT, PCS; Moore, Jim PT, PhD; Girolami, Gay L PT, PhD; Dannemiller, Lisa PT, DSc, PCS; Donaldson, Cathron PT, DPT; Boynewics, Kara PT, DPT, PhD; Carey, Helen PT, DHSc, PCS; Chase, Kris*tine Michelle PT, DPT, PCS; Hall, Amanda* PT, MPT; Jones, Maryleen PT, MPT, DHS, CLT, NCS; O'Shea, Roberta Kuchler PT, DPT, PhD; Zipp, Genevieve Pinto PT, EdD, FNAP. Movement System Diagnosis: A Consensus-Based Position for Pediatric Movement Specialists. Pediatric Physical Therapy 37(2):p 257-264, April 2025. | DOI: 10.1097/PEP.0000000000001186(*accessed on 12 May 2025).*

14. Crockett, J. L., Kim, S., von Scheven, E., Mathur, A., & Cordoro, K. (2024). Combined pediatric rheumatology/dermatology clinics: Benefits and challenges. Pediatric Dermatology. https://www.semanticscholar.org/paper/cf008107a4f95b9bba2135915*9f467c94ba5de22* (accessed on 12 May 2025).

15. Daly, M. B., Pal, T., Berry, M. P., Buys, S. S., Dickson, P., Domchek, S. M., Elkhanany, A., et al. (2021). Genetic/familial high-risk assessment: Breast, ovarian, and pancreatic, version 2.2021, NCCN clinical practice guidelines in oncology. Journal of the National Comprehensive Cancer Network, *19, 77–102. https://doi.org/10.6004/jn*ccn.2021.0001.

16. Deng, W., Hoffman, E., Stoller, J., Rubsam, M., Ku, M., Barbieri, M., Lacci, C., & Jayaraman, A. (2025). Environment Enrichment Strategies for Pre- and Post-Term Infants: A Summarized Communication From Pediatric Physical Therapists. Pediatric physical th*erapy : the official publicat*ion of the Section on Pediatrics of the American Physical Therapy Association, 37(2), 265–276. https://doi.org/10.1097/PEP.0000000000001187(accessed on 12 May 2025).

17. Eichenfield, L. F., & Ginsberg, D. N. (2016). Debates in allergy medicine: Specific immunotherapy in children with atopic dermatitis, the "con" view. CORE. https://core.ac.uk/download/323310753.pdf. Ginsberg, D. N., & Eichenfield, L. F. (2016). Debates in allergy medicine: Specific immunotherapy in children with atopic dermatitis, the "con" view. The World Allergy Organization journal, 9, 16. https://doi.org/10.1186/s40413-016-0107-2

18. Eichenfield, L. F., Ganslandt, C., Kurvits, M., & Schlessinger, J. (2015). Safety and efficacy of calcipotriene plus betamethasone dipropionate topical suspension in the treatment of extensive scalp psoriasis in adolescents ages 12 to 17 years. Pediatric dermatology, 32(1), 28–35. https://doi.org/10.1111/pde.12429Eichenfield, L., He*bert, A. A., Harper,* J. C., Baldwin, H., Bhatia, N., Stein Gold, L. S., Kircik, L., et al. (2024). Efficacy and safety of fixed-dose triple-combination clindamycin phosphate 1.2%/adapalene 0.15%/benzoyl peroxide 3.1% gel for moderate-to-severe acne vulgaris in children and adolescents. SKIN The Journal of Cutaneous Medicine. https://www.semanticscholar.org/paper/07fdc8*fb1ffa0d1a9730555702 79245c0c871576 (accessed on 12 May* 2025).

19. Goodings, A. J., & Kajitani, S. H. (2024). A biopsychosocial approach to a 6-year-old patient with impetiginized atopic dermatitis: A case report. CORE. https://doi.org/10.33178/SMJ.2024.1.9 (accessed on 12 May 2025).

20. Gupta, A. K., Polla Ravi, S., Wang, T., Faour, S., Bamimore, *M., Heath, C. R., Fallon Friedlander, S.*

(2024). An update on tinea capitis in children. Pediatric Dermatology. https://doi.org/10.1111/pde.13142.

21. Hebert, A., Browning, J., Kwong, P., Duarte, A., Price, H., & Siegfried, E. (2023). Diagnosis and management of pediatric psoriasis: An overview for pediatricians. Journal of Drugs in Dermatology, 22(8), 742–753. https://doi.org/10.36849/JDD.7324.
22. Heide, R. (2009). Clinical aspects of pediatric and adult onset mastocytosis in the skin. CORE. https://core.ac.uk/download/18511476.pdf (accessed on 12 May 2025).
23. Hidvégi, B., & Bali, G. (2018). Diagnostic and treatment strategies of dermatologists for treating morphea in Hungary. Acta Dermatovenerol Croat Treatment of morphea in Hungary 2018;26(1):21-24. https://core.ac.uk/download/212467162.pdf (accessed on 12 May 2025).
24. Khan, A., Liu, S., & Tao, F. (2025). Current trends in pediatric migraine: Clinical insights and therapeutic strategies. Brain Sciences, 15. https://doi.org/10.3390/brainsci15071015.
25. Korotkiy, V. (2024). Pharmacoeconomic analysis of different treatment methods for acne in children and adolescents. Pediatric. Journal Named After G.N. Speransky. https://www.semanticscholar.org/paper/1c3aad8b6e8ae83bb9d7023bc951884180bbbe5b (accessed on 12 May 2025).
26. Leahy, M., & Murphy, A. (2024). P30 trouble with skin: Do parents understand the impact skin conditions have on children's quality of life? British Journal of Dermatology. https://www.semanticscholar.org/paper/c6587a27fd0c095c6582e44457e3dd1e7609f059 (accessed on 12 May 2025).
27. Lopes, A., Sokolova, A., Lopes, C., & Lopes, C. (2020). Atopic Dermatitis Host and Environment Model: Revisiting Therapeutic Options. European annals of allergy and clinical immunology, 52(1), 4–14. https://doi.org/10.23822/EurAnnACI.1764-1489.125 (accessed on 12 May 2025).
28. Metin Z, Durmaz K. Effects of delivery method on skin diseases and allergy status: A cross-sectional study. Turk J Dermatol 2023;17:126-31. (accessed on 12 May 2025).
29. Meyer, A., Ogle, A., Mchugh, M., Beck, M., Lampe, A., Cluster, A., Brossier, N., et al. (2024). NURS-02. The development and implementation of skincare treatment plans and product kits for pediatric patients receiving targeted therapies that cause skin toxicity. Neuro-Oncology, 26. https://doi.org/10.1093/neuonc/noaa211.
30. Moattari, C. R., & Jafferany, M. (2021). Psychological aspects of hair disorders: Considerations for dermatologists, cosmetologists, aesthetic, and plastic surgeons. Skin Appendage Disorders, 8, 186–194. https://doi.org/10.1159/000519817.
31. Naguthevar, S., Tak, V., Khera, D., Didel, S., & Abhishek, K. S. (2025). P-934. Emerging trends and challenges in pediatric infective endocarditis: Insights from a single-center observational study. Open Forum Infectious Diseases, 12. https://www.semanticscholar.org/paper/d59d6155774effa0f3deb230349f7a9d83d184c6 (accessed on 12 May 2025).
32. Nemeh, M. N., & Hogeling, M. (2022). Pediatric skin picking disorder: A review of management. Pediatric Dermatology, 39, 363–368. https://www.semanticscholar.org/paper/ce47ab9521f270e67a6444d2b1ee9105a14e0063 (accessed on 12 May 2025).
33. Northrup, H., Aronow, M. E., Bebin, E. M., Bissler, J. J., Darling, T. N., de Vries, P. J., Frost, M., et al. (2021). Updated international tuberous sclerosis complex diagnostic criteria and

surveillance and management recommendations. Pediatric Neurology, 123, 50–66. https://doi.org/10.1016/j.pediatrneurol.2021.07.011.

34. Osman, A., Morsi, A., El-Refee, S., *& Suliman, S. (2024*). Novel PIK3R1 gene mutation associated with SHORT syndrome: A case report of a 15-year-old female. Journal of Pediatric Endocrinology & Metabolism: JPEM. https*://doi.org/10.1515/jpem-2023-0813.*

35. *Otani, I. M.*, Carroll, R. W., Yager, P., Kroshinsky, D., Murphy, S., Hornick, J. L., Akin, C., Castells, M., & Walter, J. E. (2018). Diffuse cutaneous mastocytosis with novel somatic KIT mutation K509I and association with tuberous sclerosis. Clinical case r*eports, 6(9), 1834–1840. https*:// doi.org/10.1002/ccr3.1607

36. Otmane, M., & Alaoui Ismaili, N. (2025). The pediatric neuroblastoma: Application of MIBG scintigraphy in diagnosis, staging, and follow-up–Analysis of three cases. Swiss Journal of Radiology and Nuclear Medicine. https://www.semanticscholar.org/paper/100b623602f5512f1ff520b33de068cadcb9158b (accessed on 12 May 2025).

37. Paller, A. S., Rangel, *S. M., Chamlin, S*., Hajek, A., Phan, S., Hogeling, M., Castelo-Soccio, L., et al. (2024). Stigmatization and mental health impact of chronic pediatric skin disorders. JAMA Dermatology. https://doi.org/10.1001/jamadermatol.202*4.0025.*

38. *Podwojniak, A., Fle*mming, J., Tan, I. J., Ghani, H., Neubauer, Z., & Jones, A. (2024). Cutaneous Adverse Effects From Diabetes Devices in Pediatric Patients With Type 1 Diabetes Mellitus: Systematic Review. JMIR dermatology, 7, e59824. https://doi.org/10.2196/5982*4 (accessed on 12 May 2025).*

39. *Sakız*, H., & Jencius, M. (2024). Inclusive mental health support for international students: Unveiling delivery components in higher education. Cambridge Prisms: Global Mental Health, 11. https://www.semanti*cscholar.org/paper/f3bb73*b70bc16d69265248c331c4c8b08e9c0d7e (accessed on 12 May 2025).

40. Salamanna, F., Maglio, M., Landini, M. P., & Fini, M. (2020). Body localization of ACE-2: On the trail of the keyhole of SARS-CoV-2. Frontiers in Medicine, 7. https://doi.org/10.3389/fmed.2020.594495.

41. Sastre, J., Baldrich, E. S., Armario Hita, J. C., Herráez, L., Jáuregui, I., Martín-Santiag*o, A., Ortiz de Frutos,* J., Silvestre, J. F., & Valero, A. (2020). Consensus on the Clinical Approach to Moderate-to-Severe Atopic Dermatitis in Spain: A Delphi Survey. Dermatology research and practice, 2020, 1524293. https://doi.org/10.1155*/2020/1524293 (accessed on 12 May 2025).*

42. *Schmidt, M.,* Jóhannesdóttir Schmidt, S. A., Adelborg, K., Sundbøll, J., Laugesen, K., Ehrenstein, V., & Sørensen, H. T. (2019). The Danish health care system and epidemiological research: From health care contacts to da*tabase records. Clinical Epidemiology, 11, 563*–591. https://doi.org/10.2147/clep.s179083.

43. Sengupta, A., & Wagani, R. (2024). Mindful self-compassion for psychological distress associated with skin conditions: An online intervention study. Indian Journal of Dermatology, Venereology and Leprology. https://doi.org/10.4103/ijdvl.ijdvl_520_23.

44. Skr*oza, N., Bernard*ini, N., Proietti, I., & Potenza, C. (2018). Clinical utility of ingenol mebutate in the management of actinic keratosis: perspectives from clinical practice. Therapeutics and clinical risk mana*gement, 14, 1879–1885. https://doi.org/10.*2147/TCRM.S145779 (accessed on 12 May 2025).

45. Somasundaram, A., Chiramel, M., Chapla, A., Sathishkumar, D., Athiyarath, R., Mathew, L., & Danda, S. (2025). Targeted filaggrin gene (FLG) sequencing: A pilot study among Indian children with at*opic dermatitis. Indian* Dermatology Online Journal, 16(263–269). https://doi.org/10.4103/idoj.idoj_232_24.

46. Teasdale, E., Muller, I., Sivyer, K., Ghio, D., Greenwell, K., Wilczynska, S., Roberts, A., Ridd, M. J., Francis, N., Yardley, L., Thomas, K. S., & Santer, M. (2021). Views and experiences of man*aging eczema: systematic* review and thematic synthesis of qualitative studies. The British journal of dermatology, 184(4), 627–637. https://doi.org/10.1111/bjd.19299 (accessed on 12 May 2025).

47. University of Nebraska Medical *Center. (1976). Bulletin of the University of Nebraska:* Annual Catalog of the College of Medicine, 1976–1978. https://core.ac.uk/download/268251865.pdf (accessed on 12 May 2025).

48. Vermeulen, F. M., Gerbens, L. A. A., Bosma, A. L., Apfelbacher, C. J., Irvine, A. D., Arents, B. W. M., Barbarot, S., Deleuran, M., Ei*chenfield, L. F., Manca, A., Schmitt,* J., Vestergaard, C., Wall, D., Weidinger, S., Middelkamp-Hup, M. A., Spuls, P. I., Flohr, C., & Inte*rnational TREAT Registry Taskforce (2019). TREatment of ATopic eczema (TREAT) Regis*try Taskforce: consensus on how and when to measure the core dataset for atopic eczema treatment research registries. The British journal of dermatology, 181(3), 492–504. https://doi.org/10.1111/bjd.17715

49. Vo Tuong Thao, V., Le Thi Thuy, N., Mai Thi Cam, C., Nguyen Thi Thanh, P., Le Thi Cao, N., Nguyen Thi Tra, M., & Mai Ba Hoang, A. (2021). *To investigate the pattern of pe*diatric dermatoses in dermatology clinic, Hue University of Medicine and Pharmacy Hospital. Journal of Medicine and Pharmacy. https://www.semanticscholar.org/paper/0124d4eff367827eb252240a5cd9af9d73049098 (accessed on 12 May 2025).

50. Wydya, S., Yenny, Fadilla, Y., Eka, R., & Kalisa, C. (2024). Characteristics, clinical, and trichoscopic features in pediatric patients w*ith alopecia areata: A single-center observational study at the dermatol*ogy clinic of Dr. M. Djamil General Hospital Padang. Bioscientia Medicina: Journal of Biomedicine and Translational Research eISSN (Online): 2598

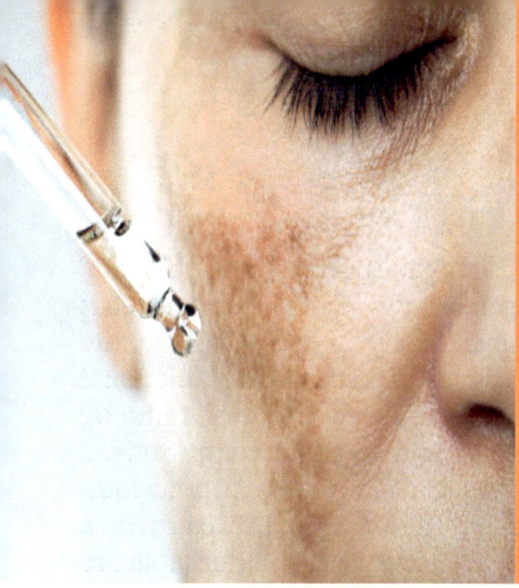

Chapter 13

GERIATRIC DERMATOLOGY

Contents

Introduction

As people age, the physiological functions of the body undergo significant changes and affect various organ systems, such as the skin. These modifications are exemplified by unique dermatological conditions that are more prevalent or pronounced in elderly persons. Geriatric dermatology strives to serve these age-associated skin changes based on the unique concerns of aging individuals. Reduced skin elasticity, decreased collagen synthesis, and impaired barrier function are among the mechanisms that contribute to conditions like xerosis, pruritus, and wound and infection susceptibility. The elderly are also more susceptible to skin malignancies due to cumulative lifetime exposure to ultraviolet (UV) radiation and hence need special prevention and screening. Understanding these physiological changes and their clinical counterparts is required to provide holistic dermatologic care tailored to older patients, especially with this population continuing to age around the world. Access to dermatological treatment is a formidable impediment for older adults that can exacerbate morbidity and mortality due to skin disease. The majority of geriatric patients would postpone dermatologic treatment because of reasons as varied as physical impairment, transportation mode challenges, absence of funds, to the perception that skin diseases are simply an aspect of aging. Studies indicate that such patients may experience challenges while accessing telemedicine platforms, which today form the backbone of modern healthcare delivery. Gender variations are also noticed, where females exhibit higher concern regarding cosmetic and aging-related skin issues, and males exhibit higher incidence and concern about skin cancers. Overcoming psychosocial and systemic obstacles is crucial in maximizing health results and ensuring equitable dermatologic treatment of the aged group (Shaw et al., 2019).

Recognition and overcoming such obstacles can significantly enhance early diagnosis and therapy of dermatological diseases in aged patients. Optimal treatment of common geriatric skin diseases, e.g., xerosis cutis (dry skin), is essential for optimal quality of life in geriatric patients. Utilization of standardized therapeutic regimens by health professionals has been demonstrated to have promising outcomes in these patients. A case in point is the use of an overall dry skin (ODS) scale for early detection and assessment of the severity of xerosis and thus facilitate targeted interventions. Patient education and interaction, through virtue of in-clinic consultations and follow-up questionnaires, improve compliance with moisturizing regimens and overall treatment outcomes. Research shows that organized interventions can reduce dry skin incidence to a significant extent while enhancing the well-being of patients. Implementation of behavior change models in patient communication also improves long-term skin care behaviors. Finally, these methods underscore the value of proactive, evidence-based dermatologic treatment centered on the vulnerabilities and needs of the elderly skin (Yao et al., 2022).

Definition and Scope of Geriatric Dermatology

Aging affects all organ systems, and the skin, as a huge organ, shows typical changes that affect health and quality of life. With age, the skin also undergoes structural and functional alterations such as reduced elasticity, thinning of the epidermis and dermis, compromised immune response, and altered repair processes. These changes present elderly individuals with a unique range of dermatologic conditions that are arguably less frequent or manifest differently in earlier age groups. As a result, geriatric dermatology thus becomes an evolving specialty dedicated to the explanation of these cutaneous changes associated with aging, both normal and abnormal. It includes diagnosis, prevention, and medical care of skin disease in aged patients with a focus on interaction between systemic aging and dermatologic presentation. The specialty does include a total approach with not just medical but also psychosocial care for health improvement in older adults. In defining the field of geriatric dermatology, proper thought must be given to the extensive variety of dermatoses which are predominantly encountered in older people. These include chronic disorders such as xerosis, pruritus, and benign neoplasias and malignant neoplasias such as basal cell carcinoma (BCC), squamous cell carcinoma, and melanoma. Additionally, age-related disease conditions such as pressure ulcers, seborrheic keratoses, and senile purpura require specialized management strategies crafted based on older patients compromised physiologic stores and comorbidities. The specialty also manages inflammatory and autoimmune conditions that present with unusual presentations due to immunosenescence. The pharmacologic subtlety and polypharmacy of older patients also point to the necessity for dermatologists to adopt a sophisticated, customized approach. Besides, telemedicine technology improvements have started to influence the specialty with remote skin examinations especially valuable for elderly patients with mobility problems (Yao et al., 2022).

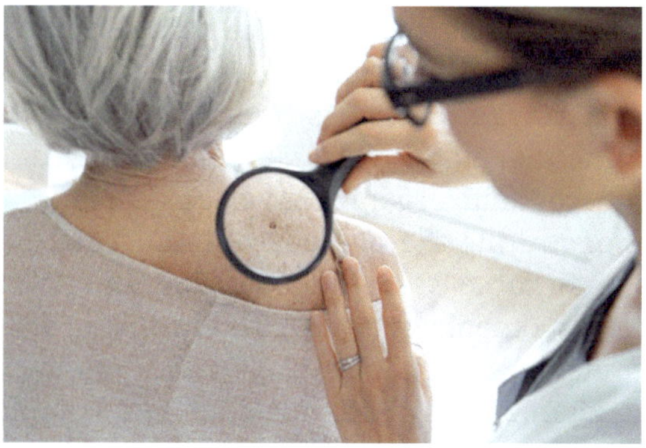

Source: MOD Dermatology. (2022). *Skin Examination with Magnifying Glass.* https://moddermatology.com/wp-content/uploads/2022/08/SkinExam.jpg.

Multidisciplinary geriatric dermatology practice is not limited to clinical practice but also includes preventive dermatology, patient education, and research tailored to the elderly. Prevention involves sun protection practices, detection of cutaneous malignancies at an early stage, and the therapy of chronic diseases that weaken skin integrity. Research aims at the elucidation of skin mechanisms of aging, rationalizing treatment modalities based on altered pharmacodynamics with aging, and encouraging the use of teledermatology in order to increase access and compliance with care (Yao et al., 2022).

Additionally, systemic comorbidities of the elderly's skin diseases, for example, cardiovascular risk and psoriasis, require multidisciplinary models of care, as advocated by guidelines that tailor treatments to the context of comorbidities. Lastly, geriatric dermatology is a living specialty, combining clinical expertise, new technology, and team-based patient care to address the complicated dermatologic needs of the elderly.

Importance of Skin Health in the Elderly

With increasing age, the physiological mechanisms in all organ systems are changed, the skin being the most apparent one. The intrinsic aging process with added extrinsic processes such as sunlight exposure and environmental toxins leads to impaired skin integrity, loss of elasticity, and barrier dysfunction. These alterations predispose older individuals to a number of dermatological disorders, which can have an adverse effect on overall health and quality of life. In the clinical setting, eczema, fungal infection, and vitiligo are also common dermatological presentations in the elderly, where there is a strong need for greater awareness as well as targeted intervention. With the increasing geriatric population all over the globe, particularly in developing nations, the occurrence of skin diseases among geriatric patients is also set to increase, hence demanding more comprehensive epidemiological data and specialized dermatological services to cater to their individual needs (Amadi et al., 2017). Recognition of skin diseases at an early stage enables appropriate control, preventing complications that can aggravate the morbidity of this vulnerable group of people. Pruritus, or chronic pruritus, is the most annoying symptom that elderly patients with this condition have to bear, and it cripples them severely when it comes to their normal functioning. Pruritic dermatoses are very common in elderly patients who come to outpatient clinics, and the literature indicates that nearly 10% of elderly patients who come to outpatient clinics have such a complaint. Chronic pruritus, apart from causing physical misery, also causes psychosocial distress by impairing the quality of sleep and reducing social activity. Its impact on quality of life, as measured by standardized instruments like the Dermatology Life Quality Index (DLQI), is often moderate to severe, hence the importance of effective treatment modalities. Apart from this, fungal infection and scabies are also usual causes of pruritus among the elderly population, which require early identification and treatment for re-achievement of normal skin and mitigation of misery (Varsha, 2023). Thus, the management of pruritus is an important part of enhancing the overall well-being of geriatric patients. As well as symptomatic control, maintenance of skin health in the elderly has widespread implications for public and healthcare system health. Increased vulnerability to infection by damaged skin barriers may result in systemic complications, increased hospitalization time, and increased healthcare expenditures. Preventive measures such as patient education in skin care, routine dermatological examinations, and utilization of gerontodermatology clinics need to be undertaken in order to prevent these risks. Geriatric complexity-specific care with physiological and psychosocial elements can improve adherence and outcomes to treatment. The crossroad of dermatology and geriatrics is about emphasizing healthy skin as a critical component of geriatric care that espouses dignity and quality of life for the elderly (Amadi et al., 2017; Varsha, 2023). In the final analysis, spending money on skincare is a testament to the investment in remedying the complex issues that come with aging.

Overview of Common Dermatological Issues in Older Adults

As a person grows old, there are many physiological alterations that make them susceptible to certain dermatological disorders. The skin's natural defense function declines with advancing age and renders the body more vulnerable to external trauma and decreased regenerative ability. Such disorders include basal and squamous cell carcinomas or non-melanoma skin cancers, which are a developing health problem. These neoplasms are most commonly found in older, light-skinned individuals and were found in about 7.2% of long-term care residents, representing a significant disease burden among geriatric nursing home residents. Precancerous actinic keratoses were found in more than 21% of the same population, and the rationale for early detection and treatment of these lesions is clear in the field of geriatric dermatology. Unfortunately, in the care home environment there is frequently limited routine dermatological screening based on resources and organizational constraints, but demonstrating the persuasive requirement for more suitable screening policies among the elderly (Akdeniz et al., 2019). Chronic pruritus is, outside malignancy, one of the ubiquitous and agonizing syndromes that are common within the elderly population and significantly impairing their quality of life. Pruritic disease research among geriatric patients establishes a prevalence rate of about 10% for outpatient patients and greater than half being chronic diseases. The complexity of pruritus as an issue among geriatric patients is further emphasized by its association with skin infections such as fungal infections and scabies, which not only exacerbate pain but also exist as difficult-to-treat situations in this vulnerable population. DLQI scores indicate a moderate to severe impact on everyday activity of patients, necessitating early recognition and proper control of pruritic states to enhance the quality of life of older patients (Varsha, 2023). Elderly skin care necessitates adopting multidisciplinary approaches that include early diagnosis, prophylactic treatment, and curative therapy. With the growing number of elderly individuals in long-term care, there should be education programs for health professionals. Utilizing the application of technological advancements such as teledermatology, dermoscopy training, and smartphone applications could bridge access and skills issues, enabling timely detection and management of common geriatric skin diseases. Moreover, the identification of lifestyle factors like smoking, which increases the risk for non-melanoma skin cancer among older individuals, can guide preventive interventions. As dermatological conditions among older individuals are usually multifactorial etiologies, assistance for primary care clinicians in dermatological assessment guarantees a more integrated strategy tailored to the individual needs of the older population (Akdeniz et al., 2019).

13.1. Aging Skin: Physiological Changes

The rate of dermal turnover gradually slows down with age and gives rise to a specific pattern of physiological alterations that constitute geriatric dermatology. There is reduced synthesis of collagen and breakdown of elastin in the dermis, which impairs the firmness and elasticity of the skin and facilitates wrinkling and sagging. The turnover rate of the epidermis is also impaired, impairing the repair capacity of the skin and leading to scars and thin, weakened epidermis. Vascular alterations also augment these effects by compromising oxygen and nutrient delivery to the skin, hence decreasing wound healing potential. These changes in general make elderly individuals more vulnerable to dermatologic issues such as eczemas, fungal dermatitis, and contact dermatitis that are observed in this group (Venus et al., 2025).

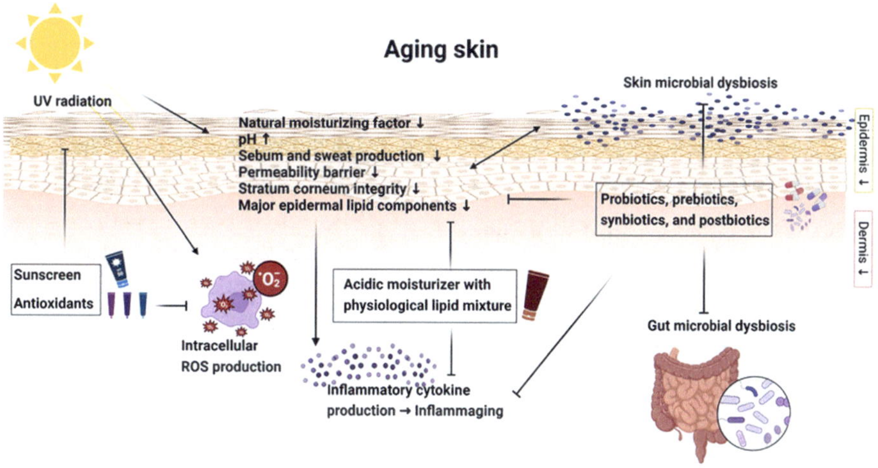

Figure 13.1. Diagrammatic overview of aging skin: skin barrier changes and intervention strategies.

Source: Woo YR and Kim HS (2024) Interaction between the microbiota and the skin barrier in aging skin: a comprehensive review. Front. Physiol. 15:1322205. doi: 10.3389/fphys.2024.1322205

It is important to understand the related physiological changes in order to formulate best diagnostic and therapeutic programs for the special needs of aged skin. Along with structural weakening, the skin's barrier function also reduces with age, increasing sensitivity to irritants and allergens. The compromised barrier is due to lipid composition changes and reduced water-holding capacity in the stratum corneum, which helps in transepidermal water loss (TEWL). Thus, aged skin is prone to dryness and pruritus, conditions which induce inflammatory responses and exacerbate dermatological disorders such as contact dermatitis. In addition, immunosenescence, or the reduction in cutaneous immune function, increases susceptibility to infection and compromises the defense mechanisms of the skin. Educational interventions were shown to induce awareness and management of disorders such as contact dermatitis in older populations, signaling the need for patient-focused interventions in the response to such physiological weakness (Hera et al., 2024). Enhancing knowledge regarding skin care can therefore act as a building block towards the maintenance of skin health in geriatric populations. Systemic health change often overlaps significantly with dermatological manifestations in elderly patients, underscoring the complexity of aging skin. Hypertension and diabetes mellitus are common comorbidities that impact skin integrity by altering microvascular perfusion and metabolism. Diabetes, on the other hand, is linked with longer fungal infections and wound healing times, complicating management of skin condition in older individuals (Venus et al., 2025). Collaboration among systemic disorders and dermatological alterations necessitates a multidisciplinary geriatric dermatological approach, whereby comprehensive assessments allow practitioners to incorporate dermatological factors against general health disorders. This combined model not only improves clinical outcomes but also the life quality of elderly patients who are afflicted by the synergistic activities of systemic aging and cutaneous aging (Figure 13.1).

13.1.1. Decreased Collagen and Elastin Production

The gradual loss of skin structure with the age factor is a step-by-step cellular and molecular process that compromises the integrity and elasticity of the skin. Among these dysfunctions, the loss of collagen and elastin fiber production within the dermal layer is particularly significant. Collagen, primarily type I, is accountable for tensile strength, while elastin is accountable for elasticity of the skin. The impaired synthesis and increased breakdown of these proteins lead to characteristic signs of aged skin, such as wrinkles, sagging, and loss of elasticity. This decrease is partially a result of the decreased activity and senescence of dermal fibroblasts, the cells responsible for the synthesis of collagen and elastin. External factors like ultraviolet (UV) radiation also further these changes by causing oxidative stress and inflammation, which further increase collagen breakdown. Therapeutic treatments that stimulate collagen and elastin production, such as microneedling, have been explored to reverse these consequences of aging by activating fibroblasts and inducing extracellular matrix remodeling (Snarskaya et al., 2023). Novel regenerative techniques have significantly expanded the therapeutic window treating the decreased collagen and elastin production of geriatric dermatology. Autologous stem cells and cultured fibroblasts offer promising skin rejuvenation options, leveraging their inherent ability for self-renewal and differentiation to restore dermal function. Adipose-derived stem cells (ADSCs), in particular, have advantages such as ease of accessibility and robust secretion of growth factors that induce collagen synthesis, angiogenesis, and antioxidant activity. Clinical trials have proved that subcutaneous administration of ADSCs increases dermal thickness and raises collagen levels, thus reversing aging structural deficiencies. Further, autologous fibroblast therapy, such as cultured dermal fibroblasts, has been approved to treat wrinkles, testifying to its efficacy to replace lost dermal elements and tighten skin with few side effects. These cell therapies show how fibroblast function targeting and extracellular matrix reconstitution can reverse age-related dermal degeneration (Mehrabani et al., 2013). The multifunctional role of fibroblasts in the maintenance of skin health and aging emphasizes their central position within geriatric dermatologic pathology owing to decreased collagen and elastin synthesis. Fibroblasts in the normal state maintain the balance of the extracellular matrix through the generation of collagens and elastin and the regulation of tissue remodeling by matrix metalloproteinases. In the aging process, such cells, however, experience replicative senescence, reducing their proliferative capacity and responsiveness to repair signals. This loss negatively affects wound healing and regeneration of the skin, resulting in cumulative damage to structure. Advanced in vitro culture techniques and cell banking have facilitated research and use of fibroblasts in cosmetic medicine, offering the potential for autologous cell therapies to rebuild the dermal niche. These approaches, which combine cellular regeneration with clinical therapies like microneedling, represent a new frontier in the reversal of dermal protein loss and management of morphological changes of aging skin (Mehrabani et al., 2013; Snarskaya et al., 2023) (Figure 13.2).

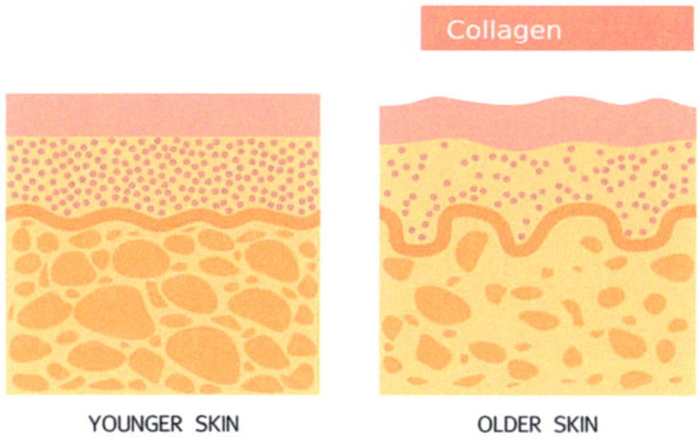

Figure 13.2. Collagen level: young and old skin.

Source: Vibrance MedSpa. (2020). *Collagen Levels in Young and Old Skin.* https://vibrancemedspa.com/wp-content/uploads/2020/04/Collagen-LevelsYoung-and-Old.jpg.

13.1.2. Changes in Skin Hydration and Barrier Function

The skin, being the first line of defense against external trauma, experiences profound physiological alterations with increasing age that impair its hydration and barrier functions. These changes are important because they affect not only the health of the cutaneous layer but also the overall well-being. Increasing age and degradation in skin barrier function are related to elevated TEWL, reduced stratum corneum hydration, and changes in pH. Recent clinical studies have examined therapeutic interventions to reverse such deterioration. A randomized controlled trial with women 60 to 90 years old, for example, showed that a senotherapeutic peptide in a topical formulation significantly enhanced skin hydration and barrier repair compared to conventional moisturizers. Such gains were objectively quantified with decreased TEWL and added skin moisture and inferred greater epidermal barrier repair processes. Additionally, participants evidenced significant subjective improvement in skin appearance, highlighting the clinical significance of focusing on skin hydration and barrier repair in aging dermatology (Zonari et al., 2025). Along with localized dermatological changes, advancing evidence demonstrates interrelations among skin barrier function and systemic inflammatory processes in aging. Impaired skin barrier function can result in increased exposure to environmental aggressors, inducing chronic low-grade inflammation that accelerates systemic aging. The above clinical trial also went on to explain that topical intervention not only enhanced cutaneous parameters but also regulated circulating cytokine profiles, lowering proinflammatory markers like IL-8. This observation suggests that the restoration of skin barrier integrity has wider implications than dermatological health and might slow biological aging. Therefore, measures promoting skin hydration and barrier resistance could be an essential part of overall geriatric treatment, with a goal not only of improving appearance but also of maintaining systemic health (Zonari et al., 2025). Such a systemic aspect of skin barrier function emphasizes the necessity to view aging skin as a multifactorial process encompassing both local and systemic influences. It is also interesting to look at barrier function changes throughout various stages of life to put into perspective the transformations that take place in the elderly. Research on neonates has demonstrated that TEWL is fairly constant during the first week of life, although skin hydration becomes progressively higher, indicating developing maturation of the skin. Further, bathing influences significantly the environmental parameters of the skin barrier, provisorily raising TEWL, which requires standard measurement techniques to account for these variations. As neonatal skin undergoes a maturation process, elderly skin typically shows the reverse trend marked by degenerative alterations and loss of moisture holding capacity. This appreciation of such contrasts elucidates that it takes specially designed interventions throughout the lifetime to achieve and maintain the optimum skin hydration and barrier homeostasis. These observations from neonatal skin research highlight the relevance of environmental and intrinsic determinants of barrier function and support the rationale for specific therapeutic approaches in geriatric patients (Figure 13.3).

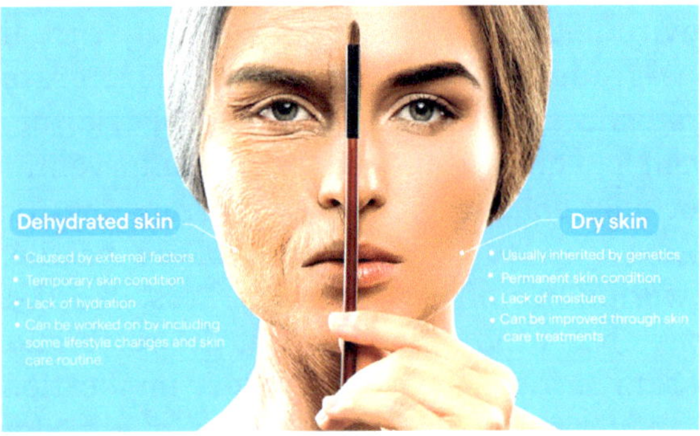

Figure 13.3. Hydrated vs. dry skin.

Source: Skin Foodie Nigeria. (2021). *Comparison Between Dehydrated Skin and Dry Skin.* https://i0.wp.com/skinfoodie.com.ng/wp-content/uploads/2021/05/Skin-foodie-HYDRATION-hydrating-skin-care-ingredients-skinfood-nigeria-diy-skincare-2-in-Skin-care-skinfoodienigeria-skinfood-1.jpeg?resize=595%2C369&ssl=1

13.1.3. Impact of Aging on Skin Healing Processes

With advancing age in the human body, there are accumulating cellular, as well as molecular, changes that have a profound effect on mechanisms of tissue repair. The largest organ, and indeed one of the earliest barriers to environmental insults, is the skin, which experiences extensive change in healing capability with age. One of the most important factors is the reduced proliferative potential of keratinocytes and fibroblasts, which reduces re-epithelialization and extracellular matrix remodeling. In addition, defective angiogenesis, an important step for the transmission of oxygen and nutrient delivery to the area of injury, weakens new vessel formation. This type of vascular regeneration reduction is proportional with lowered expression of the vascular endothelial growth factor (VEGF), a mediator of key importance in wound healing mechanisms. Novel treatments such as polydeoxyribonucleotide (PDRN) have been identified to induce angiogenesis by augmented expression of VEGF and activation of purinergic receptors, suggesting new therapeutic approaches to age-related cutaneous healing retardation (Akaberi et al., 2025). These biological data underscore the complexity of skin aging and the need for targeted intervention in geriatric dermatology. In addition to cellular senescence and angiogenic impairment, senescent skin also displays epigenetic alterations that modify patterns of gene expression relevant to repair mechanisms. More recent work highlights the role of epigenetic mechanisms, including DNA methylation and histone modification, in regulating the biological age and response to injury of the skin. Epigenetic clocks, such as Horvath's Clock, provide a mechanism for establishing biological versus chronological age, which means that biological aging can inequitably affect healing efficiency. Epigenetic clocks further suggest that interventions which target epigenetic remodeling can restore young gene expression profiles, benefiting collagen synthesis and tissue regeneration. Energy-based technologies like fraction lasers have been shown to possess potential to reverse epigenetic markers of aging in some degree and thereby enhance healing potential in older patients (Haykal et al., 2025). Elucidating these extremely complex molecular adaptations is essential towards the development of individualized dermatologic treatments against the regenerative inadequacies noted among aged skin. Aiding the underlying cellular and molecular changes, systemic geriatric cohort characteristic conditions also disrupt wound healing further, with heightened rates of chronic wounds and infection.

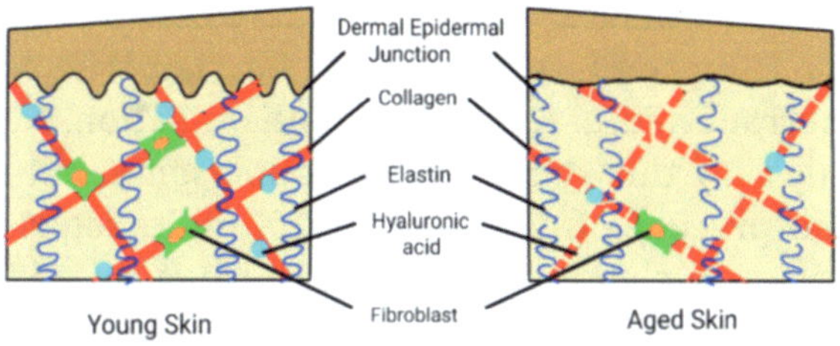

Figure 13.4. Effects of aging on wound healing.

Source: Khalid, Kamarul Ariffin, Ahmad Faris Mohd Nawi, Nuraqilah Zulkifli, Md. Abul Barkat, and Hazrina Hadi. 2022. "Aging and Wound Healing of the Skin: A Review of Clinical and Pathophysiological Hallmarks" *Life* 12, no. 12: 2142. https://doi.org/10.3390/life12122142

Diminished immune surveillance, more accurately described as immunosenescence, causes delayed inflammation necessary for the initial phases of wound repair. Concomitant age-related loss of growth factors and pro-inflammatory milieu may result in abnormally controlled matrix remodeling and scarring. Therapy with bioregulatory agents like PDRN shows elevated collagen synthesis and reduced inflammation, thus improving the quality and speed of healing in older individuals (Akaberi et al., 2025). Integrating molecular insights with epigenetic experience provides a global approach to management of impaired healing in geriatric dermatology in an orientation toward combining emerging therapeutics and precision medicine to achieve the optimal outcome in skin repair in aging individuals (Haykal et al., 2025) (Figure 13.4).

13.2. Common Dermatological Conditions in the Elderly

The integumentary system is heavily affected by aging, and this results in increased susceptibility to skin disease. Loss of the skin barrier function with age, reduction in cellular turnover, and weakened immunity are factors that are associated with elevating the incidence of dermatological conditions among the elderly. Clinically, eczema has been of special concern and tends to manifest as pruritic, erythematous plaques that can have a significant impact on quality of life. A retrospective review at a tertiary care center revealed eczema to be the single most prevalent diagnosis amongst geriatric patients and highlights its pervasiveness amongst elderly dermatology. The complex etiology of the condition, commonly seen with xerosis and external irritants, mandates broad treatment strategies taking into account the unique changes in the physiology of aging skin. Knowledge of these pathophysiologic processes is critical in formulating effective treatment regimens, particularly in the elderly (Amadi et al., 2017). Cutaneous infections are also a common issue in geriatric dermatology, once again due mainly to immunosenescence and comorbidities that disrupt host defense. Fungal infections, especially superficial mycoses, are very common in older people, frequently superimposed upon diabetes and limited mobility that facilitate moist, warm environments supporting fungal growth. They are not only a nuisance due to pain and aesthetic appeal but also because they have the potential to lead to secondary bacterial infections. Early recognition of fungal infections and application of timely antifungal treatments may prevent complications and enhance patient outcomes. In addition, regular skin checks among older persons, particularly in institutionalized settings, are important to identify and treat infections before they contribute to underlying dermatological conditions (Amadi et al., 2017). Non-melanoma skin cancers are increasingly emerging as a prominent dermatological issue among the elderly, particularly in fair-skinned individuals with high cumulative UV exposure. Actinic keratoses, which commonly precede invasive squamous cell carcinoma, are common lesions in this population and act as a sentinel marker for sun damage to the skin. Epidemiologic data highlights the increasing incidence of these neoplasms as well as related morbidity and health care expenditures. Notwithstanding this, systematic skin cancer screening within nursing home and long-term care settings remains inadequate, constrained by competing resource demands and workforce shortages. Improve early detection with teledermatology and education of primary healthcare providers to help promote timely intervention, thus decreasing the burden of advanced skin cancers in elderly populations. Preventive and diagnostic measures must be prioritized to meet this new challenge in geriatric dermatology.

13.2.1. Xerosis (Dry Skin) and Its Implications

The process of aging results in numerous physiological changes that have far-reaching impacts on skin health, with xerosis taking on epidemic proportions in the geriatric population. Alterations that include decreased function in sebaceous and sweat glands decrease the ability of the skin to retain moisture, and the skin, in turn, becomes drier and more prone to irritation. These changes are compounded by environmental influences like climate, long-term drug therapy, and underlying systemic disease, with additional compounded effects on skin barrier failure. Xerosis in the elderly is not only a matter of discomfort but as a precursor to more serious complications like pruritus and secondary infection. The complex interplay between systemic disease and skin barrier dysfunction makes the dermatologic management of careful, age-specific preventive and focused treatment for the preservation of cutaneous integrity and overall health all the more significant (Elif et al., 2025). Understanding of the clinical ramifications beyond xerosis reveals that it leads to precipitous chronic pruritus, a condition that severely affects the quality of life of elderly patients. Chronic itching or pruritus is often intimately linked with xerosis, such that the compromised epidermal barrier triggers aberrant neural reflexes and inflammation. Not only may this symptom be troublesome, but it also precedes the probability of multifactorial causes such as metabolic disturbances, side effects of drugs, or skin conditions like psoriasis, which is prevalent among elderly populations. The xerosis with pruritus calls for proper evaluation to establish contributory factors and to put in place aggressive management regimens that include emollient therapy and careful medication scrutiny in view of the high incidence of polypharmacy in the elderly management (Elif et al., 2025). Effective care of xerosis in older patients is a strategy with a combined approach whose primary objectives include hydration of skin and repair of the barrier while, at the same time, addressing comorbidities and potential pharmacological influences. Emollients form a central aspect of treatment, as they enable the re-establishment of hydration and protection from external irritation. Clinical vigilance is required, however, to safeguard against such complications as secondary infection or exacerbation of chronic inflammatory dermatoses, states which are known to have their presentations altered in elderly patients. Moreover, knowing the impact ordinary geriatric medication has on xerosis and skin dryness raises the need for interdisciplinary care involving dermatologists, primary care professionals, and pharmacists to modulate therapeutic schemes. Education about skin care maneuvers among patients and caregivers is similarly vital in stopping the risk determinants of xerosis and elderly complications (Mazan et al., 2024) (Figure 13.5).

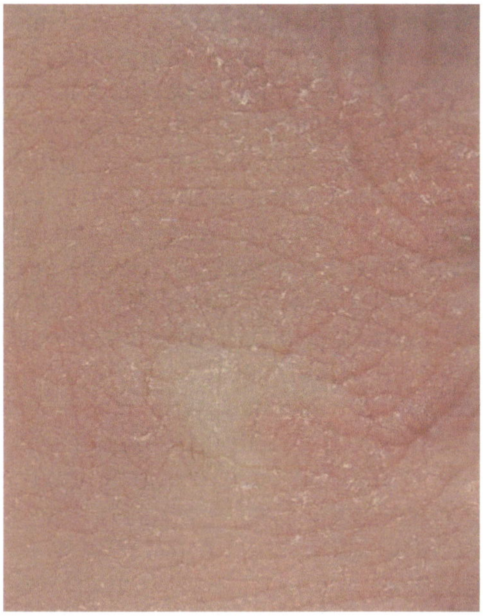

Figure 13.5. Xerosis in old age.

Source: By The original uploader was Ser Amantio di Nicolao at English Wikipedia. - Transferred from en.wikipedia to Commons by AlbertHerring using CommonsHelper., CC BY-SA 3.0, https://commons.wikimedia.org/w/index.php?curid=9493330

13.2.2. Skin Cancers: Prevalence and Types

Epidemiological patterns indicate an increased incidence of skin cancer among the elderly, especially among light-skinned populations. The trend among this age group can be explained based on total cumulative exposure to UV radiation and, therefore, compromised cutaneous repair mechanisms by the aged skin. Non-melanoma skin cancers such as BCC and cutaneous squamous cell carcinoma have become prevalent cancers among patients aged above 70 years. These cancers not only are very morbific but also highly account for healthcare costs in the elderly's inpatient care. A multicenter investigation of the actinic keratoses prevalence among institutionally elderly groups identified actinic keratoses, precancerous lesions that give rise to squamous cell carcinoma, the most common epithelial dermatosis found, highlighting the serious importance of their detection and surveillance among this high-risk population (Akdeniz et al., 2019). These findings emphasize the demographic specificity of the incidence of skin cancer in elderly populations and the need for specialized intervention strategies. All types of skin cancer express themselves differently in the elderly patient group, based on intrinsic aging processes as well as external environmental factors. BCC, as the most frequent type with its local growth and limited metastatic potential, presents as most often nodular or superficial lesions on chronically sun-exposed locations. Cutaneous squamous cell carcinoma, however, carries a higher risk for regional spread and usually precedes actinic keratoses that are indicative of chronic photodamage and cellular atypia. Melanoma, though less frequent among nursing home patients based on the current epidemiological reports, is accountable for an inordinate number of skin cancer fatalities due to virulence and metastatic capability (Akdeniz et al., 2019). Identification of these differential presentations is crucial in geriatric dermatology, where the diagnostic dilemma arises from uniform clinical presentations of benign and malignant lesions in the aged skin and restricted availability of specialist care. Even with the preventable etiology of most skin cancers, their incidence is still on the increase in the world, and it demands efficient prevention and curative models. Public health statistics project that one in five Americans will develop skin cancer, and deaths from melanoma reappear with frightening frequency. This reveals the evidence for education, early detection, and standard preventive practices like photoprotection deficits while showing the need for intervention in targeted populations of older adults whose lifetime UV exposure raises risk. Treatment modalities vary from excision to topical therapy and PDT but treatment of elderly patients also needs to be in the context of comorbidities and functional status. Geriatric dermatology thus needs to be a compromise between good cancer management and quality of life preservation, but with increasing screening programs, patient education with more aggressiveness, and incorporation of teledermatology for optimizing outcomes in this expanding population (Akdeniz et al., 2019) (Figure 13.6).

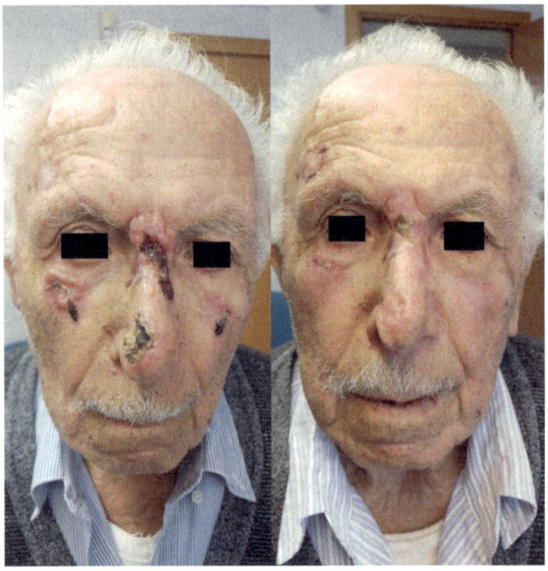

Figure 13.6. A patient with multiple facial Non-Melanoma Skin Cancer (NMsc): on the left pre-radiotherapy status, on the right -8 weeks after rT status.

Source: Calzavara-Pinton, P., Zanca, A., Venturini, M., & Sala, R. (2021). *A Patient with Multiple Facial Non-Melanoma Skin Cancers (NMSC)*. ResearchGate.

13.2.3. Pressure Ulcers and Their Management

Pressure ulcer development is one of the most important clinical problems in geriatric dermatology, intimately associated with declining skin integrity and mobility that accompanies aging. The aged patient possesses thinner subcutaneous fat and thinner dermis, which are possibly additive to his or her susceptibility to ongoing pressure and shear stress resulting in localized tissue ischemia. The association of comorbid conditions prevalent in the elderly population, like peripheral vascular disease and diabetes mellitus, also deranges microcirculation to some extent, adding to the risk of developing ulcers. The ulcers not only provide a portal of entry for infection but also have severe implications on the patient's quality of life, tending to result in prolonged hospitalization and aggravated morbidity. Management thus succeeds in imposing an interdisciplinary approach with a focus on early detection, comprehensive assessment of risk, and intervention aimed at arresting progression and promoting healing of wounds. Preventive measures continue to be paramount in the eradication of pressure ulcers among the elderly because this minimizes the morbidity load and costs incurred in hospitalization of patients with chronic wounds. The main interventions are frequent repositioning to offload pressure on at-risk areas, optimization of nutritional status to promote tissue healing, and the application of specialist pressure-relieving support surfaces such as pressure-relieving mattresses. Complexity of care is also increased by the high incidence of comorbidities and polypharmacy, both of which can slow healing and complicate treatment plans. Evidence-based guidelines put into practice have reflected improved pathways to improved outcomes, and still, there is an eye-opening gap between recommended and provided care. Such a gap identifies the necessity for more education among health professionals and system-level reform in order to facilitate consistent use of best practice in pressure ulcer prevention and treatment. Following pressure ulcer development, effective management is contingent on early detection, dead tissue removal through debridement, prevention of infection, and more recent therapeutic modalities intended to facilitate increased granulation and epithelialization. The patient's medical status as an elderly patient must be taken seriously in the determination of treatment protocols because comorbid vascular impairment or autoimmune processes can interfere with healing patterns (Mayrovitz et al., 2023). In addition, specialist wound care clinics have been said to deliver streamlined care in a manner that minimizes treatment complexity through concentration of expertise and facilitation of evidence-based practice. As evidence verifies, a structured care pathway is very conducive to healing rates and functional outcomes, testifying to the efficacy of combined multidisciplinary management of chronic wounds (Edwards et al., 2013). Finally, geriatric pressure ulcers need extensive, personalized management to maximize healing and avoid complications, with improvement in the quality of life of the patient (Figure 13.7).

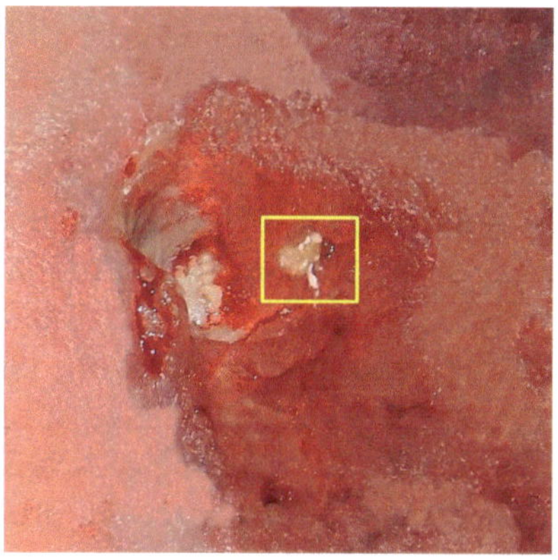

Figure 13.7. Pressure ulcer.

Source: By Noles1984 (talk) 15:45, 7 May 2008 (UTC) - Own work (Original text: self-made), Public Domain, https://commons.wikimedia.org/w/index.php?curid=10719960

13.3. Diagnosis and Assessment in Geriatric Patients

Effective evaluation and diagnosis in geriatric dermatology are based on an extremely advanced comprehension of the precise physiological alterations of aging skin. With aging, the skin suffers structural and functional changes such as impaired barrier function, deranged vascularization, and compromised immune response, thereby making clinical examination more difficult. Elderly patients also present concomitant comorbid disease and polypharmacy, whose effect can mask or mimic dermatologic disease. Thus, clinicians have to embrace an integrative approach with history of the patient in consideration, lesion morphology examination, and sensitivity towards general well-being.

Teledermatology, especially store-and-forward teledermatology (SFTD), has proved to be an effective adjunct in such a scenario. SFTD facilitates dermatologic evaluation in long-term care facilities with reduced travel burdens and quicker diagnosis, of the highest importance in the management of common skin cancers and infections in the elderly (Tian et al., 2023). The quality of clinical data and follow-up compliance remain issues requiring improvement in the assessment process. In assessing geriatric patients, it is important to include frailty and functional assessment, as well as dermatologic factors, to optimize clinical decision-making.

Frailty, which is routinely assessed using the Clinical Frailty Scale (CFS), has been a reliable predictor of mortality and course of recovery in the elderly. These general assessments encompass more than cutaneous appearance and include cognitive function and activities of daily living with implications for compliance with therapy and prognosis. The interaction between frailty and dermatologic illness is bidirectional—frail patients have compromised wound healing and susceptibility to skin infection, complicating the diagnostic process. Evidence supports the inclusion of geriatric syndromes, particularly frailty, as it improves the prognosis of elderly patients with acute disease, highlighting the importance of its inherent inclusion in dermatological evaluation models (Guidet et al., 2019).

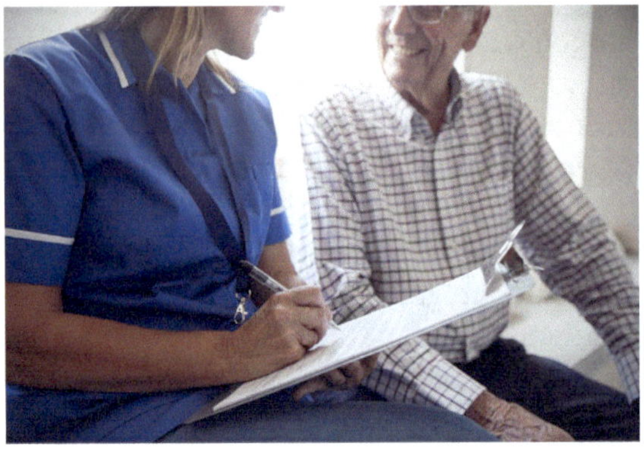

Source: CaringGivers. (2020). *Senior Man Sits with Nurse Making Notes.* https://caringgivers.com/wp-content/uploads/2020/04/senior-man-sits-with-nurse-making-notes-at-PZV45MP-1024x683.jpg.

Multidimensional assessment allows for modulated treatment planning following the patient's overall status and not solely based on single clinical indicators. Despite advancements, some of its limitations continue in the diagnosis and evaluation of skin disease in the elderly, prompting a reflective understanding of health-seeking behavior as well as compliance. Teledermatology has proved to be successful in overcoming access barriers, but rates of missing appointments for scheduled interventions continue to be an issue, limiting its overall performance (Tian et al., 2023). Moreover, cognitive impairment and physical disability secondary to the complexity of geriatric illness undermine the reliability of clinical histories and physical examination findings. Interprofessional collaboration among caregivers, geriatricians, and dermatologists is then necessary in order to achieve maximal diagnostic accuracy and continuity of care. Individualized geriatric pathways for the underlying conditions pertinent to adherence and follow-up are needed in order to guarantee optimal effectiveness of dermatologic evaluation in this high-risk population. These models of integration assist in reversing resource wastage while optimizing outcomes for patients in geriatric dermatology.

13.3.1. Unique Challenges in Diagnosing Skin Conditions

Clinical evaluation of cutaneous disease in geriatric patients is confounded by the physiologic changes associated with aging. As immune surveillance and the barrier function of the skin fail with advancing age, the presentation of cutaneous disease might not occur as in younger patients. Unpredictability from this failure could result in delay or misdiagnosis of disease, particularly distinguishing benign from malignant lesions. In addition, the presence of several dermatologic signs in one patient makes it difficult to diagnose. Polypharmacy and systemic illness among the elderly population also increase the difficulty of finding cutaneous manifestations because several drugs induce unusual rashes or exacerbate existing dermatosis. Therefore, dermatologists must take complete patient histories and interact with other departments to accurately determine causative factors. Systemic disease assessment that is coupled with dermatological examination is essential, considering the common overlap of symptomatology and comorbidity reported among aging populations (Venus et al., 2025). Adding to the challenge of making a diagnosis of skin disease in the elderly is that certain malignancies and pre-malignant lesions present insidiously. For example, differentiation of clear cell acanthoma from squamous cell carcinoma must be done by meticulous histopathological examination because of similar clinical presentation and occasional overlap. These differentiations are crucial, particularly because of their extremely dissimilar prognostic and therapeutic consequences. Rare presentations of diseases such as HPV-positive clear cell acanthoma and keratinized squamous cell carcinoma also violate conventional diagnostic guidelines.

Limited evidence highlights the importance of increased clinical suspicion and sophisticated diagnostic modalities for concomitant underlying pathologies in the elderly. The case highlights a crucial area of knowledge deficit with regard to viral contributions towards benign lesions and their corresponding association with malignancy, highlighting the importance of continued exploration to increase diagnostic certainty and therapeutic strategies in geriatric dermatology (Cuomo et al., 2024). Additionally, the age-related heterogeneity of dermatoses often coincides with socio-demographic determinants like gender and age groups and has implications on clinical presentation and diagnosis. Some dermatoses, like eczemas and fungal infections, show differential rates of prevalence based on these parameters, and standardized diagnostic models are hence difficult to develop. In addition, older age skin has diminished sensory function and decreased inflammatory response, which may slow classic signs like erythema or pruritus. Such modified presentations of symptoms often lead to underreporting or delayed medical consultation, which impedes effective diagnosis. The multifactorial pathogenesis of these diagnostic dilemmas necessitates a blend of patient education, clinical vigilance, and specific investigative strategies to effectively navigate the complex environment of geriatric skin disease (Venus et al., 2025).

13.3.2. Importance of Thorough Skin Examinations

Aging is associated with many changes in the skin that make clinical examination of the elderly complex. These very subtle changes cover the onset of skin diseases, especially malignancies. Therefore, careful clinical observation has to be used. Complete skin examination is more than mere visual inspection and involves palpation and detailed patient history, which are most important in the identification of precancerous lesions and skin cancers, which are rarely seen in the elderly. Given the endemic prevalence of skin cancer among this population, a total skin exam makes possible early detection and treatment with potential minimization of morbidity and mortality. The high prevalence of undiagnosed precursors among older patients underscores the importance of such an examination, especially given that male gender and prior history of skin cancer are strong risk factors. Utilization of these tests in the course of ordinary geriatric practice not only facilitates earlier diagnosis but also the delivery of more complete patient education and prevention programs with long-term gains in clinical outcomes (Sinikumpu et al., 2022). Within geriatric dermatology, diagnosis is further hampered by multifactorial causes of presenting issues such as chronic pruritus. The symptom is commonly a manifestation of underlying neuropathic disorders rather than dermatological or systemic processes and thus requires a multidisciplinary diagnosis. Skin examinations need to be rigorous and coordinated, separating neuropathic pruritus from dermatalogical or systemic causes based on clinical correlation with history and relevant investigations. Failing to set up the etiology promptly leads to inadequate treatment because neuropathic pruritus will defy conventional antipruritic treatment and demands subspecialty management. Dermatologists, neurologists, and other specialists need to practice in a multidisciplinary setup when examining the skin in order to make accurate diagnoses and comprehensive management that accounts for the special concerns of aged skin (Akarsu, 2023). Routine full skin checks are of paramount significance in elderly patient care, both for diagnosis of malignancy and neuropathic processes but also for recognition of benign yet potentially annoying dermatoses that are commonly present in older individuals. Immunologic changes with aging and repeated environmental injuries render individuals susceptible to numerous dermatoses, thus making them candidates for ongoing monitoring.

The total body skin examination (TBSE) is distinct to this function, being useful in the detection of precursors of skin cancer with high accuracy and evaluation of risk factors such as socioeconomic status and history of outdoor occupation. TBSE prioritization in clinical practice is particularly crucial for high-risk groups like elderly men with disproportionate skin cancer rates. Finally, the incorporation of full skin examination into standard geriatric assessment provides the highest rate of early detection, allows prompt therapeutic intervention, and promotes individualized preventive efforts, ultimately optimizing skin health outcomes in this high-risk population (Sinikumpu et al., 2022) (Figure 13.8).

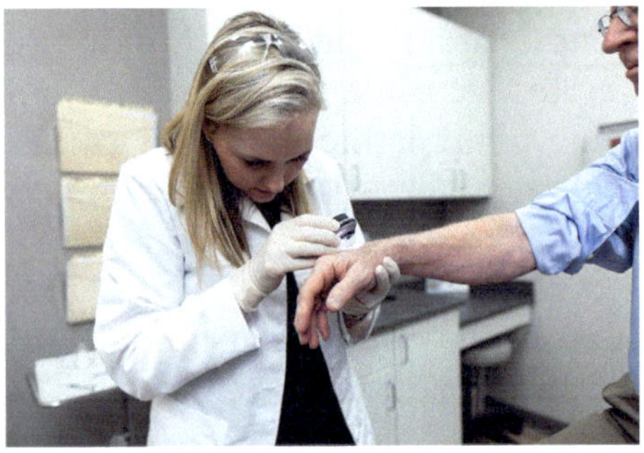

Figure 13.8. Performing skin examination in elder patients.

Source: MOD Dermatology. (2018). *Dermatologist Examining Patient's Skin with a Dermatoscope.* https://moddermatology.com/wp-content/uploads/2018/08/MG_5201-min.jpg.

13.3.3. Use of Diagnostic Tools and Technologies

Refinements in diagnostic technology have greatly improved the assessment and care of cutaneous disease among older persons. Elderly patients often demonstrate atypical presentations of the skin secondary to physiologic aging, comorbid disease, and drug therapy, which obfuscate the traditional clinical differential. High-tech imaging devices like dermoscopy and confocal microscopy have allowed the detection of subtle morphological changes that are crucial in early diagnosis, particularly in separating benign from malignant lesions. These technologies allow non-invasive testing, with reduced risk of painful biopsies in weakened patients. In addition, bringing digital health records into coordination with diagnostic imaging enables longitudinal management of chronic skin diseases common in geriatrics. Nevertheless, diagnostic precision continues to be hampered by cutaneous changes inherent in aging, and tools optimized for this population are needed. Design of age-inclusive diagnostic platforms is needed to increase detection, enable the provision of tailored interventions, and ultimately optimize dermatologic care in older adults (Voshaar et al., 2025). The arrival of artificial intelligence (AI) in dermatologic diagnosis has revolutionized prospects for geriatric patients through improved accuracy and predictability. AI-based computational algorithms are able to analyze complex imaging data to identify patterns that are not visible to the human eye, hence allowing for early detection of skin cancer and precancerous lesions. AI tools also provide real-time tracking through simulated treatment and readjustment of therapy plans in real-time, hence the provision for the changing responses typical in the care of aged skin. This customized approach is appropriate to the heterogeneity of geriatric dermatology where efficacy and tolerance to treatment are often influenced by comorbidities and polypharmacy. While these technologies foresee improved patient outcomes and satisfaction, bias in algorithms and data privacy concerns must be addressed cautiously to allow ethical and equitable use. Education of clinicians and interprofessional communication are key in the integration of AI into routine practice without compromising patient safety (Haykal, 2024). Building on the capability of newer diagnostic tests, real application in geriatric settings involves a multidisciplinary framework that can support the unique needs of older individuals.

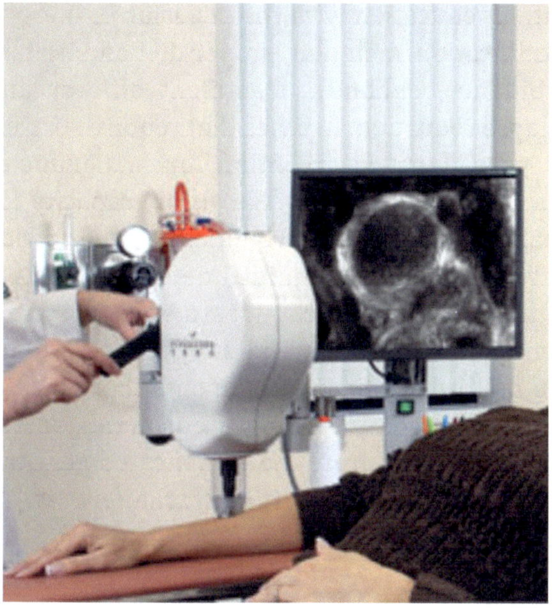

Figure 13.9. Using confocal microscopy for skin diagnosis.

Source: Illinois Melanoma Center. (2009). *Confocal Microscopy Procedure for Skin Imaging.* https://www.ilmelanoma.com/wp-content/uploads/2009/10/confocal-microscopy.jpg.

Cognitive impairment and personality disorders common among older individuals complicate symptom reporting and adherence to diagnostic practices, necessitating modifications in communication patterns and facilitative practices across clinical teams. Real-time monitoring technology has the potential to overcome these limitations by providing continuous, objective data on skin conditions, reducing reliance on patient self-report and enhancing clinical decision-making. Ethical concepts, for example, protection of autonomy and dignity—must also form the basis of introducing such technology, with establishing trust and accessibility being a priority. The integration of these diagnostic developments necessitates coordinated models of geriatric care that provide interdisciplinary communication and ensure integral management, thus maximally enhancing the quality of dermatologic treatment in the elderly (Voshaar et al., 2025) (Figure 13.9).

13.4. Treatment Options for Geriatric Dermatological Issues

The complexity of treating dermatological diseases in the elderly is that intrinsic aging processes interact with the most prevalent systemic diseases that may either aggravate skin disease or complicate treatment. Taking into account these challenges, treatment protocols should be tailored individually for consideration of impaired skin barrier function and altered pharmacokinetics that are characteristic for the elderly patient. For example, eczematous conditions, which are prevalent in this population, typically require treatment with mild moisturizers and topical corticosteroids at altered potencies and frequencies to prevent unwanted effects. Fungal infections also require careful diagnosis and judicious use of antifungal agents, particularly in patients with co-morbid diseases like diabetes mellitus, where control of infection is required but systemic treatments may be hazardous. This demand for individualized care is underscored by the necessity of integrating dermatologic treatments with worldwide management regimens addressing root systemic disease, as typified in more recent clinical series of geriatric outpatient populations (Venus et al., 2025). No less critical is the didactic value and diagnostic acumen of health providers who examine older skin diseases, and the outcome of treatment is directly determined. Research that quantified physician competence reported competent detection of malignant and benign erythematous lesions but showed poor gaps in detecting premalignant and benign hypopigmented skin conditions. Misdiagnosis typically leads to inappropriate or harmful therapy, thus the necessity for increased training and sensitivity concerning geriatric dermatology. Poor systemic antifungal therapy in conditions like subungual melanoma underscores the risk of diagnostic errors. Therefore, it is crucial to enhance the awareness of physicians about the characteristic presentation of geriatric skin disease in selecting the optimal and safest treatment modalities, preventing morbidity, and enhancing better quality of life among geriatric patients (Chanyachailert et al., 2023).

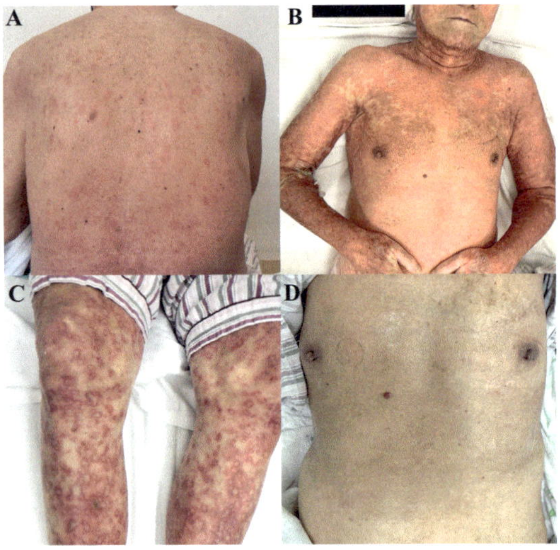

Figure 13.10. Photographs of skin lesion induced by sintilimab in an elderly patient with relapsed thymic carcinoma. (A) Rashes after the first cycle of treatment; (B, C) Rashes with blisters and skin detachment after the second cycle of treatment; and (D) Skin after recovery from severe toxic epidermal necrolysis.

Source: Yang H, Ma Q, Sun Y, Zhang K, Xing Y and Li H (2022) Case Report: Toxic epidermal necrolysis associated with sintilimab in a patient with relapsed thymic carcinoma. Front. Oncol. 12:1065137. doi: 10.3389/fonc.2022.1065137

Besides pharmacologic management, non-pharmacologic care plays a critical role in the management of dermatologic conditions among the elderly, particularly in preventing exacerbations and preserving skin integrity. Skin care regimens of repeated hydration, use of bland cleansers, and sun protection aid in maintaining skin barrier integrity and minimizing the occurrence of conditions like xerotica eczema and actinic keratosis. Secondly, patient education with the inclusion of lifestyle modification, including proper diet and irritant avoidance, enhances treatment efficacy and relapse reduction. In cases that require surgical or procedural intervention for malignancies that are typical in this age group, capacity for healing, potential comorbidities, and worldwide functional status guide decision-making. Individualized topical treatments, systemic therapy as indicated, and supportive care are the multi-disciplinary treatments that embody the paradigmatic integrated management necessary to address the complicated geriatric dermatology patient (Chanyachailert et al., 2023; Venus et al., 2025) (Figure 13.10).

13.4.1. Topical Treatments and Their Effectiveness

Advancements in dermatologic therapeutics have greatly enhanced the management of skin conditions prevalent in elderly patients. Local therapy remains a cornerstone for the management of most dermatological presentations among the elderly patients due to their localized action and fewer systemic side effects. However, the effect of such drugs is altered by the alterations with aging such as diminished epidermal barrier function, altered skin pH, and decreased cutaneous hydration, which alter drug penetration and effect. For instance, corticosteroids and calcineurin inhibitors are commonly employed in the therapy of inflammatory dermatoses, but when applied to older skin for long durations, caution needs to be exercised to prevent atrophy and absorption from the site. Furthermore, adherence to topical regimens is often hindered in this group because of physical or cognitive impairment, further compromising the therapeutic effect. Therefore, formulating topical preparations and delivery systems specifically in response to the unique physiological changes of elderly skin is essential for the optimization of treatment efficacy and patient compliance in geriatric dermatology.

Chronic inflammatory cutaneous diseases in older patients usually present complex comorbidities and demand the best possible selection of topical agents to maximize efficacy and safety. Topical immunosuppressants like cyclosporine, azathioprine, and methotrexate are used more widely in severe cases requiring systemic therapy, but local therapy is also necessary for localized disease control and prevention of systemic adverse effects (Sicras-Mainar et al., 2019). The heterogeneity of the drug regimen and the duration of the treatment observed in the clinic reflects the heterogeneity of the disorders of aged skin and patient-specific disorders. Moreover, prevalent psychiatric comorbidities encountered in this population may influence disease severity and drug responsiveness and highlight the necessity of integrated care. Regardless of hope from new biologics, cost and availability constraints render topical therapy the available first-line treatment in a large proportion of elderly patients. Therefore, tailoring such topical therapies to correct underlying pathophysiology along with patient context is necessary in order to attain maximum therapeutic benefit in geriatric dermatology. While the majority of topical dermatologic therapies are fairly innocuous, their use among elderly patients should be closely monitored due to the risk of delay in treatment and diagnosis, especially among institutionalized populations. As an example, scabies epidemics among nursing home residents highlight the problems of effective use of topical agents complicated by environmental and systemic factors (Morrison et al., 2019). The paucity of large datasets for the outcome of treatment and symptom relief for this group obstructs evidence-based recommendations and introduces heterogeneity in treatment approaches. Strong clinical trials of topical treatments have to be carried out in order to create standardized protocols considering the unique vulnerabilities of geriatric skin, including compromised immunity and frailty. Additionally, patient-reported outcomes and environmental control interventions along with pharmacotherapy can contribute to treatment effectiveness. More research in this field will allow clinicians to maximize topical treatment protocols such that effectiveness and safety can be assured for elderly patients with dermatological disorders (Figure 13.11).

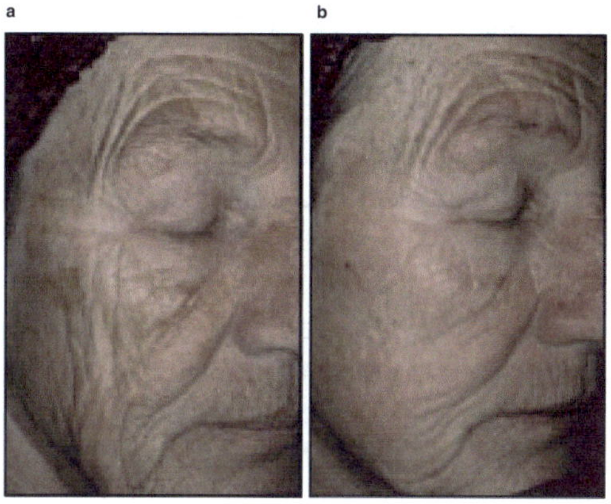

Figure 13.11. Case example of a subject treated with tretinoin emollient cream 0.05%. (a) Baseline; and (b) After 24 months of treatment.

Source: Milbauer, J., & Gilchrest, B. A. (2005). *Case Example of a Subject Treated with Tretinoin Emollient Cream 0.05%*. ResearchGate.

13.4.2. Systemic Therapies and Considerations

The management of dermatologic diseases among the elderly requires a detailed knowledge of systemic treatments, particularly because of the complexity added by the physiology of aging. Elderly patients frequently have several comorbidities and polypharmacy and the presence of these factors can increase the risk for drug-drug interactions and adverse drug reactions. For instance, drugs like methotrexate, ciclosporin, and retinoids, which are frequently utilized in psoriasis, need careful monitoring to avoid hepatotoxicity, nephrotoxicity, and other systemic toxicity. Also, changed pharmacokinetics in older persons with decreased renal excretion and hepatic metabolism necessitate dose reductions and individualized regimens to optimize therapeutic effectiveness vis-a-vis toxicity. These factors highlight the importance of customized treatment regimens for consideration of patients' general health status and simultaneous medical treatments (Nast et al., 2020). Also of significance is the utilization of thorough evaluation before starting systemic therapies in geriatric dermatology. The Rotterdam Study portrays the burden of chronic illness among the elderly population, which needs to be included in dermatological care planning (Ikram et al., 2020). Chronic hepatic, cardiac, or renal disease can significantly affect drug selection and monitoring plan, given the increased risk of this population to systemic side effects. Further, cognitive and functional decline may be an obstacle to medication adherence, requiring the involvement of caregivers and interventions.

Regular evaluation and interdisciplinary care enable clinicians to reduce risks from systemic therapy while optimizing outcomes for older patients with complex dermatologic diseases. Lastly, changing systemic treatments, such as biologics and small molecules, provide promising newer treatments for older adults but require subtle considerations of safety and long-term consequences. Drugs like adalimumab, apremilast, and more recently developed interleukin inhibitors are targeted immunomodulatory agents with potentially less systemic side effects than conventional immunosuppressants (Nast et al., 2020). However, sparse geriatric-specific data and concerns regarding immunosenescence support the need for applying with caution and strictly monitoring following treatment for the early identification of infections or cancer. Ultimately, a plan involving evidence-based recommendations, patient-centered risk assessment, and standard clinical monitoring serves as the basis for effective systemic treatment in geriatric dermatology.

13.4.3. Role of Preventive Care and Education

Aging introduces unavoidable alterations to the skin that heighten vulnerability to different dermatoses, though these conditions are not necessarily effectively controlled without preventive measures. Conditions like xerosis, eczema, and fungal infections are common in the elderly, usually triggered by environmental conditions and poor skin care habits. These conditions underscore the essential role of preventive management strategies to ensure the maintenance of skin integrity prior to the onset of severe symptoms. Instructing older patients and caregivers in correct hygiene, emollient use, and sun protection can greatly alleviate the incidence and severity of cutaneous disorders. By focusing on early detection and treatments, healthcare professionals can alleviate suffering and enhance the quality of life for members of this group, especially those living in rural areas where access to dermatologic services may be compromised (Prasad et al., 2024). This preventive strategy not only treats current skin issues but also reduces long-term sequelae that are a result of chronic dermatological pathologies. Although skin diseases are prevalent in geriatric patients, their clinical manifestations tend to diverge from those of younger patients and thus accurate diagnosis and prompt treatment may be difficult. Education and preventive care are indispensable in enabling geriatric patients to identify early warning signs and appropriate treatment modalities. For example, pruritus associated with xerosis, which is a common complaint in elderly patients, may be relieved with regular use of moisturizers and the elimination of irritants—procedures that are inexpensive and simple to apply through focused educational programs. In addition, patient education regarding the dangers of self-treatment and sun avoidance can avoid worsening benign and malignant skin tumors that are prevalent in the geriatric population. Such education promotes patient involvement and self-management, which is essential considering the complex interplay of comorbidities such as diabetes that can exacerbate dermatologic consequences (Eslavat et al., 2023). Preventive care in geriatric dermatology must include not only individual education but also wider community and healthcare system measures to optimize effectiveness. Education of primary care providers and caregivers in the subtleties of age-related skin changes guarantees early recognition and effective treatment of common dermatoses. Educational programs emphasizing foot hygiene, foot care, and regular skin examination can be particularly useful for older persons involved in agricultural or outdoor occupations, who are at higher risk because of chronic sun exposure and hard work. The incorporation of multidisciplinary care models with a focus on preventive education in addition to regular dermatologic assessment decreases the burden of disease and healthcare expenses considerably. Eventually, the development of a culture of prevention through education encourages older individuals to have healthy skin, postpones complications, and contributes to healthy aging (Eslavat et al., 2023; Prasad et al., 2024).

13.5. Psychosocial Aspects of Skin Conditions

The aging process is commonly accompanied by multiple health conditions that extend beyond physical status and impact psychological and social levels as well. Geriatric patients with dermatological diseases are commonly confronted with complex psychosocial mechanisms that can enhance the severity of their skin diseases. Dermatological conditions such as bullous diseases or psoriasis are often accompanied by psychiatric and musculoskeletal comorbidities, which also have an interaction effect on the quality of life and social function of the patients. The prevalence of these interacting comorbidities among older dermatological patients points out the reason that skin diseases cannot be treated separately. Geriatric inpatients typically possess a range of comorbidities, including cardiac, endocrine, and psychiatric comorbidities, which suggest that paradigms of dermatological management must be incorporated in the management of both the somatic and psychosocial aspects (Ansorge et al., 2022). Incorporation is vital in minimizing the overall impact of skin conditions on patients' mental well-being and adjustment to society. Depression and other psychiatric conditions are particularly prevalent in older populations with skin conditions, complicating treatment and remission. Representative cohorts of populations have, in empirical evidence, demonstrated that almost one in five older people report diagnosed dermatologic conditions, with many showing a significant proportion of concomitant symptoms congruent with depressive disorders (Guerra et al., 2014). This bidirectional association underscores the concurrent interaction between mental well-being and dermal health, noting that psychological manifestations both arise from and initiate dermatological illness. The perpetual visibility and distress of cutaneous disease may induce social avoidance, stigmatization, and self-esteem deficits in older patients, compounding loneliness and despair. These results reinforce the underpinning need to include psychiatric assessment and psychosocial intervention within routine dermatologic care among elderly populations to improve overall health outcomes (Guerra et al., 2014). Treating the psychosocial origins of dermatological conditions among elderly patients necessitates a synthesis of both clinical care beyond mere skin consultation. Multidisciplinary treatments including psychiatric screening, cognitive-behavioral therapy, and social support networks can help much in establishing patient coping and resilience. The chronic, often multifaceted nature of diseases like elderly venous insufficiency or neoplastic diseases requires not just medical therapies like Moh's surgery but also rehabilitation and psychological treatments to optimize overall well-being (Ansorge et al., 2022). Acknowledgment of the emotional burden that the geriatric dermatology patient bears enables health professionals to tailor treatments to acknowledge the emotional hurt associated with skin function and appearance. Ultimately, boosting the psychosocial component of dermatology in the elderly can enhance compliance with therapy, enhance quality of life, and reduce the cumulative effects of mental illness comorbidities.

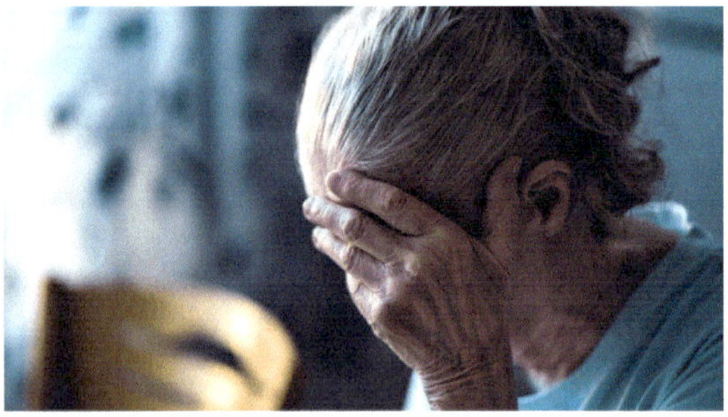

Source: Antara Senior Care. (n.d.). *Elderly Woman Covering Her Face in Distress.* https://www.antaraseniorcare.com/_next/image?url=https%3A%2F%2Fbackend.antaraseniorcare.com%2Fstatic%2Fuploads%2Fblogs%2Fblogs34cc376aa0ace80b135e5103e874c422.png&w=1200&q=75.

13.5.1. Impact of Skin Disorders on Mental Health

Aging also involves several health issues, most of which go beyond bodily discomfort and into the realm of mental wellbeing. Of these, skin ailments play a powerful but frequently overlooked role. Pruritus and eczematous disease are among the most common dermatological ailments in older age, and they do more than physically irritate. They have a strong impact on mental health as well. Chronic itching, for instance, interrupts sleep and daily functioning, causing increased stress and anxiety. The recurrence of these symptoms disrupts emotional stability and can lead to social withdrawal, thus aggravating the feelings of isolation that are commonly seen in elderly people. The effect of such skin disease on quality of life highlights the importance of identifying dermatological conditions as an essential part of mental health care in the geriatric age group (Varsha, 2023). Apart from physical manifestations, the social and aesthetic consequences of skin diseases have a powerful effect on mental health outcomes among the elderly. Most elderly patients are confronted with visible effects like xerosis, seborrheic keratosis, and psoriasis, which can lead to decreased self-esteem and issues related to body image. These issues can be even more pronounced in a group already at risk for loneliness and depression. In addition, the change in dermatological presentation among older adults can hide underlying psychological distress, making diagnosis and management difficult. The frequency of psychocutaneous disorders in this group, delusional parasitosis and other manifestations of anxiety, illustrates the complex relationship between skin disease and mental health issues (Eslavat et al., 2023). The management of these problems requires an integrated therapy modality that takes into consideration both dermatologic and psychological requirements.

The socioeconomic conditions that underlie skin disease among the elderly also exacerbate their psychological impact. Older adults often do hazardous labor or lack adequate access to health care, conditions that lead to unaddressed or under-treated skin disease. This neglect maximizes physical distress and its psychological burden, creating chronic stress and depression. Concomitant systemic diseases like diabetes not only make skin diseases more complicated but also increase the load on mental resilience. Successful intervention strategies should accordingly involve skin care education, early diagnosis, and holistic treatment plans that deal with both the physical presentation and the emotional consequences of skin diseases. In so doing, geriatric dermatology has the potential to contribute significantly towards enhancing general mental health and well-being among the elderly (Figure 13.12) (Eslavat et al., 2023; Varsha, 2023).

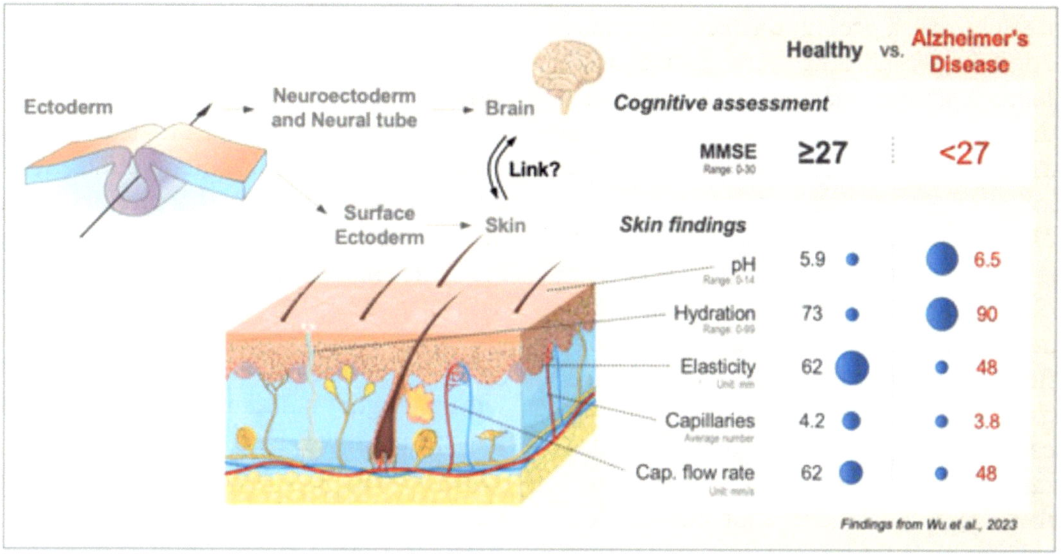

Figure 13.12. The skin-mind connection.

Source: Klostermeier S, Li A, Hou HX, Green U, Lennerz JK. Exploring the Skin Brain Link: Biomarkers in the Skin with Implications for Aging Research and Alzheimer's Disease Diagnostics. *International Journal of Molecular Sciences*. 2023; 24(17):13309. https://doi.org/10.3390/ijms241713309

13.5.2. Social Stigma and Its Effects on Elderly Patients

The complex interaction of aging and societal perceptions profoundly impacts older patients, particularly dermatology. The sight of the skin becomes a focus for social stigmatization, condemning the elderly with additional feelings of vulnerability. These dermatological changes, like wrinkles, lesions, or colorations, can be interpreted as signs of hygienic abandonment or absence of care, promoting stereotypes of older individuals as burdens or less capable. This dynamic worsens social isolation because older patients can retreat from interaction to evade stigmatization, eventually discouraging them from accessing necessary medical treatment. Societal devaluation of aging bodies, which has roots in different cultures and political systems throughout history, is a symptom of wider systemic problems. Significantly, trends in global aging policy, such as those driven by Maltese activism at the United Nations, have heightened awareness of these issues but thus far have not completely addressed the age-related stigma complexities of healthcare settings (Chirchop & Formosa, 2012). As such, stigma continues to act as a hindrance to optimal dermatological care for geriatric patients. The psychological impact of stigmatization among older patients goes beyond exteriorized embarrassment, penetrating deeply into mental well-being and treatment adherence. Chronic, visible skin diseases frequently lead to triggering or exacerbation of anxiety and depression in the aging population, making clinical outcomes more challenging. Stigmatization also results in a loss of self-esteem, causing some older patients to hide signs or ignore follow-up visits, thus resulting in delayed diagnosis and treatment. In geriatric dermatology, such reticence is especially troublesome since numerous skin diseases are signs of underlying systemic diseases that need early treatment. Clinicians need to be aware that in addition to clinical findings, the psychosocial impact of stigma has a profound effect on patient participation. Understanding these psychosocial aspects leads to greater empathy and integrated care with improved trust and communication. Such sensitivity is consistent with global public health policy targeting enhanced quality of life among older populations and the dismantling of damaging stereotypes (Chirchop & Formosa, 2012). Reducing social stigma necessitates comprehensive approaches including education, compassionate clinical practice, and policy change targeting aging populations. Dermatologists have a significant role in combating negative attitudes by facilitating patient dignity and individualized care, which can eliminate marginalization feelings. Moreover, public health campaigns that aim to make aging and its dermatological effects commonplace may eliminate societal prejudices, thus motivating geriatric patients to seek early treatment. Online media and images, such as those featured in contemporary medical archives, highlight the role of representation and visibility in reforming public opinion about aging skin. At the systemic level, policies inspired by global aging frameworks call for enhanced support systems that acknowledge and address stigma as a determinant of healthcare access. Through these combined efforts, geriatric dermatology can improve both clinical outcomes and social integration for elderly individuals, transforming stigma from a barrier into an opportunity for greater inclusion.

13.5.3. Importance of Support Systems and Counseling

Care for the multifaceted dermatological requirements of the elderly goes beyond immediate clinical management and includes psychological and emotional care. Most geriatric dermatoses, including chronic skin conditions or cancers, can severely impact the quality of life, resulting in anxiety, depression, and social isolation. In such patients, formal support systems and professional counseling are pivotal. They provide patients with an outlet to voice concerns and learn coping skills, which can ultimately enhance treatment plan adherence and overall outcomes. The inclusion of psychosocial interventions in dermatological treatment of older adults maximizes therapeutic effectiveness by recognizing the complex interaction between mental and skin health, thus promoting patient resilience in dealing with chronic or progressive skin diseases.

This integrated method is consistent with changing standards of care that focus on patient-centered care (Latzka et al., 2023). In addition, support systems, such as family and peer group support, offer critical emotional support that can counteract perceptions of loneliness prevalent among older patients with apparent dermatological conditions. Counseling specifically for this group of patients must take age-specific issues like cognitive impairment or sensory loss into account, which otherwise could interfere with proper communication and mental health care. With the inclusion of specialized counseling in the practice of geriatric dermatology, healthcare clinicians encourage improved self-management and facilitate early notification of symptoms, which are essential in diseases that need constant monitoring or complicated therapeutic regimens. This multidimensional care improves the patient's capacity to cope with the psychological weight of long-term diseases, thus preserving dignity and autonomy despite worsening skin diseases (Nast et al., 2020). Integrating support systems and counseling into geriatric dermatology practice also allows early detection of psychosocial stressors that may worsen dermatological disease severity, such as stress-related flare-ups typical in psoriasis or eczema. Counseling empowers patients by educating them regarding their diseases, which eliminates myths and establishes realistic expectations regarding the outcome of treatment, thus avoiding frustration and improving coping. Support groups also ensure continuity of care by connecting patients with community resources and social interaction, which minimizes isolation and enhances mental well-being. Finally, such holistic care models highlight the necessity of addressing both physical and emotional aspects of skin disease in the elderly population and ensuring treatments are not only clinically effective but also psychologically beneficial (Latzka et al., 2023; Nast et al., 2020).

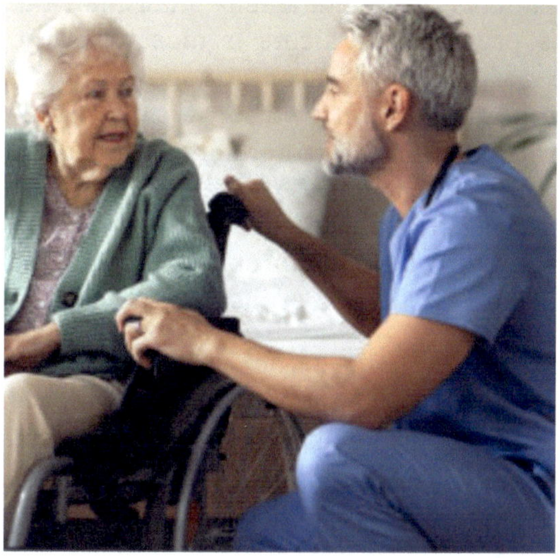

Source: Hope Hospice. (2023). *Caregiver Providing Toileting Assistance to Elderly Woman in Wheelchair*. https://www.hopehospice.com/wp-content/uploads/2023/10/toileting-assistance_FB-250x250.jpg.

13.6. Research and Advances in Geriatric Dermatology

The process of aging induces complex physiological changes across the integumentary system that demand sophisticated investigation of dermatological disease in the elderly. Recent studies highlight the rising occurrence of non-melanoma skin cancer (NSCLC) in the ageing population, a condition which emphasizes the need for sophisticated diagnostic and therapeutic care targeted to their individual clinical profiles. Evidences show there is a rising trend in incidences of NSCLC everywhere globally, as the older population is disproportionately affected through cumulative accumulation of UV exposure and aging-immunosenescence. Results emphasize the urgency for age-adjusted clinical protocols that address the complexity of management of skin carcinomas in older adults. Current research supports an integrated approach to geriatric dermatology, encompassing patient-specific factors, comorbidities, and psychosocial factors to optimize therapeutic outcomes and quality of life (Aleksandra et al., 2024). The new paradigm supports a shift towards precision medicine in dermatologic oncology for the elderly. Pharmacological advances have also been at the forefront of advancing geriatric dermatology, particularly through drug form design improvement towards the management of age-related medication adherence challenges. Oral drug delivery through orodispersible tablets is one of the key advances that facilitate more convenient delivery of drugs to patients who are elderly and frequently experience dysphagia or other swallowing diseases. These oral dissolution formulations are quickly soluble in the mouth without the need for water, thus improving therapy compliance and improving bioavailability of dermatological medicines. These technologies are especially suited for drugs that require repeated dosing for the management of chronic dermatoses or opportunistic infections prevalent in older skin. The employment of natural super disintegrants in tablet forms is a classic illustration of how pharmaceutical science is optimizing both the pharmacokinetic and patient-centered characteristics of dermatologic therapeutics, thereby enhancing safety, efficacy, and tolerability profiles in geriatric patients (Kumar, 2016). Recent geriatric dermatology research further advocates for interprofessional care and personalized treatment models to cope with the complex relationship between skin aging and disease processes in the body. Therapeutic navigation requires multidisciplinary teamwork among geriatricians, dermatologists, pharmacologists, and caregivers to develop personalized care plans. Moreover, improvements in molecular immunology and biology are elucidating the pathophysiologic substrate of cutaneous disease in older adults so that interventions can now be specifically directed with fewer adverse effects. On the horizon are future developments based on incorporating new diagnostics, such as biomarker analysis and imaging technology, along with patient-reported outcomes to maximize therapeutic effect. Lastly, current research work attempts to optimize clinical decision-making and improve general care of cutaneous diseases in the elderly, with a balance between medically effective therapy and maintenance of quality of life (Aleksandra et al., 2024).

13.6.1. Current Trends in Dermatological Research

With an aging world population, new approaches in dermatological research are essential in addressing the unique challenges presented by geriatric patients. New studies emphasize the integration of new technologies that improve the diagnosis and treatment of age-related skin diseases. Among them, AI has emerged as a powerful tool, with capabilities greater than those of traditional clinical methods. Artificial intelligence -powered systems are increasingly being used to analyze complex dermatological images, enabling earlier and more precise diagnosis of cancerous lesions and chronic skin diseases prevalent in the elderly. This technology evolution not only provides improved treatment results but also attempts to minimize clinical processes, so that dermatologic treatment is more convenient and effective for aged patients who typically suffer from complex skin issues due to additive environmental and bodily stress. Hence, AI is a giant leap towards making the care specific to the needs of the aging skin (Godase, 2025). In addition to the diagnostic advances, recent research in geriatric dermatology explores how AI can further help enhance therapy modalities, particularly concerning tailored treatment protocols. Computer programs possessing the capacity to integrate massive datasets allow for assessing individual patient histories, genetic factors, and environmental exposures to inform bespoke interventions to promote maximum skin health among older individuals. This precision medicine is most relevant in the treatment of chronic wounds, pressure ulcers, and pigmentary disorders ubiquitous in geriatric patients. Furthermore, AI in cosmetic dermatology, though less traditionally prioritized in the geriatric context, has been very promising in improving aesthetic problems, which greatly influence the quality of life and mental health of the elderly.

These developments represent a general trend toward the application of AI to the treatment of both medical and cosmetic problems, as part of an integrated strategy for geriatric skin care and expanding research frontiers (Godase, 2025). Apart from clinical and treatment purposes, the modern age of dermatological research in geriatrics also underscores the importance of AI-based dermatopathology. The introduction of deep learning algorithms like CNNs has revolutionized microscopic examination, facilitating quicker and more precise detection of pathological alterations in skin biopsies. This is particularly important in the elderly, whose skin biopsies are likely to harbor superimposing pathologies resulting from cumulative aging and comorbidities. AI-dermatopathology enhances accuracy, reduces inter-observer disagreement, and accelerates pathologic evaluation, thereby facilitating timely clinical decisions. Concurrently with technical advancements, research also offers solutions to bridging the issues of image quality preservation, data privacy, and management of computational resources, all critical for the practical application of these technologies in geriatric dermatology clinics. Combined, these developments foretell a future where smart systems play a crucial role in improving the elderly's dermatology (Figure 13.13).

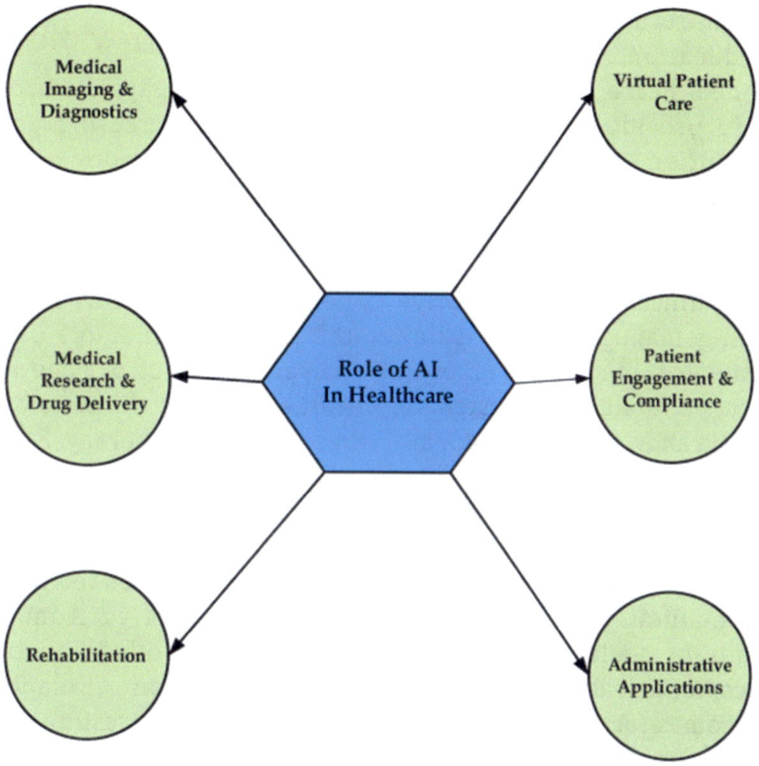

Figure 13.13. The schematic diagram shows the hypothetical use of machine learning algorithms to help dermatologists diagnose lesions to make appropriate clinical decisions.

Source: Al Kuwaiti A, Nazer K, Al-Reedy A, Al-Shehri S, Al-Muhanna A, Subbarayalu AV, Al Muhanna D, Al-Muhanna FA. A Review of the Role of Artificial Intelligence in Healthcare. *Journal of Personalized Medicine*. 2023; 13(6):951. https://doi.org/10.3390/jpm13060951

13.6.2. Innovations in Treatment and Technology

Innovations in the dermatologic treatment of aging have gone on to embrace new technologies that address the complexities of skin in old age. Among them is medical laser therapy, which has been shown to possess the capacity to cause skin regrowth alongside superficial enhancement. Recent evidence indicates that laser treatment initiates epigenetic modifications like DNA methylation and histone acetylation that reprogram gene expression that controls collagen synthesis and cellular repair. Such molecular reprogramming of the skin improves its healing and rejuvenating capacity long-term, with promising outcomes in the treatment of wrinkles, scars, and pigmentation abnormalities prevalent in geriatric patients. Through the targeting of discrete layers of the skin, lasers induce controlled damage that induces natural repair cascades, regulated via epigenetic mechanisms.

These advances signal a trend toward therapies that engage the skin's biology at the genetic level, providing long-term clinical outcomes to address the particular needs of aged skin (Haykal et al., 2025). Along with these treatment innovations, dermatological use of social media and digital platforms has revolutionized patient engagement and education, especially for the elderly. Today, healthcare providers are using social media to provide individualized dermatologic information, deliver distant consultation sessions, and build patient-provider relationships, thereby increasing access for the elderly with potential mobility problems. This new form of digital healthcare improves early diagnosis and ongoing management of skin conditions using telemedicine and online follow-ups, filling gaps in conventional care systems. In addition, social media allows for professional networking and continuing education among dermatologists to lead to further dissemination of technological innovations and best practices in geriatric dermatology. Acknowledging the significance of maintaining digital and conventional methods of health care makes technological advancements lead to significant improvements in outcomes for elderly patients (Farsi, 2021). In the future, individualized dermatological care based on breakthroughs such as precision laser treatments and epigenetic profiling is becoming an emerging frontier in geriatric practice. Through the examination of patient-specific epigenetic markers, doctors are able to tailor laser parameters and concurrent treatments to maximize dermal regeneration and minimize complications like post-inflammatory hyperpigmentation. Moreover, AI programs are being created to decode complex genetic and epigenetic information, providing predictive analysis of treatment response and allowing dynamic modification of therapeutic plans. Such integration enables a transition from a one-size-fits-all model to very individualized treatment addressing the heterogeneity of the aging process. The convergence of epigenetics, sophisticated laser technologies, and digital technologies therefore holds promise for a new age of geriatric dermatology, as breakthroughs interact synergistically to transform skin health and well-being (Farsi, 2021; Haykal et al., 2025).

13.6.3. Future Directions for Geriatric Dermatology

With the demographic drift of a global population towards age increasing, geriatric dermatology is now all the more confronted to identify innovative strategies specifically tuned into the extremely unique physiological transformations of the aged skin. Future research must emphasize personalization of treatment that transcends the complex trade-off of comorbidities and polypharmacy of old age that exerts a potent influence over dermatologic well-being and responsivity to therapy. Further, the integration of emerging studies on adaptogenic agents holds the potential for enhancing skin resilience and transcending age-associated deterioration by modulating neuroendocrine-immune regulation. The drugs, derived from traditional medical systems, may offer holistic benefits through their stimulation of adaptive stress response and potentially arresting pre-mature skin aging and overall dermal youthfulness. Therefore, the convergence of dermatology with gerontology and pharmacology in a multi-aspect concept may change preventive and therapeutic practices, encouraging increased quality of life among aging patients through targeted biological interventions (Panossian et al., 2020). Advances in technology for digital health provide novel opportunities in treating dermatological conditions among the elderly. The availability of wearable sensors and smartphone apps allows continuous tracking of skin health parameters, allowing patients to take an active role in skin care and early detection of pathologies. Yet the uptake of such digital self-management tools also requires a balancing act for the doctor-patient relationship, as clinicians are tasked with incorporating patient-generated information into clinical processes without undermining the individualized attention necessary for older adults. Bridging the divide between technologically facilitated autonomy and professional health counseling demands frameworks that integrate data fusion to support effective and safe decision-making. Emphasizing collaborative digital literacy and patient education can enhance compliance and responsiveness to dermatologic therapy, and thus subsequent models of care can be evidence-based and participatory (Fiske et al., 2020). In the future, application of systems pharmacology and network pharmacology approaches to research in geriatric dermatology promises to shed light to a larger extent on molecular and cellular processes of skin aging and disease manifestation among the elderly. This is because, in this methodology, synergistic drug combinations not present with the conventional single-drug studies may be identified, in addition to novel therapeutic targets. By going back to and validating ancient medicinal practices using rigorous scientific examination, clinicians may add the therapeutic armamentarium to botanicals and adaptogens tailor-made for stress-related and age-related dermatologic diseases. The path ahead is hence an integrative model combining the newest biomedical technologies with holistic concepts to develop multifactorial therapies tailored to personalized treatment of multifactorial etiologies of skin aging in geriatric patients (Panossian et al., 2020).

CLOSER LOOK

Clear Cell Acanthoma

Clear cell acanthoma is an uncommon, benign epidermal tumor marked by a slowly growing, pink to brown papule or nodule, frequently with a "stuck-on" appearance and a wafer-like scale collarette. It is most often found on middle-aged to elderly patients, typically on the lower extremities but may occur elsewhere. Although dermoscopy can be helpful in diagnosis, a skin biopsy is usually necessary for identification.

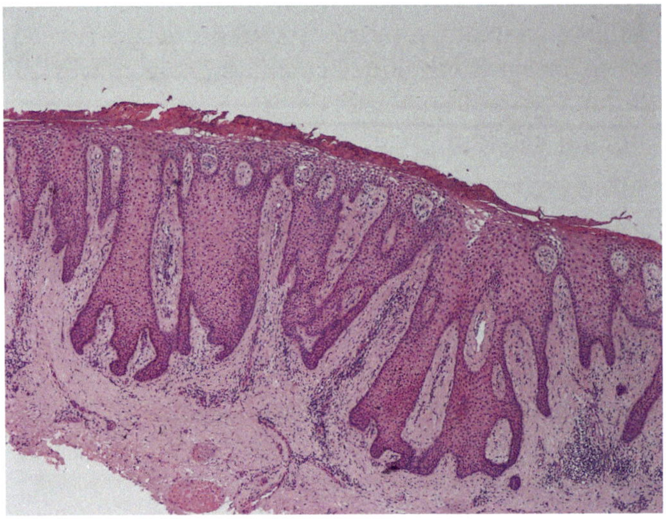

Source: By LWozniak&KWZielinski - Own work, CC BY-SA 3.0, https://commons.wikimedia.org/w/index.php?curid=11141172

- **Key Features of Clear Cell Acanthoma**
  - **Appearance:** A slowly growing, pink to brown, dome-shaped papule or nodule.
  - **Location:** Typically occurs on the lower extremities, but can also be present on the trunk, forearm, face, inguinal region, and in rare instances, the nipple and areola.
  - **Clinical Presentation:** Typically asymptomatic, but may be pruritic or bleed following trivial trauma.
  - **Dermoscopy:** Dermoscopy demonstrates a characteristic pattern with glomerular or dotted vessels in a "pearl necklace" or "string of pearls" pattern.
  - **Histology:** Histologically, it exhibits an intra-epidermal well-demarcated proliferation of glycogen-rich keratinocytes.
  - **Prognosis:** Clear cell acanthoma is benign and has an excellent prognosis.
  - **Treatment:** Small lesions need not be treated, whereas larger lesions can be excised.
- **Diagnosis**

- **Clinical Examination:** The lesion's characteristic appearance can serve as a clue, but in most cases, a skin biopsy is required to diagnose.
- **Dermoscopy:** Dermoscopy may help in diagnosis by showing the characteristic "pearl necklace" pattern.
- **Histopathology:** Histological study establishes the diagnosis through demonstration of typical intra-epidermal proliferation of glycogen-containing keratinocytes.

- **Differential Diagnoses**
  - **Pyogenic Granuloma:** Dermoscopy can be used to differentiate between the two.
  - **Amelanotic Melanoma:** Dermoscopy and histology are required to exclude melanoma.
  - **Traumatized Hemangioma:** Dermoscopy can differentiate between the two.
  - **Squamous Cell Carcinoma:** Histology is essential to differentiate between clear cell acanthoma and squamous cell carcinoma.
  - **Bowen's Disease:** Dermoscopy and histology are required to differentiate between the two.
  - **Seborrheic Keratosis:** Dermoscopy can differentiate between the two.
  - **Psoriasis:** Histology and dermoscopy are required to distinguish between the two.

SUMMARY

With the increased aging population worldwide, geriatric dermatology is under increased stress that requires advanced-level clinical skills and increased empathy. Skin diseases in the elderly are complicated not just by physiological aging but also by polypharmacy and comorbidities, which require meticulous drug management. A significant proportion of older patients receive potentially inappropriate drugs that have the potential to worsen dermatologic disease or impede skin healing (Abdulla et al., 2025). Therefore, incorporation of comprehensive geriatric assessment and multi-professional collaboration becomes essential in the prevention of side effects and enhancing skin health outcomes. The integration of such strategies guarantees that dermatological treatment is not done in isolation but considers the larger picture of overall geriatric well-being, with a focus on efficacy and safety in the treatment process for this susceptible group in particular. Clinical training and education are also essential to improving the dermatologic care of the elderly. In spite of the intricacy in skin disease in the aged, the experience with dermatology in training can advance future clinicians' confidence and ability in managing such diseases (Malik et al., 2025). Practical learning formats like live patient demonstrations have proved to be very helpful in reinforcing core knowledge, and making students ready for actual applications in dermatological work. Such training also promotes appreciation of dermatology as a subspecialty, potentially satisfying the demand for more specialists who serve geriatric populations. With a sound training foundation, health systems can produce clinicians proficient in addressing the dermatologic needs of older patients sensitively and professionally. Lastly, management of the dermatologic problems of older adults demands multi-disciplinary effort balancing judicious pharmacologic management, superb clinical training, and a knowledge of aging physiologic processes. Inappropriate medication in older adults is a high-profile target for policy and practice reform aimed at reducing harm and maximizing skin function (Abdulla et al., 2025). Parallelly, the development of dermatology clerkships can equip emerging healthcare professionals to provide more informed and empathetic care to this population (Malik et al., 2025). Collectively, these initiatives will eventually lead to better clinical outcomes and quality of life in geriatric patients, hence validating the utmost significance of developing geriatric dermatology in both research and practice contexts.

The changing trend in the delivery of healthcare supports the necessity of general definitions and parameters of models of geriatric care, and this has significant consequences for the care of dermatologic diseases in older people. The integration of medical specialist and generalist care in acute geriatric community hospitals represents a new model of managing complex needs in older people, including their skin. By refining admission criteria to such care environments, clinicians can be assured of delivering age-targeted interventions along with dermatologic management for elderly patients with comorbidities. The emphasis points to multidisciplinary care as the ideal way of tackling the aging skin complexities of increased susceptibility, risk of infection, and chronic wounds, which call for specialist competencies and practice environments (Kroeze et al., 2024). These advances highlight the dynamic interplay between paradigms of geriatric and dermatologic care in the elderly. Education is also critical to developing the exemplary practice of geriatric dermatology, especially in undergraduate medical education. The described heterogeneity of education in geriatric medicine nationwide, in spite of national guidelines, indicates patchwork that corrodes general awareness of the special dermatologic phenomena of the elderly. Standardization and revision of these courses will be required to prepare future clinicians with the information and skills to make accurate diagnoses and manage and treat age-related dermatologic diseases properly. Highlighting newer teaching methods adaptable to population changes and fresh medical exigencies will ensure greater preparedness of medical graduates, essential when the global population is growing older and geriatric skin diseases are becoming common and complex (Kupis et al., 2024). Education reform, thus, becomes an integral part of serving as the door to development in geriatric dermatology. The integration of healthcare delivery innovation and education reforms offers a broader platform for managing the complexities of geriatric dermatology. Care model fine-tuning seeks to maximize patient outcomes via differentiated admission criteria and multidisciplinary interventions, while curriculum integration seeks to deliver capable practitioners who are able to manage skin conditions among the elderly. Both aspects respond to an imperative requirement to cater to population trends toward longer longevity and the resulting increase in geriatric dermatological disease. Integrating changes in clinical practice into educational development, the specialty can better treat elderly patients' complex needs with care that is holistic to body and skin. This holistic outlook ultimately improves older adults' quality of life through improved dermatological treatment.

KEY TERMS FROM THIS CHAPTER

- Angiogenesis
- Collagen
- Elasticity
- Malignant neoplasias
- Overall dry skin
- Pruritus
- Senile purpura
- Tensile strength
- Xerosis cutis
- Autologous stem cells
- Cultured fibroblasts
- Geriatric dermatology
- Metabolism
- Polydeoxyribonucleotide
- Quality of life
- Skin cancers
- Transepidermal water loss
- Benign neoplasias
- Diabetes mellitus
- Hypertension
- Microvascular perfusion
- Pressure ulcers
- Seborrheic keratoses
- Teledermatology
- Xerosis

REFERENCES

1. Abdulla, M. F., Obaid, F. E., Moaket, O. S., & Alawainati, M. A. (2025). Potentially inappropriate medications for geriatric patients in Bahrain: Prevalence, predi*ctors, and implica*tions for practice. BMC Geriatrics, 25. https://www.semanticscholar.org/paper/8eb5d8d04a5c42affd6943d82528bc5ae36f638f (accessed on 12 May 2025).
2. Akaberi S M, Sharma K, Ahmadi-Ashtiani H R, Hedayati M, Polydeoxyribonucleotide in Skincare and Cosmetics: Mechanisms, Therapeutic Applications, and Advancements Beyond Wound Healing and Anti-aging.J Skin Stem Cell.2025;12(1):e159728.https://doi.org/10.5812/jssc-159728.(accessed on 12 May 2025).
3. Akarsu, S. (2023). Neuropathic Pruritus: An Underrecognized and Often Misdiagnosed and Difficult to Treat Medical Condition. IntechOpen. doi: 10.5772/intechopen.110825 (accessed on 12 May 2025).
4. Akdeniz, M., Hahnel, E., Ulrich, C., Blume-Peytavi, U., & Kottner, J. (2019). Prevalence and associated factors of skin cancer in aged nursing home resid*ents: A* mu*lti*center prevalence study. PloS one, 14(4), e0215379. https://doi.org/10.1371/journal.pone.0215379(accessed on 12 May 2025).
5. Amadi, E. S., Bellgam, H. I., & Pepple, E. R. (2017). The prevalence and pattern of dermatological disorders among elderly patients in a tertiary hospital in South-South Nigeria. https://core.ac.uk/download/478392291.pdf (accessed on 12 May 2025).
6. Ansorge, C., Miocic, J. M., & Schauer, F. (2022). Skin diseases in hospitalized geriatrics: a 9-year analysis from a Univ*ersity Dermatology Center in German*y. *Ar*chives of dermatological research, 314(5), 427–437. https://doi.org/10.1007/s00403-021-02244-9Morrison, E. J., Middleton, J., Lanza, S., Cowen, J. E., Hewitt, K., Walker, S. L., Nicholls, M., Rajan-Iyer, J., Fletcher, J., & Cassell, J. A. (2019). Do we know how scabies outbreaks in residential and nursing care homes for the elderly should be managed? A systematic review of interventions using a novel *approach to assess eviden*ce *qu*ality. Epidemiology and infection, 147, e250. https://doi.org/10.1017/S0950268819001249
7. Chanyachailert, P. ., Pattanaprichakul, P. ., Bunyaratavej, S. ., Leeyaphan, C. ., Pongkittilar, B. ., *Sereeaphinan, C. ., & Stockman, D. . (2023)*. Evaluation of Clinical Knowledge Regarding Geriatric Skin Conditions among Thai Physicians. Siriraj Medical Journal, 75(1), 1–6. https://doi.org/10.33192/smj.v75i1.260522(accessed on 12 May 2025).
8. Chirchop, J., & Formosa, M. (2012). Revisiting Labour History. https://www.um.edu.mt/li*brary/oar/handle/123456789/105577(acc*essed on 12 May 2025).
9. Cuomo, R., Rozen, W. M., Pentangelo, P., Ceccaroni, A., Alfano, C., & Seth, I. (2024). Human Papillomavirus-Associated Giant Clear Cell Acanthoma and Squamous Cell Carcinoma: A Rare Case Report and Literature Review. Journal of clinical medicine, 13(9), 2482. https://doi.org/10.3390/jcm13092482(accessed on 12 May 2025).
10. Edw*ards, H., Finlayson, K., Co*urtney, M., Graves, N., Gibb, M., & Parker, C. (2013). Health service pathways for patients with chronic leg ulcer*s: identifying effective* pathways for facilitation of evidence based wound care. BMC health services research, 13, 86. https://doi.org/10.1186/1472-6963-13-86 (accessed on 12 May 2025).

11. Eslavat, S., Vemu, D., Kunti, S., Naik, P., & Ramadas, K. (2023). A clinic epidemiological study of geriatric dermatoses. EUREKA: Health Sciences. https://www.semanticscholar.org/paper/5f4733d71d853b787ee580d8e3bc8d82304a0879 (accessed on 12 May 2025).

12. Eslavat, S., Vemu, D., Kunti, S., Naik NM, P., & Ramadas, K. (2023). A clinicoepidemiological study of geriatric dermatoses. EUREKA: Health Sciences, (3), 46-57. https://doi.org/10.21303/2504-5679.2023.003007 (accessed on 12 May 2025).

13. Farsi, D. (2021). Social media and health care, part I: Literature review of social media use by health care providers. Journal of Medical Internet Research, 23, e23205. https://doi.org/10.2196/23205.

14. Fiske, A., Buyx, A., & Prainsack, B. (2020). The double-edged sword of digital self-care: Physician perspectives from Northern Germany. Social Science & Medicine, 260, 113174. https://doi.org/10.1016/j.socscimed.2020.113174.

15. Gisondi, P., Fargnoli, M. C., Amerio, P., Argenziano, G., Bardazzi, F., Bianchi, L., Chiricozzi, A., et al. (2022). Italian adaptation of EuroGuiDerm guideline on the systemic treatment of chronic plaque psoriasis. Italian Journal of Dermatology and Venereology, 157. https://doi.org/10.23736/s2784-8671.21.07132-2.

16. Godase, P. (2025). Artificial intelligence driven skin analysis tool: Current trends in cosmetic and cosmeceuticals. International Journal for Research in Applied Science and Engineering Technology. International Journal for Research in Applied Science & Engineering Technology (IJRASET) ISSN: 2321-9653; IC Value: 45.98; SJ Impact Factor: 7.538 Volume 13 Issue IV Apr 2025- Available at www.ijraset.com (accessed on 12 May 2025).

17. Guerra, S. G. (2014). Affections dermatologiques et troubles dépressifs: Leur association chez les personnes âgées du Québec. CORE. https://core.ac.uk/download/51333942.pdf (accessed on 12 May 2025).

18. Guidet, B., de Lange, D. D., Boumendil, A., Leaver, S., Watson, X., Boulanger, C., Szczeklik, W., et al. (2019). The contribution of frailty, cognition, activity of daily life and comorbidities on outcome in acutely admitted patients over 80 years in European ICUs: The VIP2 study. Intensive Care Medicine, 46, 57–69. https://www.semanticscholar.org/paper/d7cb5d0afb377ab15e2ec792c960fbce72cb4d7b (accessed on 12 May 2025).

19. Haykal, D. (2024). Emerging and pioneering AI technologies in aesthetic dermatology: Sketching a path toward personalized, predictive, and proactive care. Cosmetics. https://www.semanticscholar.org/paper/e4be2d230ab1f25c6fad5c53961b52c502f2ddf9 (accessed on 12 May 2025).

20. Haykal, D., Flament, F., Mora, P., Balooch, G., & Cartier, H. (2025). Unlocking Longevity in Aesthetic Dermatology: Epigenetics, Aging, and Personalized Care. International journal of dermatology, 10.1111/ijd.17725. Advance online publication. https://doi.org/10.1111/ijd.17725(accessed on 12 May 2025).

21. Haykal, D., Will, F., Cartier, H., & Dahan, S. (2025). Epigenetic modifications and the role of medical lasers in enhancing skin regeneration. Journal of Cosmetic Dermatology, 24. https://doi.org/10.1111/jocd.16780.

22. Hera, R. E., Damayanti, Lilik Djuari, & Ema Qurnianingsih. (2024). The Role of Health Education on the Level of Knowledge of Contact Dermatitis in the Elderly. Berkala Ilmu Kesehatan Kulit

Dan Kelamin, 36(3), 184–190. *https://doi.org/10.20473/bikk.V36.3.*2024.184-190(accessed on 12 May 2025).

23. Ikram, M. A., Brusselle, G., Ghanbari, M., Goedegebure, A., Ikram, M., Kavousi, M., Kieboom, B. C. T., et al. (2020). Objectives, design and main findings until 2020 from the Rotterdam Study. European Journal of *Epidemiology, 35, 483–517. https://*doi.org/10.1007/s10654-020-00640-5.
24. Kroeze, E., de Groot, A. J., Smorenburg, S. M., Mac Neil Vroomen, J. L., Van Vught, A., & Buurman, B. M. (2024). A case vignette study to refine the target group *of an intermediate care model: The acute ger*iatric community hospital. European Geriatric Medicine, 15, 977–989. https://www.semanticscholar.org/paper/bec9ac206d021a1a3af81bf6b1380d64b06c8808 (accessed on 12 May 2025).
25. Kumar, V. (2016). Formulation and evaluation of meclizine HCl orally dispersi*ble tablets by usi*ng natural super disintegrants. 2, 53–80. https://www.semanticscholar.org/paper/030f194a50ecc2ec3db6e8671567716e02aabd63 (accessed on 12 May 2025).
26. Kupis, R., Perera, I., Targowski, T., Gąsowski, J., & Piotrowicz, K. (2024). Is geriatric medicine teaching homogeneous? The *analysis of geriatric medicine cour*ses at Polish undergraduate medical programmes. European Geriatric Medicine, 15, 1523–1532. https://www.semanticscholar.org/paper/c70f8f8b10a316de16828d41f4b5d642e5c1198f (accessed on 12 May 2025).
27. Latzka, J., Assaf, C., Bagot, M., Cozzio, A., Dummer, R., Guenova, E., Gniadecki, R., et a*l. (2023). EORTC consensus reco*mmendations for the treatment of mycosis fungoides/Sézary syndrome–Update 2023. European Journal of Cancer, 195, Article 113343. https://doi.org/10.1016/j.ejca.2023.113343.
28. Malik, S., Akhtar, A., Ejaz, H., Anwar, A., Tahir, M., & Sadiq, S. (2025). Exploring the students' perspective: Unveiling insights into dermatology clerkship in undergraduate medical students. Pakistan Armed Forces Medical Journal. https://www.semanticscholar.org/paper/313b191a45db00630f8223af317833771942d21c (accessed on 12 May 2025).
29. Mayrovitz, H. N., Wong, S., & Mancuso, C. (2023). Venous, *Arterial, and Neuropathic Leg* Ulcers With Emphasis on the Geriatric Population. Cureus, 15(4), e38123. https://doi.org/10.7759/cureus.38123(accessed on 12 May 2025).
30. Mazan, P., Lesiak, A., Skibińska, M., Rynkowska-Kidawa, M., Bednarski, I., Sobolewska-Sztychny, D*., **Noweta, M., et al. (2024).*** Pruritus prevalence and characteristics in care and treatment facility and geriatric outpatient clinic patients: A cross-sectional study using standardized pruritus questionnaires. Advances in Dermatology and Allergology, 41, 463–472. https://*www.semanticscholar.org/paper/c7*928d95afea1a9ed566c4d43dd6b904fbf12b58 (accessed on 12 May 2025).
31. Mehrabani, D., & Manafi, N. (2013). Role of cultured skin fibroblasts in aesthetic and plastic surgery. World Journal of Plastic Surgery, 2, 2–5. https://www.semanticscholar.org/paper/0*772024625a252d094f7aa6c6780b947e7a91ed1 (*accessed on 12 May 2025).
32. Nast, A., Smith, C., Spuls, P. I., Avila Valle, G., Bata-Csörgõ, Z., Boonen, H., de Jong, E. M. G. J., et al. (2020). EuroGuiDerm guideline on the systemic treatment of psoriasis vulgaris–Part 1: Treatment and monitoring *recommend*ations. Journal of the European Academy of Dermatology and Venereology, 34, 2461–2498. https://doi.org/10.1111/jdv.16915.
33. Nikam, B., Deokar, N. P., & Varsha, J. (2023). Pruritic dermatoses among the elderly: Impact on

quality of life and implications for geriatric dermatology. Journal of advanced Zoology Volume 44Issue S-2Year 2023Page 509:518. CORE. https://core.ac.uk/download/588567104.pdf.

34. Oude Voshaar, R. C., & van Dijk, S. V. (2025). New horizons in personality disorders, from neglect to necessity in geriatric care. Age and Ageing, 54. https://www.semanticscholar.org/paper/f191cf2c0bc266a4c893b7a64f5e1fe12c1bb5f2 (accessed on 12 May 2025).

35. Panossian, A., Efferth, T., Shikov, A. N., Pozharitskaya, O. N., Kuchta, K., Mukherjee, P. K., Banerjee, S., et al. (2020). Evolution of the adaptogenic concept from traditional use to medical systems: Pharmacology of stress- and aging-related diseases. Medicinal Research Reviews, 41, 630–703. https://doi.org/10.1002/med.21743.

36. Pirozhnikova A.A., Stetsyuk M.V., Kudrevich K.A., Abdurakhmanova E.E., Umerova A.I., Tamasyan E.G., Kovali D.Yu., Tovmasyan K.A., Filipova V.A., Diarova A.A., Nemirova O.V., Bagdasaryan A.A., Shadiev Kh.-A.A. The current state of the issue of diagnosis and treatment of non-melanoma skin cancer in elderly patients. Clinical review for general practice. 2024; 5 (12): 56–66 (In Russ.). DOI: 10.47407/kr2024.5.12.00538

37. Prasad A M, Lalitha C, Babu A R, A clinical study of Geriatric dermatoses at Tertiary care center in South India. IP Indian J Clin Exp Dermatol 2024;10(1):19-22 (accessed on 12 May 2025).

38. Sadhwani, V. N., Vithalani, N. J., Dani, A., & Hasani, R. J. (2025). Clinical pattern of dermatological diseases in geriatric patients: A cross-sectional study from Central India. Cureus, 17. https://www.semanticscholar.org/paper/f00100a32d20dd40d7aae125e3502739830200f9 (accessed on 12 May 2025).

39. Shaw, R. (2019). Assessing the Dermatological Healthcare Needs of Today's Geriatric Population; A Nation-Wide Behavioral Analysis. https://open.bu.edu/bitstream/2144/38724/7/Shaw_bu_0017N_14964.pdf (accessed on 12 May 2025).

40. Sicras-Mainar, A., Navarro-Artieda, R., & Armario-Hita, J. C. (2019). Severe Atopic Dermatitis In Spain: A Real-Life Observational Study. Therapeutics and clinical risk management, 15, 1393–1401. https://doi.org/10.2147/TCRM.S226456 (accessed on 12 May 2025).

41. Sinikumpu, S. P., Jokelainen, J., Keinänen-Kiukaanniemi, S., & Huilaja, L. (2022). Skin cancers and their risk factors in older persons: a population-based study. BMC geriatrics, 22(1), 269. https://doi.org/10.1186/s12877-022-02964-1 (accessed on 12 May 2025).

42. Snarskaya, E., & Bykanov, A. S. (2023). Efficacy of transdermal microneedling redermalization with high-molecular-weight hyaluronic acid and sodium succinate in the correction of postacne scars. Russian Journal of Skin and Venereal Diseases. https://www.semanticscholar.org/paper/bc44229d8566b82173227b7935ef196eb8ce039e (accessed on 12 May 2025).

43. Tanaka, F., Hayashi, C., Iida, M., Shinya, K., & Futamura, M. (2024). Changes in Skin Barrier Function in Neonates: Daily Variation and Impact of Bathing. Pediatric dermatology, 41(6), 1099–1105. https://doi.org/10.1111/pde.15772(accessed on 12 May 2025).

44. Tian, Y., Hirsch, G., Skayem, C., Thomas, E., Hua, C., David, J., Chosidow, O., et al. (2023). Evolution and challenges of store-and-forward teledermatology for skin diseases of elderly in long-term care facilities: Results of a 5-year analysis. Journal of the European Academy of Dermatology and Venereology, 37. https://www.semanticscholar.org/paper/d58afd7cd1619ff3f764da2b3b618b6317787e6e (accessed on 12 May 2025).

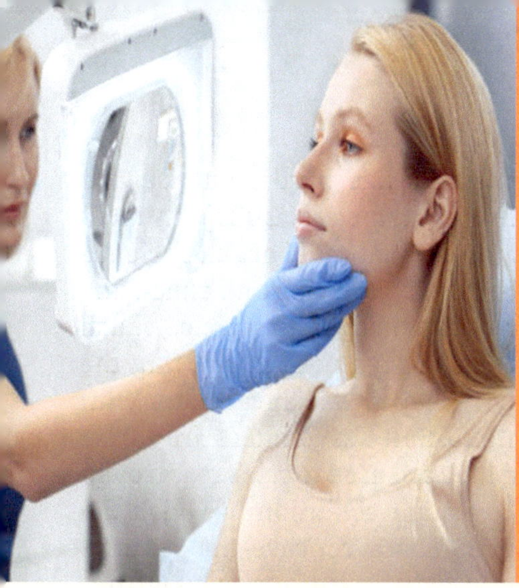

Chapter 14

COSMETIC AND PROCEDURAL DERMATOLOGY

Contents

Introduction

Medicine has advanced a great distance, taking dermatology outside its former limits. Modern treatments now combine skin wellness with a splash of aesthetic flair, and most patients today desire not only to correct skin problems but also to enhance their appearance. This concept, which beauty and healing can go hand in hand—has led to less traumatic procedures and new, creative approaches. Treatments today range from anti-aging signs to particular skin conditions, addressing both repairing the skin and enhancing its appearance. All of this implies that physicians require a certain type of know-how and training specific to these new procedures, always with safety and long-term health in mind. Combining the tried-and-true fundamentals of skin care with the newest aesthetic tricks is not necessarily easy. Many of these cosmetic treatments that are not surgical occur in private clinics rather than traditional teaching hospitals, creating a training gap. In most situations, teachers have intervened to create postgraduate courses that integrate the necessary medical background, practical capabilities, and ethical awareness. They tend to promote a type of learning that supports questioning and improvising on the spot—developing an inquiring, hands-on attitude towards new treatment methods. By structuring the training on major concepts and incorporating examinations of actual competence, these courses enable confidence in doctors' and practitioners' ability to provide treatments in a manner that is safe for patients with varying needs (Kumar et al., 2021). With further evolution of cosmetic and procedural dermatology and its growing popularity, formal education and routine training are even more necessary. A rigorous curriculum not only prepares doctors for technical rigor, but it also goes a long way toward developing the kind of professional spirit and ethical base that is necessary for patient-centered care. Methods like objective structured practical examinations (OSPE) and objective structured clinical examinations (OSCE) now act as standards for testing whether an individual has mastered required procedures. This transition represents a move from an informal, experience-based art to a scientifically supported discipline. Ultimately, evidence-based training protocols open the door to enhanced patient safety, enhanced clinical outcomes, and a strong foundation for future innovation in cosmetic and procedural dermatology (Kumar et al., 2021).

Definition of Cosmetic Dermatology

Dermatology itself has evolved and branched off into various niches throughout the years. Cosmetic dermatology, for instance, is not merely about identifying a skin issue—it is all about sprucing up your look through treatments that leave you feeling rejuvenated. Rather than exclusively concentrating on the diagnosis of skin sickness, this arm focuses on toning, softening, and enhancing day-to-day looks. Procedures here span from non-invasive adjustments to lightly invasive approaches designed to smooth out signs of aging, correct discoloration, and even recontour facial features. Physicians now frequently require special training in these non-surgical procedures, learning through programs that emphasize hard evidence and critical thinking (Kumar et al., 2021). In most instances, it is a combination of art and science in action, committed to restoring and enhancing a patient's self-confidence. At its essence, much of cosmetic dermatology is about reviving the skin and subtly reshaping facial contours with minimal downtime. Soft tissue fillers are a case in point—often they are used to relax tear trough deformities, a frequent condition in which the lower eyelid area has a concave appearance. With precision, releasing measured quantities of filler with instruments such as cannulas, practitioners can restore lost volume and restore equilibrium among facial features naturally. Current research has yielded, in the majority of instances, perceptible enhancements after undergoing these treatments, with decreases in hollowness, less noticeable hyperpigmentation, and fewer wrinkles. These findings emphasize that accuracy is crucial in preventing undesirable side effects, getting to the heart of cosmetic dermatology's mission to hone appearance without sacrificing functionality and safety (Bernardini et al., 2024). Another compelling aspect is the intersection of cosmetic dermatology with procedural dermatology, merging both non-surgical and surgical solutions to improve the way we appear. Training for these experts now tends to blend rigorous theoretical lessons with copious amounts of hands-on practice—think organized practical exams that put skill to the test. These educational models typically correlate with international needs assessments, indicating where additional training is necessary and encouraging more homogeneous learning in aesthetic medicine. The industry's expansion naturally follows changing patient expectations and technological innovations that increase the availability of more customized treatment options. As a whole, cosmetic dermatology has emerged as a multidisciplinary field where evidence-based practice intersects with a form of creative, nearly artisanal, practice of skin care (Kumar et al., 2021).

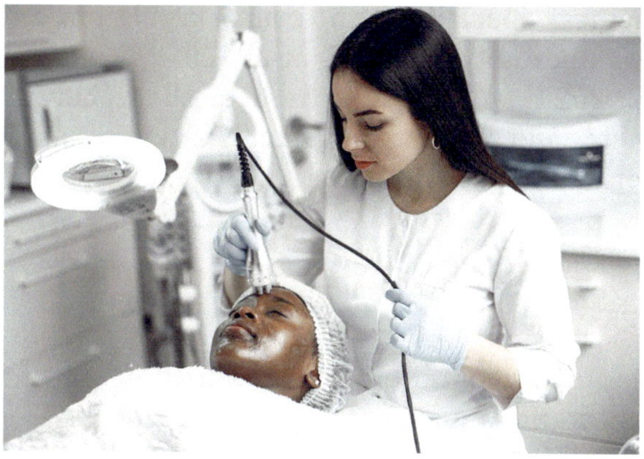

Source: APT Injection Training. (2022). *Injection Training Procedure.* https://aptinjectiontraining.com/wp-content/uploads/2022/06/Featured.jpg.

Importance of Dermatological Procedures

Today's medical advances in health and technology have totally changed the way we approach skincare. Physicians today can do so much more than simply cure diseases; now they also treat cosmetic adjustments that can enhance self-esteem and influence the way people interact socially. Skin treatments now combine repairing medical conditions with appearance enhancement, and this combination addresses both physical health and, essentially, emotional well-being. Increasingly varied roles in skin surgery uncover some quite complicated work; however, there is a great deal of variability in who gets trained to do what and under how much supervision, and that can significantly alter patient outcomes (Eddy & Duffy, 2019). Standardizing the training is regarded as being central to ensuring care is both safe and effective—not just for cosmetic gain but to maintain high overall clinical standards. The hype about aesthetic skin procedures illustrates how much needs have changed in recent times. Most people now prefer less aggressive techniques that rejuvenate looks without the long downtime or excessive risk that traditional surgery used to pose. Consider chemical peels, laser zapping, fillers, and even microneedling—each of these treatments promises its own type of lift, be it imparting youthful radiance to skin or healing a persistent condition. Their regular utilization truly emphasizes the importance of having good procedural know-how, including what to do beforehand and afterward to reduce risks and achieve optimal outcomes (Madnani et al., 2022). Ultimately, these treatments are not merely about appearing better; they are important tools in enhancing daily life by integrating components of well-being and aesthetics. It is not just about the aesthetic advantages, however—they are lifesavers as well. Rapid biopsies, excising a questionable area, or performing specialized procedures can detect serious conditions early, particularly in hard-to-find conditions like skin cancer where timing is critical. This combination of cosmetic and medical purposes demonstrates just how multifaceted these procedures have become. It is essential that doctors and nurse surgeons receive the proper training so that patient safety and good care remain at the forefront (Eddy & Duffy, 2019). As the industry continues to advance, these treatments continue to merge the science and art of skincare, improving not just appearance but safeguarding general skin health and well-being.

14.1. Historical Background

Cosmetic and procedural dermatology have developed in tandem with the way that medical training progresses. Years ago, most of these procedures occurred in feature, unorthodox environments—clearly far removed from the typical teaching hospital environment, and it was difficult to establish a standard for acquiring the knowledge and demonstrating the proficiency. Initially, most practitioners picked things up through an apprenticeship experience, without a formal, evidence-based curriculum. Today, there is a discernible trend: postgraduate education, which emphasizes not only technical expertise but also the art of thought, is becoming the new standard. In general, this shift combines scientific competence with aesthetic practice, committing to care that is both safe and effective. Evidence in favor of established curricula and instruments such as OSPE and OSCE (Kumar et al., 2021) has supported these reforms, creating a paradigm shift in the teaching and practice of dermatology. Regulation by regulatory systems has also influenced the discipline over time. Contemporary healthcare is not governed by a single rule that fits all but by a knotty combination of laws designed to safeguard patients and maintain professional standards. Consider the Ontario example—self-regulatory organizations have strict guidelines to walk a tightrope of scope of practice, education, and disciplining. Yes, those systems occasionally encounter roadblocks with professional self-interest and power struggles. Disputes regarding delayed investigations and patchy enforcement of educational standards underpin that There is still a call for balanced regulation, where competence and ethics converge. Most often, such frameworks must evolve as dermatology changes, balancing new technologies with efforts to cover up loopholes (Ghimire et al., 2018). In the years that have passed, the discipline gradually and inevitably came to appreciate evidence-based practice and quality control by systematized means. Initially, aesthetic procedures were dispersed throughout different environments, and without consistent regulation, patient results could seriously vary. Slowly, however, the medical profession learned that solid, evidence-based curricula and full regulatory policies were necessary. Over the past few decades, schools, regulatory bodies, and practitioners have increasingly coalesced, sometimes in surprising combinations—to establish standards for training and practice. These collaborative initiatives, seeking to minimize skill gaps and maintain patient safety at the forefront, have propelled the discipline from a mosaic of methods to a well-defined medical specialty with formal regulation and accountability (Ghimire et al., 2018; Kumar et al., 2021). The past is used to shape current trends and presumably dictates where cosmetic dermatology is headed.

14.1.1. Evolution of Dermatological Practices

Medical technology and shifting patient expectations have literally turned skin care on its head in the last few decades. The doctors used to primarily concern themselves with identifying and treating skin problems, but today the discipline has expanded to encompass a whole list of cosmetic alterations aimed at enhancing both looks and self-esteem. New, less invasive methods—methods that typically focus on safety and efficiency—have been a major contributing factor in increasing the popularity of cosmetic dermatology. Non-surgical repairs such as botulinum toxin injections and dermal fillers are increasingly popular, providing treatments that can be safely accomplished even away from conventional hospital complexes. Nevertheless, establishing a default training plan for these new approaches is no easy task, considering the combination of treatment areas and the frenetic pace of technology updates; in most instances, evidence-based curriculum is paramount to maintaining high standards (Kumar et al., 2021). Skin care education has been forced to adapt to these changes by combining well-established practices with new approaches. Training modules these days balance traditional techniques with newer approaches, so that practitioners do not forget the fundamentals while acquiring new tricks. Curriculum revisions of late tend to rely heavily on practical exams and clinical tests, particularly those specialized in cosmetic treatments, an effort that not only enhances a doctor's talent but also attempts to fill gaps created by a majority of treatments occurring outside the conventional hospital universe. Broadly, equipping residents with critical thinking and an inquiring mind is essential, thereby enabling them to deal with the complexities of cosmetic procedures safely and ethically. A formalized postgraduate pathway thus assists in bridging the technology leaps with real-world preparedness, protecting both patient outcomes and professional integrity (Kumar et al., 2021). On another level, the dynamic dermatology of today reflects an increasing convergence of the medical and the cosmetic, reflecting the wider concepts of beauty and health today. The blend necessitates a more integrated approach that combines rigorous, evidence-based clinical practice with the attention that is attuned to each patient's cosmetic aspirations.

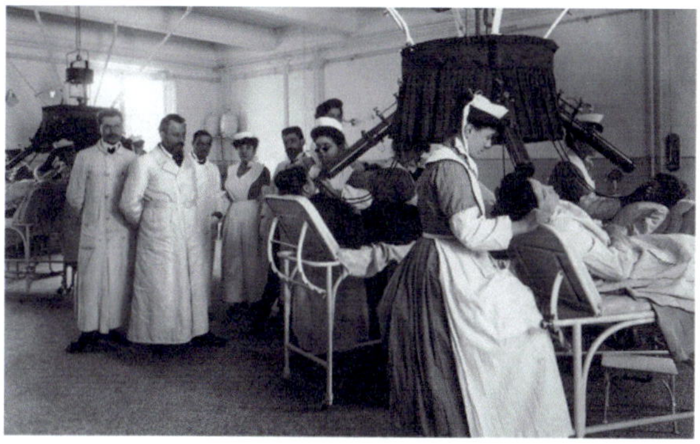

Figure 14.1. Pellizzari and his staff at the Institute Fotoradioterapico of Florenc.

Source: OAText. (n.d.). *Historical Medical Treatment Using Early X-ray Therapy Devices*. https://oatext.com/img/GOD-S1-011-3.jpg.

With tech marching forward, we are likely to see everyday procedures relying on innovations like laser therapies, microneedling, or even regenerative treatments—opening up new possibilities left and right. Sharing fresh insights through accessible, high-quality resources, be it in specialized newsletters or digital platforms, naturally feeds into the ongoing professional growth and awareness of cutting-edge practices. In total, all these factors give an idea of a dynamic, constantly changing era in dermatology wherein flexibility and constant adaptability are the keys to serve the changing demands of the patients as well as professionals (Kumar et al., 2021) (Figure 14.1).

14.1.2. Key Milestones in Cosmetic Dermatology

Cosmetic dermatology has gone a new way with methods that address challenging skin problems such as scarring. Consider microneedling, for instance, it achieves this by inflicting small, controlled punctures on the skin such that collagen is naturally stimulated and healing is nudged along but the top layer remains relatively intact.

This technique has generally proved effective in atrophic acne scars, consider rolling and boxcar types, albeit whose effect can be truly disparate. Research indicates that performing a few sessions with tools like the dermapen can improve general skin appearance while reducing recovery time and undesirable side effects. It is even used near delicate areas like the periorbital region, which truly demonstrates its versatility (Sivaranjani et al., 2019). This trend indicates treatments that do not penetrate too deeply but are still a significant punch. Not surprisingly, the field did not evolve out of new therapies alone but was also driven by an increasing demand for greater training and education. In the past, most non-surgical aesthetic procedures were performed in private clinics with no formal teaching mechanisms for postgraduate physicians. Aware of this, there have been recent attempts that result in curricula that combine practical practice with critical thinking through enquiry-based models, broadly speaking, much-needed overhauling of training techniques. Methods such as objective structured practical examinations (OSPE) and objective structured clinical examinations (OSCE) now introduce a level of rigor and reliability to these courses. This evolution assists in guaranteeing that practitioners are able to maintain pace with contemporary practices and paves the way for continuous innovation and patient safety (Kumar et al., 2021).

It is, in the majority of situations, a great leap forward in the professionalization of aesthetic care. Another significant change in the field is the trend toward combining various treatment techniques that are customized for the particular kind of scar or skin ailment under consideration. Whereas microneedling is a standout for rolling and boxcar scars, other types of marks, such as ice-pick scars, tend to require the mixed approach, such as employing submission in conjunction with a trichloroacetic acid peel to achieve maximum results. This requirement for dual treatments speaks to the multifaceted process of repairing the skin and reminds us that one technique may not suit all cases. Apart from treating scars, these new procedures have the added benefits at times, such as reducing seborrhea and smoothening the skin, which extends cosmetic dermatology beyond mere scar repair and towards a more holistic skin health goal. These wide-ranging, patient-specific approaches, imperfect though they may be, show the active and continuously developing aspect of the specialty (Sivaranjani et al., 2019) (Figure 14.2).

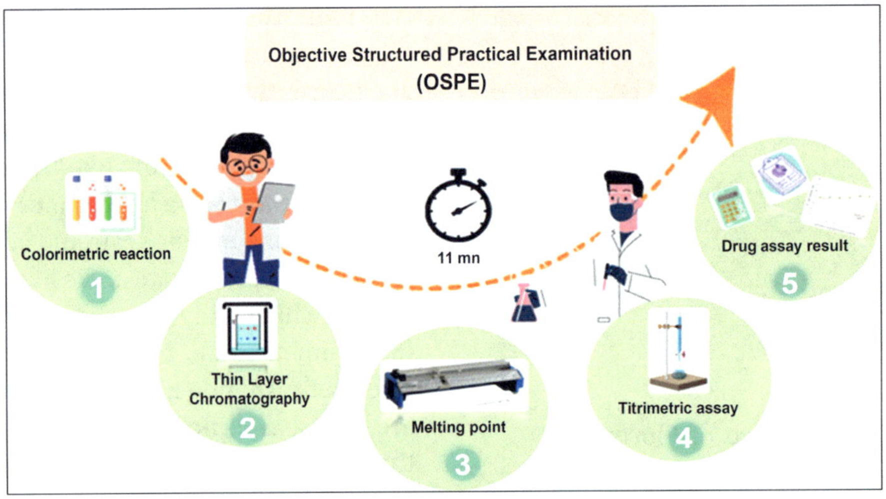

Figure 14.2. Objective structured practical examinations (OSPE).

Source: Benrejeb, H., Marzouk, A., Mnif, F., Ghachem, A., & Amri, H. (2024). *Objective Structured Practical Examination (OSPE) for Pharmaceutical Analysis: A New Approach to Improve Students' Learning Experience*. American Chemical Society.

14.1.3. Influence of Technology on Dermatological Advancements

Over the past few decades, dermatology transformed greatly due to new technologies that subtly rearrange the way physicians practice. High-tech imaging and digital skin-examination techniques allow clinicians to identify problems, from small harmless markings to possible cancers, with almost unparalleled precision. When electronic records become combined with artificial intelligence (AI), treatment plans and patient follow-ups become more natural, customized to individual patients' needs. This fusion of tech and clinical know-how has created a movement towards procedures that not only perform well but also appear better, indicative of a shift towards care that is more patient-focused (Nova Southeastern University, 2014). Finally, all these advances have become the foundation of today's procedural and cosmetic skin care. Even surgical procedures are not spared in this technology-based change—surgeries themselves have had quite an overhaul. Consider, for instance, micrographic Mohs surgery; it illustrates how technology can increase the efficacy of treatment while conserving healthy tissue and reducing scarring. By depending upon microscopic examination throughout the excision of cancers (particularly basal and squamous cell cancers), practitioners combine surgical skill with technical precision. New methods, such as utilizing immunostaining, for instance, are used to identify tumor edges with greater distinctness, which tends to result in fewer procedures and enhanced cosmetic outcomes.

There is a delicate tightrope walk here between killing all the cancer and preserving as much healthy skin as possible, a step that tends to increase the quality of care and patient satisfaction (Perkowska et al., 2024). In most instances, Mohs surgery is an excellent case in point for how technology can lead the way in advancing dermatology. Outside of surgery, non-surgical cosmetic procedures have also been revolutionized by technology. Laser, radiofrequency, and even ultrasound gadgets now address wrinkles, pigmentation, and scars with less downtime and greater safety. Frequently, the devices are modified to fit what each patient requires, resulting in more customized and successful results. It is this combination of acutely diagnostic tools and precisely targeted therapies that best shows how much these technologies have opened up the possibilities in cosmetic dermatology. Ultimately, such equipment not only enhances how procedures are conducted but also raises the standard of care overall—plainly establishing tech's indispensable place in the contemporary practice of dermatology (Nova Southeastern University, 2014).

14.2. Common Cosmetic Procedures

Dermatologic treatment has transformed significantly of late. Non-surgical cosmetic treatments are now in the limelight ; they provide an exit from complicated surgeries sans long recovery periods and risky factors that were attached to classic procedures earlier. See, procedures such as chemical peels and laser treatments have emerged as favorites among many, dealing with everything from patchy pigmentation to resurfacing the skin. In most cases, though, being able to perform these treatments safely is not something you pick up in standard medical classes; it calls for extra, specialized training. The techniques are tricky and the range of tools is huge, so having a more formal training setup can really help ensure both skill and safety. There is a push to integrate evidence-based, postgraduate training in nonsurgical facial aesthetics into mainstream medical education – one that could potentially enhance practitioner confidence as well as patient trust (Kumar et al., 2021). In the realm of cosmetic treatments, a whole range of choices such as dermal fillers, microneedling radiofrequency, and derma rollers are all on the menu. These are just wonderful for rejuvenating the skin, helping increase collagen, smoothing out skin texture, and even restoring lost volume — often with immediate results. However, since these procedures span such a broad spectrum of treatments, they require not only technique but also a good understanding of the care pre- and post-procedure. Clinical standards generally identify that correct patient checks, product selection, and following safety protocols are the keys to achieving those cosmetic objectives. In most instances, being on top of new developments is critical, where every process from beginning to end is as seamless and secure as possible (Madnani et al., 2022). Throughout the globe, the increased demand for cosmetic dermatology is making it apparent: our resident training programs must be upgraded. Surveys of both mentors and those in training frequently indicate a unanimous call for more formalized, supervised programs – perhaps approximately a year long – to properly prepare clinicians for solo work. Ideally, such programs would combine a little theory, some hands-on workshops, and lots of guided practice, which together establish competence as well as confidence. In general, bringing medical education in sync with the dynamic world of aesthetic dermatology is not merely about keeping pace with the latest trends; it is a good approach to enhancing patient safety and satisfaction in the long term (Kumar et al., 2021).

14.2.1. Botox and Its Applications

Cosmetic and procedural dermatology has evolved a great deal—signs of aging and some medical conditions are being treated quite differently now. Botox, which initially was utilized for conditions such as spasmodic dysphonia and hyperhidrosis, now makes an appearance every day in aesthetic centers. It acts by inhibiting the release of acetylcholine at the point where nerves interface with muscles (Kerna et al., 2024). It temporarily relaxes facial muscles, ironing out wrinkles and relaxing expression lines without resorting to major surgery. The increased popularity of Botox, in part, reflects our ongoing pursuit of a youthful appearance—media photographs, social acceptance, all contributing their share, which has pushed it into the realm of regular cosmetic treatment. Its application both in beauty and functional treatments truly demonstrates how dermatology today bridges several disciplines (Kerna et al., 2024). The appeal of Botox is not just that it minimizes wrinkles—it has become a frequent visitor to a more diverse combination of cosmetic treatments such as chemical peels, laser procedures, and dermal fillers. These various treatments are frequently mixed together to restore the skin, enhance its texture, and generally lift its appearance. Even with more choices available, physicians simply have to get it right on who is the ideal candidate, learn the technique, and monitor care pre- and post-treatment to avoid undesirable problems. This sort of well-rounded procedure not only attempts to maximize the potential of Botox but also prioritizes patient safety and satisfaction. In the meantime, increasing practitioner awareness is critical, particularly where cosmetic dermatology is thriving (Figure 14.3).

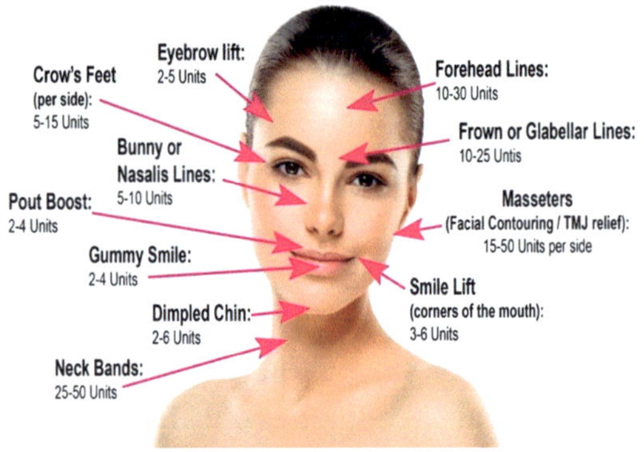

Figure 14.3. Site for Botox injections.

Source: Ravichandran, S. (2021). *Site for Botox Injections.*

In addition to appearing good, Botox is also revealing another ability to relieve some psychological and neurological issues. Recent research suggests that, in many instances, it may be able to soothe signs of depression, anxiety, and even body dysmorphic disorder—perhaps by adjusting the feedback between muscles and nerves that directs our emotions (Kerna et al., 2024). They even speak of using it for pain management and for temporomandibular joint disorder, extending its conventional application. Even though these new possibilities are intriguing, they raise concerns such as equal access, obtaining really informed consent, and ethical issues in cosmetic as well as procedural treatment. Continued investigation into patient outcomes and long-term safety will be instrumental in ironing out guidelines and enhancing the manner in which numerous specialties converge in dermatology (Kerna et al., 2024) (Figure 14.4).

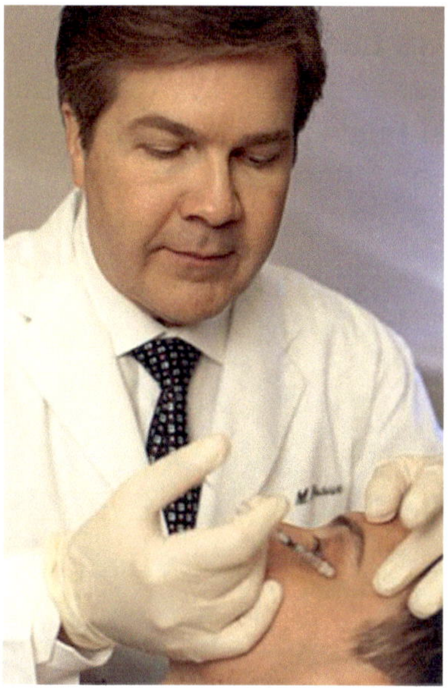

Figure 14.4. Botulinum toxin being injected in the human face.

Source: Braun, M. (2010). *Dr. Braun Performs a Botox Injection*. Wikimedia Commons.

14.2.2. Dermal Fillers and Their Uses

The latest imaging developments have revolutionized the field for cosmetic dermatology. Ultrasound, for instance, is not merely an added device—it is now an option of choice when it comes to dermal fillers. This noninvasive examination allows physicians not only to view the top skin but also the layers below in real-time, even tracing out the arteries to ensure avoiding complications like artery blockages. Rather than operating off of a static picture, practitioners now receive a dynamic perspective that is easier to use to place fillers safely and even handle any hiccups through guided solutions like employing low-dose hyaluronidase. For the most part, this live mapping not only individualizes the appearance of each patient but also improves safety and provides an added layer of legal protection. Essentially, ultrasound is increasingly regarded as essential in cosmetic procedures, supporting the notion that prevention is half the battle (Haykal et al., 2023).

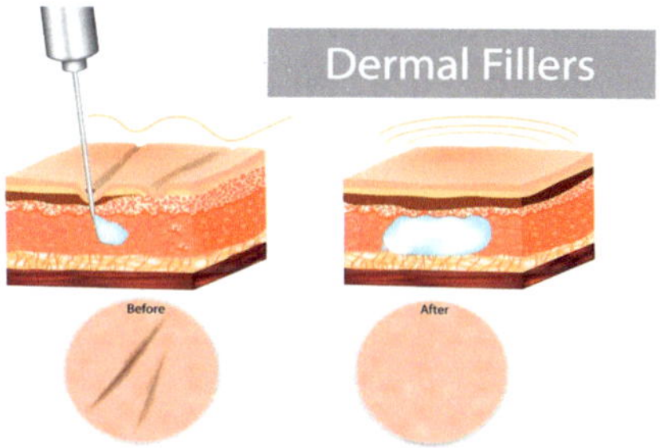

Figure 14.5. Dermal fillers.

Source: Dreamstime. (n.d.). *Dermal Fillers (Soft Tissue Fillers) Illustration.* https://thumbs.dreamstime.com/b/dermal-fillers-soft-tissue-also-known-as-injectables-176161130.jpg.

Facial rejuvenation is all about restoring lost volume as a result of aging, and fillers are at the center of that endeavor. As you understand, soft tissues gradually shrink, and we have many ways to reverse that—skeletal onlay grafts, subcutaneous volumizers, or simply dermal fillers. Each of these has differing durability and invasiveness; newer filler formulations have even made available customized treatments for younger patients or those who want less invasive repairs. It is quite crucial to get a good diagnosis of atrophic layers first because dermal fillers do best when volume loss is more superficial. Conversely, when aging is more severe, pairing fillers with longer duration implants or grafts may be the wiser option (Figure 14.5).

In general, having a good understanding of filler behavior and its viscoelastic nature assists practitioners with planning treatments that are just right for an individual (Newman, 2009). At times, adding volume is not even the goal—the intention is to refine the entire facial contour and texture as well. Dermal fillers mix with the skin to restore smooth curves that look youthful, erase fine lines, and even out facial imbalances in a manner that looks natural. Their minimally invasive nature renders them a favorite among people seeking gentle yet impactful enhancements without surgery. Additionally, combining imaging techniques such as ultrasound ensures that important structures are spared, further enhancing the placement procedure. Continuous refinement of filler materials translates to longer longevity and more symbiotic coexistence with soft tissues. These innovations highlight how beneficial and all-around versatile dermal fillers have become in modern facial rejuvenation procedures (Newman, 2009; Haykal et al., 2023) (Figure 14.6).

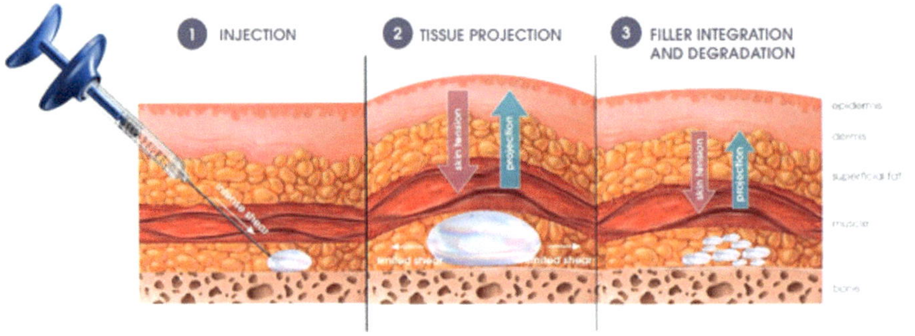

Figure 14.6. Dermal fillers areas.

Source: Flégeau K, Jing J, Vantou C, Brusini R, Bourdon F, Faivre J. Strengthening the Key Features of Volumizing Fillers: Projection Capacity and Long-Term Persistence. *Pharmaceutics*. 2023; 15(11):2585. https://doi.org/10.3390/pharmaceutics15112585

14.2.3. Chemical Peels and Skin Resurfacing

Recent advances in skin treatments have opened up new avenues for improving both the texture and appearance of our skin. Chemical peels and overall skin resurfacing, both now standard in cosmetic procedures, a accomplish this by peeling off the old, damaged outer layers, which then stimulates collagen production and assists new skin cells in moving in. It is not simply a matter of ironing out fine lines or evening out color; these procedures can also take care of more stubborn problems such as actinic keratosis. Scientists have explored how various methods, including the use of trichloroacetic acid, stack up in actual clinical practice, at times discovering that cryotherapy tends to end up surpassing chemical peels for particular lesions (Lai et al., 2018).

Such apples-to-apples comparisons, more often than not, really bring home the point of placing patient care and sound evidence at the forefront of the process. Making the choice between a chemical peel and other resurfacing procedures is not always black and white. It usually comes down to the fabric of the lesion being treated, the type of skin the patient has, and even whether or not there are overall quality-of-life issues involved. In a nutshell, although a chemical peel induces a deliberate skin injury that triggers regrowth, laser methods can better isolate tiny segments of the skin such as chromophores, which may be a better option for congenital or even acquired spots. For instance, in the case of facial congenital melanocytic nevi, physicians will at times need to make a choice between removing lesions surgically or using the laser to gain both function and beauty. Research, in most instances, emphasizes that with children as patients the entire picture—the psychological and social aspects as well as the clinical—must be catered to when devising treatment (Lai et al., 2018). This balanced approach truly identifies how patient-specific considerations are taking center stage in contemporary cosmetic dermatology. Despite the popularity of these procedures, stringent safety measures are still indispensable to prevent complications such as hyperpigmentation, scarring, or infection. Prolonged inspection of a patient's skin and health record before the procedure, followed by conscientious wound care and UV protection afterward, all serve to keep things on the straight and narrow. There is also constant innovation in application techniques and the chemical formulations employed, which means treatments can be more individually customized. Comparing cryotherapy with chemical peels for a condition such as actinic keratosis, it would appear evident that the most appropriate option is one that weighs up evident clinical advantages, tolerance of the patient, and what means are available (Sabir & Ridha, 2019).

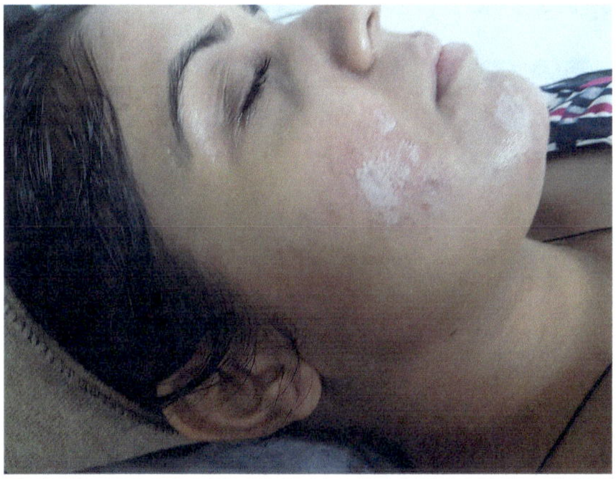

Figure 14.7. Depth penetration of chemicals peels.

Source: By NewAgeAesthetics - Own work, CC BY-SA 4.0, https://commons.wikimedia.org/w/index.php?curid=131619177

The combination of innovative clinical knowledge with personalized care plans continues to be central to effective cosmetic and procedural dermatology practice (Figure 14.7).

14.3. Surgical Dermatology

The fast-paced development of medical technology has rocked dermatology, particularly surgery where it is all about getting it right in terms of both function and appearance. Surgical dermatology is now combining techniques to cure health ailments and enhance looks simultaneously, addressing increased demands for repairs that are functional and aesthetically pleasing as well. It even incorporates methods from fields such as plastic surgery and otolaryngology, which makes a ton of new treatment avenues available. For instance, facial plastic surgery now includes things like eyelid lifts, nose reshaping, and even small vascular reconstructs that address deformity while providing a renewed appearance. Additionally, additional tools such as injectable fillers and lasers provide an added bonus to the results, making this field dynamic and on the move (Chuang et al., 2016). Consider congenital melanocytic nevi, for example—those birthmarks can be any size and mark, even right on the face or neck. Those cases tend to compel physicians to intervene early, in part due to issues of appearance and in part because of risks to health. Most commonly, incising the mark out or laser therapy are the treatments of choice. However, the absence of firm, evidence-based guidelines means there is an actual need for studies that balance not only the clinical repairs but the patient's overall well-being. New studies are already attempting to close that gap by assessing the sense of life after a procedure, moving care toward being properly patient-centered (Lai et al., 2018). Merging surgical removal with state-of-the-art laser therapies is another indicator of the movement toward less invasive cosmetic procedures with good results but less lost time. Surgical dermatology relies on exacting techniques to excise both perilous and benign skin lesions, fill in deformities, and enhance the overall texture of the skin – all of which tend to make patients happier. Advances such as microvascular reconstruction demonstrate that the specialty can restore both function and shape, particularly after setbacks such as tumor excisions or trauma. This combination of repair and improvement truly distinguishes surgical dermatology as a vital field that continues to advance through new technology and collaboration across specialties, ultimately expanding treatment possibilities and improving outcomes (Chuang et al., 2016).

14.3.1. Mohs Surgery for Skin Cancer

It is difficult to treat skin cancer, primarily because you must eliminate every last particle of the tumor while sacrificing as little healthy tissue as possible. With areas where function and appearance are paramount, like around the face or neck—Mohs micrographic surgery has become a go-to choice for cases such as basal cell and squamous cell carcinomas. It does this by cutting out the cancer gradually; every cut is analyzed under a microscope to ensure no cancer remnant persists. This step-by-step approach maximizes cure rates and minimizes cosmetic problems, which is very important for delicate locations (Perkowska et al., 2024). Merging fresh technology with surgical expertise has truly shaken things up in skin cancer treatment. Consider hyperspectral imaging, for example—it is a new technology providing a quick computer-assisted scan of tumor margins that may fall through the cracks with routine examinations. For the most part, while Mohs continues to head the list for nasty or fuzzy tumor margins, hyperspectral imaging can identify hidden spreads often not seen by regular dermoscopy. Yes, this technology does not want to replace Mohs, but it certainly offers useful additional clues for optimal surgical planning and patient selection, all of which can result in optimal outcomes both cosmetically and oncologically (Salmivuori, 2020). When deciding what treatment to use, physicians must balance how well the treatment will work versus how natural it will look. Mohs surgery manages to balance these concerns quite well—it combines high cure rates with the aim of leaving natural skin intact, so fewer scars and a better appearance. Less invasive choices such as photodynamic therapy (PDT), although they win brownie points for minimal invasiveness and good first impressions, tend to clear out fewer cancer cells; that is why they are typically used in lower-risk situations. The special precision of Mohs in verifying and clearing margins of tumors provides it with a significant advantage, particularly where tumors occur in sensitive anatomical locations. Its precise accuracy and low recurrence chances highlight why it occupies such an important position in dermatologic cancer management (Salmivuori, 2020; Perkowska et al., 2024) (Figure 14.8).

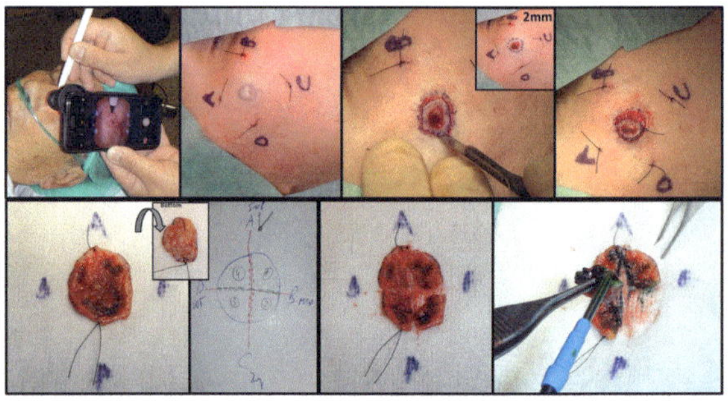

Figure 14.8. Stages in Mohs micrographic surgery, identification and marking of the lesion with a pen, assisted by a dermatoscope or a microscope. Tumor debulking and first excision stage assisted by a map. The specimen is cut into smaller quadrants whose cutting edges are color-coded according to a map.

Source: Miot, H. A. (2020). *Stages in Mohs Micrographic Surgery: Identification and Marking of the Lesion with a Pen*. ResearchGate.

14.3.2. Cosmetic Surgical Procedures (e.g., Facelifts)

Medical science has been on a gradual march, remodeling the way we cope with aging and, specifically, skin rejuvenation. These days, people are pursuing that youthful sheen, and facelifts have taken a place in routine dermatology. They modify things by relocating droopy tissue and shaving off surplus skin, essentially, moving around what is lost over time to restore a more youthful appearance. Conventional surgery now frequently blends with less disruptive tricks, on average, to provide good outcomes with a faster recovery.

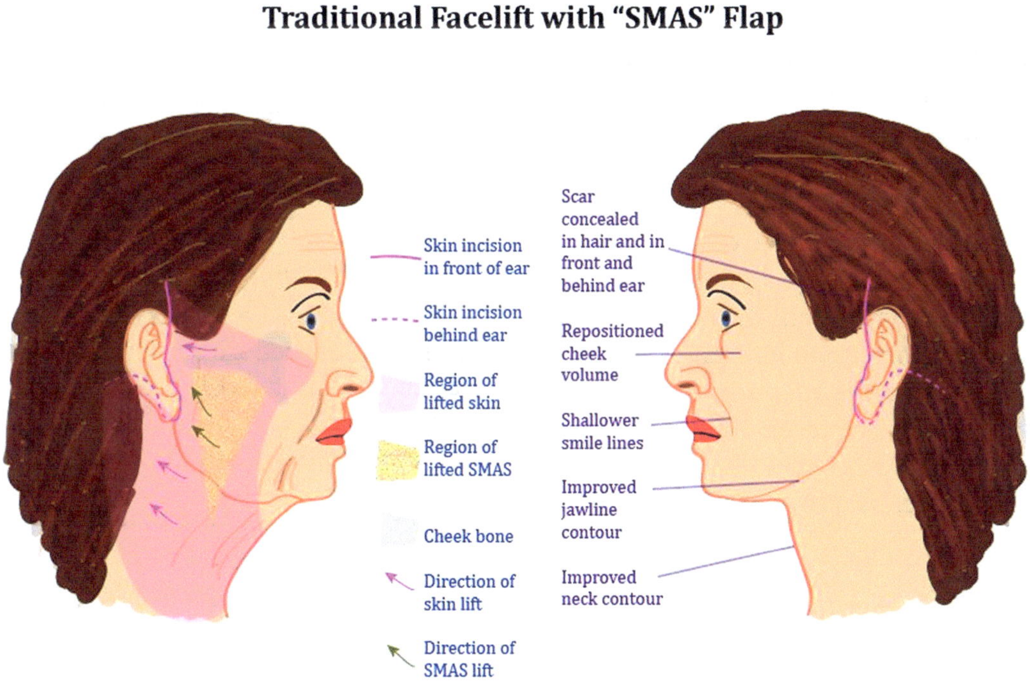

Figure 14.9. Traditional facelifts with "SMAS" flap.

Source: West County Plastic Surgeons. (n.d.). *Traditional Facelift with "SMAS" Flap.* https://westcountyplasticsurgeons.wustl.edu/images/facelift-standard.jpg.

The trend indicates procedures that are fashioned somewhat more for each individual's requirements, not merely for a good appearance but for safety as well. Procedures such as fat grafting and resorbable threads, for example, introduce still more diversity in what dermatologists can perform (Portilla et al., 2024). Apart from the technical aspects, there is an entire psychological aspect of undergoing cosmetic work that is worthy of examination. Societal preoccupation with staying youthful drives many, but all individuals do not enter these surgeries with the same intentions or emotional preparation. As it happens, how people approach and recover from a facelift or like treatment can significantly influence their satisfaction level—perhaps more so than the procedure itself. Physicians have to measure these emotions, frequently visiting preop to identify who may be at risk of being less satisfied with the outcome. Most of the time, knowing why somebody is interested in cosmetic treatment helps the entire care team deliver a more comprehensive treatment, covering the body and psyche (Castle et al., 2006). On the practical side, everyday clinics are now combining old-school cosmetic surgery with newer, minimally invasive skin techniques. Facelifts still hold their ground as a go-to method, yet there is a growing mix of additional procedures that either boost the main work or give a hand to patients who are reluctant or simply not suited for a full surgery. Consider Ultherapy, for instance, a noninvasive procedure that employs concentrated ultrasound to stimulate collagen, and thread lifts that utilize materials such as polydioxanone and polylactic acid to lift tissues discreetly, without requiring plenty of downtime. These new possibilities allow physicians to craft plans that can be added up progressively, sometimes forestalling a heavy surgery or even complementing it. In effect, the entire sector has moved into a range of options driven by continuous innovation and shifting patient preferences (Portilla et al., 2024) (Figure 14.9).

14.3.3. Scar Revision Techniques

Scar recovery is not easy and at times requires a very specific method, particularly when scars bother your body or even weigh on your mind. Contemporary cosmetic skin care has, in recent years, advanced with some surprising techniques that do not merely camouflage scars but attempt to reconstruct the skin from the inside out. You may find choices ranging from full-on surgical excision with re-stitching to more subtle, less drastic methods that coax the skin to heal itself. For most, a technique known as platelet-rich plasma (PRP) therapy is becoming increasingly popular; it essentially harvests your own growth factors and cytokines to stimulate cell activity and provide collagen with a reboot, smoothing out texture and tone. This type of advancement hints at a transition to regenerative medicine - overall, it is less about camouflaging imperfections and more about restoring normal function (Suruchi et al., 2018). It creates more options for doctors and patients who want enduring enhancements. Laser procedures also enter the equation when it comes to treating pigmentation variations, irregular thickness, or lopsided contours in scars. Fractional lasers, for instance, create small areas of channeled heat, inducing a repair response that loosens up scar tissue and tones down redness. The accuracy of these devices is fairly impressive; mereka can target scars, whether they are too prominent or too indented, without disrupting the skin around them. When these treatments are paired with methods such as microneedling or chemical peels, you have a sort of patchwork approach that works really well for individual needs. These combined strategies quietly remind us that individualized care can make a big impact in cosmetic dermatology (Editorial Office, 2016). That being said, not all scars or all individuals fit a one-size-fits-all solution.

In general, it is all a matter of thoroughly examining the scar characteristics, skin type and general health of the person before selecting a strategy. Surgical approaches remain viable for chronic contractures or significantly elevated scars, and such treatments are usually coupled with aftercare to reduce the likelihood of things recurring. In contrast, non-surgical corrections hope to enhance the look while minimizing recovery time and risk—good news for those not excited about surgery. New therapies such as PRP and other concepts for regeneration foretell a world in which scar revision is more than merely playing with the look; it is truly about the recovery of function. Continuing research and clinical trials will be expected to continue to hone these methods, making them safer and more effective still, which, after all, is what patients today expect (Suruchi et al., 2018) (Figure 14.10).

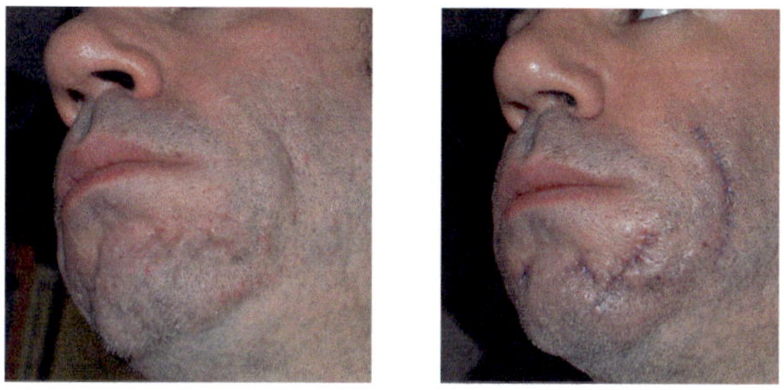

Figure 14.10. Scar revision: before and after.

Source: By Themeparkphoto, CC BY-SA 3.0, https://commons.wikimedia.org/w/index.php?curid=10001504

14.4. Non-Surgical Treatments

Dermatology has been trending toward non-surgical solutions over the last few years. You see, treatments such as laser procedures, chemical peels, and injectables, botulinum toxin or dermal fillers, for example, can work miracles without the massive recovery time and big risk that comes with traditional surgery. These treatments typically equate to less downtime, fewer complications, and, all in all, lower expenses. It is very much a big deal, though, that any choice regarding these treatments considers the overall condition of the patient, particularly in pediatric situations where each move can influence quality of life significantly. An example is laser treatment that has gained traction for conditions such as congenital melanocytic nevi in children, which both minimizes the physical burden and emotional distress at critical development periods (Lai et al., 2018). Ethical considerations emerge big time when younger patients are involved. The pressure behind cosmetic alterations often accompanies a whole package of psychological and emotional baggage that must be cautiously checked—tools such as the Derriford Appearance Scale (DAS-59) are utilized, for example, to determine exactly how much distress a person is experiencing over his or her appearance. Most times, this scale assists in ensuring that any choice to undergo cosmetic treatment is one that has its roots firmly in the best interest of the patient and not based on whim or external pressure. Across multiple sessions, clinicians and counselors work together to penetrate to the root of what is driving the adolescent and if they really understand what informed consent is. This type of care prevents us from performing procedures that are technically possible but ethically problematic, particularly when they begin creeping into the arena of pursuing an "ideal beauty" as opposed to addressing actual problems (Luca et al., 2018). What it comes back to, fundamentally, is the motivation in cosmetic dermatology: to make things as minimally invasive as possible. Surgical alternatives only become sensible when they resolve overt physical issues, defects that can influence social interactions, self-image, and every day functioning. For instance, procedures to correct such things as protruding ears or benign spots on the skin demonstrate that achieving a good balance of hard clinical results with ethical consideration is important. A combination of specialists—psychologists, dermatologists, and even relatives—frequently collaborate to implement plans that address wellness comprehensively rather than surface changes. Really, these non-invasive techniques are not only about appearing more attractive; they can be key in making someone feel emotionally balanced and more comfortable being around others, as long as the treatments are carried out to strict clinical and ethical criteria (Lai et al., 2018; Luca et al., 2018).

14.4.1. Laser Therapy for Skin Conditions

Laser treatment has truly started to rock skin treatments. Contemporary laser machines, say that reliable 675 nm LLLT, utilize red light to address everyday problems such as aging skin and pigment abnormalities without needles.

Studies tend to indicate that this wavelength induces collagen remodeling, which subsequently softens texture and fades wrinkles. It has also been utilized for melasma, acne vulgaris, and even for stretch marks, all with a rather low risk profile (Rahib et al., 2025). Sometimes it seems like the old-fashioned ways are just no competition for these new-fangled methods. Then there are the strange case of 1927 nm fractional thulium lasers. In contrast to certain older methods, these devices combine ablative with nonablative characteristics, incorporating techniques that both abrade and recontour skin tissue at once.

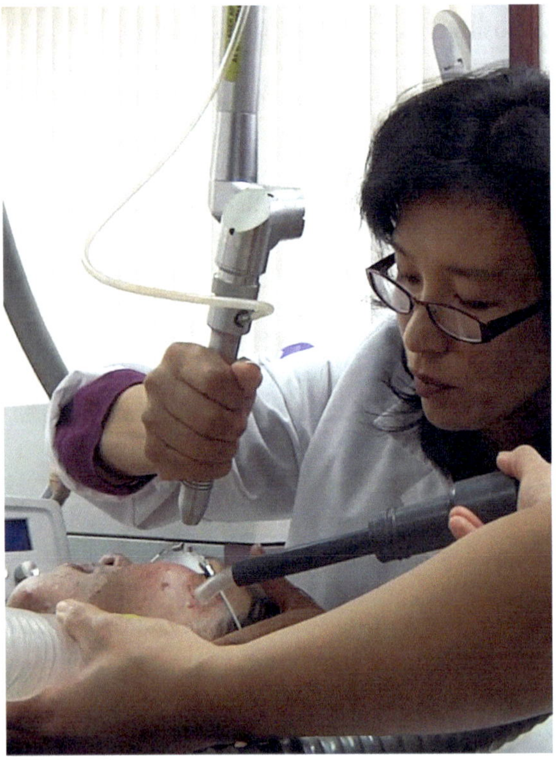

Figure 14.11. Laser skin resurfacing.

Source: By SurgicalPhotos - Own work, CC BY-SA 4.0, https://commons.wikimedia.org/w/index.php?curid=41991649

These machines are more likely to encourage cell regeneration, eliminate persistent pigment, and even stimulate collagen formation. Various studies have reported melasma and scarring improvements, with patients usually having shorter healing times and less side effects than with lasers such as Er: YAG and Alexandrite. Yes, additional clinical trials are necessary to truly hammer out the optimal treatment protocols (Mariana et al., 2025). Taking the big picture into consideration, laser treatment these days is not merely about fast fixes—patient safety and satisfaction are paramount. Several practitioners now tailor their protocols according to the particular laser wavelength as well as individual patient considerations, at times integrating laser sessions with other treatments to target several skin problems simultaneously. Early experience is promising, but still needed are more extensive clinical studies to establish firm guidelines, particularly as new devices continue to appear. Ultimately, this active, noninvasive modality fits well with contemporary dermatolocial principles of maximizing aesthetics while minimizing risks (Mariana et al., 2025; Rahib et al., 2025) (Figure 14.11).

14.4.2. Microdermabrasion and Its Benefits

Non-surgical cosmetic procedures just keep getting better, providing a whole array of new means to revitalize skin and deal with various dermatological anomalies. Microdermabrasion, for example, has become a popular shortcut since it smoothes out roughness and enhances looks without requiring much lost time. , it softly exfoliates off the outer layer of old skin with tiny abrasive pieces or even a diamond wand tip—this serves to get the skin to regenerate itself and allow creams or serums penetrate more smoothly. In the majority of cases, this process initiates collagen growth and accelerates cell turnover, which will smooth out fine wrinkles, minor scars, and discoloration. The outcome is a considerably fresher appearance with fewer variations, something that is behind its widespread application both in cosmetic procedures and in more clinical dermatology. Its safety and wide compatibility are some of the biggest selling points of microdermabrasion; it is effective even on people whose skin is a little more sensitive to harsh treatments. Instead of risking redness or scarring like deeper treatments could, this treatment tends not to have those types of complications, so it is a practical choice for anyone who wants steady, subtle changes without an extensive recovery time. It is also a treatment that can be done in repeated sessions, making it easy to do ongoing improvements of the skin without compromising the natural barrier. In most cases, microdermabrasion is not merely aesthetics; it may also complement acne treatment regimens, reducing both the frequency and severity of flare-ups (Nojek et al., 2024).

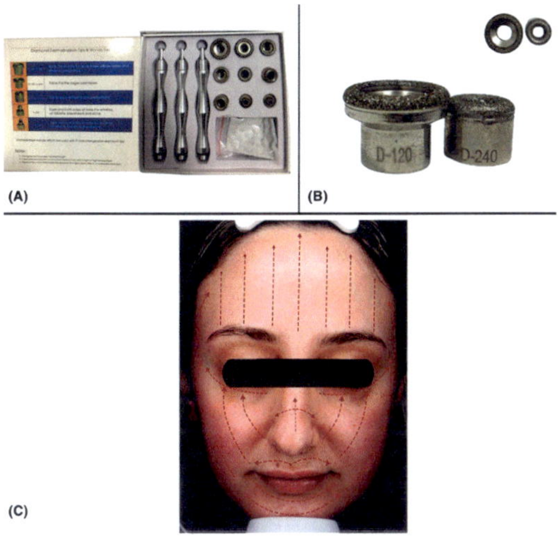

Figure 14.12. (A) Microdermabrasion wands and tip set; (B) Close up view of attachable tips; and (C) Direction of wand movements on the face.

Source: Alhammadi, A. H., & Alnaqbi, K. A. (2024). *Microdermabrasion Wands and Tip Set; Close-Up View of Attachable Tips; Treatment Area Markings.* ResearchGate.

Its adaptability and simplicity make it truly shine in current skincare regimens. That being said, to reap its true benefits, a little extra caution prior to and following microdermabrasion is necessary to prevent complications and enhance healing. Dermatologists tend to emphasize, in general, that healed skin needs to be protected from excessive sun and provided the appropriate moisturizers to restore its barrier (Madnani et al., 2022). It is also important to take into account every individual's skin type and conditions so that the treatment environment can be adjusted for optimal results. Placed deliberately into a general scheme of skin care, microdermabrasion is a convenient instrument in the arsenal of minimally invasive aesthetic procedures, enhancing the looks with relatively little danger, and maintaining high patient satisfaction when combined with appropriate follow-up (Figure 14.12).

14.4.3. Light Therapy for Acne and Pigmentation

Dermatological therapies today turn increasingly towards alternatives that do not include invasive methods. Light therapy, for instance, has risen in popularity as a means of addressing skin concerns such as acne and irregular pigmentation. Rather than a stubborn pill regimen, this type applies select wavelengths of light to push the skin's natural processes into function. In the case of acne, specific rays trigger photochemical reactions that reduce sebum production, knock out bacterial colonies, and calm inflammation. Concomitantly, fine-tuning light exposure subtly modifies the behavior of melanocytes, which can ideally correct both over- and under-pigmented surfaces. These non-surgical alternatives appear to combine efficacy with safety and are an organized substitute for conventional drugs that dermatologists are eager to prescribe (Sy & Jusuf, 2024). All in all, light therapy is emerging as a convenient adjunct to skin care, particularly where appearance is paramount. A controlled trial lends support to employing a combination of blue and red lights to treat more difficult cases of acne. In one experiment with patients having severe acne vulgaris, individuals who received 415 nm blue light as well as

633 nm red light for 12 weeks experienced marked improvements. The outcomes were unambiguous: both red inflamed pimples and less symptomatic lesions decreased in the count. In this case, blue light tends to function as an antibacterial punch against *Cutibacterium acnes*, and red light appears to soothe inflammation and accelerate skin healing, albeit with some experiencing mildly parched lips in the process. These changing treatment intervals in most instances reflect a general good safety and efficacy and indicate that combination light therapies may complement system drugs such as isotretinoin (Thuy et al., 2024) quite well. Light therapy is not solely for acne, however; it is getting a nod for pigmentation concerns as well. Low-level laser treatment (LLLT) has generated a bit of interest for its odd property of modulating the behavior of melanocytes, aiding, for example, in diseases such as vitiligo.

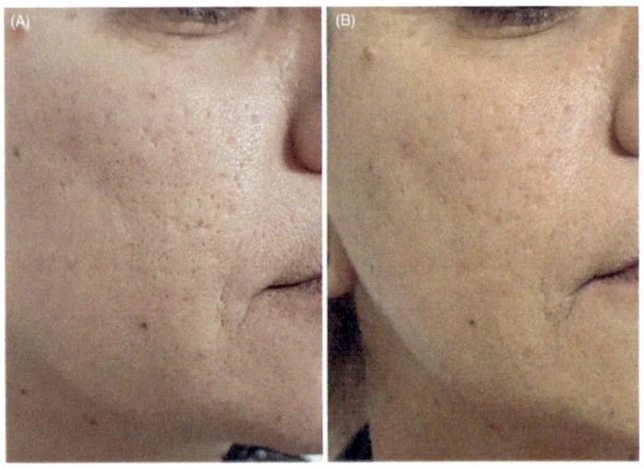

Figure 14.13. Treatment of acne scars with fractional laser (two sessions). (A) Before treatment; and (B) after treatment.

Source: Miot, H. A. (2020). *Treatment of Acne Scars with Fractional Laser – Two Sessions: (A) Before Treatment; and (B) After Treatment.* ResearchGate.

By mildly activating these color cells, LLLT promotes repigmentation as well as ameliorating the actions of UV radiation that exacerbate hyperpigmentation. This non-surgical approach, which provides an excellent balance between safety and fewer side effects, sets the bar high for what cosmetic dermatology can deliver today (Sy & Jusuf, 2024). Light therapy is increasingly making its presence felt not merely in ironing out surface problems but also in altering the cellular response that counts in skin disorders (Figure 14.13).

14.5. Patient Considerations

Patients' safety and comfort in cosmetic and skin treatments depend on meticulous planning beforehand as well as during the procedure. Pain management, particularly, is always at the top of one's mind—patients' stress and pain can quickly send the entire process awry. Anesthesia is not universal—it takes only a cream to do the trick at times, while a local injection or regional block is necessary at others, depending on each individual's characterestics. Children and elderly individuals, especially, require additional vigilance because threats such as delayed healing, unforeseen allergic responses, or even systemic toxicity can creep in. Newer strategies such as microneedle patches and *cryoanesthesia* now suggest improved pain control with reduced side effects, and on some occasions, individualizing anesthesia with suggestions from genetic and proteomic information may indeed provide even more acutely precise management tactics (Rahib et al., 2024). Children pose their own set of issues to these procedures—preventing them from ending up with permanent scars or emotional distress is a necessity. In a less invasive variation, newer technology such as line-field confocal optical coherence tomography (LC-OCT) has entered the scene. This approach, which provides high-resolution images, can frequently reduce the necessity of awkward biopsies, a relief, particularly for an anxious child. Research indicates that, overall, applying LC-OCT increases diagnostic confidence by over 20%, resulting in easier but wiser treatment plans for kids (Cappilli et al., 2023).

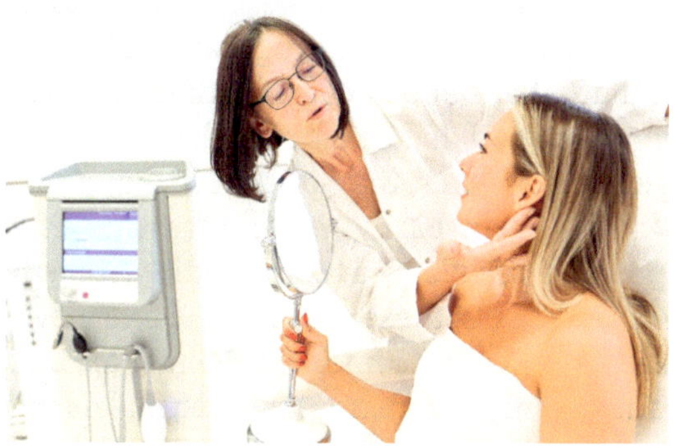

Source: APT Injection Training. (2024). *Aesthetic Consultation Before Treatment.* https://aptinjectiontraining.com/wp-content/uploads/2024/10/28.png.

It is a trend that gently supports consideration of both body and mind when treating the pediatric demographic. A large portion of the process is controlling what patients anticipate and ensuring they know what to expect. Individuals tend to enter with individual, oftentimes very subjective, visions of beauty that have to align with practical results; otherwise, disillusionment can enter the picture. Careful consultations—where there is an honest discussion of risks, potential complications, and recovery periods, particularly if there are pre-existing factors that may interfere with healing, are most important. The mind plays a part here as well; concerns regarding body image and underlying psychological factors can determine if a procedure is going to work well or not. Integration of sound pain management, diligent diagnosis, a touch of emotional support, and honest-to-goodness chats creates a holistic approach that enhances safety, comfort, and total satisfaction along the entire dermatologic journey (Cappilli et al., 2023; Rahib et al., 2024).

14.5.1. Importance of Consultation and Assessment

Cosmetic and procedural dermatology is not all about learning fancy procedures ; it all starts with that very first, thorough conversation. Physicians pay close attention to a patient's skin, their medical history information, and precisely what they want, even before any procedure is done. This initial step not only serves to customize the treatment to individuals but also provides an opportunity to ensure that what they hope for is really achievable. In most instances, an awareness of what can safely be achieved versus what a patient fantasizes about prevents subsequent disappointments and issues. Avoiding that full-fledged initial talk could translate into bypassing significant issues, such as concealed skin issues, previous treatments that were not satisfactory, or even hints of existing psychological issues. Such early interactions instill trust and facilitate open lines of communication vital for safe cosmetic treatment (Buljan et al., 2010). Observing emotional and mental indicators as early on as possible is also essential. A few patients, for example, may have excessively high expectations or even present symptoms of body dysmorphic disorder, so their discontent will be more related to a warped sense of self than to how well a treatment works. When these warnings are not detected, it can cause multiple procedures that never correct the problem, cumulatively adding up in both risk and ethical nightmares. That is why physicians are aided by an attentive, empathetic check-in—of careful dialogue combined with a keen eye. Inserting minor steps such as photography or recording detailed consent records will serve as a safety net for the patient and the physician (Buljan et al., 2010). Currently, non-surgical aesthetic treatments are gaining popularity, and that trend has driven training into a more formatted track. With procedures creeping into private clinics, schools now implement uniform courses and formal examinations, OSCE, to ensure each practitioner is proficient. It is not unusual, these days, for advanced courses to incorporate hands-on patient assessments, establish achievable objectives, and even map out those inevitable bumps along the road. Emphasis on comprehensive initial consultations are the key to effective cosmetic dermatology. Correspondingly, advancing educational standards supports fostering a climate where excellence and true patient care are inseparable (Figure 14.14).

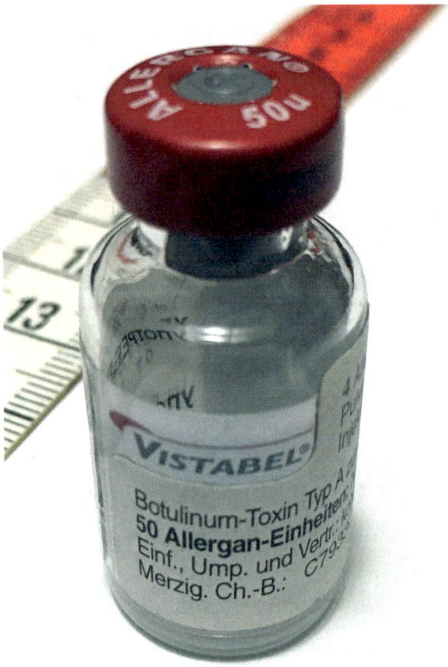

Figure 14.14. Consultation with a dermatologist.

Source: By Pittigrilli - Own work, CC BY 4.0, https://commons.wikimedia.org/w/index.php?curid=150531994

14.5.2. Risks and Side Effects of Procedures

Cosmetic skin treatments have evolved significantly and draw increasing numbers of patients, but they still have their share of bumps along the way. Chemical peels and laser treatments may look easy, but physicians must be careful to watch closely for the small risks that they carry. At times, a patient will only get a little redness or swelling that dissolves quickly, but other times more serious things such as scarring or discoloration of the skin develop—rare, yet enough to require attentive follow-ups before proceeding. Each patient's skin and background make the case its own unique puzzle, challenging practitioners to formulate plans specifically for them. Aftercare, also mentioned, is not an afterthought; a bit of forgetfulness after the procedure happens all too quickly can easily exacerbate side effects or prolong recovery, and the skill with which a doctor knows these risks can quite literally dictate the final outcome (Madnani et al., 2022). Treating younger patients, however, makes things complicated. Consider congenital melanocytic nevi because those birthmarks seen at birth are a great example. Surgery and laser removal, the standard recourse for eliminating them, have their own special challenges. Kids' skin, as a rule, is even more sensitive, and whatever mark shows up, be it scar tissue or an untidy area left on display, can strike not only the skin but the self-confidence too. The reality that we do not have good, quality-of-life-oriented guidelines only complicates decision-making, with every option (surgery with its potential anesthesia hiccups and scarring or lasers that may not get everything sorted out) presenting a mixed bag of functional and aesthetic issues. In all but the most straightforward situations, this delicate dance requires additional research to truly unravel the subtle trade-offs at play (Lai et al., 2018). Even with all these advancements, chasing that ideal look through skin procedures is not without its hiccups, after all, our bodies have a mind of their own. Issues like infections, allergic responses, or simply a delayed recovery can emerge whether you are looking at fillers, microneedling radiofrequency, or something else entirely. This means that sticking to clean techniques and performing proper patient screening (no shortcuts, really) remains crucial. In addition to that, a practitioner's expertise is key; natural differences in competence mean that a bit of added expertise can frequently ward off complications. It comes down to managing a balance between striking the cosmetic target and avoiding side effects, with pre-procedure consultations and careful work on hands, follow-up checks, and everything else all contributing.

Missing out on any part of that puzzle can damage not only safety but also satisfaction overall, really highlighting how technique and risk are always kind of in a dance with each other in aesthetic dermatology (Madnani et al., 2022).

14.5.3. Psychological Impact of Cosmetic Treatments

How you perceive yourself tends to dictate whether or not you will attempt cosmetic procedures, and it is heavily connected with your emotional health. Many individuals opt for these surgeries just to ease that internal conflict of not liking how they look, sometimes expecting it to also enable them to mingle better socially and be more positive inside. , getting to what is behind those decisions is important for anyone in cosmetic dermatology, particularly because teenagers can be particularly susceptible to society's glitzy ideals, which might predispose them to have sky-high, unrealistic expectations. That is the reason why lots of docs make a point to look out for a patient's overall emotional state and underlying motives before proceeding. Scales such as the DAS-59 may really come in handy in determining who would really benefit mentally from the changes and who would be at more risk (Luca et al., 2018). Most times, this sort of close examination is intended to lead decisions towards a more balanced mental health and not necessarily for a good-looking face. Cosmetic treatments do not simply repair what you see in the mirror; they tend to have a ripple effect into many areas of life—your mood, your confidence, and even your quality of life. Studies generally indicate that when chosen well and performed ethically, these treatments can raise self-esteem, alleviate social anxiety, and assist in bettering relationships at a personal level. A lot of patients feel a new boost of confidence after their procedures, as if the physical transformation and state of mind are positively reinforcing one another. That being said, not everyone gets happy about it—if complications arise or the end result is not what they had envisioned, it can bring on more angst. Pre-procedure discussions and the establishment of realistic expectations are most important here because achieving a proper balance between the psychological advantages and downsides avoids treatments inadvertently exacerbating any underlying psychological issues or contributing to dangerous body image disorders (Luca et al., 2018). Ongoing research continues to trickle in regarding just how patients perceive these cosmetic procedures, providing further understanding of the psychological aspect of cosmetic surgery. Reviews do not just speak about the clinical safety of procedures, such as abobotulinumtoxinA injections—but also present patient anecdotes about enhanced self-view and improvement in mood. Often, strong satisfaction scores are accompanied by perceivable benefits in the way individuals perceive themselves, which supports the argument that, if employed cautiously, these interventions can yield a beneficial mental return. Nonetheless, there are periodic hiccups, such as the infrequent development of neutralizing antibodies or other adverse effects that may indirectly alter a subject's psychological state, keeping clinicians vigilant with frequent check-ins along the way. The combination of solid clinical skills and a healthy dose of psychological check-ins is still essential to achieving the optimal outcome while minimizing risks.

14.6. Ethical Considerations

Procedural and cosmetic dermatology is booming today, and with it, an ugly array of ethical dilemmas that truly deserve scrutiny. Most individuals seeking aesthetic solutions tend to be influenced by social pressures, consider media photos and social network ideals, and that makes it difficult to determine whether or not a procedure is medically required or simply an elective fashion choice. That haze places physicians in the difficult position of attempting to do good and avoid harm. Often, the pressure for treatments such as BOTOX is not simply about appearing more pleasing; it can connect to more fundamental issues like body dysmorphic disorder or depression, blurring exactly what constitutes appropriate informed consent. Physicians must ensure patients understand both the risks and realistic outcomes, so they do not inadvertently exploit or worsen existing mental health concerns. Even though injectables have proven safe over time, that long safety record does not let us off the hook when it comes to ethical responsibility, especially when it is about protecting vulnerable groups and addressing uneven access and expectations (Kerna et al., 2024). Taking a step back, the ethical issues go beyond a single treatment. Most of these procedures occur in private clinics instead of academic institutions, where, by and large, standardized technical and ethical education are absent. This discrepancy can translate into uneven care and even hazardous interventions, pointing to why establishing robust, evidence-based postgraduate programs is of such significance. Combining authentic critical thinking and inquiry learning can equip emerging practitioners to manage the sensitive duties of this domain more effectively. Practically oriented evaluations that challenge manual skills as well as ethical judgment are the best way to maintain high standards and protect patient safety (Kumar et al., 2021). Equitable access provides another dimension of concern. Socioeconomic disparities, cultural prejudices, and racial differences all influence who receives these treatments and how they are viewed, tending to reinforce established social hierarchies.

Providers must be attuned to these forces, striving to avoid discriminatory behaviors while honoring diverse values and expectations held by patients. Being transparent with benefits, risks, costs, and boundaries is absolutely necessary to enable everyone to make educated decisions. In addition, the business-oriented aspect of cosmetic procedures sometimes conflicts with true patient care. In the end, adherence to principles of justice, respect for persons, and firm professional responsibility is what governs ethical practice in this rapidly evolving cosmetic and procedural dermatology environment (Kumar et al., 2021; Kerna et al., 2024).

14.6.1. Informed Consent in Dermatological Procedures

Frank, honest communication is at the top of any medical procedure, particularly with skin treatments where being pleasing to the eye is paramount. Any procedure such as hyaluronic acid fillers has issues that accompany it; patients must understand that complications, even fairly uncommon conditions such as vascular occlusion, can arise.

Defining these risks is not mere paperwork—it is to create trust in an honest sense. Physicians, therefore, need to be sure enough to talk about these issues without beating around the bush so patients can know what they are getting themselves into. They also need to ensure people receive the detail of aftercare and are able to work out, even if a bit dim-witted sometimes, when something is not quite right, which eventually increases both safety and overall success (Sanders, 2024). Sorting out what patients want can get messy and complicated. Although chemical peels, Botox injections, and laser resurfacing sound easy on paper, a lot of clients walk away with unrealistically high expectations, sometimes driven by problems such as body dysmorphic disorder. Catching it early is really crucial because if the expectations are not met, if they are unrealistic, it could contribute to dissatisfaction, possible legal confusion, or even a rupture in the doctor-patient conversation. More often than not, consent should not be merely a paper notice but probe why someone wants the treatment and assist in establishing goals that get increasingly concrete. Taking detailed notes, such as before-and-after photos, introduces an element of transparency and can prevent everyone from cursing themselves with hindsight (Buljan et al., 2010).

Subject Information and Consent Form

A Phase 3, Double-Blind, Placebo-Controlled Study of Maintenance Pemetrexed plus Best Supportive Care versus Best Supportive Care Immediately Following Induction Treatment with Pemetrexed + Cisplatin for Advanced Non-Squamous Non-Small Cell Lung Cancer

Qualified Investigator:	[Insert name and contact information]
Sub-Investigator(s):	[Insert name(s) and contact information, if required]
Sponsor:	**Eli Lilly Canada Inc.**

Introduction

You are being invited to take part in a research study *(also called a clinical trial)*. This research will study a drug known as pemetrexed (Alimta®). It is your choice if you want to be in this study or not. Research studies are different from regular care. Research studies are ways of finding out new information that might help other people with similar conditions or illnesses to yours. This form explains why we are doing the study, and how the treatment that is being offered to you is different from regular care. It tells you what will happen during the study. It also tells you about any inconvenience, discomfort or risk with this study. It also gives you a complete description of the treatment offered. This information will help you decide whether you wish to be part of the study.

What Is The Purpose of The Study?

The main reason for doing this study is to help answer the following research question:

- Whether the administration of pemetrexed as a maintenance treatment will improve upon therapy you initially received (pemetrexed in combination with cisplatin) and will prevent your cancer from growing or recurring.

Who Can Take Part In The Study?

To take part in this study you must have the diagnosis of unresectable, locally advanced, stage IIIB or stage IV, non-squamous non-small cell lung cancer. The study doctor or study staff has discussed with you the requirements for being in this study. It is important that you are completely honest with the doctor and staff about your health history. You should not take part in this study if you do not meet all requirements.

You cannot participate in this study if:

- You have an active infection or other serious condition such as cardiac disease
- You have had another malignant cancer less than five years ago
- You take aspirin or aspirin like medication that you are unable to stop taking for a few days during each cycle of therapy
- You are unable or unwilling to take folic acid, vitamin B12 and dexamethasone or other corticosteroids medication.
- You have had a yellow fever vaccination within the last 30 days or plan to have it.

Figure 14.15. Informed consent.

Source: By Eli Lilly and Company - other parties that are summarized here: https://creativecommons.org/licenses/by/3.0/ . - Thomas Krohn", CC BY 3.0, https://commons.wikimedia.org/w/index.php?curid=28301481.

Dermatologists are not in it to obtain a signature—they are there to put patients first by truthfully presenting both the pluses and the minuses of the procedure. In the majority of cases, good training in these cosmetic procedures means they are prepared to deal with any curveballs and present complicated things in ways that are not, you know, all over the place. Securing the proper type of informed consent, one supported by thorough interactions and visual signs, establishes shared understanding and genuinely honors an individual's right to make decisions. It not only prevents legal issues from arising but also adheres to a fundamental virtue of honesty, ensuring what is done is in accordance with what patients expect and require in terms of safety. Ultimately, informed consent in cosmetic dermatology is a dynamic, constantly changing process that serves both patient welfare and the professional integrity of the practitioners (Buljan et al., 2010; Sanders, 2024) (Figure 14.15).

14.6.2. Marketing and Representation in Cosmetic Dermatology

Today's cosmetic dermatology is being redefined by marketing that quietly sets the stage for how patients perceive their choices. Social media updates, celebrity endorsements, and targeted-to-you advertisements assist in raising the profile of non-surgical aesthetic treatments in a manner that is both new and, in a word, a little bit like a tale of youth and beauty told especially for you. It is not just about hyping the new technology; it is also about spinning an aspirational story that can connect with a wide audience. There is also that pesky issue of maintaining ethicality ; advertisements should not exploit weaknesses or promote unattainable ideals, particularly because many of these treatments are being performed outside the standard clinical environments. For the most part, openness about how well treatments work and what risks they involve goes hand-in-hand with good patient education and informed consent, which in turn preserves both clinical credibility and consumer confidence (Kumar et al., 2021). More than slick campaigns, how people receive representation goes a long way toward making cosmetic dermatology truly accessible. Historically, marketing materials have kept to one very specific concept of beauty, excluding varied skin tones and cultural looks. Such a limited perspective may deter prospective patients and even limit studies targeting multiple needs. Recently, however, an effort has been made to shake things up—commercials now include a more diverse spectrum of ethnicities and age groups while also targeting procedures to varying skin needs. Expanding representation not only addresses equity but also appears to enhance outcomes of treatment when care is culturally sensitive. This practice emphasizes that providers must relate to a growing patient population of greater diversity, creating a practice that feels inclusive and effective (Nova Southeastern University, 2014). Education and training are also closely intersecting with these representation and marketing shifts in cosmetic dermatology. New postgraduate programs in non-surgical aesthetics have emerged to bridge deficits caused by less structured traditional training, outfitting clinicians with research-based expertise and ethical guidelines. These courses promote critical thinking, inquiry-based learning, and a blend of assessment modalities so that practitioners are better able to manage pressures of marketing-driven expectations. And, to boot, they stress cultural awareness and sensitivity to varied patient needs, which inevitably carries over to how treatments are marketed and communicated. When sound training is married to ethical marketing and more robust representation, the entire industry can improve its standards, gain more public confidence, and improve patient safety and satisfaction (Kumar et al., 2021).

14.6.3. Addressing Unrealistic Expectations

Cosmetic and procedural dermatology is getting a lot of attention these days, with more and more patients inquiring about it due to the onslaught of photos and information online. Individuals tend to be caught up by online hype, sometimes expecting overnight, perfectly-posed results that never come true. Patients are inclined toward shortcuts that are inspired by those perfect posts on social media, even though these depictions never typically represent normal outcomes. This type of disconnect in comprehension can make people feel disappointed even when treatments are effective from a medical perspective. That is why dermatologists must speak honestly with patients, providing genuine, evidence-based information about what to anticipate, the dangers involved, and how results may vary between individuals. Implementing pre-procedure consultations that include mental preparedness and achievable expectations can truly smooth out expectations and increase satisfaction in aesthetic skin care practice (Dhillon et al., 2024). Apart from effective communication, clinicians must also remember that non-medical factors significantly contribute to influencing what patients want. Today, energy devices and injectables are sprouting up everywhere, hyped sometimes with higher promises of rejuvenation and wholesale change. For example, non-surgical vulvovaginal rejuvenation is frequently promoted for both functional and cosmetic benefits, even though there is not much long-term safety information or standard recommendations to be found. Quite a number of patients will end up imagining drastic alterations based on these advertising brochures and videos, only to be disillusioned when the changes are modest or temporary. In all instances, this implies dermatologists must offer balanced, scientifically grounded perspectives on such new treatments—noting the existing boundaries of scientific evidence and even certain legal problems (Dhillon et al., 2024). This candid, thoughtful response not only preserves professional integrity but also reaffirms trust between physicians and patients. Digital technology, while it has its advantages, has proven to be a double-edged sword in the context of influencing expectations in cosmetic and procedural dermatology. Social media sites readily disseminate knowledge and enable physicians to communicate with patients, but they also advance idealized beauty standards that may seem unattainable. The availability of effortless, high-gloss, highly produced content tends to blur the distinction between natural results and manipulated visuals, clouding what patients believe can be done. Dermatologists must intervene—not only to teach, but also to softly disabuse of myths that could create unrealistically high expectations. Finding that balance between embracing digital communication and maintaining realistic patient expectations takes continuous adjusting, tact, and occasionally a touch of creative nuance. A considerate approach to such platforms can go a long way in helping patients have a more realistic view of their dermatologic treatment (Tiara & Saraswati, 2023).

CLOSER LOOK

Skin Resurfacing

Skin resurfacing, particularly lasers, is designed to revitalize skin by eliminating injured outer layers and inducing the formation of new collagen, resulting in smoother, more youthful-looking skin. This procedure can treat a number of conditions such as wrinkles, scars, sun spots, and impaired skin tone.

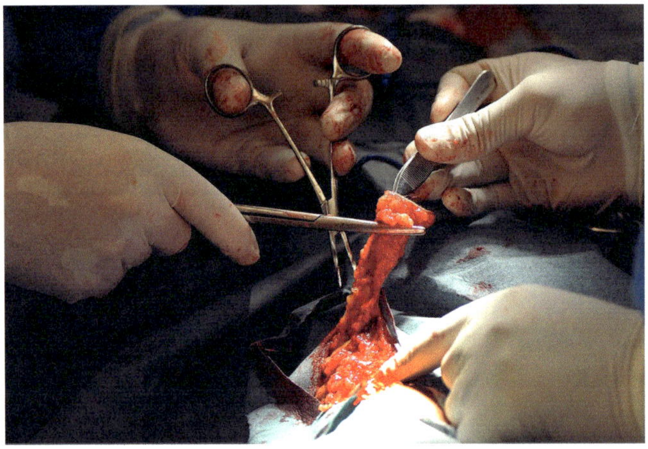

Source: By Senior Airman Kenneth Holston - https://www.dvidshub.net/image/256992/burn-victim-treated-kandahar, Public Domain, https://commons.wikimedia.org/w/index.php?curid=57461867

- **How It Works**
    - **Ablative Lasers:** Focused streams of light energy boil off the surface skin layers, leaving healthy new skin exposed, and inducing collagen formation.
    - **Non-Ablative Lasers:** Induce collagen synthesis without eliminating the skin's surface, commonly used for mild skin issues such as fine lines and wrinkles.
    - **Mechanical Resurfacing:** Refers to mechanical exfoliation with a tool to remove the top layers of skin.
- **Advantages**
    - **Better Skin Texture and Color:** Exfoliates off dead skin layers and encourages the growth of new, healthy skin cells.
    - **Less Wrinkles and Fine Lines:** Stimulates collagen growth, filling wrinkles and making skin smoother overall.
    - **Reduces Scars and Discoloration:** Fades acne scars, surgical scars, and pigmentation problems such as sunspots and age spots.
    - **Tightens Skin:** Encourages the production of collagen and elastin, resulting in tighter, more youthful skin.
    - **Treats Sun Damage:** Reverses the consequences of years of sun damage, including premature aging and pigmentation.

- **Considerations**
  - **Ablative Lasers:** They may have a longer recovery and can take more than one session to show the best results.
  - **Non-Ablative Lasers:** Generally fewer treatments, and less down time.
  - **Selecting Appropriate Treatment:** An expert professional's consultation is needed to decide on the best course of treatment for specific skin issues and objectives.
  - **Possible Side Effects and** Risks: These may consist of redness, swelling, peeling, and in some individuals, scarring or pigment alterations, so it is a good idea to go over these with your practitioner.

SUMMARY

Cosmetic and procedural dermatology have truly changed the way we look after our skin. Beauty is not about looks anymore; it is now inextricably linked with treatments that are both safe and effective. Today, you can see non-surgical procedures entering postgrad training, and with that, evidence-based education proves that it can improve both patient safety and procedural know-how. Organized learning such as this constructs vital skills and even reminds practitioners about doing what is right by their patients. In some sense, these shifts not only improve clinical outcomes but also keep ethics at the forefront, marrying new concepts with a sense of duty (Kumar et al., 2021). Diagnostic equipment and continuous training are equally important in this profession, primarily due to the fact that the earlier the problems are identified, the improved the recovery of the patient is likely to be.

Consider dermoscopy training sessions, for example—such practical sessions have proven to achieve more precise lesion examinations than a basic bare-eyed glance. Yes, the outcomes at times highlight areas that still require a little altering, but these programs emphasize the ever-present necessity of reexamining and refining diagnostic procedures for detecting melanomas more quickly. Adding these hands-on, research-based sessions truly demonstrates how continual professional development can hone both technical competence and overall quality of care (Armstrong et al., 2011). Ultimately, cosmetic and procedural dermatology is a specialty in which innovative methods intersect rigorous education and savvy diagnostics. Thoroughly designed courses and advanced training are the pillars that enable clinicians to provide care that is safe, effective, and , by and large, patient-centered. Although recent evidence indicates training and diagnostic accuracy have undergone significant advancements, research continued along with ongoing modifications continue to be essential as newer clinical issues arise. In the end, relying on an evidence-based method facilitates a culture of accountability and excellence while ensuring the practice continues to advance responsibly to improve both esthetic outcomes and skin health (Armstrong et al., 2011; Kumar et al., 2021).

Hyaluronic acid dermal fillers are on a roll in cosmetic dermatology these days, with cool innovations but also some pesky issues. A major concern is that at times blood vessels can become obstructed, a nasty event that can result in severe damage if not detected immediately. Practitioners must be sharp, and training sessions have proven that they indeed learn the tricks to manage such complications. For instance, utilizing a basic Plan-Do-Study-Act cycle as an educational tool has facilitated the increase in comfort and skill levels, with end-of-training evaluations being much better than they initially were. In the majority of situations, it would appear that an added bit of education can go very far in maintaining these risks under control, reminding practitioners of the heavy responsibility they carry in patient care (Sanders, 2024).

At the same time, the world of cosmetic dermatology is also trying to figure out how to mesh non-surgical aesthetic procedures with formal medical training. You will often find these NSA procedures happening in private clinics, away from the usual hospital training grounds. Because of that, some evidence-based postgraduate courses have popped up, built from systematic reviews and worldwide needs checks. These programs place a heavy emphasis on thinking critically, practical learning, and combining good information with actual professional ethics. They even employ practical exams, such as those objective structured clinical assessments—to assist in honing both the skills and ethics required in this area. This creates a move towards attempting to organize some sense into what previously was a fairly spotty education system (Kumar et al., 2021). These changes demonstrate genuine improvement in the safety and dependability of cosmetic dermatology. When physicians are better able to detect and address problems such as vascular occlusion, patients fare better. With curricula becoming less fractured and more considered, there is a resounding drift towards aligning pragmatic know-how with good ethical standards, making sure that the profession is keeping up with its runaway changes (Kumar et al., 2021; Sanders, 2024).

KEY TERMS FROM THIS CHAPTER

Chemical peels	Diagnostic tools	Fillers
Laser	Laser zapping	Microneedling
Mohs micrographic surgery	Photodynamic therapy	Pigmentation
Platelet-rich plasma (PRP) therapy	Radiofrequency	Scars
Supervised programs	Trichloroacetic acid	Wrinkles

REFERENCES

1. Armstrong, A. (2011). Dermoscopy: An Evidence-Based Approach for The Early Detection of Melanoma. https://core.ac.uk/download/80548511.pdf (accessed on 12 May 2025).

2. Bernardini, F. P., Skippen, B., Cetto, R., Calomeni, M., Cotofana, S., Urso, S. U., Paternostro, F., & Hartstein, M. E. (2025). Bridging the Gap Rather Than Filling the Entire Valley-Anatomic Insights When Treating the Medial Infraorbital Region. Journal of cosmetic dermatology, 24(1), e16582. https://doi.org/10.1111/jocd.16582(accessed on 12 May 2025).

3. Buljan, M., & Šitum, M. (2010). Kako zaštititi liječnika od nerealnih očekivanja pojedinih klijenata u korektivnoj dermatologiji? https://core.ac.uk/download/14451788.pdf (accessed on 12 May 2025).

4. Cappilli, S., Guerriero, C., Iacoangeli, A., Verzì, A., Cinotti, E., Suppa, M., Peris, K., et al. (2023). Utility of line-field confocal optical coherence tomography in the pediatric population. Italian Journal of Dermatology and Venereology, 158(3), 197–204. https://www.semanticscholar.org/paper/c2ab1929abdba101cc3cca2d62ccdd3355e25ae0 (accessed on 12 May 2025).

5. Castle, D. J., & Honigman, R. (2006). Aging and Cosmetic Enhancement. https://core.ac.uk/download/pdf/8296058.pdf.

6. Chuang, J., Barnes, C., & Wong, B. J. F. (2016). Overview of Facial Plastic Surgery and Current Developments. Surgery journal (New York, N.Y.), 2(1), e17–e28. https://doi.org/10.1055/s-0036-1572360 (accessed on 12 May 2025).

7. Cohen, J. L., & Scuderi, N. (2017). Safety and patient satisfaction of abobotulinumtoxinA for aesthetic use: A systematic review. https://core.ac.uk/download/98346025.pdf Cohen, J. L., & Scuderi, N. (2017). Safety and Patient Satisfaction of AbobotulinumtoxinA for Aesthetic Use: A Systematic Review. Aesthetic surgery journal, 37(suppl_1), S32–S44. https://doi.org/10.1093/asj/sjx010 (accessed on 12 May 2025).

8. Eddy, L., & Duffy, R. (2019). A study of the skills, education and qualifications of nurses performing dermatological surgery in the United Kingdom. Dermatological Nursing: The journal of the British Dermatological Nursing Group, 18(4), 10-15. https://bdng.org.uk/dn/Editorial Office. (2016). JSD Volume 1, Issue 3 full issue. https://core.ac.uk/download/193166657.pdf (accessed on 12 May 2025).

9. Ghimire, K. M., & Lemmens, T. (2018). Regulation of Health Professions in Ontario: Self-Regulation with Statutory-Based Public Accountability. https://core.ac.uk/download/268313402.pdf (accessed on 12 May 2025).

10. Haykal, D., Cartier, H., Benzaquen, M., Damiani, G., & Habib, S. M. (2023). The growing importance of ultrasonography in cosmetic dermatology: An update after the 23rd IMCAS Annual World Congress (2022). Journal of cosmetic dermatology, 22(1), 222–225. https://doi.org/10.1111/jocd.15503 (accessed on 12 May 2025).

11. Islam, R. K., & Khachemoune, A. (2025). Exploring the potential of the emerging 675 nm laser across diverse skin pathologies: a comprehensive review. Journal of cosmetic and laser therapy : official publication of the European Society for Laser Dermatology, 27(1-2), 39–42. https://doi.org/10.1080/14764172.2025.2468496(accessed on 12 May 2025).

12. Islam, R. K., Tong, V. T., Robicheaux, C., Tageant, H., Haas, C. J., Kline, R. J., & Islam, K. N. (2024). The impact of anesthesia on dermatological outcomes: A narrative review. Cureus,

16. https://www.semanticscholar.org/paper/8e56fe6bcf52fd98948309e41ac01c50cfc4322b (accessed on 12 May 2025).

13. Kerna*, N. A., Carsrud, N. V.,* Ngw*u*, D. C., Holets, H. M., Flores, J. V., Pruitt, K. D., Chawla, S., Chawla, V. S., Senat, A. J. B., Nwachukwu, D., Akuma, O. M., & Azi, C. I. (2024). BOTOX's Mechanism, Diversity Considerations, and Therapeutic Potential in Cosmetic, Medical, and Dental Practice. European Journal of Medical and Health Research, 2(3), 154-165. https://doi.org/10.59324/ejmhr.2024.2(3)

14. Kumar, N., & Rahman, E. (202*1). Global needs-assessment for a postgraduate program on nonsurgic*al facial aesthetics. https://core.ac.uk/download/477687156.pdf (accessed on 12 May 2025).

15. Kumar, Narendra; (2021) Design, Development and Implementation Framework for a Postgraduate Non-Surgical Aesthetics Curriculum. Doctoral thesis (Ph.D), UCL (University College London)

16. Lai, Y. (2018). Comparing Congenital Melanocytic Nevus Treatment Effect on Children's Health-Related Qua*lity of Life. https://core.ac.uk/download/475688229.pdf (accessed on 12 May 2025).*

17. Madnani, N *et* al. (2022). Expert opinion on pre- and post-procedure care in aesthetic dermatology. Int J Res Med Sci. 2022 Apr;10(4):991-1000. https://core.ac.uk/download/539912253.pdf (accessed on 12 Ma*y 2025).*

*18. Mutia Fadhila Sy, & Jusuf, N. K. (2024). Use of Low Level Laser in Cosmet*ic Dermatology. Cermin Dunia Kedokteran, 51(6), 352–356. https://doi.org/10.55175/cdk.v51i6.991(accessed on 12 May 2025).

19. Newman J. (2009). Review of soft tissue augmentation in the face. Clinical, cosm*etic and investigational dermatology, 2, 141–150. https://doi.org/10.2147/ccid.s3631Nova Southeastern U*niversity, "Academic Impressions, 2014" (2014). Newsletters. 8. https://nsuworks.nova.edu/hpd_cdm_newsletters/8Sabir, Hawar & Ridha, Intiha. (2019). Comparative Study of Cryotherapy versus Trichloroacetic Acid Chemical Pe**els in the Treatment of Actinic Kerat**osis. UKH Journal of Science and Engineering. 3. 59-63. 10.25079/ukhjse.v3n1y2019.pp59-63. (accessed on 12 May 2025).

20. Nojek, P., Pawlik, W., Zimonczyk, M., Zawół, M., Błaszczyński, G., & Nowotarska, A. (2024). Effective*ness of different acne treatment methods: a comparison of pharmacological, procedural and natural therapies.* Journal of Education, Health and Sport, 71, 55977. https://doi.org/10.12775/JEHS.2024.71.55977 (accessed on 12 May 2025).

21. Perkowska, K., Kaźmierczak, A., Izdebska, W., Sornek, P., Borkowska, A., Kiełb, A., ... Stanek, J. (2024). Mohs Micrographic Surgery – what the gold *standard* in dermatologic surgery offers us. A Literature Review. Quality in Sport, 18, 53925. https://doi.org/10.12775/QS.2024.18.53925 (accessed on 12 May 2025).

22. Portilla, A. S. P., Portilla, C. S. P., Palacios, G. S. G., Rodríguez, B. S. P., Castillo, S. G. A., Espin, N. E. P., & Pita, G. P. M. (2024). The integration of surgical and dermatological techniques in the treatment of cutaneous aging: multidisciplinary approaches and clinical outcomes - a comprehensive systematic review of current literature. International Journa*l of Research in Medical Sciences, 12(5), 1659–1667. https://doi.org/10.18203/2320-6012.ijrms2024094*3 (accessed on 12 May 2025).

23. Salmivuori, M. (2020). New Options for Non-invasive Imaging and Non-invasive Treatment of Skin Cancers. (Tam*pere University Dissertations - Tampereen yliopist*on väitöskirjat; Vol. 245). Tampere University. http://urn.fi/URN:ISBN:978-952-03-1541-2(accessed on 12 May 2025).
24. *Sanders, Ge*nny, "A bundle of care for prevention, early recognition, and treatment of hyaluronic acid dermal filler associated vascular occlusion" (2024). Doctor of Nursing Practice Papers. Paper 168. Retrieved from https://ir.library.louisville.edu/dnp/168
25. Sardinha, M. da S., & Monteiro, M. S. de S. B. (2025). Evaluation of the safety and efficacy *of the thulium 1927 laser in aesthetic health: An integrative review. Journal of* Cosmetic and Laser Therapy: Official Publication of the European Society for Laser Dermatology. https://www.semanticscholar.org/paper/fda15a16dcbc5d529ebc0b1be9632f1c3c22f293 (accessed on 12 May 2025).
26. Sivaranjani, J. (2019). Percutaneous collagen induction in the treatment of atrophic acne scars using an automated micro*needling device: A novel approach.* CORE. https://core.ac.uk/download/235670538.pdf (accessed on 12 May 2025).
27. Suruchi, G., Shweta, M., & Chandi, G. (2018). T*he Wonder Tool Platelet Rich Plasma in Cosmetic Dermatology, Trichology and Hair Transplant. InTech. doi:* 10*.5772/intechopen.70287*
28. Tiara Aman*na A*mandita & Hastika Saraswati, (2023). Current role of social media in aesthetic plastic surgery: Why plastic surgeons must take concern? https://orcid.org/0000-00*03-4949-9255. https://core*.ac.uk/download/648128993.pdf (accessed on 12 May 2025).
29. Vergallo, G. M., Marinelli, E., Napoletano, S., Di Luca, N. M., & Zaami, S. (2018). Ethics and/or Aesthetics? Reflections on Cosmetic Surgery for Adolescents. ¿Ética o Estética? Reflexiones sobre la Cirugía Estética en Adolescentes*. Cuadernos de bioeti*ca : revista oficial de la Asociacion Espanola de Bioetica y Etica Medica, 29(96), 177–189. (accessed on 12 May 2025).

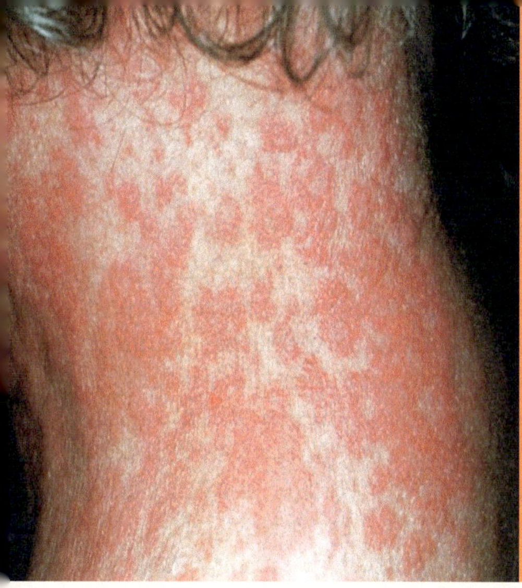

Chapter 15

DERMATOLOGIC EMERGENCIES AND TREATMENT

Contents

Introduction

Skin diseases can worsen quickly, overloading patients and medical professionals when they seek medical attention as emergencies. Such situations call for immediate identification and treatment since delays can lead to severe morbidity or death. Dermatologic emergencies include several acute skin conditions with high systemic involvement or large area skin injury. Of these, Stevens-Johnson Syndrome (SJS) and Toxic Epidermal Necrolysis (TEN) are potentially life-threatening reactions usually caused by drugs, while erythroderma and necrotizing fasciitis are extensive skin inflammation and infection that mandate immediate attention. Careful attention to the pathophysiology, early clinical presentation, and treatment priorities is essential for effective management. Emergency and primary care doctors therefore need to be able to diagnose these conditions early in order to implement life-saving interventions and arrange specialty care. The presentation of dermatologic emergencies is frequently overlapping with other systemic diseases, making diagnosis tricky. SJS and TEN, for instance, have epidermal necrolysis and detachment resulting in extensive denuded areas of skin and predisposing to infection and fluid loss. Erythroderma, on the other hand, is generalized erythema and scaling that can be caused by exacerbations of chronic skin diseases or drug reactions. Necrotizing fasciitis is characterized by rapidly advancing soft tissue infection with out-of-proportion pain and usually associated with systemic toxicity. Proper distinction relies on thorough history-taking, physical examination, and laboratory testing. Early identification is critical since the treatment modalities are vastly different; whereas immunomodulation and supportive care are central for SJS/TEN, antibiotics and aggressive debridement are key in necrotizing fasciitis (Alsudairy et al., 2023).

Family physicians and emergency responders' roles go beyond primary diagnosis to coordinated care and early referrals. Because of the infrequent but severe nature of dermatologic emergencies, their identification may take experience with atypical clinical presentations and warning signs of impending deterioration. In addition to their immediate stabilization, i.e., fluid resuscitation, control of infection, multidisciplinary approaches, including dermatology, surgery, and intensive care specialists, are enhancing outcomes. Furthermore, the education of front-line providers in terms of risk factors, typical precipitants like certain medications or infections, and preventive measures enhances the capacity for early intervention. The inclusion of comprehensive musculoskeletal and systemic assessments, recommended in rheumatological clinical practice, might also assist in identifying complex presentations and systemic involvement characteristic of some dermatologic emergencies (Adaskevich, 2016). Therefore, increased clinical awareness and an organized approach continue to be the pillars for optimal management of these acute, life-threatening dermatologic emergencies.

Definition and Significance of Dermatologic Emergencies

The clinical environment of medicine frequently includes conditions that require immediate and decisive action to avoid irreversible damage or death. Some of these are dermatologic emergencies, a class of acute dermatoses by rapid evolution and potentially lethal outcome. The emergencies, including SJS, TEN, erythroderma, and necrotizing fasciitis, go beyond being merely dermatologic in presentation, with systemic involvement and complex pathophysiology. Recognition of their presentation is an imperative to distinguish them from milder forms of dermatoses, since delays in diagnosis and treatment may result in severe morbidity, such as widespread skin loss, secondary infection, and multi-organ failure. Awareness of definition and subtleties of these conditions is a cornerstone for both dermatologists and general practitioners, emphasizing their fundamental role in inter-specialty care and emergency handling. This background knowledge is a prerequisite for successful therapeutic approaches that have the potential to significantly impact patient outcomes (Adaskevich, 2016). Furthermore, the importance of dermatological emergencies is highlighted by their high mortality and the complex medical management they require. For example, SJS and TEN are serious mucocutaneous reactions mainly caused by drug exposure, inducing extensive epidermal necrosis and detachment with a similar appearance to severe burns. The severity of these syndromes is not only due to acute skin necrosis but also the involvement of the systemic circulation, such as dehydration, imbalance of electrolytes, and sepsis, requiring careful fluid management and infection prevention in specialized critical care units.

Although erythroderma may be an expression of chronic dermatoses at times, it takes on an urgent quality when it causes extreme changes in thermoregulation and barrier function. Therefore, these conditions require immediate multidisciplinary management including supportive care, etiological therapy, and close observation.

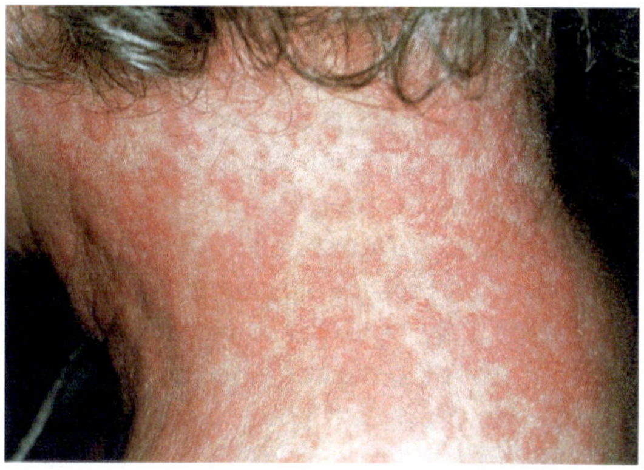

Source: Clinical Advisor. (2018). *10 Dermatologic Emergencies You Should Know About*. https://www.clinicaladvisor.com/wp-content/uploads/sites/11/2018/12/3dresssyndrome_1491634-860x591.jpg.

The seriousness of such emergencies is compounded in clinical practice as a result of their unpredictable course and difficulty with early detection, reinforcing the essential role of specialist perception and intervention. The importance of early recognition and therapy of skin emergencies transcends the short-term clinical process to the overall context of healthcare systems and patient quality of life. The acute disorders, if improperly treated, can lead to long-term physical deformities, psychological scars, and extensive healthcare utilization in terms of lengthy hospitalization and intensive care management. In addition, the heterogeneous etiologies and variable presentations of such diseases as necrotizing fasciitis, an aggressively spreading soft tissue infection with high mortality, require a high level of suspicion and violent surgical and medical treatment to stop progression. Education and awareness about dermatologic emergencies encourage early referral to referral centers and enable integration of multidisciplinary teams such as dermatologists, critical care specialists, and infectious disease specialists, which are crucial for maximal survival and functional recovery. This highlights the delicate integration between rapid clinical judgment and one-stop care, using emphasis on the irreplaceable role of comprehension of dermatologic emergencies in contemporary clinical practice (Adaskevich, 2016).

Overview of Common Conditions: SJS, TEN, Erythroderma, and Necrotizing Fasciitis

Among the dermatologic emergencies, there are some conditions that are major threats because of their quick progression and potentially lethal consequences. SJS and TEN are severe mucocutaneous reactions caused by medications or infections in most cases. Both conditions present with extensive epidermal necrosis and detachment, but vary in severity; SJS occurs in less than 10% of the body surface area (BSA) and TEN occurs in more than 30%. Clinically, the patient manifests with painful rash, blistering, and mucosal lesions, which are capable of impairing vital functions like vision and respiration. Prompt identification and management of these syndromes are important, necessitating supportive care in intensive units and, in most cases, discontinuation of causative agents. Pathogenesis involves a multifaceted immune-mediated process resulting in keratinocyte apoptosis, and understanding this stresses the role of immunological factors in management planning. Unlike SJS and TEN, erythroderma is an extensive inflammatory cutaneous disease with more than 90% body surface erythema and scaling. It often develops from pre-existing dermatoses, drug eruption, or malignancy and can lead to systemic morbidity such as fluid loss, disturbance in thermoregulation, and secondary infection. Erythroderma is caused by generalized redness, exfoliation, and edema and needs thorough evaluation to determine underlying etiology. Its focus on stabilizing patients, treatment of the etiology, and prevention of complications via careful skin care and vigilance, as well as the possibility of coexistence or similarity with other forms of severe dermatologic emergencies, requires differential diagnostic skill. The serious morbidity it carries places an emphasis on prompt intervention in order to prevent the development and systemic extension this disease so frequently takes. Necrotizing fasciitis is a highly aggressive soft tissue infection characterized by extensive necrosis of subcutaneous tissue and fascia. The fulminant bacterial infection, most commonly polymicrobial, requires emergency surgical debridement in addition to broad-spectrum antibiotics to avoid mortality. Clinical presentation early in the course can be subtly benign, with out-of-proportion pain and edema, progressing rapidly to systemic toxicity, septic shock, and multi-organ failure. Underlying diabetes or immunosuppression predisposes to susceptibility. In contrast to the largely immunologic epidermal necrosis of SJS and TEN, necrotizing fasciitis is characterized by direct microbial invasion with toxin-induced tissue damage, underlining different therapeutic imperatives. Early diagnosis and multifaceted aggressive management are critical because delayed recognition severely compromises the prognosis. Effective management of this calamitous dermatologic emergency requires balance between clinical alertness and surgical preparedness (Adaskevich, 2016).

Importance of Timely Diagnosis and Treatment

Prompt clinical identification most frequently is the key initial step towards better outcomes in patients with dangerous dermatologic emergencies like SJS and TEN. Both are initially characterized by minor but characteristic mucocutaneous signs easily misdiagnosed, causing a delay in treatment. Early discrimination from minor cutaneous reactions or infectious causes enables rapid intervention and removal of the causative agents, which dramatically limits development. In addition, initiation of supportive care within intensive facilities reduces complications such as sepsis and multi-organ failure. Early identification by frontline health workers, particularly within primary health and emergency facilities, is crucial because these clinicians are usually the first contact for acute presentations (Alsudairy et al., 2023). The therapeutic window becomes narrow more sharply with increasing epidermal detachment, emphasizing the importance of early diagnosis and simultaneous management to minimize morbidity and mortality. The course of treatment for necrotizing fasciitis and erythroderma also depends on rapid and firm clinical intervention. Necrotizing fasciitis has a rapid course, usually within hours, causing destruction of skin, fat, and fascia, necessitating immediate surgical debridement with broad-spectrum antibiotics. Tardive diagnosis may result in irreversible tissue loss and systemic toxicity, necessitating early suspicion and diagnosis. Likewise, erythroderma with widespread erythema and scaling requires early evaluation to uncover the causes of drug reaction, malignancy, or exacerbation of psoriasis. Inadequate early recognition of these acute dermatologic disorders can cause precipitating systemic complications like fluid imbalances and infection, extending the duration of hospital stay and healthcare expenses. Therefore, early diagnosis not only has a direct effect on patient survival but also maximizes resource use in healthcare systems, further supporting the value of clinician alertness and prompt action (Alsudairy et al., 2023). In addition to immediate life-saving interventions, early treatment and diagnosis are critical in preventing long-term consequences and enhancing quality of life for those suffering from such dermatologic emergencies. For example, patients who survive SJS/TEN frequently suffer from permanent ocular injury, scarring, or psychosocial morbidity, which can be reduced by early ophthalmologic evaluation and rehabilitation measures instituted in the acute setting. The use of multidisciplinary care with rheumatologists and dermatologists further increases diagnostic specificity and therapeutic specificity, especially when comorbidities obscure presentations. Furthermore, early intervention measures provide prompt initiation of immunomodulatory or biologic therapy where appropriate, preventing disease progression. Globally, the liaison between prompt diagnosis with specific treatment protocols is invaluable to gaining the best clinical results, underscoring its pivotal position within the management structure of cutaneous emergencies.

15.1. Stevens-Johnson Syndrome (SJS)

The acute presentation of severe dermatologic disorders in emergency departments requires immediate diagnosis and proper intervention in order to avoid significant morbidity and mortality. Of these, SJS is an acute medical emergency that is marked by epidermal detachment and acute mucocutaneous necrosis, often induced by drug eruption. SJS is characterized clinically by prodrome of flu-like symptoms, followed by blistering skin eruptions and mucosal lesions, which differentiate it from milder dermatoses. The widespread epidermal involvement disrupts the barrier, making the patients highly susceptible to secondary infections, fluid imbalance, and sepsis. Initial treatment focuses on early identification and cessation of the causative agent along with supportive management in intensive care units. Insight into the pathophysiology of SJS in the form of its immunologic mechanisms as well as risk factors helps clinicians provide individualized treatment approaches that may check the progression and enhance outcomes in these critically ill patients. Hospitalization rates and clinical severity markers highlight the emergent nature of SJS in dermatology emergencies. Urban tertiary care center retrospective reviews indicate that SJS accounts for a large percentage of inpatient cutaneous diseases. Patients with SJS, unlike milder forms of dermatoses, often present with generalized blistering pain along with mucosal ulcers that make outpatient treatment inappropriate. These characteristics are strongly associated with the requirement for sophisticated wound care, pain management, and multidisciplinary treatment to manage systemic complications. Furthermore, the acute presentation and expedited course typical of SJS require greater alertness on the part of emergency clinicians to facilitate dermatology consultation and begin proper systemic therapy in a timely manner. This evidence highlights how differentiating clinical factors can guide triage decisions, ultimately ensuring that patients with SJS receive timely, specialized treatment to reduce morbidity (Jack et al., 2011). Advancements in therapeutic approaches for SJS have converged on immunomodulatory methods that aim to attenuate the underlying immune-mediated epidermal destruction. Immune-based therapies such as checkpoint inhibitors have transformed oncology but highlight the risk of immune-related adverse events, one of which is severe cutaneous reactions such as SJS. Their management involves immediate recognition and discontinuation of offending agents, along with immunosuppressive treatment strategies such as corticosteroids or intravenous immunoglobulin (IVIG). Furthermore, the intersection of these therapies with dermatologic emergencies requires detailed supportive care and multidepartment coordination to maximize outcomes. Emergency physicians are therefore required to keep abreast of changing treatment horizons and their concomitant dermatologic implications to be able to manage SJS's complex clinical presentations efficiently and adopt evidence-based, interdisciplinary management strategies (Long et al., 2020) (Figure 15.1).

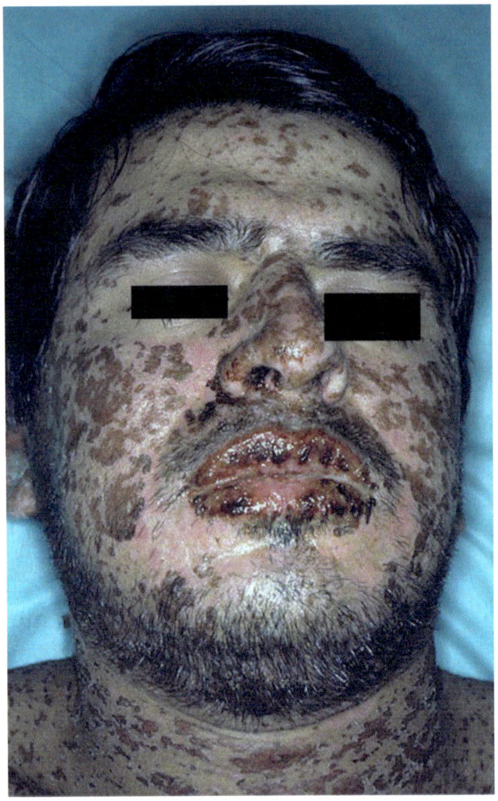

Figure 15.1. Man with characteristic skin lesions of Stevens–Johnson syndrome.

Source: Wikipedia contributors. (n.d.). *Stevens-Johnson Syndrome.* https://upload.wikimedia.org/wikipedia/commons/5/58/Stevens-johnson-syndrome.jpg.

15.1.1. Definition and Pathophysiology of Stevens-Johnson Syndrome (SJS)

The complex interplay of immune mechanisms underlies many severe dermatologic emergencies, necessitating a thorough understanding of their pathophysiology to optimize treatment strategies. SJS is a rare but life-threatening mucocutaneous reaction, predominantly induced by adverse drug responses. It presents with widespread epidermal necrosis and detachment, along with mucous membrane erosion. The immunopathogenesis involves cytotoxic T cells and natural killer cells releasing granulysin and other cytotoxic proteins, which induce keratinocyte apoptosis. This mechanism leads to the typical epidermal sloughing and inflammation in SJS. Although drugs like anticonvulsants and antibiotics are frequent culprits, the immune response in SJS has mechanistic similarities with immune-related adverse events occurring in checkpoint inhibitor therapy, which emphasizes the new immunologic paradigms applicability relevant to dermatologic emergencies (Long et al., 2020). The clinical presentation of SJS mirrors its pathophysiology, characterized by distant systemic compromise that makes it difficult to manage and predict. After an inciting drug or infection, cytotoxic lymphocytes are activated, which recognize drug-related peptides presented by keratinocytes and result in extensive apoptosis.

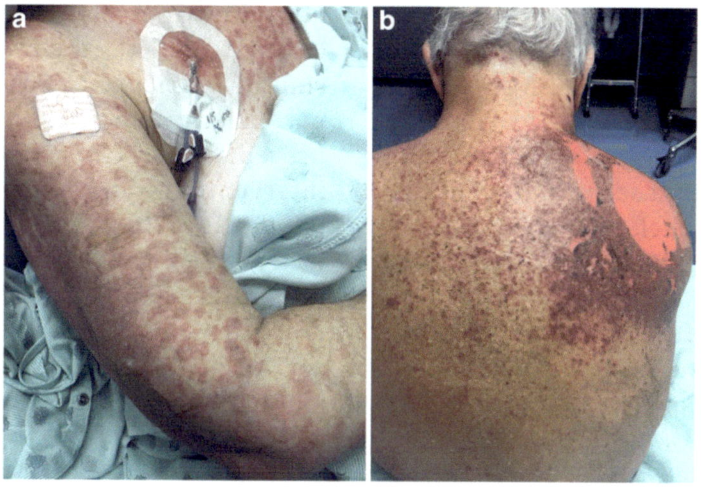

Figure 15.2. A Stevens-Johnson syndrome with blisters developing in atypical targetoid papules. b Erosion and denuded skin in fully evolved Stevens-Johnson syndrome.

Source: Rahnama-Moghadam, S., & Tillmann, H. (2018). *DILI Associated with Skin Reactions*. Current Hepatology Reports.

This immunologic attack weakens the skin's barrier function, makes the patient susceptible to secondary infections, and induces a systemic inflammatory response syndrome (SIRS). The condition worsens over time, exposing patients to severe complications like sepsis, multiorgan failure, and late sequelae like scarring and ocular injury. It is critical to understand these molecular and cellular mechanisms to ensure early diagnosis and intervention to prevent morbidity, in line with the significance of meticulous clinical assessment methodology in autoimmune and inflammatory diseases with overlapping pathology features (Adaskevich, 2016). Pathophysiologically, the epidermal necrosis of SJS illustrates the catastrophic effects of immune dysregulation, differentiating it from other dermatologic emergencies in both clinical presentation and therapeutic management. In contrast to erythroderma or necrotizing fasciitis, SJS occurs mainly due to apoptotic mechanisms initiated by a hypersensitivity response, emphasizing the importance of immediate withdrawal of the causative agent. Furthermore, the immune mediation of SJS entails distinct molecular targets, such as Fas-FasL interactions and perforin-granzyme mechanisms, which provide plausible directions for targeted therapy with ongoing research. The finer immunologic understanding derived from SJS improves the overall perspective of dermatologic emergencies, promoting the necessity of multidisciplinary management to deal with cutaneous and systemic implications equally effectively (Long et al., 2020) (Figure 15.2).

15.1.2. Common Triggers and Risk Factors

Understanding the etiology that leads to dermatologic emergencies is important in order for appropriate diagnosis and treatment to be as effective as possible. For SJS and TEN, among the main triggers are adverse drug reactions to antibiotics, anticonvulsants, and nonsteroidal anti-inflammatory drugs. These reactions tend to trigger an abnormal immune response, causing extensive epidermal necrosis. Infections such as Mycoplasma pneumoniae are also major contributors, particularly among the younger population. The complex etiology of such triggers renders early identification challenging, with a high degree of dependence on the clinician to carefully evaluate patient history and drug exposure. Furthermore, genetic susceptibility factors, including certain HLA alleles, have been shown to contribute to heightened susceptibility to these severe reactions. Knowledge of these factors enables early detection and intervention, which is crucial considering the accelerated course and high mortality of these disorders (Alsudairy et al., 2023). Erythroderma, which is widespread erythema and scaling of much of the body surface, arises largely from pre-existing skin diseases such as psoriasis or drug-induced cutaneous hypersensitivity reactions. Chronicity or sudden onset of such precipitants determines the severity of erythroderma. Systemic drugs like sulfonamides and antiepileptics have been commonly associated with erythrodermic presentations. Underlying malignancies and immune dysregulation also contribute to the pathogenesis, making the skin even more susceptible. The environmental elements involved, such as exposure to irritants or allergens, can exacerbate the cutaneous inflammation associated with erythroderma. A recognition of these risk elements not only facilitates early diagnosis but also guides therapeutic interventions that address both the skin features and the systemic consequences of this potentially fatal illness (Badia et al., 2020). Necrotizing fasciitis, a virulent soft tissue infection, often occurs after trauma, surgery, or disruptions in skin integrity, which offer portal sites of entry for pathogens. Immunocompromised conditions, such as diabetes mellitus, malignancy, and chronic kidney disease, increase the risk significantly by weakening host defenses. Bacterial pathogens, such as Group A Streptococcus and polymicrobial flora, synthesize toxins that enhance tissue destruction. Protracted diagnosis resulting from the nonspecific presentation of early symptoms is a frequent cause of enhanced morbidity and mortality. The interaction among these risk factors underlines the importance of increased clinical suspicion in such at-risk individuals, particularly individuals with recent invasive procedures or chronic disease. Preventative interventions and timely management rely on the identification of these predisposing factors to minimize the destruction caused by this operative emergency (Badia et al., 2020; Alsudairy et al., 2023).

15.1.3. Clinical Presentation and Symptoms

The development of dermatologic emergencies tends to be heralded by nonspecific symptoms that can quickly advance, making timely diagnosis challenging. SJS and TEN patients usually present with flu-like prodromal illness manifested by fever, malaise, and sore throat preceding the typical mucocutaneous lesions. The lesions start as erythematous macules and progress to tender blisters and extensive epidermal detachment. The widespread skin necrosis of TEN, with over 30% of the body surface area (BSA) involved, is a more severe expression than SJS, where less than 10% of the BSA is involved. Mucosal involvement, particularly of the oral, ocular, and genital mucosae, characterizes these disorders, an indication of the overall severity of the disease. This evolution requires early diagnosis and management to avoid complications like secondary infection and multi-organ failure (Alsudairy et al., 2023). Erythroderma, another important dermatologic emergency, has a characteristic clinical presentation of generalized erythema and scaling of more than 90% of the BSA. The patient typically presents with systemic signs and symptoms such as fever, chills, and malaise, indicative of the intense inflammatory nature of the disease. The skin looks diffusely red, inflamed, and can be edematous or lichenified in chronic presentations. The diffuse involvement of the skin compromises the skin barrier function, predisposing to fluid and electrolyte imbalance, thermoregulatory disturbances, and secondary infection. Accurate identification of the underlying causes, from drug reactions to cutaneous T-cell lymphoma, is important to address specifically. Timely identification of erythroderma's typical presentations is potentially life-saving since late treatment is associated with extensive morbidity (Badia et al., 2020). Necrotizing fasciitis, on the other hand, has a rapidly advancing infection that primarily starts with localized pain out of proportion to physical examination findings. Early presentation consists of erythema, warmth, swelling, and pain at the site of involvement, usually with systemic toxicity in the form of fever, tachycardia, and hypotension. With progression of infection, skin changes progress to blistering, ecchymosis, and eventual necrosis with crepitus sometimes felt because of subcutaneous gas formation. The distinguishing feature of necrotizing fasciitis is the early destruction of fascia and subcutaneous tissue, which results in SIRS and multiorgan failure if left untreated. Early clinical subtlety necessitates that clinicians have heightened suspicion to allow for immediate surgical debridement and antimicrobial therapy (Alsudairy et al., 2023).

15.2. Toxic Epidermal Necrolysis (TEN)

The dermatologic emergency clinical scene comprises conditions that advance at a fast rate and need to be urgently addressed to prevent widespread morbidity and mortality. Of these, TEN manifests as one of the most serious presentations, with broad epidermal separation and involvement of the mucous membranes. TEN pathophysiology is most often an immune-mediated process triggered by pharmacological agents that results in extensive keratinocyte apoptosis. Early clinical presentation generally presents with prodromic symptoms of fever and malaise, followed by sudden onset of painful, erythematous macules that coalesce and become large bullous lesions. This severe clinical presentation requires rapid identification by clinicians to allow early initiation of supportive management in specialty centers to avoid complications of sepsis and multi-organ failure. The urgency in the management of TEN corresponds with more general dermatologic emergency principles, all of which place emphasis on the paramount importance of early diagnosis in order to maximize outcomes for the patient (Falodun & Ogunbiyi, 2010).

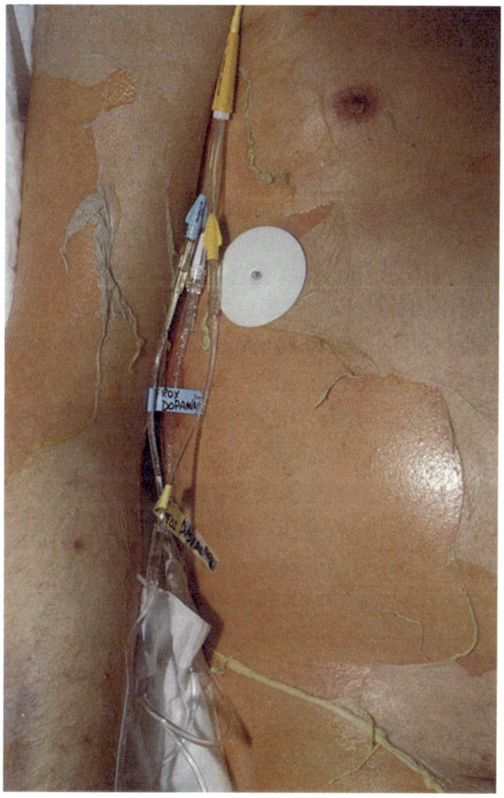

Figure 15.3. Toxic epidermal necrolysis.

Source: Wikipedia contributors. (n.d.). *Toxic Epidermal Necrolysis.* https://upload.wikimedia.org/wikipedia/commons/a/ae/Toxic-epidermal-necrolysis.jpg.

Diagnosis for TEN combines clinical assessment with histopathological verification from skin biopsy. Differential diagnosis carefully needs to rule out other blistering diseases that may simulate TEN, including staphylococcal scalded skin syndrome (SSSS) or autoimmune blistering disease.

The physical examination is important, with a positive Nikolsky's sign—exfoliation caused by mild rubbing of the skin, a characteristic hallmark. Remarkably, TEN's pathogenesis is largely drug-induced, with frequent offenders being anticonvulsants, sulfonamides, and nonsteroidal anti-inflammatory agents. Nonetheless, instances of idiopathic TEN or due to trivial trauma, i.e., burns, have been reported, underlining the broad range of potential causes and the importance of careful patient history taking.

Identifying atypical presentations is life-saving, since delay in diagnosis substantially raises the risk of mortality (Parker & Berkeley, 2010). TEN management is by nature multidisciplinary, with emphasis on the withdrawal of the causative agent and intensive supportive therapy to correct fluid and electrolyte disturbances, wound management, and secondary infection prophylaxis. Admission to intensive care or a burn unit is frequently indicated by the extent of epidermal loss and systemic involvement. Adjunctive therapeutic approaches, such as immunomodulatory therapy with IVIG or corticosteroids, are still controversial but can be of value in selected instances.

The risk of complications, particularly sepsis and respiratory failure, necessitates close monitoring and infection control practices. Finally, early detection and aggressive treatment strategies follow prescribed protocols for dermal emergencies that prioritize rapid action to minimize skin failure and increase survival rates in TEN patients (Falodun & Ogunbiyi, 2010) (Figure 15.3).

15.2.1. Definition and Differentiation from Stevens-Johnson Syndrome (SJS)

The clinical picture of severe cutaneous adverse reactions is multifaceted, with the need for clear definitions to inform effective treatment plans. SJS is defined as a rare but potentially life-threatening hypersensitivity reaction that is most commonly caused by medications or infections. It is associated with epidermal necrosis and mucocutaneous involvement, affecting less than 10% of the BSA. This delineation is critical, as the extent of skin detachment will directly affect diagnosis and management strategies. SJS is distinguished from its worse-appearing twin, TEN, largely based on the extent of epidermal separation, with TEN characterized by greater than 30% BSA. These diseases are a continuum of severity rather than strictly distinct entities, thus the value of careful clinical evaluation to detect early lesions and predict development. It is important to distinguish SJS from other dermatological emergencies like erythroderma or necrotizing fasciitis because they have different pathophysiology and treatment needs. Erythroderma, or exfoliative dermatitis, usually occurs as diffuse erythema involving greater than 90% BSA with scaling and possible systemic symptoms but without the SJS's full-thickness epidermal necrosis. Conversely, necrotizing fasciitis is an aggressively progressive bacterial infection with massive destruction of soft tissue, systemic toxicity, and a distinctly different etiology from the immune-mediated disease process of SJS. Accurate clinical assessment augmented by histopathological examination differentiates SJS, thereby allowing for proper intervention since misdiagnosis can retard essential therapies and exacerbate the course of patients who present with emergencies in the skin.

The subtle diagnosis of SJS and its separation from overlapping dermatologic disorders often depend on clinical presentation and histopathology. Although skin biopsy is the gold standard for diagnosis, clinical criteria like the degree of mucosal involvement, nature of target lesions, and presence of systemic symptoms give critical diagnostic hints. Notably, SJS is largely an immune-mediated process of keratinocyte apoptosis in response to cytotoxic T-cells, as opposed to erythroderma, which frequently arises from chronic inflammatory or neoplastic conditions.

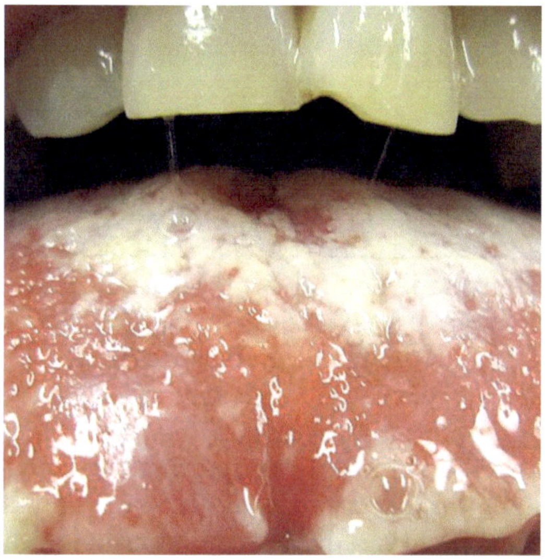

Figure 15.4. Stevens-Johnson syndrome (SJS) and toxic epidermal necrolysis (TEN).

Source: By James Heilman, MD - Own work, CC BY-SA 3.0, https://commons.wikimedia.org/w/index.php?curid=14772523

Understanding this pathophysiological difference plays a key role in the modulation of therapeutic strategies including immunosuppressive therapy, which bears very little resemblance to the antimicrobial and surgical treatments necessary for necrotizing fasciitis. Combining multi-disciplinary knowledge, backed by comprehensive patient assessment procedures, maximizes diagnostic precision and streamlines management models of these overlapping cutaneous disasters (Adaskevich, 2016) (Figure 15.4).

15.2.2. Etiology and Associated Medications

The etiology of severe cutaneous emergency conditions frequently entails complex interactions between environmental and immunologic factors, requiring meticulous examination of possible etiologic agents. SJS and TEN, as a case in point, occur predominantly as idiosyncratic drug reactions, indicating the pivotal role played by specific pharmacologic agents in initiating these near-fatal states. Sulfonamide antibiotics, antiepileptics like carbamazepine and phenytoin, and nonsteroidal anti-inflammatory drugs (NSAIDs) are well-documented to have associations with these syndromes. The underlying immunologic process is usually a T-cell-mediated cytotoxic reaction against drug-related antigen-expressing keratinocytes leading to extensive epidermal necrosis. The identification of the causative drug is mandatory since prompt discontinuation is essential to prevent further progression of disease. This complex interaction between drug exposure and immune system response emphasizes the importance of clinicians exercising caution with the use of known high-risk medications to avoid abrupt dermatologic crises. Besides drug-induced immunologic responses, erythroderma covers a wider etiologic spectrum with the involvement of both primary dermatologic disorders and systemic diseases. Frequent precipitants are exacerbations of existing dermatoses like psoriasis and atopic dermatitis (AD), drug hypersensitivity reactions, and even neoplasia is like cutaneous T-cell lymphoma. Drugs involved in erythroderma tend to overlap with those involved in SJS/TEN, most notably anticonvulsants and antibiotics, which solidifies the role of pharmacologic agents as an important etiologic factor. In contrast to the largely immune-cytotoxic pathophysiology of SJS/TEN, erythroderma's pathology often includes generalized inflammation and disruption of skin barrier function, resulting in diffuse erythema and scaling. Identifying drug-related etiologies continues to be crucial to successful management because the removal of the offending agent often prompts clinical improvement. Therefore, complete medication histories and familiarity with inciting drug suspects are cornerstones to the treatment of erythroderma and preventing its progression to more aggressive outcomes (Adaskevich, 2016). Necrotizing fasciitis, although largely infectious in etiology, also shows multifactorial etiology affected by comorbidities of the patient and sometimes by drugs that alter immune function.

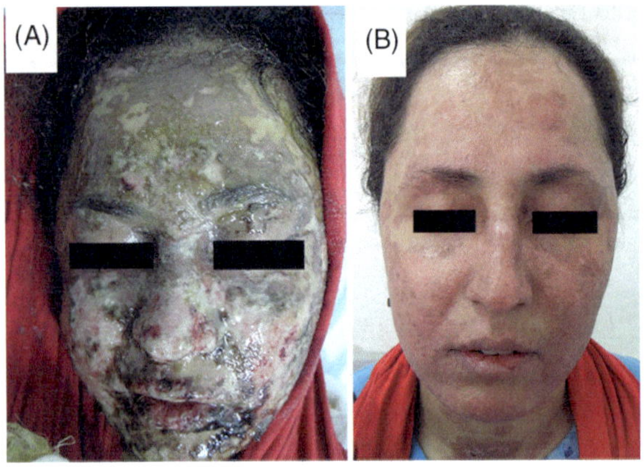

Figure 15.5. A case of toxic epidermal necrolysis (TEN). (A) Before treatment; and (B) Excellent improvement after symptomatic treatment only.

Source: Aboutaleb, D. A. E., El-Sayed, A. M., Ghabesha, A. A., & Hassan, S. B. (2020). *Severe Cutaneous Adverse Drug Reactions: Incidence, Clinical Patterns, Causative Drugs and Modalities of Treatment in Assiut University Hospital, Upper Egypt*. Dermatologic Therapy.

This rapidly advancing soft tissue infection usually occurs due to polymicrobial invasion, such as group A Streptococcus, anaerobes, and Gram-negative rods, gaining entry through breaks in the integrity of the skin. Immunosuppressive therapy, including corticosteroids or chemotherapy agents, can make patients susceptible to invasive infections by suppressing host defense. Further, more recent surgery or trauma providing portals for bacterial invasion complicates susceptibility. While treatment continues to center around antibiotics, the prior use of certain medications potentially compromises by interfering with immune response or masking clinical early signs. An understanding of this complex etiology highlighting microbial agents and medication effects informs therapeutic interventions correctly and averts death in necrotizing fasciitis (Barrera et al., 2011) (Figure 15.5).

15.2.3. Clinical Features and Progression of the Disease

The development of SJS and TEN usually starts with nonspecific prodromal symptoms like fever, malaise, and sore throat, which may precede the typical mucocutaneous presentation. Painful erythematous macules early on progress rapidly to blistering, with extensive epidermal detachment, having a similar appearance to widespread burns. These dermatologic emergencies involve the skin and various mucosal surfaces like oral, ocular, and genital mucosa, causing extreme pain and secondary complications. Histopathologically, features like necrotic keratinocytes and lymphocytic exocytosis have been described to be significantly evident in severe cutaneous adverse reactions in contrast to milder variants like maculopapular exanthema. High serum granulysin concentrations, particularly among SJS/TEN patients, are positively correlated with the severity of the disease, pointing towards its utility as a biomarker for monitoring disease progress (Jacquline et al., 2018). Such molecular markers offer insights into immunopathogenesis and can possibly direct therapeutic interventions at the appropriate time. The clinical course of erythroderma is characterized by generalized erythema and scaling of more than 90% BSA, leading to severe systemic consequences. First, patients have localized dermatitis, which quickly progresses to generalized erythema, significant edema, and desquamation. This widespread dermal investment interferes with the barrier function of the skin, making patients vulnerable to electrolyte disturbances, infections, and thermoregulatory disturbances. Although erythroderma can have multiple etiologies, such as underlying dermatoses, drug eruptions, or malignancies, its progressive nature necessitates early identification and treatment to prevent morbidity. Clinical findings usually show the involvement of particular anatomical locations, including scrotum and labium majora, typical of nonvenereal dermatoses of the genitalia, highlighting the need to rule out infectious etiologies to prevent misdiagnosis (Maalik et al., 2015). Prompt dermatologic evaluation is necessary because of the possible systemic effects. Necrotizing fasciitis is characterized by destructive soft tissue infection with a significant impact on deeper subcutaneous tissues and fascial planes. The illness classically progresses with disproportionate, severe pain in the absence of overt cutaneous evidence early in the process, succeeded by fast-progressive edema, erythema, and necrosis of the skin. Systemic toxicity is frequent and presents as hypotension, fever, and multi-organ failure, frequently requiring immediate surgical intervention. Clinically, fulminant development of necrotizing fasciitis mimics other cutaneous emergencies but must be rapidly differentiated due to its unique pathophysiologic process and the urgency of treatment. Unlike presentations of the same in erythroderma or SJS/TEN where epidermal detachment is dominant, necrotizing fasciitis is characterized by widespread fascia destruction, and it requires multidisciplinary interventions. These clinical features and stages across dermatologic emergencies are important to understand to maximize timely diagnosis and enhance patient outcomes.

15.3. Erythroderma

The demonstration of widespread skin involvement in acute dermatologic emergencies usually makes it difficult for clinicians to arrive at a clinical diagnosis and management, requiring immediate attention to clinical features differentiating such severe conditions from each other. Erythroderma by virtue of generalized erythema and scaling involving more than 90 % of the BSA is an acute dermatologic emergency because it has the potential for systemic complications like fluid imbalance, thermoregulatory abnormality, and secondary infection. In contrast to SJS and TEN, which are mainly characterized by epidermal detachment and mucous membrane involvement, erythroderma most often develops from flare-ups of pre-existing dermatoses, drug reactions, or malignancies.

Early recognition is crucial because it is related to severe morbidity and mortality and should be evaluated with thorough assessment encompassing patient history, laboratory examination, and skin biopsy if needed to rule out other blistering disorders. Prompt stabilization of the patient's systemic status, in combination with targeted dermatologic treatment, is critical in avoiding progression and secondary complications (Alsudairy et al., 2023). In treating erythroderma, clinical intervention needs to go beyond dermatologic symptoms to include the systemic sequelae resulting from the compromised skin barrier. Excessive inflammation and exfoliation result in elevated insensible water loss, severe protein loss, and increased susceptibility to infection, which add to patient morbidity. Thus, supportive care in the form of fluid and electrolyte repletion, temperature control, and nutrition, similar to burn care, is highlighted in the guidelines for treatment. Elimination of the causative factor, as may be achieved by withdrawal of a culprit drug or management of underlying dermatoses such as psoriasis or AD, is key to clinical resolution. In addition, the approach to erythroderma frequently involves interdisciplinary coordination, such as dermatology, infectious disease, and critical care consultation, to achieve the best outcomes. This integrated approach highlights the importance of early diagnosis and intervention in erythroderma as a cutaneous emergency (Alsudairy et al., 2023). In spite of an improved understanding and management, erythroderma continues to pose challenges in clinical practice because of its variability and threat of quick deterioration if not adequately treated. Differentiation of erythroderma from other conditions with similar symptoms such as SJS/TEN and necrotizing fasciitis is paramount since therapeutic managements and prognoses are vastly different. Current research emphasizes the importance of thorough musculoskeletal and systemic assessments when erythroderma develops in patients with rheumatologic diseases, recognizing that systemic inflammation can worsen skin disease and complicate management. Further investigation into biomarkers and new therapeutics is required to further improve diagnostic specificity and patient outcomes. The combination of early supportive management with specific interventions continues to be the mainstay of managing erythroderma within the overall context of dermatological emergencies (Figure 15.6).

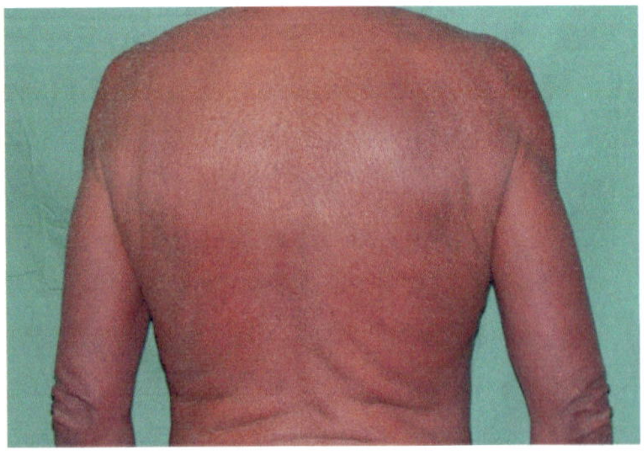

Figure 15.6. Erythroderma.

Source: The Dermatology Specialists. (2013). *Erythroderma.* https://www.thedermspecs.com/wp-content/uploads/2013/04/Erythroderma.png.

15.3.1. Definition and Classification of Erythroderma

The complexity of dermatologic emergencies warrants a clear comprehension of conditions that present with extensive skin involvement, one of them being erythroderma. Frequently characterized by diffuse erythema and scaling, erythroderma is a severe cutaneous reaction that involves over 90% of the BSA. In contrast to more focal dermatoses, its systemic effects are significant and include fluid and electrolyte imbalance as well as susceptibility to infections. Because of its widespread skin presentation, erythroderma needs prompt clinical identification and treatment different from other dermatologic emergencies such as SJS or TEN, which are mainly characterized by epidermal detachment. Knowledge about erythroderma's definition in the larger scheme of dermatologic emergencies enables clinicians to order differential diagnoses based on importance and appropriate intervention, emphasizing the unique pathophysiology in contrast to necrotizing fasciitis and other dermatological conditions (Adaskevich, 2016). The etiology-based classification of erythroderma determines the therapeutic approach and prognostication. Erythroderma is generally divided into primary and secondary forms. Primary erythroderma is the manifestation of underlying dermatoses like psoriasis, AD, or cutaneous T-cell lymphoma, indicating chronic skin disease exacerbations. Secondary erythroderma is usually drug-related and is caused by systemic drugs or toxins. Infectious and idiopathic forms also aid in the classification scheme. This etiologic stratification is important because not only does it affect the management of the patient but also decides on possible systemic complications related to the etiology. In addition, the classification helps in distinguishing erythroderma from other conditions of severe cutaneous reactions such as SJS/TEN, which are essentially immunologically mediated hypersensitivity phenomena and not chronic inflammatory conditions (Barrera et al., 2011). Clinically, erythroderma represents a dermatologic emergency due to its systemic sequelae, but its heterogeneous nature demands a nuanced approach to classification and treatment. Recognizing the extent and source of erythroderma is essential, as its presentation frequently overlaps with other dermatologic crises, complicating immediate diagnosis. The condition's classification hinges on a multidisciplinary evaluation that may include biopsy, serologic tests, and a comprehensive drug history. Such comprehensive evaluation distinguishes erythroderma from other syndromes, allowing for targeted therapies and supportive care measures that treat both cutaneous harm and systemic risks. Here, erythroderma ranks with SJS, TEN, and necrotizing fasciitis as an acute condition in need of immediate intervention owing to the risk of life-threatening complications (Adaskevich, 2016).

15.3.2. Causes and Underlying Conditions

The precipitating factors for dermatologic emergencies like SJS and TEN are also multisegmental, frequently involving immune-mediated responses mainly triggered by drugs. Medications such as anticonvulsants, sulfonamides, and allopurinol are commonly involved, highlighting drug hypersensitivity as a key player in these adverse cutaneous drug reactions. Besides drugs, infections, particularly *Mycoplasma pneumoniae*, have been implicated as precipitating factors, particularly among children. Pathophysiology entails an abnormal immune reaction where cytotoxic T cells cause extensive keratinocyte apoptosis, resulting in massive epidermal detachment. Genetic susceptibility, especially specific HLA alleles, additionally regulates vulnerability, emphasizing a balance between environmental factors and host susceptibility. Elucidation of such causes is crucial in early detection and prevention to curtail the significant morbidity and mortality seen in SJS and TEN. Underlying systemic diseases have a key contributory role in the etiology of erythroderma, usually complicating the clinical course. Chronic dermatoses such as psoriasis and eczema can develop into erythroderma when triggered by infections, drug eruptions, or withdrawal of therapy. In addition, hematologic malignancies, such as cutaneous T-cell lymphoma, commonly present with erythroderma as a presenting feature, indicative of neoplastic infiltration of the skin. The generalized inflammation and epidermal hyperplasia lead to widespread disruption of the skin barrier, making patients susceptible to secondary infections and metabolic derangements. Immune dysregulation, most likely associated with cytokine imbalances, is the substrate for these events, making it important to carry out extensive diagnostic workup to determine underlying etiologies. The multifactorial pathogenesis of erythroderma requires an extensive management strategy that targets both primary etiologies as well as systemic involvement to enhance patient outcomes.

Causes	Frequency (%)
Psoriasis	11 (36.6)
Eczema	8 (26.7)
Drug-induced erythroderma	5 (16.7)
Colloidan baby	1 (3.3)
Pityriasis rubra pilaris	1 (3.3)
Idiopathic	4 (13.3)

Figure 15.7. Causes of erythroderma.

Source: Aboutaleb, D. A. E., El-Sayed, A. M., Ghabesha, A. A., & Hassan, S. B. (2020). *Severe Cutaneous Adverse Drug Reactions: Incidence, Clinical Patterns, Causative Drugs and Modalities of treatment in Assiut University Hospital, Upper Egypt*. Dermatologic Therapy.

Necrotizing fasciitis, an aggressive soft tissue infection, occurs primarily as a result of polymicrobial invasion secondary to trauma, surgery, or comorbid conditions like diabetes mellitus and immunosuppression. Infection results in extensive fascial and subcutaneous tissue necrosis due to bacterial exotoxins and an aggressive host inflammatory response. Although Group A Streptococcus is a major pathogen, anaerobic and facultative synergism usually complicates the infectious environment. Invasive infections illustrate how local predisposing factors, such as breaches in the skin, unite with systemic vulnerabilities, such as peripheral vascular disease, to increase risk. Pathogenesis is based on microvascular thrombosis and resulting tissue ischemia, amplifying tissue damage. Early recognition of these underlying conditions is essential, since delays in diagnosis greatly elevate mortality rates. Successful treatment relies on early surgical debridement and wide-spectrum antimicrobial therapy, with choice guided by the causative pathogens, underlining the complexity of this skin emergency (Adaskevich, 2016) (Figure 15.7).

15.3.3. Symptoms and Systemic Effects

The cutaneous manifestations of dermatologic emergencies tend to extend far beyond the superficial cutaneous lesions, involving a variety of systemic symptoms that have profound effects on outcomes in patients. For example, in SJS and TEN, patients most often have prodromal flu-like symptoms in the form of fever, malaise, and sore throat before the pathognomonic mucocutaneous erosions appear. These initial systemic signs of widespread immune stimulation are often followed by tender erythematous macules and massive epidermal detachment. Systemic involvement is not limited to the cutaneous system; mucosal surfaces such as the oral cavity, eyes, and genitalia may be involved and cause serious complications like conjunctivitis and respiratory insufficiency. These emergent signs require prompt identification and treatment, as the systemic immune response is responsible for the associated high morbidity and mortality (Jacquline et al., 2018). In erythroderma, a cutaneous emergency represented by diffuse erythema and scaling of the skin more than 90% of the BSA, systemic repercussions come from both the widespread cutaneous inflammation and from the physiological insult of skin barrier dysfunction. Patients usually present with symptoms of high fever, chills, lymphadenopathy, and hemodynamic instability signs, indicative of a systemic inflammatory response. The impaired skin barrier makes these patients susceptible to greater transepidermal water loss (TEWL), thermoregulatory incompetence, and secondary infection, which exacerbate the systemic complications. The metabolic needs also increase in response to the skin's increased turnover and inflammatory process, usually causing hypoproteinemia and nutritional impairment. Therefore, erythroderma is a multisystem condition that demands immediate multidisciplinary management for resolving cutaneous instability in conjunction with systemic derangements (Jacquline et al., 2018). Necrotizing fasciitis is characterized by rapidly evolving soft tissue destruction and systemic toxicity, reflecting the profound systemic consequences usually preponderant to the initial localized infection. Early symptoms involve severe pain out of proportion to apparent skin change, fever, tachycardia, and hypotension, precursors to incipient septic shock. The infection progresses rapidly along fascial planes, causing extensive tissue necrosis and intense inflammatory reactions that are capable of resulting in multi-organ failure. Systemic involvement is reflected by laboratory abnormalities such as leukocytosis, elevated C-reactive protein (CRP), and metabolic acidosis. Mortality rates are high if not treated by immediate surgical intervention and aggressive supportive therapy. This virulent character highlights the utmost importance of timely diagnosis and holistic treatment protocols targeting both cutaneous destruction and the systemic inflammatory cascade (Badia et al., 2020).

15.4. Necrotizing Fasciitis

It is important to appreciate the need for urgency of some dermatologic diseases within clinical practice, particularly where initial signs are insidious but may advance rapidly to life-threatening processes. Necrotizing fasciitis is an example of one such emergency described by a rapidly spreading infection that kills skin, fat, and tissue covering muscles. The early presentations may be mimicking benign cellulitis or soft tissue infections of minor nature, so they are prone to misdiagnosis. But the rapid course, frequently with excruciating pain out of proportion to physical findings, systemic toxicity signs, and discoloration of the skin, should prompt clinicians to a more profound, invasive process. Early recognition in primary care or emergency settings is crucial, as delays markedly escalate morbidity and mortality. Family doctors and emergency medicine specialists should therefore be able to differentiate necrotizing fasciitis from milder dermatologic disorders to make timely interventions (Alsudairy et al., 2023). Such watchfulness can be the difference between survival and devastating consequences. The pathophysiologic basis of necrotizing fasciitis is polymicrobial infection, most commonly by Group A Streptococcus, Staphylococcus aureus, and anaerobic bacteria, resulting in hypoperfusion and necrosis of tissue by exotoxin production and ischemia. Its clinical course may change over a matter of hours, with SIRS and multi-organ failure if left untreated. The diagnosis is dependent on a high degree of suspicion supplemented by the clinical picture and laboratory evidence like raised white blood cell count, hyponatremia, and lactic acidosis. Imaging techniques such as MRI or CT scans might be helpful in outlining fascial involvement, but surgical exploration is the diagnostic and therapeutic gold standard. Management requires emergent operative debridement in conjunction with broad-spectrum antibiotics and supportive critical care. Multidisciplinary coordinated care is necessary, and operative intervention is often required repeatedly, along with intensive monitoring of the patient, emphasizing the severity of this dermatologic emergency (Kellen et al., 2018). Among dermatologic emergencies, necrotizing fasciitis is unique because of its virulent nature and requirement for urgent intervention. Unlike more benign dermatologic conditions like SJS or erythroderma, necrotizing fasciitis presents a dilemma to clinicians by presenting first as less severe infections and thus holding off treatment. Education and awareness form an important foundation for healthcare providers to enhance early detection and intervention rates. Referral to specialist centers for surgical treatment and intensive care is frequently indicated. Moreover, technological improvement in wound management, reconstructive surgery, and adjuvant therapies such as IVIG has played a role in better outcomes but cannot supplant the need for early diagnosis. Necrotizing fasciitis is a serious juncture of dermatology and emergency medicine that stresses the need for prompt, firm action in saving life and limb (Alsudairy et al., 2023; Kellen et al., 2018) (Figure 15.8).

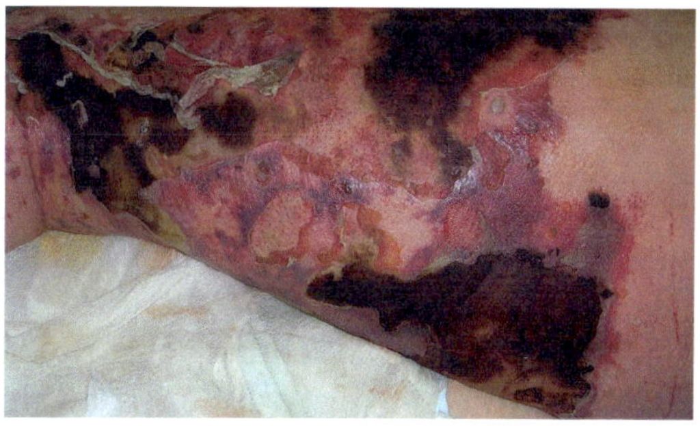

Figure 15.8. Person with necrotizing fasciitis. The left leg shows extensive redness and tissue death.

Source: Wikipedia contributors. (n.d.). *Necrotizing Fasciitis, Left Leg.* https://upload.wikimedia.org/wikipedia/commons/thumb/6/6a/Necrotizing_fasciitis_left_leg.JPEG/1024px-Necrotizing_fasciitis_left_leg.JPEG.

15.4.1. Definition and Types of Necrotizing Fasciitis

The dermatologic emergency spectrum includes a variety of severe conditions which require timely recognition and treatment. Of these, necrotizing fasciitis is a highly virulent soft tissue infection that involves accelerated destruction of subcutaneous tissue and fascial planes. Misdiagnosed in the initial presentation because of the nonspecific nature of the presenting symptoms, the condition progresses rapidly with resultant systemic toxicity and possible mortality if not treated promptly. Necrotizing fasciitis is clinically characterized by extensive necrosis of the fascia and overlying tissues, often with associated exquisite pain disproportionate to the extent of visible skin findings. An understanding of the pathophysiology and clinical presentation is important in distinguishing it from other dermatologic emergencies such as SJS or TEN, which are characterized mainly by epidermal detachment as opposed to deep tissue necrosis. These differences highlight the need to identify necrotizing fasciitis within the general rubric of skin emergencies in order to allow early surgical and medical intervention (Adaskevich, 2016). Necrotizing fasciitis is generally divided into several categories according to microbial etiology and clinical presentation. Type I, the most frequent, is a polymicrobial infection usually consisting of aerobic and anaerobic bacteria like Bacteroides species and Enterobacteriaceae that synergistically cause tissue damage. Type II is due to monomicrobial infections, most commonly group A Streptococcus, leading to expedited disease progression as well as systemic toxicity. Type III necrotizing fasciitis occurs less frequently with marine animals such as *Vibrio vulnificus*, whereas Type IV is fungal. Each category has its own particular difficulty concerning diagnosis and treatment, making it imperative that the underlying causative agents be known for directing antibiotic treatment in addition to surgical debridement. The distinction of these subtypes is paramount because of differences in clinical presentation, risk factors, and patient outcome, which underscore the importance of correct categorization in the emergency dermatologic context (Barrera et al., 2011). In practice, emergency clinicians must identify the varied presentations within necrotizing fasciitis in a multidisciplinary context that balances clinical suspicion with laboratory and imaging findings. Patients can first present with erythema, edema, and severe pain, commonly followed by systemic symptoms of fever and hypotension.

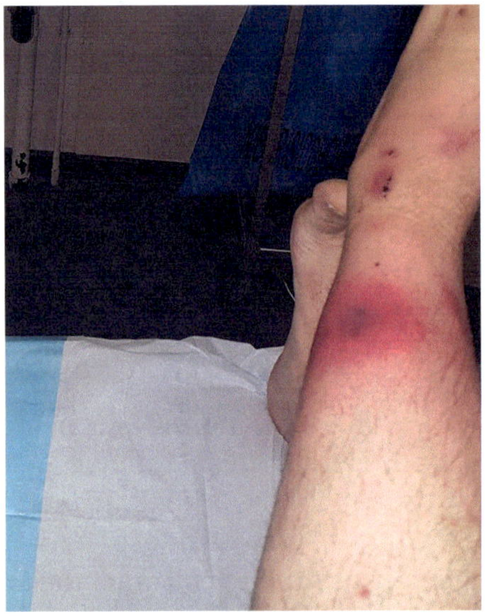

Figure 15.9. Early symptoms of necrotizing fasciitis. The darker red center is going black.

Source: Wikipedia contributors. (n.d.). *Early Symptoms of Necrotizing Fasciitis (NF)*. https://upload.wikimedia.org/wikipedia/commons/thumb/b/bd/Early_symptoms_of_NF.jpg/800px-Early_symptoms_of_NF.jpg.

The early development of skin discoloration, bullae, and necrosis is usually indicative of advanced disease and mandates urgent surgical consultation. Early laboratory markers such as a rising white blood cell count, CRP, and serum creatinine help to estimate severity but are not specific. Imaging modalities such as MRI and CT scans give clear information regarding the degree of fascial involvement, which helps in making therapeutic decisions. The addition of this integral diagnostic approach increases early identification and control of necrotizing fasciitis from other dermatological emergencies such as SJS, TEN, and erythroderma, which have other clinical and pathological presentations (Adaskevich, 2016) (Figure 15.9).

15.4.2. Risk Factors and Common Pathogens

The development of dermatologic emergencies is based on a variety of predisposing factors, frequently enhancing severity, and complicating the clinical course. Immunocompromised conditions, either resulting from HIV infection, malignancy, or iatrogenic immunosuppression through chemotherapy and immunosuppressive therapy, dramatically enhance vulnerability to serious cutaneous adverse reactions such as SJS and TEN. Genetic susceptibility, specifically particular human leukocyte antigen (HLA) alleles, has been associated with increased risk for such conditions after exposure to particular drugs, such as anticonvulsants, sulfonamides, and nonsteroidal anti-inflammatory agents. In addition, underlying systemic illness, like autoimmune disease, can augment cutaneous involvement via dysregulated immunity. Awareness of these risk factors allows clinicians to individualize prevention and early therapy to prevent further progression and death in these acute dermatologic syndromes. Necrotizing fasciitis, on the other hand, has a characteristic set of risk factors largely attributed to compromises in skin integrity and concurrent systemic susceptibilities. Trauma, surgical cutaneous lesions, or primary dermatologic processes offer portals of entry for bacteria that inhabit soft tissue planes. Diabetes mellitus, peripheral vascular disease, or chronic renal failure are conditions that have compromised immune protection and reduced tissue perfusion, setting the stage for uncontrolled spread of infection. The most common implicated pathogens are group A Streptococcus (*Streptococcus pyogenes*), Staphylococcus aureus, both methicillin-resistant and sensitive, and polymicrobial combinations featuring anaerobes and facultative bacteria. These pathogens commonly produce virulence factors that promote deep tissue necrosis and systemic toxicity, calling for emergent surgical and antimicrobial treatment. Knowledge of these risk factors provides early identification and aggressive treatment essential for lowering mortality rates for necrotizing fasciitis. Erythroderma, defined by extensive erythema and scaling covering over 90% of the BSA, frequently results from varied etiologies with particular pathogenic correlations. Exacerbations of preexistent dermatoses like psoriasis or AD, drug reactions, and malignancies such as cutaneous T-cell lymphoma are common precipitating causes. Infectious causes can also play a role, especially when secondary bacterial colonization or viral infections complicate the clinical scenario. Although Staphylococcus aureus commonly colonizes the erythrodermic skin to superinfect, the pathogenesis of this condition most often involves complicated immune dysregulation culminating in epidermal barrier disruption. Determination of these risk factors and the contribution of microbial pathogens is important in directing supportive therapy as well as specific antimicrobial treatment to ensure better outcomes in a condition that is often complicated by systemic involvement. (Adaskevich, 2016).

15.4.3. Clinical Signs and Urgency of Treatment

Early identification of clinical signs in dermatologic emergencies is paramount due to the risk of rapid systemic involvement and death. In disorders such as SJS and TEN, an early presentation may be flu-like with subsequent rapidly evolving painful eruption involving mucous membranes. The characteristic epidermal peeling and extensive erythema indicate widespread skin barrier compromise, threatening fluid loss and infection hazard that needs to be addressed urgently. Likewise, the ongoing fever, change in mental status, and hypotension in these patients suggests SIRS progression, calling for urgent intensive care intervention. Recognition of such early clinical signs is critical to ensure timely offending agent discontinuation, supportive management, and specialist consultation, highlighting the need for clinicians to have a high suspicion in high-risk patients (Adaskevich, 2016). Clinical manifestations like generalized erythema involving over 90% of body surface area and scaling and pruritus should be thoroughly evaluated in the management of erythroderma since this syndrome may evolve to life-threatening situations. The skin's basic functions, such as thermoregulation and barrier defense, are compromised in erythroderma, resulting in a heightened predisposition to infection, fluid, and electrolyte disturbances.

Treatments of the highest priority in urgent situations target the detection of underlying etiologies, ranging from drug reactions to malignancy, and onset of supportive treatments like fluid management, nutritional supplementation, and infection control. The high level of epidermal involvement in erythroderma requires close monitoring for systemic complications such as sepsis or heart failure, highlighting the high importance of early diagnosis and intervention (Adaskevich, 2016). Necrotizing fasciitis involves one of the most intense dermatologic emergencies, with clinical presentations usually initially mild but progressing very quickly to intense pain out of proportion with physical findings, erythema, edema, and skin and underlying fascial plane necrosis. Systemic signs such as fever, tachycardia, and hypotension portend severe sepsis or septic shock, which are treated with prompt surgical debridement along with broad-spectrum antibiotics.

The time window for effective treatment in necrotizing fasciitis is limited; delay significantly raises mortality. Prompt recognition is made difficult by the fact that initial presentation simulates cellulitis, emphasizing the need for diagnostic vigilance and aggressive intervention to avoid extensive tissue damage and multi-organ failure.

15.5. Diagnostic Approaches

Early recognition of dermatologic emergencies requires a subtle strategy integrating clinical acumen with quick assessment instruments. Patients who present in emergency departments usually have overlapping signs like extensive erythema, blistering, or necrosis, which can mask the diagnosis unless carefully defined. A detailed patient history, including recent drug exposure and antecedent infections, is a cornerstone of differentiating SJS and TEN from other acute dermatoses. For example, mucous membrane involvement and rapid epidermal detachment are characteristic features necessitating urgent diagnosis. Definitive histopathologic evidence by diagnostic skin biopsies, which are invasive, may show typical patterns like full-thickness necrosis of the epidermis of TEN. It is crucial that emergency and family physicians have a high index of suspicion to instigate early intervention since delay can hugely enhance morbidity and mortality in presentations such as SJS/TEN (Alsudairy et al., 2023). Concomitantly, erythroderma calls for a methodical diagnostic process because of its heterogeneous etiologies, including drug reactions to systemic diseases such as cutaneous T-cell lymphoma. Clinicians need to make differentiating erythroderma from the other causes of widespread inflammation of the skin a priority with thorough examination and focused laboratory workup. Blood studies, such as complete blood counts (CBCs) and inflammatory markers, aid in discerning systemic involvement, while skin biopsies uncover such fine points as lymphocytic infiltration, which can lead to specific diagnoses. The diagnostic process also gains from the inclusion of imaging tests in suspecting systemic complications, including malignancies and infections that are usually associated with widespread skin involvement. A multidisciplinary assessment due to the complexity of erythroderma guarantees that the underlying cause is correctly diagnosed and treated without delay (Adaskevich, 2016). Necrotizing fasciitis poses a clearly emergent diagnostic challenge due to the speed at which it progresses and its potentially fatal outcome.

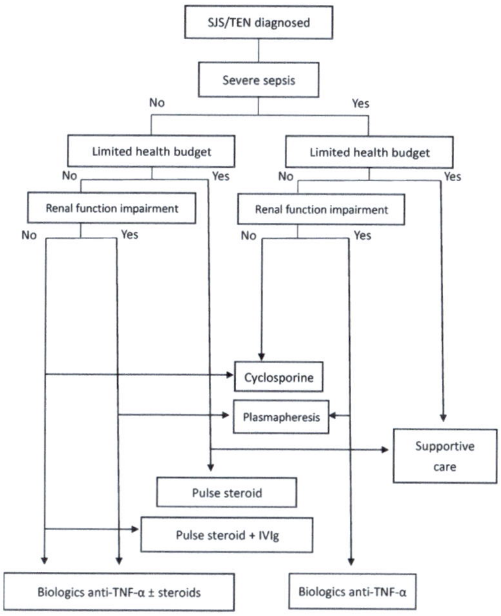

Figure 15.10. Algorithm for choosing systemic treatments for Stevens-Johnson syndrome (SJS) / toxic epidermal necrolysis (TEN).

Source: Chang, H. C., Wang, T. J., Lin, M. H., & Chen, T. J. (2022). A review of the systemic treatment of Stevens–Johnson syndrome and toxic epidermal necrolysis. *Biomedicines, 10*(9), 2105.

Early clinical suspicion is paramount, usually precipitated by disproportionate pain, swelling, erythema, and systemic symptoms like fever or sepsis. The diagnostic imaging of magnetic resonance imaging (MRI) and computed tomography (CT) aids early detection through delineation of involvement of the fascial plane, but final diagnosis rests upon surgical exploration. Laboratory markers, like increased white blood cell count and CRP levels, identify inflammatory activity but are nonspecific. Immediate biopsy and microbiological cultures direct targeted antimicrobial therapy and surgical debridement. Consultation of surgical and dermatology specialists creates a holistic diagnostic approach, maximizing patient outcomes in this high-risk emergency (Alsudairy et al., 2023) (Figure 15.10).

15.5.1. Clinical Evaluation and History Taking

Precise clinical assessment is the pillar in the approach to dermatologic emergencies like SJS, TEN, erythroderma, and necrotizing fasciitis. With the high morbidity and fast pace of these conditions, proper and systematic history and physical examination are the top priorities for clinicians. Determination of the development and evolution of the symptoms, recent drug use, infections, or systemic symptoms may direct early diagnosis and intervention. Specifically, a thorough question about recent drug use is essential because some medications are commonly incriminated as causative agents for SJS and TEN. Concurrently, the assessment should be directed toward systemic evidence of sepsis and multi-organ disease, which frequently accompany these catastrophic skin diseases. This general clinical context enables professionals to differentiate from these emergencies other dermatologic or systemic diseases that can simulate their presentations, hence enabling timely and proper management. In history taking, a full review of the patient's medical history including previous dermatologic illness, immune status, and co-occurring diseases is unavoidable. For instance, erythroderma can occur secondary to underlying dermatoses or hematologic malignancies, and hence recognizing these associations both influences diagnosis as well as therapeutic approaches. Precise attention to the chronology of symptoms, for instance, the rate of progression of skin detachment, distribution of lesions, and mucosal involvement, can further narrow the differential diagnosis. Systemic symptoms such as fever, malaise, and respiratory distress should also be noted by the clinician to detect potential complications. Securing a precise drug history and recent infection record is crucial because increasingly, the evidence points toward an underlying drug-induced hypersensitivity reaction as the cause of many dermatologic emergencies such as SJS and TEN. Furthermore, evaluation for possible risk factors like genetic tendencies or underlying immunosuppression raises clinical suspicion and directs investigations further. Physical examination augments history taking in that it captures vital visual and palpable details regarding the nature and severity of cutaneous involvement. Essential clinical findings such as epidermal detachment, Nikolsky sign, and detection of necrotic tissue assist in confirming diagnoses and impact immediate management choices. In necrotizing fasciitis, detection of signs including out-of-proportion pain, edema, and erythema with progressive progression can lead to immediate surgical intervention. Complete systemic examination is also crucial to assess airway patency, hydration, and organ function since these conditions are often multisystem in their impact. Such thorough evaluation calls for a multidisciplinary method and integration of clinical competencies, emphasizing the need for specific examination methods outlined in rheumatology and dermatology literature (Adaskevich, 2016). Therefore, merging in-depth history-taking with targeted physical assessment is the foundation for proper diagnosis and successful treatment planning in dermatologic emergencies.

15.5.2. Laboratory Tests and Imaging Studies

The diagnostic process for severe dermatologic emergencies such as SJS and TEN relies heavily on targeted laboratory tests to confirm clinical suspicions and assess systemic involvement. Initial evaluations typically include CBCs to detect leukocytosis or anemia, which may indicate infection or systemic inflammation. Serum electrolyte panels are vital to identify imbalances caused by fluid losses through extensive skin denudation. Liver and renal function tests are also regularly checked since the organs often undergo secondary insult as a result of the extensive system involvement present in such conditions. Skin biopsies, even though not laboratory investigations in themselves, yield histopathological evidence, showing necrotic keratinocytes and subepidermal bullae typical of SJS/TEN and hence lead to precise diagnosis and planning of treatment. In erythroderma, extensive laboratory tests are essential in distinguishing the condition from other dermatological as well as systemic disorders. With erythroderma's multi-etiology involving drug reactions, malignancies, or flare of underlying dermatoses, laboratory tests aim to evaluate the overall systemic condition and etiology of the patient. CBC may demonstrate anemia or eosinophilia, which is helpful in favoring an allergic or neoplastic cause. Inflammatory parameters like erythrocyte sedimentation rate (ESR) and CRP are performed to assess the extent of systemic inflammation. Liver function tests and kidney function tests screen for organ failure commonly seen in severe erythroderma. These tests guide the urgency and manner of intervention, enabling clinicians to customize therapies for the best outcomes of their patients. Necrotizing fasciitis is a surgical urgency necessitating immediate imaging studies to augment clinical assessment for early diagnosis and treatment. Although laboratory studies like white blood cell count elevation and CRP are markers of the severity of infection, imaging studies offer essential anatomic information. Ultrasound is useful in rapidly detecting fluid or gas in soft tissues indicative of the necrotic process. CT scans provide images of greater resolution, defining fascial plane engagement and degree of tissue destruction, thus informing surgical debridement planning. MRI is particularly useful in uncertain cases because of its excellent soft tissue differentiation. Combined, these laboratory and imaging strategies provide timely, precise necrotizing fasciitis diagnosis, enhancing the chances of successful therapy and survival (Adaskevich, 2016) (Figure 15.11).

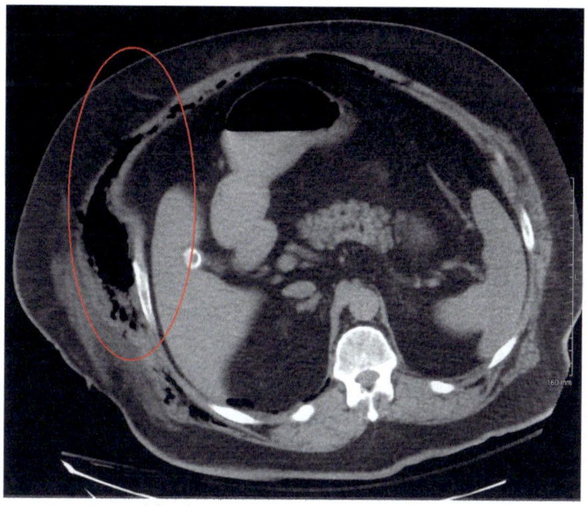

Figure 15.11. Necrotizing fasciitis producing gas in the soft tissues as seen on a CT scan.

Source: Wikipedia contributors. (n.d.). *CT Scan Showing Necrotising Fasciitis with Gas in Soft Tissues.* https://upload.wikimedia.org/wikipedia/commons/thumb/f/fb/Pnecrotisingfasc.png/800px-Pnecrotisingfasc.png.

15.5.3. Differential Diagnosis Considerations

Appropriate evaluation in dermatologic emergencies involves differentiation among conditions sharing overlapping clinical presentations. For example, SJS and TEN are both characterized by mucocutaneous blistering and epidermal detachment, but the degree of skin involvement and systemic features dictate differentiation. Equally valuable is discrimination from extreme drug reactions like erythroderma, which shares broad erythema and scaling but generally does not have the necrotic detachment of the epidermis seen in SJS/TEN. The inability to accurately identify the pathology may result in a delay of important interventions, highlighting the importance of careful clinical evaluation in conjunction with histopathological diagnosis whenever possible. Differential diagnosis, thus, depends on relating clinical presentation to patient history in the form of recent drug exposure, infection, or underlying systemic diseases to allow for appropriate management strategies. Differentiating necrotizing fasciitis from other cutaneous emergencies poses added challenges because of its aggressive soft tissue destruction and speedy course. In contrast to SJS, TEN, or erythroderma, necrotizing fasciitis involves mainly deeper fascial planes and subcutaneous tissue, usually preceded by out-of-proportion pain and systemic toxicity. Presenting signs can mimic cellulitis or acute soft tissue infection, making early recognition difficult. Imaging studies like MRI or CT may reinforce suspicion with evidence of gas in soft tissues or fascial swelling, but definitive diagnosis depends on surgical exploration and tissue biopsy. Differentiation is important because necrotizing fasciitis requires emergent surgical debridement with concomitant broad-spectrum antibiotics compared to the largely supportive or immunomodulatory treatments used in SJS, TEN, or erythroderma (Adaskevich, 2016). Interdisciplinary evaluation improves diagnostic accuracy, particularly in cases that are unclear. Mimicking conditions should be considered, as autoimmune blistering diseases, severe cutaneous adverse reactions, and infectious causes can mimic the presentation of SJS, TEN, erythroderma, or necrotizing fasciitis. For instance, pemphigus vulgaris and bullous pemphigoid are characterized by blistering and erosions but generally have more chronic courses and characteristic immunopathologic features. SSSS likewise can cause epidermal peeling that mimics SJS/TEN but tends to preferentially involve infants and young children and tends to spare mucous membranes. Erythroderma requires exclusion of underlying exacerbated dermatoses such as psoriasis or cutaneous lymphoma, which determine treatment. Multidisciplinary diagnostic approach, including dermatopathology, microbiology, and laboratory markers, is still essential to precisely distinguish among these entities and maximize patient outcomes (Barrera et al., 2011).

15.6. Treatment Strategies

Proper management of cutaneous emergencies like SJS and TEN requires prompt identification and supportive treatment to prevent morbidity and mortality. Stabilization is generally achieved with fluid resuscitation and wound management similar to burns, with a focus on avoiding secondary infection and maintaining electrolytes. Withdrawal of suspected offending agents is critical, as these conditions most commonly arise from drug reactions. Adjunct treatments, such as systemic corticosteroids and IVIGs, are also contentious but used in certain clinical environments to alter the immune response. Multidisciplinary coordination between dermatology, intensive care, and infectious disease specialists improves treatment results. Early intervention and individualized supportive interventions are paramount, underlining the importance of rapid diagnosis and appropriate referral patterns in primary care, as the syndromes progress rapidly and have the potential for systemic involvement (Alsudairy et al., 2023). Necrotizing fasciitis necessitates an aggressive, multi-modal treatment regimen because of its rapid progression and high mortality rate. Surgical removal of dead tissue by debridement is the foundation of therapy and should be done urgently to stop infection from spreading. Empirical broad-spectrum intravenous antibiotics are started before targeted therapy after culture results, treating polymicrobial infection typical of the disease. Supportive therapy in an intensive care unit is directed at hemodynamic stabilization, pain management, and treatment of sepsis or organ dysfunction. Adjunctive treatments, such as hyperbaric oxygen therapy, have been investigated but are still adjunctive and not primary treatments. Prompt diagnosis and treatment starting from the primary care level can impact prognosis significantly, emphasizing the awareness of family physicians regarding dermatological emergencies (Alsudairy et al., 2023). Erythroderma poses specific challenges in treatment that focus on the identification and control of underlying causes, which are usually aggravations of pre-existing dermatoses, infections, or drug reactions. Supportive therapy seeks to reestablish skin barrier integrity and control symptoms like pruritus, desquamation, and fluid imbalance. Hospitalization in severe cases may be required to maximize monitoring and apply systemic therapies such as corticosteroids or immunosuppressants after establishing the etiology. Due to the wide range of clinical presentations and potentially life-threatening complications like thermoregulatory instability or secondary infection, proper diagnosis followed by directed treatment is crucial. Family physicians and dermatologists need to work together to follow guidelines and provide continuity of care, ultimately leading to better outcomes in this at-risk population (Alsudairy et al., 2023).

15.6.1. General Management Principles for Dermatologic Emergencies

Management of dermatologic emergencies must be approached from various directions, but above all, prioritizing the quick diagnosis and stabilization of the patient's condition. The initial assessment must involve the airway, breathing, and circulation since, in the course of severe skin diseases such as SJS and TEN, common complications include sepsis, acute respiratory distress, or fluid imbalance. Prompt recognition of the precipitant, typically drug-related, and removal of causative agents are essential to avoid aggravation of the course. Supportive management is a key intervention, above all the correction of fluid and electrolytes, the prevention of infection, and preservation of skin integrity through wound management similar to that applied in burns. Multidisciplinary team involvement with input from dermatologists, intensivists, and infectious disease specialists optimizes outcomes through the provision of holistic care that envisions and manages systemic complications that are commonly part of these disorders (Adaskevich, 2016). Having stabilized the acute episode, attention is then devoted to individualized therapeutic strategies designed to modulate the underlying inflammatory or infectious processes unique to each dermatologic emergency. In situations such as necrotizing fasciitis, surgical debridement with aggressive resection and broad-spectrum intravenous antibiotics are critical to stop advancing tissue destruction and systemic toxicity. In erythroderma, however, careful assessment of the inciting cause—drug-related, infectious, or malignancy-associated, is the determinant for treatment options such as corticosteroids or immunosuppressive agents. Intensive monitoring for complications like secondary infection, metabolic derangement, and organ system failure is critical throughout the course of treatment. Treatment strategies highlight close attention to nutritional care and pain control, their essential influence on healing and patient comfort (BARRERA ET AL., 2011). Beyond clinical care, useful general principles highlight early communication and recording, patient teaching, and psychosocial intervention, since dermatologic emergencies cause excessive distress and long-term sequelae. Drawing sharp lines of communication between healthcare providers guarantees up-to-date information and care coordination, which can be critical in rapidly advancing diseases such as SJS/TEN and necrotizing fasciitis. Recording medication history, clinical data, and treatment outcomes makes it possible to continually monitor and implement secondary prevention measures. In addition, patient and family education regarding disease prognosis, possible complications, and signs of recurrence is important for optimizing prognosis and follow-up compliance. The incorporation of psychological support services also responds to the emotional trauma that follows visible skin loss and disfigurement, highlighting the comprehensive nature of dermatologic emergency management (Adaskevich, 2016).

15.6.2. Specific Treatments for Stevens-Johnson Syndrome (SJS) and Toxic Epidermal Necrolysis (TEN)

The treatment of SJS and TEN constitutes a multi-component strategy with the goal of stopping disease advancement while maintaining the functions of essential organs. Immediate treatments focus on the instantaneous withdrawal of the causative drug, which is critical in order not to perpetuate epidermal destruction. Supportive care is the mainstay, frequently requiring hospitalization in intensive care or specialized burn units for extensive loss of skin. Fluid resuscitation, electrolyte management, and prevention of infection are emphasized to restore homeostasis and minimize the risk of mortality. Wound management tactics employ practices similar to those in burn treatment, using non-adherent dressings and careful monitoring to avoid secondary infection. Pain management and nutrition further have an impact on the patient outcome, ensuring a total therapeutic program individualized according to patient requirements and the extent of the epidermal separation. These foundational measures set the stage for adjunctive therapies aimed at modifying the immune response. Emerging treatment modalities focus on immunomodulation to mitigate the intense inflammatory cascade characteristic of SJS and TEN. Systemic corticosteroids have been traditionally employed due to their potent anti-inflammatory effects. However, their usage remains controversial, given conflicting evidence surrounding efficacy and risks of infection. IVIG therapy is another adjunct, acting by neutralization of Fas ligand-induced keratinocyte apoptosis, which is central to disease pathology. In addition to some reports implying benefits in preventing epidermal detachment and speeding recovery, inconsistencies in clinical trial findings have prevented universal acceptance. Other immunosuppressants, including cyclosporine, look promising by inhibiting T-cell mediated cytotoxicity and possibly lowering mortality rates. Nevertheless, no individual immunotherapy has established clear superiority unequivocally and therefore calls for personalized choice within multidisciplinary treatment platforms. Current discoveries regarding immune-mediated toxicities due to cancer treatment provide insight directly applicable to the management of SJS and TEN. Immune checkpoint inhibitors (ICIs), in transforming oncologic therapy, also can cause emergent dermatologic immune-related adverse events mimicking or enhancing existing conditions such as SJS/TEN. The dynamic pharmacovigilance evidence stresses the importance of timely detection and intervention to prevent these complications (Raschi et al., 2020; Long et al., 2020). This shift highlights the general principle that immune system modulation can be a double-edged sword that needs to be carefully balanced. Learning from immune-oncology directs future possibilities, such as targeted biological therapies against selected inflammatory mediators participating in epidermal necrolysis. These precision medicine strategies could enhance therapy by blunting detrimental immune activation and maintaining important host defenses and, ultimately, improve the management of these catastrophic dermatologic emergencies.

15.6.3. Management of Erythroderma and Necrotizing Fasciitis

Successful management of erythroderma requires an immediate and thorough diagnostic workup since the condition tends to portend a systemic or dermatologic underlying pathology. Clinicians will need first to stabilize the patient by resuscitating fluid and electrolyte deficits, considering the large-surface skin involvement that predisposes to TEWL as well as to infection. Supportive care is characterized by careful observation for evidence of secondary infections, which may progress to septicemia, particularly in patients with predisposing comorbid conditions like diabetes mellitus and anemia. The therapeutic approach is usually centered on the identification and withdrawal of any causative agents, especially in drug-induced scenarios, alongside the use of systemic corticosteroids or immunosuppressants based on the underlying etiology. Multidisciplinary care that includes dermatology, infectious disease, and critical care improves outcomes because specialized units are better equipped to handle the complexity of this potentially deadly emergency (Skayem et al., 2024). Having this coordinated approach is important, considering the propensity of erythroderma to result in extensive skin barrier disruption, which requires scrupulous infection control watchfulness (Pătrașcu et al., 2024). Necrotizing fasciitis, an aggressive soft tissue infection, necessitates prompt identification and treatment to minimize mortality. Treatment focuses on early aggressive surgical debridement of dead tissue along with empirical broad-spectrum antibiotic therapy to cover polymicrobial pathogens such as Staphylococcus aureus, Pseudomonas aeruginosa, and Gram-negative bacilli. Advanced diagnosis depends frequently on the accumulation of clinical manifestations such as extreme pain that is not proportionate to physical examination findings, systemic toxicity, and spreading erythema and edema. Adjunctive therapy involves hemodynamic intervention and vigilant monitoring for septic shock. Comorbid conditions such as chronic heart failure or immune suppression can be potent disease accelerators, making individualized care plans essential. Multimodal therapy also incorporates wound care principles and may find advantages in hyperbaric oxygen, though this is adjunctive. The immediacy of surgical treatment, along with aggressive antimicrobial and supportive therapy, forms the foundation of successful necrotizing fasciitis treatment (Adriana-Ionela et al., 2024; Skayem et al., 2024). Erythroderma and necrotizing fasciitis both highlight the critical importance of dermatologic emergency skills enabled by organized healthcare networks and advanced care delivery systems. Teledermatology services, specifically urgent store-and-forward programs, have become instrumental in maximizing patient triage and allowing expedient expert consultation without the necessity for face-to-face referrals to specialized dermatologic emergency facilities. Such a model has been efficacious in the management of critical cutaneous emergencies, such as erythroderma and necrotizing fasciitis, through prompt diagnosis and initiation of treatment. In addition, these telemedicine sites promote the preservation of scarce healthcare resources as well as the reduction of avoidable hospital consultations, especially during periods of increased patient flow and limited manpower (Skayem et al., 2024) (Figure 15.12).

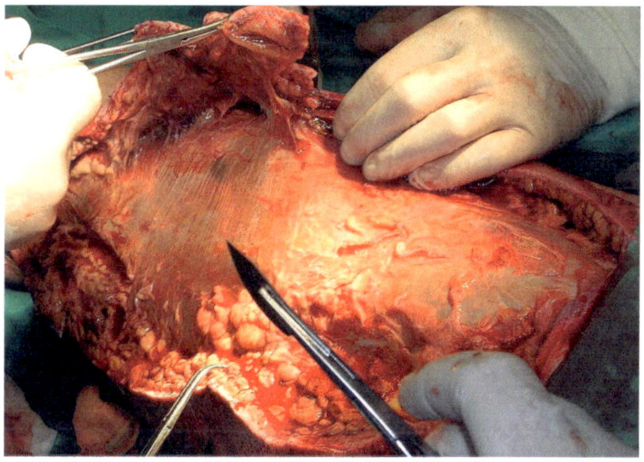

Figure 15.12. Necrotic tissue from the left leg surgically removed.

Source: Wikipedia contributors. (n.d.). *Surgical Debridement of Necrotizing Fasciitis in the Left Leg.* https://upload.wikimedia.org/wikipedia/commons/thumb/7/73/Necrotizing_fasciitis_left_leg_debridement.JPEG/1024px-Necrotizing_fasciitis_left_leg_debridement.JPEG.

CLOSER LOOK

ACUTE MUCOCUTANEOUS NECROSIS

Acute mucocutaneous necrosis, including SJS and TEN, is a serious, life-threatening illness that is caused by extensive skin and mucous membrane destruction, usually induced by drugs. The disease includes epidermal necrosis, separation of the skin, and painful mucous membrane erosions, especially in the mouth, eyes, and genitals.

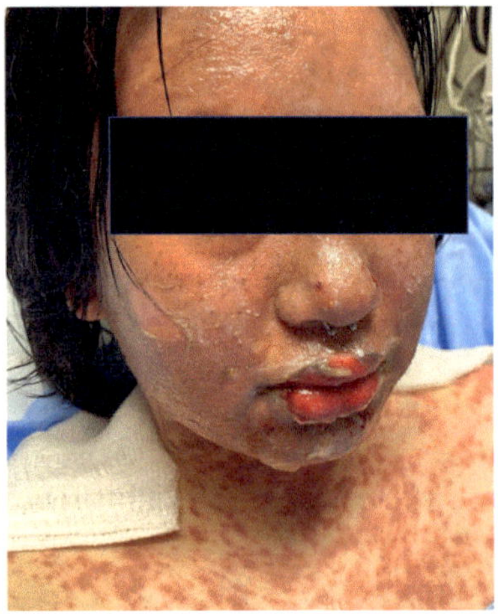

Source: Frantz R, Huang S, Are A, Motaparthi K. Stevens–Johnson Syndrome and Toxic Epidermal Necrolysis: A Review of Diagnosis and Management. *Medicina*. 2021; 57(9):895. https://doi.org/10.3390/medicina57090895

Key Features of Acute Mucocutaneous Necrosis

- **Causes:** Although SJS/TEN may be idiopathic, they are most often drug-induced, with anticonvulsants, NSAIDs, and sulfonamides being common offenders. Infections also precipitate the condition.
- **Symptoms:**
  - **Prodrome:** Prodromal symptoms are fever, upper respiratory tract symptoms (rhinitis, cough), and conjunctivitis.
  - **Skin Lesions:** Erythematous macules, dusky and tender, break out and extend rapidly to form flaccid blisters and sheet-like epidermal detachment.
  - **Mucosal Involvement:** Profound erosions and ulcerations of oral, ocular, and genital mucous membranes are frequent, inducing pain and discomfort with eating, swallowing, and vision.
- **Epidermal Detachment:** Epidermal detachment is the hallmark of SJS/TEN and may be an inapparent feature in SJS (less than 10% of BSA) and a prominent feature in TEN (more than 30% of BSA).

- o **Overlap:** There is a range of severity between SJS and TEN, with an overlap (10–29% epidermal detachment) being a specific diagnostic entity.
- o **Complications:** SJS/TEN may have severe complications involving infections, fluid and electrolyte disturbances, and renal and respiratory distress.
- o **Histopathology:** Histopathologically, SJS/TEN is characterized by complete-thickness keratinocyte necrosis, with subepidermal vesiculation in later stages.

Ø **Diagnosis**

- Clinical diagnosis is mainly based on typical skin and mucosal lesions, and a history of putative causative exposures.
- Histopathology can be supportive, but clinical findings are usually sufficient for diagnosis.

Ø **Treatment**

- Supportive Care: The major treatment emphasis is on supportive care, such as wound care, fluid and electrolyte balance, nutritional support, and pain control.
- Pharmacologic Management: Multiple drugs, such as IVIGs, systemic corticosteroids, and other immunomodulators, are utilized to regulate the immune response and decrease inflammation, but their effectiveness is controversial.
- Early Treatment and Diagnosis: Early detection and timely intervention are important to enhance patient outcomes.

SUMMARY

The intricacies associated with the treatment of dermatologic emergencies like SJS, TEN, erythroderma, and necrotizing fasciitis necessitate multidisciplinary management for maximal benefit for the patient. These emergencies present with commonalities in clinical presentation that may pose a hindrance to early diagnosis and treatment, necessitating timely identification. Emergency physicians and primary care physicians have an important role to play in the early recognition of subtle dermatologic signs before they advance to life-threatening phases. The use of evidence-based treatment algorithms and supportive care interventions profoundly impacts survival and late morbidity. Furthermore, recognition of the pathophysiologic processes responsible for these emergencies promotes clinical acumen and therapeutic specificity. An overarching strategy that involves immediate diagnosis, removal of causative agents, and fluid therapy is the backbone of effective care, emphasizing the need for increased clinical awareness (Alsudairy et al., 2023). Despite technical advances in diagnostic methods and therapeutic modalities, the morbidity and mortality from these severe cutaneous emergencies are still high, and research and education continue to be needed. The infrequency of disorders such as SJS and TEN tends to delay referrals and lead to less-than-optimal care, and greater awareness among physicians is desirable. Bringing current literature into clinical practice guidelines allows for earlier recognition and individualized therapy with a diminution in the complication burden. Multidisciplinary teamwork, such as with dermatologists, intensivists, infectious disease specialists, and rheumatologists, is required for complete management, particularly in complicated cases where there is systemic involvement. Increased training and facilities in emergency conditions can enhance initial evaluation, whereas continuous medical education keeps frontline workers up to date with current trends in therapeutic policies (Adaskevich, 2016). Finally, the treatment of dermatologic emergencies like SJS, TEN, erythroderma, and necrotizing fasciitis requires immediate diagnosis and management protocol to reduce the associated high risk of these disorders. Early detection and treatment not only reduce death but also avoid long-term sequelae that drastically impact patients' quality of life. Future initiatives need to address knowledge gaps between healthcare professionals via focused education programs and the establishment of uniform protocols. Improvement of communication channels between primary care and specialist services will also improve clinical results. Finally, the synthesis of multidisciplinary treatment, evidence-based therapies, and research advances will further develop the specialty, with enhanced prognosis and safety for these critical dermatologic emergencies (Alsudairy et al., 2023).

The complex management of dermatologic emergencies like SJS, TEN, erythroderma, and necrotizing fasciitis requires an in-depth understanding of their pathophysiology, clinical presentation, and treatment modalities. They usually have overlapping features of extensive cutaneous involvement and systemic complications, which may impede timely diagnosis and cause delays in life-saving measures. Early recognition remains a cornerstone, particularly in distinguishing between SJS and TEN based on involved BSA, as their mortality rates vary significantly. Supportive care tailored to prevent secondary infections, fluid loss, and organ dysfunction is critical in all four conditions. Additionally, collaboration among multidisciplinary teams enhances patient outcomes by addressing the dermatological pathology alongside systemic effects, emphasizing the importance of a comprehensive clinical approach. At the center of treatment approaches is the identification and removal of causative pathogens, particularly drug precipitants, which are the most common precipitating factors in SJS and TEN. Adjunct therapies, although variably supported, consist of immunomodulatory agents like IVIG or corticosteroids, whose function remains being critically assessed. In erythroderma, therapy is aimed at correction of the underlying cause, whether inflammatory, infectious, or neoplastic, with stabilization of skin barrier function. Necrotizing fasciitis requires immediate aggressive surgical debridement combined with broad-spectrum antibiotics to prevent fascial necrosis and systemic spread. An appreciation of these differentiated yet intertwined management principles highlights the significance of the early intervention combined with patient-specific factors, such as comorbidities and immune status, to maximize prognosis in these dermatologic emergencies. All in all, management of the clinical intricacies of SJS, TEN, erythroderma, and necrotizing fasciitis demands not only swift diagnosis and supportive therapy but also ongoing developments in therapeutic interventions to enhance survival rates. Including organ system evaluations, as stressed in rheumatological literature, concords with the multidisciplinary management needed for these conditions (Adaskevich, 2016). Despite the presence of evidence-based guidelines, the diversity of clinical presentation dictates individualized care plans that consider each patient's specific pathophysiological status and complications. Ultimately, increased clinical awareness, continued research, and interprofessional cooperation continue to be critical to both the enhancement of the understanding and treatment of such severe dermatologic emergencies, minimizing mortality, and enhancing the quality of life for the involved patients.

KEY TERMS FROM THIS CHAPTER

- Antibiotics
- Anticonvulsants
- Body surface area
- Corticosteroids
- Erythroderma
- Fluid resuscitation
- Granulysin
- Hospitalization
- Immunomodulation
- Intensive care specialists
- Necrotizing fasciitis
- Stevens-johnson syndrome
- Supportive care
- Toxic epidermal necrolysis

REFERENCES

1. Adaskevich, V. P. (2016). Skin diseases and sexually transmitted infections. *A-25 Skin Diseases and Sexually Transmitted Infections : handbook / U.P.* (accessed on 12 May 2025).
2. Alsudairy, Najlaa & Aljuhani, Razan & Alhassan, Zahraa & Alharbi, Abdulmajeed & Alshammari, Hamdan & Alshammari, Hamoud & Almalki, Abdullah & Alasmari, Saeed & Alduhailan, Yousef & Alshmri, Mohmed & Alneami, Afnan & Mansur, Sahar & Alhuthayli, Abdulaziz & Alsahli, Hajar. (2023). Dermatological Emergencies in Family Medicine: Recognition, Management, and Referral Considerations. Journal of Advanced Zoology. 44. 10.53555/jaz.v44i5.3389.
3. Alsudairy, N. M., Aljuhani, R. A. F., Alhassan, Z. A. J., Alharbi, A. S. A., Alshammari, H. S. A., Alshammari, H. M. F., Almalki, A. S. O., et al. (2023). Dermatological emergencies in family medicine: Recognition, management, and referral considerations. *Journal of Advanced Zoology, 44*(5), 3389. https://doi.org/10.53555/jaz.v44i5.3389.
4. Raschi, E., Gatti, M., Gelsomino, F., Ardizzoni, A., Poluzzi, E., & De Ponti, F. (2020). Lessons to be Learnt from Real-World Studies on Immune-Related Adverse Events with Checkpoint Inhibitors: A Clinical Perspective from Pharmacovigilance. *Targeted oncology*, *15*(4), 449–466. https://doi.org/10.1007/s11523-020-00738-6 (accessed on 12 May 2025).
5. Babu, A. N. M. (2015). A clinical study of non-venereal genital dermatoses. *CORE*. https://core.ac.uk/download/235667095.pdf (accessed on 12 May 2025).
6. Parker, J. R., & Berkeley, R. P. (2010). Toxic epidermal necrolysis from a cigarette burn. *The western journal of emergency medicine*, *11*(2), 205–207.
7. Long, B., Brém, E., & Koyfman, A. (2020). Oncologic Emergencies: Immune-Based Cancer Therapies and Complications. *The western journal of emergency medicine*, *21*(3), 566–580. https://doi.org/10.5811/westjem.2020.1.45898Badia, M., Casanova, J. M., Serviá, L., Montserrat, N., Codina, J., & Trujillano, J. (2020). Dermatological Manifestations in the Intensive Care Unit: A Practical Approach. *Critical care research and practice, 2020*, 9729814. https://doi.org/10.1155/2020/9729814
8. Jack, A. R., Spence, A. A., Nichols, B. J., Chong, S., Williams, D. T., Swadron, S. P., & Peng, D. H. (2011). Cutaneous conditions leading to dermatology consultations in the emergency department. *The western journal of emergency medicine*, *12*(4), 551–555. https://doi.org/10.5811/westjem.2010.4.1653
9. Falodun, O., & Ogunbiyi, A. (2010). Dermatological emergencies: Current trends in management. *CORE*. Annals of Ibadan Postgraduate Medicine. Vol.4 No2 Dec.,2006 https://core.ac.uk/download/478397283.pdf (accessed on 12 May 2025).
10. Jose, J. (2018). A pilot study of serum granulysin in drug-induced exanthems and severe cutaneous adverse reactions (SCARs). *CORE*. https://core.ac.uk/download/235668525.pdf (accessed on 12 May 2025).
11. Kellen, R., & Berlin, J. M. (2018). Dermatology emergencies. *Journal of the Dermatology Nurses' Association, 10*, 164–173. https://doi.org/10.1097/jdn.0000000000000394.
12. Barrera, Roberto et al. (2011). Preparedness and response for Chikungunya virus introduction in the Americas. Pătraşcu, A. I., Vâţă, D., Temelie-Olinici, D., Mocanu, M., Guguluş, D. L., Marinescu, M., Stafie, L., et al. (2024). Skin lesions with loss of tissue and cutaneous-onset

sepsis: The skin infection–sepsis relationship. *Diagnostics, 14*(6), 659. https://doi.org/10.3390/diagnostics14060659.

13. Skayem, C., Drahy, F., Hirsch, G., Hua, C., & Duong, T. A. (2024). Expertise in dermatologic emergencies: Real-world study on in-person vs. teledermatology emergencies in a reference center. *JDDG Journal der Deutschen Dermatologischen Gesellschaft, 22*, 1272–1274. https://doi.org/10.1111/ddg.15475.

INDEX

C

D

N

O

P

T

U

V

W

X

Y